THE FACTS ON FILE ENCYCLOPEDIA OF

HEALTH AND MEDICINE

IN FOUR VOLUMES:
VOLUME 4

THE FACTS ON FILE ENCYCLOPEDIA OF

HEALTH AND MEDICINE

IN FOUR VOLUMES:
VOLUME 4

An Amaranth Book

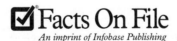
☑ Facts On File
An imprint of Infobase Publishing

To your health!

The information presented in *The Facts On File Encyclopedia of Health and Medicine* is provided for research purposes only and is not intended to replace consultation with or diagnosis and treatment by medical doctors or other qualified experts. Readers who may be experiencing a condition or disease described herein should seek medical attention and not rely on the information found here as medical advice.

The Facts On File Encyclopedia of Health and Medicine in Four Volumes: Volume 4

Facts On File, Inc.
An imprint of Infobase Publishing
132 West 31st Street
New York NY 10001

Produced by
Amaranth Illuminare
PO Box 573
Port Townsend WA 98368

Library of Congress Cataloging-in-Publication Data

The Facts on File encyclopedia of health and medicine / Amaranth Illuminare and Deborah S. Romaine.
p. ; cm.
"An Amaranth book."
Includes index.
ISBN 0-8160-6063-0 (hc : alk. paper)
1. Medicine—Encyclopedias. 2. Health—Encyclopedias.
[DNLM: 1. Medicine—Encyclopedias—English. 2. Physiological
Processes—Encyclopedias—English. WB 13 R842f 2006] I. Title:
Encyclopedia of health and medicine. II. Romaine, Deborah S., 1956- III.
Facts on File, Inc. IV. Title.
R125.R68 2006
610.3—dc22
2005027679

Facts On File books are available at special discounts when purchased in bulk quantities for businesses, associations, institutions, or sales promotions. Please call our Special Sales Department in New York at (212) 967-8800 or (800) 322-8755.

You can find Facts On File on the World Wide Web at http://www.factsonfile.com

Text design and typesetting by Rhea Braunstein, RB Design
Cover design by Dorothy Preston

Printed in the United States of America

VB RB 10 9 8 7 6 5 4 3 2 1

This book is printed on acid-free paper.

CONTENTS
VOLUME 4

FOREWORD

A big part of my role as a physician is educating my patients about their health. I take as much time as each person needs to explain prevention measures, test results, and treatment options. I encourage questions. But in the moment, sitting there in my office, most people do not yet know what to ask me. By the time questions flood their thoughts, they may be back at work or at home.

Numerous events and circumstances can challenge health, and we all need to know what actions we can take to keep ourselves healthy as well as to obtain appropriate treatment for health conditions that do affect us. Knowledge empowers all of us to make informed and appropriate decisions about health care. Certainly there is no shortage of reference material. Yet there is *so* much information available today! Even for physicians, it is challenging to keep up. How can you get to the core of what you want to know, reliably and to the level of detail you need?

The Facts On File Encyclopedia of Health and Medicine is a great resource for up-to-date health information presented in a manner that is both comprehensive and easy to understand no matter what your level of medical knowledge. The encyclopedia organizes entries by body system. The progression of body systems—and entries—throughout the encyclopedia presents topics the way you think about them.

Going beyond this basic structure, however, is another layer of organization that particularly appeals to me, which is a comprehensive structure of cross references that integrates entries across body systems. After all, your body functions in an integrated way; so, too, should a reference series that discusses your body's health. Not very much that happens with your health affects one part of your body in isolation from other body structures and functions. Your body attempts to compensate and adjust, often without your awareness, until it can no longer accommodate the injury or illness. The symptoms you bring to your doctor may reflect this compensation, for example frequent headaches that point not to brain tumor (as many people fear but is very rare) but to eye strain or muscle tension or sometimes to hypertension (high blood pressure).

In my medical practice I emphasize integrative health care, embracing the philosophy that health exists as the intricate intertwining of the body's many systems, structures, and functions. So, too, does the care of health. I received my medical degree from Tufts University School of Medicine in Boston, an institution noted for remaining at the forefront of the medical profession. I also completed clinical programs in Mind-Body Medicine at Harvard University, Integrative Medicine at the University of Arizona School of Medicine, and Medical Acupuncture at the University of California-Los Angeles (UCLA). I am a board-certified obstetrician-gynecologist, a board-certified clinical nutritionist, and a licensed acupuncturist. I see patients in my practice in Cincinnati, Ohio; I teach, I lecture, and I frequently go on television and radio to talk about health topics. In each of these areas, I encourage people to think about their health and health concerns from an integrative perspective. When you understand your health from multiple dimensions, you can better understand what to do to keep yourself as healthy as possible.

I wish you the best of health for all of a long, satisfying life. But when the time comes that you must make decisions about medical care, I want you to have the knowledge to make informed choices that are right for you. Whether you start here and move on to more specialized resources or locate all the information you need within these four volumes, you will find *The Facts On File* *Encyclopedia of Health and Medicine* to be a most valuable reference resource.

—**Maureen M. Pelletier, M.D., C.C.N.,**
F.A.C.O.G.

HOW TO USE
THE FACTS ON FILE ENCYCLOPEDIA OF HEALTH AND MEDICINE

Welcome to *The Facts On File Encyclopedia of Health and Medicine*, a four-volume reference set. This comprehensive resource is an indispensable reference for students, allied health professionals, physicians, caregivers, lay researchers, and people seeking information about health circumstances and conditions for themselves or others. Entries present the latest health concepts and medical knowledge in a clear, concise format. Readers may easily accumulate information and build a complete medical profile on just about any health or medical topic of interest or concern.

A New Paradigm for the Health and Medical Encyclopedia

As the art and science of health and medicine continues to evolve, with complex and elegant discoveries and new techniques, medications, and treatments emerging all the time, the need has arisen for a new paradigm for the encyclopedia of health and medicine—a rethinking of the old, and increasingly outmoded, presentations. Carefully researched and compiled, *The Facts On File Encyclopedia of Health and Medicine* offers many distinguishing features that present readers and researchers with an organization as up-to-date and compelling as the breakthrough information its entries contain.

Recognizing the current emphasis on presenting a truly integrative approach to both health and disease, *The Facts On File Encyclopedia of Health and Medicine* organizes content across volumes within a distinctive format that groups related entries by body system (for example, "The Cardiovascular System") or by general health topic (for example, "Genetics and Molecular Medicine"):

- **Volume 1** presents the sensory and structural body systems that allow the body to engage

with its surroundings and the external environment.

- **Volume 2** presents the cell- and fluid-based body systems that transport nutrients, remove molecular wastes, and provide protection from infection.

- **Volume 3** presents the biochemical body systems that support cellular functions.

- **Volume 4** presents topics that apply across body systems (such as "Fitness: Exercise and Health") or that address broad areas within health care (such as "Preventive Medicine").

- The appendixes provide supportive or additional reference information (such as "Appendix X: Immunization and Routine Examination Schedules").

Following Research Pathways

The Facts On File Encyclopedia of Health and Medicine's organization and structure support the reader's and researcher's ease of use. Many encyclopedia users will find all the information they desire within one volume. Others may use several or all four of the encyclopedia's volumes to arrive at a comprehensive, multifaceted, in-depth understanding of related health and medical concepts and information. Researchers efficiently look up information in *The Facts On File Encyclopedia of Health and Medicine* in several ways.

Each section's entries appear in alphabetical order (except the entries in Volume 4's "Emergency and First Aid" section, which are grouped by type of emergency). The researcher finds a desired entry by looking in the relevant volume and section. For example, the entry for **acne** is in Volume 1 in the section "The Integumentary System" and the entry for **stomach** is in Volume 3 in the section "The Gastrointestinal System." The researcher can also consult the index at the back of the volume to locate the entry, then turn to the appropriate page in the volume.

Terms that appear in SMALL CAPS within the text of an entry are themselves entries elsewhere in *The Facts On File Encyclopedia of Health and Medicine*. Encyclopedia users can look up the entries for those terms as well, for further information of potential interest. Such SMALL CAPS cross references typically provide related content that expands upon the primary topic, sometimes leading the user in new research directions he or she might otherwise not have explored.

For example, the entry **hypertension** is in the section "The Cardiovascular System." The entry presents a comprehensive discussion of the health condition hypertension (high blood pressure), covering symptoms, diagnosis, treatment options, risk factors, and prevention efforts. Among the numerous SMALL CAPS cross references within the hypertension entry are the entries for

- **retinopathy**, an entry in the section "The Eyes" in Volume 1, which discusses damage to the eye that may result from untreated or poorly managed hypertension
- **blood pressure**, an entry in the Volume 2 section "The Cardiovascular System," which discusses the body's mechanisms for maintaining appropriate pressure within the circulatory system
- **stroke** and **heart attack**, entries in Volume 2's "The Cardiovascular System" about significant health conditions that may result from hypertension
- **kidney,** an entry in the section "The Urinary System" in Volume 3, which discusses the kidney's role in regulating the body's electrolyte balances and fluid volume to control blood pressure
- **atherosclerosis, diabetes, hyperlipidemia,** and **obesity**, entries in the sections "The Cardiovascular System" in Volume 2, "The Endocrine System" in Volume 3, and "Lifestyle Variables: Smoking and Obesity" in Volume 4, and all of which are health conditions that contribute to hypertension

Following the path of an encyclopedic entry's internal cross references, as shown above, can illuminate connections between body systems; define and apply medical terminology; reveal a broad matrix of related health conditions, issues, and concerns; and more. The SMALL CAPS cross references indicated within the text of encyclopedic entries lead encyclopedia users on wide-ranging research pathways that branch and blossom.

At the end of the entry for **hypertension** a list of cross references gathered in alphabetical order links together groups of related entries in other sections and volumes, such as **smoking cessation** in Volume 4's "Lifestyle Variables: Smoking and Obesity," to provide specific, highly relevant research strings. These *see also* cross references also appear in SMALL CAPS, identifying them at a glance. Encyclopedia users are encouraged to look here for leads on honing research with precision to a direct pathway of connected entries.

So, extensive cross-references in *The Facts On File Encyclopedia of Health and Medicine* link related topics within and across sections and volumes, in both broad and narrow research pathways. This approach encourages researchers to investigate beyond the conventional level and focus of information, providing logical direction to relevant subjects. Each cross-referenced entry correspondingly has its own set of cross references, ever widening the web of knowledge.

Using the Facts On File Encyclopedia of Health and Medicine

Each section of the encyclopedia begins with an overview that introduces the section and its key concepts, connecting information to present a comprehensive view of the relevant system of the human body or health and medical subject area. For most body systems, this overview begins with a list and drawings of the system's structures and incorporates discussion of historic, current, and future contexts.

Entries present a spectrum of information from lifestyle factors and complementary methods to the most current technologic advances and approaches, as appropriate. Text that is set apart or bold within an entry gives an important health warning, or targets salient points of interest to add layers of meaning and context. Lists and tables collect concise presentations of related information for easy reference.

Each type of entry (mid-length and longer) incorporates consistent elements, identified by standardized subheadings:

- *Entries for health conditions and diseases* begin with a general discussion of the condition and its known or possible causes and then incorporate content under the subheadings "Symptoms and Diagnostic Path," "Treatment Options and Outlook," and "Risk Factors and Preventive Measures."

- *Entries for surgery operations* begin with a general discussion of the procedure and then incorporate content under the subheadings "Surgical Procedure," "Risks and Complications," and "Outlook and Lifestyle Modifications."

- *Entries for medication classifications* begin with a general discussion of the type of medication and its common uses and then incorporate content under the subheadings "How These Medications Work," "Therapeutic Applications," and "Risks and Side Effects."

- *Entries for diagnostic procedures* begin with a general discussion of the test or procedure and then incorporate content under the subheadings "Reasons for Doing This Test," "Preparation, Procedure, and Recovery," and "Risks and Complications."

Entries in Volume 4's section "Emergency and First Aid" are unique within the orientation of *The Facts On File Encyclopedia of Health and Medicine* in that they feature instructional rather than informational content. **These entries do *not* replace appropriate training in emergency response and first aid methods.** Rather, these entries provide brief directives that are appropriate for guiding the actions of a person with little or no first aid training who is first on the scene of an emergency.

Each volume concludes with a complete, full index for the sections and entries within the volume. Volume 4 of *The Facts On File Encyclopedia of Medicine* contains a comprehensive index for all four encyclopedia volumes that researchers can use to quickly and easily determine which volumes contain desired sections or entries.

The Facts On File Encyclopedia of Health and Medicine in Four Volumes

PREFACE TO VOLUME 4

Volume 4 of the four-volume *The Facts On File Encyclopedia of Health and Medicine* is unique in its organization and presentation of content. The sections of Volume 4 extend across body systems and medical disciplines to look at the larger picture of health and health care. Though the entries in these sections cover a broad spectrum of information, the thread that connects all of these sections is the individual's participation, through lifestyle choices and informed decisions, in his or her health and health care.

Preventive Medicine

The protection of a population's overall health, particularly measures to maintain health and prevent health problems, is a major emphasis. The section "Preventive Medicine" examines efforts and initiatives intended to reduce the general risks for injury or illness. Entries present both personal and community-based perspectives.

Alternative and Complementary Approaches

The section, "Alternative and Complementary Approaches" explores methods based in other systems of health care such as acupuncture and herbal remedies. Entries present the methods within the framework of how they fit within the Western medicine model common in the United States, with cross references to comparable Western approaches discusses in entries elsewhere in *The Facts On File Encyclopedia of Health and Medicine*.

Genetics and Molecular Medicine

In April 2003 an international, cross-disciplinary team of scientists completed the human genome sequence, unraveling for the first time the structure of human existence. The section "Genetics and Molecular Medicine" entries look at research that uses the map of the human genome to explore new pathways for understanding disease and illness. Through this new knowledge lies hope for preventing many of the health conditions common today.

Drugs

Pharmaceutical therapies are the basis for treatment of many health conditions, from infections to cardiovascular disease to cancer. The section "Drugs" contains entries that discuss the types of medications doctors use to treat a wide range of health conditions. Entries cover classifications of prescription drugs as well as over-the-counter products and include cross references to alternative remedies.

Nutrition and Diet

Nutrition (what the body requires to fuel its functions) comes from diet (the foods people eat). Dietary choices affect nutrition, and consequently health, in ways that can support health and lower the risk for disease. The entries in this section discuss the major categories of nutrients and explain how dietary choices affect the body's functions.

Fitness: Exercise and Health

Fitness reflects a personal choice to engage in activities that maintain the body's strength, flexibility, and mobility to support optimal health. Many researchers consider physical *in*activity to be the leading factor in the development of chronic health conditions such as hypertension (high blood pressure), diabetes, and obesity. The entries in this section discuss the correlation between regular physical activity and key health conditions as well as present information about how physical activity affects the body.

Human Relations

Humans are social beings. Yet many social interactions are ones not necessarily chosen, such those within school and work environments. The entries here present discussions of behavior issues, with an emphasis on understanding the influence of diverse backgrounds and personal experiences.

Surgery

Surgery is the treatment of choice for hundreds of health conditions. The section "Surgery" presents entries about general topics such as anesthesia and surgery benefits and risks. Entries about specific operations appear in the relevant body system section. For example, the entry for appendectomy (surgery to remove the appendix) appears in the section "The Gastrointestinal System."

Lifestyle Variables: Smoking and Obesity

Cigarette smoking and obesity (extreme overweight) are the leading lifestyle factors that contribute to serious health conditions such as cardiovascular disease, diabetes, and cancer. In this section *The Facts On File Encyclopedia of Health and Medicine* presents entries about the health effects of smoking and obesity within the context of lifestyle choices that are within the reach of every individual to control.

Substance Abuse

Substance abuse, including alcoholism, is a significant health concern in the United States. The entries in this section discuss commonly abused substances, including their short-term and long-term effects on health. There are also entries about treatment approaches and programs.

Emergency and First Aid

The section "Emergency and First Aid" stands apart from all other sections in the *Facts On File Encyclopedia of Health and Medicine*. Entries here provide instructional content and are organized by type of emergency, presenting the most basic information for the person who has no medical knowledge or training and who happens to be first on the scene of a medical emergency (first responder). Entries are concise and directive, with cross references to information-based entries throughout the four volumes of the encyclopedia.

Appendixes and Cumulative Index to Volumes 1-4

A dozen appendixes that provide supplemental information bring Volume 4 to a close. Volume 4 also contains a comprehensive "Cumulative Index" for the entire four-volume *Facts On File Encyclopedia of Health and Medicine*.

PREVENTIVE MEDICINE

The medical discipline of preventive medicine covers the gamut of measures, individual and societal, that can reduce the occurrence of illness and injury. Physicians who practice in preventive medicine may be infectious disease specialists, community health specialists, and occupational health specialists. Preventive medicine is also a mainstay of most other medical specialties, notably family practice, internal medicine, and pediatrics. The research field of epidemiology studies trends in and risks for illness and injury and explores methods for reducing health risks. Epidemiologists and preventive medicine practitioners work closely together.

This section, "Preventive Medicine," presents an overview discussion of preventive medicine concepts and entries about preventive health measures and the public health dimensions of illness and injury. The entries in this section focus on the larger picture of how illness and injury affect the health and well-being of communities and populations. Entries in other sections of *The Facts On File Encyclopedia of Health and Medicine* provide detailed content about the causes, symptoms, diagnosis, treatment, and outlook for specific infections and diseases. Cross-references link the entries to one another.

Traditions in Preventive Medicine History

Early cultures and medical systems had their unique variations on preventing illness and INFECTION. There is some evidence of guidelines for sanitation and public health practices in ancient Macedonia, and the ruins of ancient Rome's intricate aqueducts and sewage canals remain today. But for the most part the premise of public health is relatively modern, emerging after a flurry of scientific discoveries in the 19th century that revealed the pathogenesis (origin and progression) of infection and disease. Key to these discoveries were the observations of physicians such as Ignaz Philipp Semmelweis, who was the first to make the connection that doctors carried the infection of childbirth FEVER from one patient to another through blood on their hands and cloth-

ing, and the experiments of scientists such as Joseph Lister, Louis Pasteur, and Robert Koch, whose discoveries proved the existence of microbes and the value of antisepsis in preventing the spread of infection. Their work further led to the development of antibiotics and vaccines.

These three factors—antisepsis, antibiotics, and vaccines—forever changed the perceptions and patterns of disease throughout the world and are among the most significant breakthroughs in medical history. In less than half a century these discoveries dramatically reduced the occurrence and severity of many diseases that had for millennia been the leading causes of death: tetanus, ANTHRAX, SMALLPOX, CHOLERA, TYPHOID FEVER, DIPHTHERIA, PERTUSSIS, POLIOMYELITIS, SYPHILIS, bacterial PNEUMONIA, bacterial wound infections, INFLUENZA, and TUBERCULOSIS. Though death due to infection after CHILDBIRTH is rare in the United States today, until the early 20th century childbirth fever (puerperal fever) was a leading cause of death among women of childbearing age. From 1900 to 1999, maternal death in childbirth declined 99 percent in the United States.

EFFECTS OF VACCINATION

- eradication of SMALLPOX in the United States in 1967 and worldwide in 1977
- near eradication of MEASLES in the United States in 1998
- near eradication of POLIOMYELITIS in the United States in 2000

Public Health

Improvements in COMMUNITY SANITATION, such as sewage and garbage control, in the late 19th and early 20th centuries further contained diseases spread through close contact reduced pest and vermin infestation and the resultant diseases, including the much dreaded "black death," plague. Cities and towns focused effort on maintaining clean and safe drinking water supplies, decreasing waterborne illnesses. The home refrigerator debuted in 1913 and quickly replaced the icebox as the standard for food storage, dramatically decreasing FOODBORNE ILLNESSES.

Doctors and others began to recognize, by the start of the 20th century, the extent to which community and personal cleanliness influenced health and illness. Poor ventilation and overcrowded living and working conditions, especially in densely populated cities, encouraged rampant and rapid spread of infectious diseases. In 1900 pneumonia, tuberculosis, and GASTROENTERITIS together were to blame for a third of all deaths in the United States. Annual influenza outbreaks could kill entire families, even communities, within weeks. In cities, infections caused the deaths of nearly a third of infants before their first birthdays.

With clean water standards came assurances that bathing would no longer be the source of illness but rather could be the guardian of health. Public officials began to extol the virtues of frequent HAND WASHING and daily, or at least weekly, bathing. Between 1920 and 1937 illnesses and deaths from waterborne infections such as cholera and typhoid fever plummeted, and by 1950 were nearly nonexistent. Health officials also encouraged opening windows and getting fresh air, measures that helped dilute the concentration of airborne pathogens such as viruses and BACTERIA and reduce opportunities for infection to occur. In 1944 the US Congress passed the Public Health Service Act that established a consistent framework for public health laws, standards, and procedures throughout the United States.

Life expectancy A key measure of public health and the effectiveness of disease-prevention efforts is LIFE EXPECTANCY. A child born in 1900 could expect to live to age 47. A child born in 1950, the dawn of the golden era of preventive health care, could expect to live nearly half again as long, to

age 68. These children were the first who also could expect to grow up without experiencing the CHILDHOOD DISEASES that claimed the lives of one in five children in their parents' generation.

Epidemics and pandemics Epidemics and pandemics strike fear in the hearts of health experts and individuals alike. Epidemics are extensive but localized outbreaks of illness or infection. Pandemics are worldwide outbreaks. Despite vaccination efforts, annual influenza epidemics sicken millions and cause the deaths of 30,000 Americans. Health experts believe basic preventive measures such as frequent hand washing and appropriate SNEEZE/COUGH ETIQUETTE, combined with more comprehensive vaccination, could prevent most of these infections.

The Spanish influenza epidemic of 1918, the worst pandemic of modern history, claimed the lives of half a million Americans and more than 20 million people worldwide. It also provided much learning for public health officials about how, and how quickly, such infections spread. Health experts have used this knowledge to develop mechanisms and systems to detect and report outbreaks that have pandemic potential. Such efforts could not entirely prevent, though did help contain, influenza pandemics in 1957 (the Asian flu) and 1968 (the Hong Kong flu). They did, however, allow early detection and containment of small outbreaks of avian influenza in 2000 and 2004, and of the deadly SEVERE ACUTE RESPIRATORY SYNDROME (SARS).

Motor vehicle safety A uniquely modern-day public health issue is motor vehicle safety. Coming into its own in the early 1900s, the automobile wasted little time acquiring notoriety. By the time Henry Ford set the standard for the "everyman" car, MOTOR VEHICLE ACCIDENTS had already claimed more than 40,000 lives. By the 1960s, motor vehicle accidents accounted for more than 40,000 deaths each year. Measures such as structural integrity requirements, seat belts, and airbags have held motor vehicle deaths steady near that level since 1998.

Individual Health Factors

The recognition that PERSONAL HYGIENE—frequent hand washing and daily or at least weekly bathing—could prevent the passing of disease from one person to another was a milestone in preventive medicine. Until the early 20th century even doctors did not often wash their hands, not even between seeing patients. This was largely a function of ignorance. Until Lister, Koch, Pasteur, and others demonstrated the existence of bacteria and their causal relationship to infection, doctors and others simply did not know their hands carried the agents of disease. Health experts today believe that frequent hand washing could prevent 90 percent or more of the infections that occur.

THE US CENTERS FOR DISEASE CONTROL AND PREVENTION'S (CDC'S) 10 MOST SIGNIFICANT PUBLIC HEALTH ACHIEVEMENTS OF THE 20TH CENTURY

control of infectious diseases
decline in deaths from heart disease and STROKE
FAMILY PLANNING
FLUORIDATION of drinking water
healthier mothers and babies
motor-vehicle safety
recognition of TOBACCO use as a health hazard
safer and healthier foods
safer workplaces
vaccination

Source: CDC, MMRW Weekly, April 2, 1999, 48(12):241–243.

Health discoveries in the 1950s and 1960s began to connect lifestyle habits with health and disease. The landmark surgeon general's report of 1964 established the scientific correlation between cigarette smoking and LUNG disease, notably lung CANCER. Research explored the roles of nutrition and exercise in preventing disease and even in the early 1960s issued recommendations for daily "calisthenics" to maintain the physical health of the body. Fast food (available in restaurants and from grocery stores) changed EATING HABITS and body weight, and health experts noted alarming rises in CARDIOVASCULAR DISEASE (CVD) and type 2 DIABETES.

In 1900 heart disease was the fourth leading cause of death in the United States; by 1977 it had become, and today remains, number one. Though infections such as HIV/AIDS and HEPATITIS remain significant threats to personal and public health, the greatest challenges are now those that are nearly exclusively within the realm of individual control. Health promotion emphasizes community-based as well as individual preventive efforts that target modifiable risk factors for injury, illness, and dis-

ease. Recommendations for individual preventive health measures emphasize nutritious eating habits and daily exercise, urge SMOKING CESSATION, promote IMMUNIZATION, and encourage routine health screenings for early detection and treatment of disease. Health experts believe lifestyle modifications—reduction of personal health risks—could eliminate as much as 90 percent of acquired heart disease as well as 95 percent of type 2 diabetes (a leading cause of heart disease).

KEY PERSONAL HEALTH FACTORS

ALCOHOL use	cigarette smoking
EATING HABITS	occupational and recreational
physical inactivity	safety
safer sex practices	seat belt and helmet use
substance abuse	

Contemporary Issues and Challenges

Preventive medicine specialists acknowledge the many challenges of controlling or eliminating the factors that result in the health conditions that are most significant at present. Despite the truly phenomenal strides in health care that have occurred in the past 50 years, the emphasis within the American health-care structure remains on treating disease. Factors that influence the success of prevention measures include cultural and generational perceptions, literacy and non-English-speaking populations, aging of the US population, access to care and mechanisms of care delivery, and disparities among population groups.

Cultural and generational perceptions Perceptions about health screening, preventive care, and even treatment for diagnosed health conditions differ among cultures and age groups. Older generations may hold to beliefs that one goes to the doctor only when ill or injured, stemming from limited access and affordability that typified health care before the emergence of health insurance. Ethnic groups may be suspicious of Western medicine and its intrusive nature or find conventional medical practices at odds with spiritual or religious beliefs. CULTURAL AND ETHNIC HEALTH-CARE PERSPECTIVES and GENERATIONAL HEALTH-CARE PERSPECTIVES greatly influence compliance with public health recommendations, affecting groups that are particularly vulnerable to health conditions, such as cardiovascular disease or infections such as hepatitis and tuberculosis, that current preventive measures target.

Literacy A key platform of public health education efforts is the presentation of information through written materials such as posters, hand-out informational sheets, brochures, and display placards. Some studies suggest that up to two thirds of English-speaking individuals lack the functional literacy level to understand the content of these materials, complete health and risk assessment tools such as surveys and questionnaires, or follow written care instructions after procedures such as surgery. In regions where there are high concentrations of non-English-speaking populations, health education materials and basic health questionnaires are often available in the dominant languages of such populations. However, most people who do not understand materials the doctor gives them will not say so.

Aging of the US population In 1900, less than 4 percent of the American population—3 million people—was over the age of 65. In 2000, 35 million Americans, nearly 13 percent of the population, were age 65 and older, a 10-fold increase over the span of a century. By 2030 the US Bureau of the Census projects that 30 percent of the population—70 million people—will be over age 65. Given the rise in the frequency of health conditions such as cancer, cardiovascular disease, and diabetes as well as the conditions relatively specific to the older population such as ALZHEIMER'S DISEASE and PARKINSON'S DISEASE, the potential demand for health-care services may quadruple. Efforts to reduce the likelihood for preventable health conditions takes on increasing significance within this scenario.

Access to care and mechanisms of delivery Though 85 percent of Americans have private or public health insurance, 15 percent do not. In a delivery model predicated on insurance as primary payer, insurance coverage determines access to care. People who do not have health insurance have difficulty receiving health-care services and often are then more seriously ill when they do receive care. Health experts worry that lack of access to appropriate health-care services, including preventive measures such as immunization, increases the risk for outbreaks of infectious diseases. Of particular concern are SEXUALLY TRANSMIT-TED DISEASES (STDS), tuberculosis, hepatitis, and HIV/AIDS, all of which have significant public health ramifications.

Breakthrough Research and Treatment Advances
At the start of the 20th century doctors marveled at the notion that living organisms so small only the magnification of a microscope revealed their existence caused the many diseases that ravaged entire populations. Perhaps the most profound breakthrough in preventive medicine at the start of the 21st century is the mapping of the HUMAN GENOME. Within reach, and in various stages of research and development, are "smart" drugs that target specific substances in the body and pharmacogenomic products that will "turn off" predisposing genetic factors for diseases such as HYPERTENSION (high BLOOD PRESSURE), diabetes, and certain cancers. GENE THERAPY holds the promise of manipulations that may end diseases such as CYSTIC FIBROSIS.

No longer the venue of science fiction is the field of molecular medicine, in which doctors can redirect cell function. In 2001, after 10 years of intensive research, a multidisciplinary team of scientists finished decoding the human genome. The unprecedented achievement revealed startling and revolutionary insights into the functions of the human body. The offshoot Microbial Genome Program, initiated in 1994, continues to unravel the genetic encoding of the organisms that function at the most foundational level of organic existence. In the space of a century, medicine has come from identifying the existence of the MICROBE to understanding the most intimate details of its functions.

Yet even as technology ushers health care into the 21st century and beyond, the challenges of the previous century linger. Infectious illnesses, though different from those that plagued earlier generations, remain at the forefront of preventive medicine. The first Nobel Prize in Medicine or Physiology was awarded to Emil von Behring in 1901 for discovering the cause of one of the time's most deadly diseases, diphtheria. The 1997 award went to Stanley Prusiner for his discovery of another new pathogen, the infectious PRION. The most rampant infection in the world, HIV/AIDS, remains incurable. Preventive medicine is on a new, yet familiar, path as the current millennium moves forward.

accidental injuries Accidental injuries, also called unintentional injuries, claim more than 100,000 lives each year and are the fifth leading cause of death in the United States. Accidental injuries account for nearly half of childhood deaths. Accidental injuries further account for more than 90 million health-care provider (ambulatory medical care) visits annually, 10 million of which are for injuries to children. Many accidental injuries are preventable.

KEY PUBLIC HEALTH MEASURES
TO REDUCE ACCIDENTAL INJURIES

boating safety regulations	building occupancy
building sprinkler systems	regulations
carbon monoxide detectors	child-resistant container laws
emergency exit requirements	fire codes
fireworks restrictions	flammability standards
playground safety standards	product labeling requirements
seat belt, child restraint,	smoke detectors
and helmet laws	structural building codes
traffic speed limits	vehicle safety standards

Major Causes of Accidental Injuries

There are numerous causes for accidental injuries. MOTOR VEHICLE ACCIDENTS lead them, accounting for 40 percent of those deaths. Poisoning and falls each account for 15 percent. Other common causes of accidental injuries include choking, fires, recreational activities, and fireworks.

Motor vehicle accidents Motor vehicle accidents are the leading cause of death for those between the ages of 2 and 33, resulting in more than 40,000 deaths each year. Motor vehicle accidents also account for nearly 3 million injuries for which people seek medical care each year. People between ages 15 and 25 years and over age 74 years are at highest risk for injury or death in motor vehicle accidents. The three most significant factors in motor vehicle accident injuries and deaths are:

- Improper restraints—nearly three fourths of those who die in motor vehicle accidents are not wearing seat belts or secured in child seats and are thrown from the vehicle in the accident.

- ALCOHOL use—alcohol use is involved in 40 percent of fatalities and 7 percent of accidents overall.

- Excessive speed—speeding contributes to a third of all motor vehicle accidents, though is a disproportionate factor among male drivers between the ages of 16 and 20.

Up to a third of motor vehicle accidents involve combinations of these factors, greatly increasing the likelihood of injury or death.

Poisoning Accidental poisoning accounts for 14,500 deaths and 500,000 injuries that require medical attention each year. More than 60 percent of poisonings are among children under the age of 14. Children under the age of 4 account for two thirds of poisonings in children. Poisoning from common OVER-THE-COUNTER (OTC) DRUGS such as acetaminophen (Tylenol), aspirin, and iron supplements can occur with as few as six or eight tablets, depending on the body weight, age, and health status of the person. Other common sources of poisoning among children are prescription medications that adults, particularly grandparents and older caregivers, are taking. Chronic lead poisoning occurs in children exposed to high levels of lead such as are present in leaded paints applied before 1978.

Falls More than 14,200 people lose their lives in falls each year, nearly two thirds of whom are

5

age 65 and older. About 7.5 million people require medical attention for accidental injuries received in falls, Falls account for nearly a third of medical visits for accidental injury and are most frequent among those under age 14 (2.3 million) and over age 60 (1.8 million). Child walkers (wheeled chairs prewalking children can push around with their feet) and stairs account for the greatest number of falls among young children. Among older adults, stairs, irregular surfaces, and items such as throw rugs present the most common falling hazards, particularly when lighting is poor as when getting up at night to go to the bathroom. Medication side effects such as drowsiness and balance disturbances often are contributing factors to falls among older adults.

Choking   Choking is a significant risk among the very young, the very old, and those who have temporary or long-term SWALLOWING DISORDERS. Choking accounts for 4,200 deaths each year as well as nearly 600,000 medical care visits. Two thirds of choking episodes involve food. Balloons, coins, and candy are also choking hazards for children.

Fires   Nearly 4,000 people lose their lives in residential fires each year, most of whom die from inhaling toxic gases and smoke (ASPHYXIATION) rather than BURNS. Health-care providers treat another 500,000 people a year for burns received in residential fires, about half of which are serious enough to result in lifelong disability.

Recreational activities   Recreational activities result in 5 million injuries that require medical attention each year. Water activities are the most lethal, accounting for 4,000 deaths annually, with 25 percent of them among children. Basketball, football, and baseball collectively account for the highest number of injuries resulting from participation in structured athletic activities, nearly 1 million per year. Bicycling accidents account for about 500,000 injuries and 800 deaths annually. Each year playground injuries send more than 200,000 children for medical care and over 2 million adults require medical attention for injuries related to overexertion.

Fireworks   Though fireworks are illegal in most federal, state, and municipal jurisdictions, fireworks account for more than 9,000 injuries that require medical attention each year. Injuries tend to concentrate in the weeks around the Fourth of July and New Year's Day celebrations. Children are at greatest risk for injuries due to fireworks, two thirds of which are burns. Cuts to the face, fingers, and hands, as well as traumatic AMPUTATION of fingers and vision-threatening EYE injuries, occur most commonly.

Health Consequences of Accidental Injuries

Though many people fully recover from the injuries they receive, some experience residual consequences that may include extended or lifelong disability. Among the most significant of such consequences are

- TRAUMATIC BRAIN INJURY (TBI)
- SPINAL CORD INJURY
- loss of limbs, fingers, and toes
- extensive scarring and disfigurement
- VISION IMPAIRMENT

Even short-term recovery, such as from fractures, burns, and lacerations, disrupts regular activities such as school and work.

Preventive Measures

Many, if not most, accidental injuries are preventable through measures that require little extra effort. Often people are unaware of the risks of their behaviors or believe their participation is not enough to expose them to such risks; for example, driving only a few blocks to the store without wearing a seat belt or turning attention away from a child in a swimming pool to answer the telephone. Overall, however, 90 percent of unintended injuries occur in or within two miles of home.

Key preventive measures among children, for whom accidental injuries carry high risk of serious disability or death, include requiring use of appropriate safety gear and supervision when participating in recreational activities. Health experts estimate that proper helmet use could prevent 80 percent of the 800 deaths and thousands of serious head injuries that result from bicycle accidents, most of which do not involve collisions with motor vehicles, among children and adults alike. Properly worn helmets reduce the risk of head injury by 80 percent when using skate-boards, roller skates, and inline skates as well as for downhill skiing and horseback riding.

Taking small bites and chewing food thoroughly before swallowing are important measures to prevent choking in children and adults. Many older adults use "scheduled DOSE" medication containers that may not be child resistant. A significant portion of poisonings among children occurs when children get into their grandparents' medications. Many medications have coatings that make them taste sweet, giving children the impression that they are candy.

KEY PERSONAL MEASURES
FOR PREVENTING ACCIDENTAL INJURIES

- wear seat belts and place children under 60 pounds in appropriate child safety seats in the back seat
- wear a helmet when riding a bicycle or horse, downhill skiing, and wheeled skating, and other appropriate safety gear for sports and athletic activities
- store medications in their original labeled containers, with childproof lids or caps, and in locked cabinets or drawers
- install handrails and lighting for stairways and hallways, and use child gates or child locks to block access to stairs, kitchens, bathrooms, garages, and other hazardous areas
- install handrails in showers and baths, especially for the elderly
- install smoke detectors and put in fresh batteries every six months
- install car horns or buzzers that operate while the vehicle is in reverse

See also ATHLETIC INJURIES; DOMESTIC VIOLENCE; FRACTURE; HEAVY-METAL POISONING; HEIMLICH MANEUVER; HIP FRACTURE IN OLDER ADULTS; NOISE EXPOSURE AND HEARING; OCCUPATIONAL HEALTH AND SAFETY; POISON PREVENTION; VIOLENCE.

antibiotic prophylaxis   A DOSE or brief course of ANTIBIOTIC MEDICATIONS before invasive dental, surgical, or diagnostic procedures for people who have had certain HEART operations or who have certain heart conditions to help prevent bacterial ENDOCARDITIS (INFLAMMATION and INFECTION of the heart). Doctors may, though do not always, suggest antibiotic prophylaxis for people who have other heart conditions as well as certain IMMUNE DISORDERS, HIV/AIDS, type 1 DIABETES, active CANCER,

and women in LABOR who are group B-strep positive or with prolonged rupture of membranes.

Bacterial endocarditis is a serious infection that can result in permanent damage to the heart, especially the heart valves, or in death. The heart valves are particularly vulnerable to bacteria cultures that establish themselves in their tissues. This risk increases when there are abnormalities of blood flow through the heart that can allow blood to slow or stagnate in the heart's chambers, or when there is damage to the valves that prevents normal movement. Invasive procedures, particularly in the MOUTH (such as tooth extraction or root canal) and gastrointestinal tract, which are rich in natural BACTERIA, provide opportunity for bacteria to enter the bloodstream and travel to the heart.

The typical regimen is a single large dose of an antibiotic one hour before the procedure, usually taken by mouth. The recommended antibiotic is amoxicillin or cephalexin, azithromycin, or clarithromycin for people who are allergic to penicillin. People who are already taking prophylactic antibiotics for other purposes should let their doctors or dentists know; the health-care practitioner will likely choose a different antibiotic for specific prophylaxis to appropriately target the potential classification of bacteria.

ANTIBIOTIC PROPHYLAXIS ADVISED

When Any of These Conditions Exist

cardiopulmonary shunt	cyanotic CONGENITAL HEART DISEASE
HEART TRANSPLANTATION	hypertrophic CARDIOMYOPATHY
mitral valve prolapse with regurgitation	previous bacterial ENDOCARDITIS
	prosthetic heart valve
RHEUMATIC HEART DISEASE	uncorrected congenital heart malformations

Before Any of These Procedures

CARDIAC CATHETERIZATION	CYSTOSCOPY
gastrointestinal ENDOSCOPY	periodontal surgery
placement of bands for braces	prophylactic professional dental cleaning
root canal	surgery (laparoscopic or open)
tissue biopsy	tooth extraction

Though numerous studies suggest the value of antibiotic prophylaxis, none definitively supports or refutes it, giving rise to some disagreement among health-care providers as to whether it truly lowers the risk for bacterial endocarditis. However, the American Heart Association, the American Dental Association, the Infectious Diseases Society of America, the American Academy of Pediatrics, and the American Society for Gastrointestinal Endoscopy jointly recommend antibiotic prophylaxis in specific circumstances.

See also IMMUNODEFICIENCY; VALVULAR HEART DISEASE.

antismoking efforts The US health community has targeted cigarette smoking since the landmark 1964 surgeon general's report, *Smoking and Health: Report of the Advisory Committee to the Surgeon General of the Public Health Service,* formally identified the connections between smoking and health conditions such as LUNG CANCER, laryngeal CANCER, and chronic BRONCHITIS. A single sentence from the 387-page document summarized what was to become a major preventive health emphasis in the United States for the ensuing decades: "Cigarette smoking is a health hazard of sufficient importance in the United States to warrant appropriate remedial action."

At the time of the 1964 surgeon general's report, 70 million Americans were smokers. The US Centers for Disease Control and Prevention (CDC) reports the number of current smokers remains fairly stable at about 46.2 million, 8.6 million of them becoming ill as a result each year. Health experts project that more than half of people who continue to smoke, about 25 million, will die of smoking-related diseases. Antismoking efforts have a two-prong focus:

1. Encourage people never to start smoking.
2. Encourage people who do smoke to stop, no matter how long they have been smoking.

These efforts emphasize coordinated educational approaches among schools, youth organizations, community organizations, sports and athletic organizations, and health-care providers. As well, a number of class-action lawsuits against TOBACCO companies have forced payments from them to fund health care for smoking-related chronic illnesses and antismoking efforts. General practice guidelines for physicians include screening for tobacco use and recommendation of SMOKING CESSATION methods for people who do smoke.

KEY ANTISMOKING EFFORTS
- intensive education of youth through the schools, advertising, community programs, celebrity advocates, and other targeted approaches
- effective and accessible SMOKING CESSATION methods
- strong warning labels on cigarette packages
- stringent enforcement of age-restricted access to TOBACCO products
- prohibition of smoking in the workplace, public buildings and venues, and other indoor locations

The 1964 report that first linked cigarettes and cancer and subsequent surgeon general's reports on smoking and health are available on the CDC's Web site (www.cdc.gov/tobacco/sgr/index.htm).

See also CANCER PREVENTION; LIFESTYLE AND HEALTH; SMOKING AND CANCER; SMOKING AND CARDIOVASCULAR DISEASE; SMOKING AND HEALTH; TOBACCO USE OTHER THAN SMOKING.

birth defects More than 150,000 infants born each year in the United States have structural or functional abnormalities present at birth, ranging from mild to severely debilitating or fatal. Substances and circumstances that can cause birth defects are teratogenic. Some birth defects, notably FETAL ALCOHOL SYNDROME (FAS) and those that occur as a SIDE EFFECT of medications, are entirely preventable. GENE mutations, some of which are hereditary mutations and many of which are spontaneous or isolated mutations, cause many birth defects. The risk for the genetic condition DOWN SYNDROME (trisomy 21), a chromosomal disorder, rises with the mother's age, the only birth defect doctors know for certain does so. Many other birth defects are not preventable, however, and may not be detectable before birth.

The risk for many other birth defects correlates to exposures during PREGNANCY, such as to the viral infections RUBELLA (German measles), CYTOMEGALOVIRUS (CMV), and CHICKENPOX, and to the parasitic INFECTION TOXOPLASMOSIS. These infections can cause mild to significant birth defects, ranging from congenital CATARACT and HEARING LOSS to HEART malformations. Avoiding these exposures prevents any consequential damage to the developing FETUS.

Teratogenic Medications

Doctors widely prescribed the DRUG thalidomide in the 1950s and early 1960s as a treatment for MORNING SICKNESS until they discovered the high incidence of limb deformities associated with its use. Thalidomide marked a turning point in public awareness about the teratogenic hazards of medications as well as in research efforts to identify those hazards. Numerous medications can cause

birth defects. The US Food and Drug Administration (FDA), which regulates drug approval and use in the United States, assigns pregnancy categories to medications to help doctors and women assess the risks of using the medications during pregnancy. These categories are

- pregnancy category A: medications for which numerous clinical studies have shown no adverse effects in pregnancy
- pregnancy category B: medications for which animal studies have shown no adverse effects or for which there are limited studies
- pregnancy category C: medications for which there are no studies to indicate either safety or hazard during pregnancy
- pregnancy category D: medications for which clinical studies demonstrate risk to the developing fetus, although the benefits to the mother of the medication may outweigh the risks to the fetus
- pregnancy category X: medications for which clinical studies demonstrate clear evidence of damage to the developing fetus

Doctors generally consider pregnancy category A and B medications safe for women to use during pregnancy, though approach the use of pregnancy category C medications with caution. Women who are pregnant or planning pregnancy should thoroughly discuss benefits and risks with their doctors before taking or continuing to take category D medications and should never take pregnancy category X medications. Pregnant women should check with their doctors or pharmacists about any medications they are taking when they become

COMMON BIRTH DEFECTS

Birth Defect	Health Risk to Infant	Preventive Measures
cleft defects (craniofacial clefts)	negligible with reconstructive surgery difficulty nursing, eating, and with speech when uncorrected	possibly folic acid supplementation GENE mutations have been identified
FETAL ALCOHOL SYNDROME (FAS)	mild to moderate physical deformities, mental retardation, and BEHAVIORAL DISORDERS	abstinence from ALCOHOL during PREGNANCY is fully preventive

genitourinary defects
  EPISPADIAS
  HYPOSPADIAS
  KIDNEY deformities
	negligible with reconstructive surgery
	absence of both kidneys is usually fatal
		none known
		gene mutations have been identified

INFECTION
  CHICKENPOX
  CYTOMEGALOVIRUS (CMV)
  MEASLES
  RUBELLA
  TOXOPLASMOSIS
  HERPES
	mild to severe deformities, depending on gestational age at time of infection
	blindness
		vaccination for measles, rubella, and chickenpox prior to pregnancy
		avoid contact with cat feces (such as through cleaning litter boxes or handling dirt outdoors) and with uncooked meat to prevent toxoplasmosis
		frequent HAND WASHING to reduce risk for infectious diseases in general

major HEART defects
  hypoplastic left heart syndrome (HLHS)
  tetralogy of Fallot
  transposition of the great arteries (TPA)
	significant, with high risk for death
	lifelong complications remain even with successful surgery
	these defects are the leading reason for heart transplantation in children
		none known
		comprehensive PRENATAL CARE for early detection and treatment planning; infant will require emergency treatment at birth
		gene mutations have been identified

minor heart defects
  ATRIAL SEPTAL DEFECT (ASD)
  PATENT DUCTUS ARTERIOSUS (PDA)
  VENTRICULAR SEPTAL DEFECT (VSD)
	negligible with appropriate treatment (usually surgical repair)	none known
		comprehensive prenatal care for early detection and treatment planning
		gene mutations have been identified

NEURAL TUBE DEFECTS
  anencephaly
  SPINA BIFIDA
	significant
	anencephaly is always fatal
	spina bifida often causes deformity and lower body PARALYSIS, including loss of bowel and BLADDER function
		folic acid supplementation before CONCEPTION through the first 28 days of pregnancy cuts risk in half
		many health experts recommend all women of childbearing age take folic acid supplements (400 micrograms per day)
		gene mutations have been identified

COMMON TERATOGENIC MEDICATIONS

Medication	Taken to Treat	Kinds of Birth Defects
Pregnancy Category X Medications		
antimetabolitic CHEMOTHERAPY drugs (aminopterin, cytarabine, methotrexate, methyl aminopterin)	CANCER	craniofacial anomalies, anencephaly, absence of kidneys, HEART malformations risk highest in first trimester
danazol (Danocrine)	ENDOMETRIOSIS, FIBROCYSTIC BREAST DISEASE, hereditary ANGIOEDEMA	PSEUDOHERMAPHRADITISM
finasteride (Propecia, Proscar)	male pattern baldness (Propecia), BENIGN PROSTATIC HYPERTROPHY (BPH) (Proscar) *pregnant women are at risk if they handle the pills*	malformation of male GENITALIA
flurazepam (Dalmane)	SLEEP DISORDERS	isolated cleft palate
lovastatin (Mevacor)	HYPERLIPIDEMIA	SPINA BIFIDA
retinoic acid, isotretinoin (Accutane)	severe ACNE	craniofacial anomalies, heart malformations, limb deformities, LIVER malformations highest risk in early first trimester
temazepam (Restoril)	sleep disorders	isolated cleft palate
triazolam (Halcion)	sleep disorders	isolated cleft palate
thalidomide (Thalomid, Synovir)	HANSEN'S DISEASE (leprosy), AIDS-related wasting disease (cachexia)	severely shortened or missing long bones in the arms and legs
warfarin (Coumadin)	blood clots (preventive)	constellation of birth defects commonly referred to as fetal warfarin syndrome multiple skeletal deformities and malformations occur with exposure in early first trimester CENTRAL NERVOUS SYSTEM damage occurs with exposure in second and third trimesters
Pregnancy Category D Medications		
angiotensin-converting enzyme (ACE) inhibitor medications (benazepril, captopril, enalapril, fosinopril, lisinopril, moexipril, ramipril, trandolapril)	HYPERTENSION	KIDNEY deformities or absence of kidneys, limb contractures, patent ductus arteriosus (PDA) risk highest in second and third trimesters

Medication	Taken to Treat	Kinds of Birth Defects
angiotensin II receptor antagonist medications (losartan, valsartan, candesartan, irbesartan)	hypertension	heart malformations, kidney deformities or absence of kidneys, widespread organ damage risk highest in third trimester
cimetidine (Tagamet)	GASTROESOPHAGEAL REFLUX DISORDER (GERD), PEPTIC ULCER DISEASE	NEURAL TUBE DEFECTS
phenytoin (Dilantin)	SEIZURE DISORDERS	constellation of birth defects commonly referred to as fetal phenytoin syndrome craniofacial anomalies, deformities of the hands and feet, rib deformities
sulfasalazine (Azulfidine)	INFLAMMATORY BOWEL DISEASE (IBD), especially ulcerative COLITIS	neural tube defects
valproic acid (Depakene)	seizure disorders	craniofacial anomalies, spinal deformities

pregnant and before taking any new medications during pregnancy. The risk for teratogenic effects may increase when a woman takes multiple medications, even when those medications are pregnancy category A and B classifications.

Prenatal Care

PRENATAL CARE lowers the risk for many birth defects. Folic acid (folate) supplementation significantly reduces the risk for NEURAL TUBE DEFECTS such as SPINA BIFIDA and also improves blood GLUCOSE (sugar) control in women who have diabetes. Doctors recommend folic acid supplementation beginning before CONCEPTION when possible, and especially for women who are or have been taking oral contraceptives (birth control pills), which lower folic acid even further. Maternal blood tests for rhesus (Rh) factor and ALPHA FETOPROTEIN (AFP), ULTRASOUND, and in utero diagnostic procedures such as CHORIONIC VILLI SAMPLING (CVS) and AMNIOCENTESIS can detect many birth defects before birth, allowing the mother and her health-care provider to make decisions and appropriate preparations. Other prevention efforts target educating women of childbearing age about the benefits of folic acid supplementation and prenatal care, as well as the risks of behaviors such as alcohol consumption during pregnancy.

KEY MEASURES FOR PREVENTING BIRTH DEFECTS
- folic acid supplementation for all women of childbearing age, whether or not they are pregnant or planning PREGNANCY
- comprehensive PRENATAL CARE during pregnancy
- no alcohol consumption during pregnancy or when attempting to conceive
- vaccination before pregnancy for RUBELLA, CHICKENPOX, MEASLES
- GENETIC COUNSELING when known hereditary conditions exist in either parent or a previous child was born with birth defects

See also ABORTION; CEREBRAL PALSY; CHROMOSOMAL DISORDERS; CLEFT PALATE/CLEFT PALATE AND LIP; CONGENITAL ANOMALY; GENETIC DISORDERS; INHERITANCE PATTERNS.

building-related illness A health condition that arises as the result of problems within a structure, such as an office, school, or home. The US Environmental Protection Agency (EPA) defines a building-related illness (also called a BRI) as one that

- causes clinically observable symptoms and signs, such as COUGH and FEVER, that extend beyond the length of time a person spends in the building

- doctors can diagnose as a specific condition
- requires correction of an identifiable problem within the building

Building-related illnesses include

- LEGIONNAIRES' DISEASE, a type of PNEUMONIA that results from bacterial contamination of building heating and air-conditioning systems
- upper respiratory illnesses due to toxic molds and fungi
- asbestos-related lung disease
- radon-induced LUNG CANCER
- BRONCHITIS, ASTHMA, chronic LARYNGITIS, pneumonia, CHRONIC OBSTRUCTIVE PULMONARY DISEASE (COPD), and cancers resulting from exposure to ENVIRONMENTAL CIGARETTE SMOKE or industrial chemicals

Doctors diagnose and treat building-related illnesses as they would similar illnesses arising from other causes. Because exposure and illness are often chronic, recovery may take extended time. Contemporary building codes and practices help prevent many of the circumstances that cause building-related illnesses, though INDOOR AIR QUALITY remains a significant concern.

See also ASBESTOSIS; ASPERGILLOSIS; LUNGS; RADON EXPOSURE; SICK BUILDING SYNDROME.

C

cancer prevention CANCER claims more than 500,000 lives each year in the United States, and nearly nine million Americans are cancer survivors. Yet all cancers related to TOBACCO use and excessive ALCOHOL consumption are preventable, and cancer experts believe lifestyle changes could prevent a third or more of most other cancers.

The first correlation between a controllable external factor and the development of cancer occurred more than a century ago with the observance that cigarette smokers died younger than nonsmokers. Researchers have since linked cigarette smoking to nearly a dozen types of cancer, notably lung, laryngeal, esophageal, STOMACH, pancreatic, colorectal, prostate, and BREAST cancers as well as myeloid LEUKEMIA. Over the past 40 years scientists have established numerous connections between other external factors and different types of cancer. Many cancer prevention efforts today target those connections, most of which are lifestyle factors. Lifestyle factors associated with an increased risk for many types of cancer include

- tobacco use (particularly cigarette smoking)
- no regular physical exercise
- EATING HABITS that favor high-fat, low-fiber, and low fruit and vegetable consumption
- OBESITY
- excessive alcohol consumption

Though the links between cancer and some lifestyle factors are less than finite, health experts believe lifestyle modifications to minimize the roles of these factors may play in causing cancer could reduce the development of new cancers by about a third and are beneficial for health overall. Some cancers occur as a consequence of chronic INFECTION, such as LIVER CANCER that results from chronic HEPATITIS. Avoiding hepatitis through vaccination and appropriate preventive practices eliminates the cancers it might otherwise cause.

Other cancer prevention efforts target early detection of precancerous and cancerous conditions through screening methods. Early detection allows the highest success for treatment. Nearly all CERVICAL CANCER results from infection with HUMAN PAPILLOMAVIRUS (HPV), which is transmitted sexually, and nearly all COLORECTAL CANCER arises from intestinal polyps. Screenings that detect precancerous conditions, such as intestinal polyps (COLONOSCOPY) and cervical DYSPLASIA (PAP TEST), permit doctors to intervene before the circumstance evolves into one of cancer.

Some health experts advocate taking supplements of antioxidants (such as vitamin C and vitamin E), and in particular COENZYME Q10, to boost the body's ability to resist cancerous growth. Clinical research studies of coenzyme Q10 suggest various health benefits for this potent antioxidant, though to date those investigating the cancer-fighting capabilities of other antioxidants have failed to demonstrate such effect. Consuming substances that decrease inflammatory markers, such as fish oils and aged garlic, may also have preventive benefit.

See also CANCER RISK FACTORS; CERVICAL INTRAEPITHELIAL NEOPLASIA (CIN); LIFESTYLE AND HEALTH; SCREENING FOR CANCER.

cardiovascular disease prevention CARDIOVASCULAR DISEASE (CVD) is the leading cause of death and disability among Americans. It accounts for nearly a million deaths each year and disables as many as 20 million people, limiting their capabilities for work and recreational activities. More than 60 million Americans live with some form of CVD.

SCREENING FOR EARLY DETECTION OF CANCER

Type of Cancer	Routine Screening*
BREAST CANCER	monthly BREAST SELF-EXAMINATION (BSE) annual breast examination from health-care provider annual MAMMOGRAM for women beginning at age 40 years
CERVICAL CANCER	PAP TEST every one to three years beginning with the start of sexual activity or at age 18
colorectal CANCER	annual FECAL OCCULT BLOOD TEST (FOBT) beginning at age 50 in combination with one of the following: • flexible sigmoidoscopy every five years OR • double-contrast BARIUM ENEMA every five years OR • COLONOSCOPY every 10 years
oral cancer (lips and structures of the MOUTH)	annual dental examination
OVARIAN CANCER	annual pelvic examination
PROSTATE CANCER	annual DIGITAL RECTAL EXAMINATION (DRE) to palpate the PROSTATE GLAND for growths beginning at age 45 annual PROSTATE-SPECIFIC ANTIGEN (PSA) blood test beginning at age 50
SKIN CANCER	regular self-examination of all SKIN surfaces skin examination by dermatologist every three to five years after age 40
TESTICULAR CANCER	monthly TESTICULAR SELF-EXAMINATION physician examination with every routine physical for men between the ages of 15 and 35

*For people who have no greater than normal risk for developing cancer. Those who have increased risk because of personal or family health history should follow the recommendations of their physicians.

Yet health experts believe that nearly 90 percent of acquired CVD is preventable. Though people commonly perceive CVD, also called HEART disease, as a condition affecting older adults, its genesis is often in ADOLESCENCE. Some research studies have found early-stage ATHEROSCLEROSIS and CORONARY ARTERY DISEASE (CAD) in teenagers whose lifestyles are sedentary and feature EATING HABITS high in fast foods.

Age and heredity are primary factors in the development of cardiovascular disease. It is not, at present, possible to do much to change their effects on the cardiovascular system. Doctors consider them fixed (immutable) risk factors that

affect every person to some degree. Even in the presence of these risks, however, cardiovascular disease remains primarily the evolution of lifestyle and behavior. These are modifiable (mutable) risk factors; it is possible to change them and thus the influences they exert on the development of cardiovascular disease. Cigarette smoking, OBESITY, lack of regular physical exercise, and eating habits are the leading factors that result in acquired (noncongenital) heart disease. Accordingly, personal prevention efforts target these habits. Key among such efforts are

• SMOKING CESSATION programs

FORMS OF CARDIOVASCULAR DISEASE

ANEURYSM	ANGINA PECTORIS
ARRHYTHMIA	ATHEROSCLEROSIS
BUNDLE BRANCH BLOCK	CARDIOMYOPATHY
cerebral vascular disease	CONGENITAL HEART DISEASE
(STROKE)	CORONARY ARTERY DISEASE (CAD)
ENDOCARDITIS	HEART ATTACK
HEART FAILURE	HYPERLIPIDEMIA
HYPERTENSION	INTERMITTENT CLAUDICATION
ISCHEMIC HEART DISEASE (IHD)	LONG QT SYNDROME
MYOCARDITIS	(LQTS)
PERICARDITIS	PERIPHERAL VASCULAR DISEASE
primary PULMONARY	(PVD)
HYPERTENSION	RAYNAUD'S SYNDROME
RHEUMATIC HEART DISEASE	SICK SINUS SYNDROME
VALVULAR HEART DISEASE	WOLFF-PARKINSON-WHITE
	SYNDROME

- WEIGHT LOSS AND WEIGHT MANAGEMENT programs

- nutrition and dietary education that emphasizes eating habits high in fruits, vegetables, and whole grain products with fewer highly processed and fried foods

- encouraging daily physical exercise through education and activities organized through schools, workplaces, and community organizations

- cholesterol screening with lifestyle modifications and lipid-lowering medications, as appropriate, to maintain healthy levels, and aggressive therapeutic interventions for people who have high blood cholesterol

- BLOOD PRESSURE checks to detect and treat HYPERTENSION

- DIABETES screening programs, as CVD is a leading complication of diabetes and many of the same lifestyle factors contribute to both health problems

Medical interventions can further reduce the effects of lifestyle factors to lower the risk for cardiovascular disease. These interventions may include lipid-lowering medications to reduce CHOLESTEROL BLOOD LEVELS, antihypertensive medications to lower blood pressure, anti-arrhythmia medications to regulate the beating of the heart, and CORONARY ARTERY BYPASS GRAFT (CABG) to replace arteries supplying the heart with blood that are clogged with vascular debris (arterial plaque).

Prevention guidelines established in 2004 take the preventive role of medications a step further, recommending that most people who have heart attacks take a "statin" medication afterward to prevent subsequent heart attacks. Statins belong to the HMG-CoA reductase inhibitor family of drugs that came into widespread use in the 1990s as lipid-lowering medications. Extensive longitudinal studies (studies over time involving varied populations) conducted in several countries, including the United States, demonstrated the further ability of statins to significantly reduce the risk for heart attack in people who have already experienced one or more heart attacks, even when blood cholesterol levels are within heart-healthy ranges.

Because many people do not know they have cardiovascular disease until they have heart attacks or strokes, statin therapy becomes a significant preventive measure for future heart conditions. However, statins deplete COENZYME Q10, an important antioxidant that has powerful anti-inflammatory actions. Taking a coenzyme Q10 supplement while on statin therapy helps restore this vital substance. Many people also benefit from ASPIRIN THERAPY, which provides a mild anticoagulant effect to reduce the risk for blood clots.

LEARN THE WARNING SIGNS OF HEART ATTACK AND HOW TO RESPOND

Health experts recommend that all adults learn the warning signs of HEART ATTACK and become trained in CARDIOPULMONARY RESUSCITATION (CPR). Schools, fire departments, community organizations, and health agencies typically offer CPR classes for minimal or no fee.

Though some studies suggest consumption of red wine lowers the risk for heart disease, most doctors recommend minimizing ALCOHOL consumption overall because of other health risks (such as LIVER disease). Foods that are high in the B vitamins, vitamin C, and vitamin E contain natural antioxidants that help counter the destructive consequences of accumulated metabolic waste (oxidants). Many doctors recommend the nutritional supplement coenzyme Q10, which several studies have shown can improve the ability of cells to resist damage and to repair themselves. Cardiovascular disease prevention is a comprehensive process that encompasses numerous facets of lifestyle and physiology. The more risk factors an individual can control, the greater the preventive benefit.

KEY MEASURES FOR PREVENTING CARDIOVASCULAR DISEASE

- Do not smoke.
- Get 30 to 45 minutes of exercise daily.
- Eat appropriate portion sizes.
- Eat more fruits, vegetables, and whole grains and fewer processed and fried foods.
- Get regular BLOOD PRESSURE and blood cholesterol level checks.

See also AGING, CARDIOVASCULAR CHANGES THAT OCCUR WITH; ANTIOXIDANT; DIET AND CARDIOVASCULAR HEALTH; LIFESTYLE AND HEALTH; MEDICATIONS TO TREAT CARDIOVASCULAR DISEASE; NUTRITIONAL NEEDS; PHYSICAL EXERCISE AND CARDIOVASCULAR HEALTH; RISK FACTORS FOR CARDIOVASCULAR DISEASE.

childhood diseases   Until the advent of vaccines in the middle of the 20th century, infectious childhood diseases such as DIPHTHERIA and PERTUSSIS (whooping cough) were the leading cause of death among children under age 18. Vaccinations have virtually eliminated some communicable diseases such as SMALLPOX (for which doctors no longer routinely administer vaccinations) and POLIOMYELITIS.

ROUTINE CHILDHOOD VACCINATIONS

CHICKENPOX	DIPHTHERIA
Haemophilus influenzae type b (Hib) pneumonia	hepatitis A
	hepatitis B
INFLUENZA (the flu)	MEASLES
MUMPS	PERTUSSIS (whooping cough)
pneumococcal pneumonia	
POLIOMYELITIS	RUBELLA (German measles)
tetanus	

Because of vaccination programs, most Americans born after 1970 have not experienced the infectious childhood diseases that caused illness for their parents as children. Some vaccinations are combination products, such as MMR (MEASLES, MUMPS, RUBELLA) and DTP (diphtheria, tetanus, pertussis). Some vaccinations confer lifelong IMMUNITY (protection from INFECTION) while others require periodic booster vaccines.

There is some concern that the mercury in thimerosal, used to preserve some vaccines, exposes young children to levels of mercury that far exceed established guidelines. In 1999 a number of US health agencies joined forces to urge development of thimerosal-free vaccines, which are now available for most vaccines recommended for children age 6 years and younger. Efforts continue to reduce or eliminate thimerosal in all vaccines. Parents should ask for their children to receive thimerosal-free vaccines. When this is not possible, parents should ask for children to receive single-agent rather than combination vaccinations to reduce mercury exposure as much as possible. For nearly all children the benefits of vaccination far outweigh the potential risks associated with mercury exposure.

Children who do acquire the infectious disease rather than receive the vaccination also develop immunity, though the course of the disease can include serious complications and exposes countless other people to infection as well. Measles can cause severe HEARING LOSS, mumps can result in male sterility, and HEPATITIS can cause LIVER failure. Rubella and chickenpox (also called varicella) can cause BIRTH DEFECTS in unborn children whose mothers get the disease in PREGNANCY.

See also HEAVY METAL POISONING; PREVENTIVE HEALTH CARE AND IMMUNIZATIONS.

community sanitation   Some of the most far-reaching improvements in public health have arisen not from laboratory experiments or technological discoveries but rather from the mundane aspects of everyday life. Community health DRINKING WATER STANDARDS, sewage treatment and disposal, and garbage collection and disposal influence health and LIFE EXPECTANCY as much as any medical intervention.

Ancient Rome provides the earliest archaeological evidence of the understanding of these correlations. The city's design featured elaborate networks of aqueducts (water conduits), public toilets and baths, and sewage drainage systems.

These infrastructures established and maintained separation among living areas, clean water, and waste management. Though perhaps implemented as much as for aesthetic purposes as for health reasons, the health benefits of such separations were clear to ancient Romans who wrote about them, such as Marcus Vitruvius Pollio (90–20 B.C.E.) who wrote extensively about Roman architecture and engineering.

Not until the 19th century and its many discoveries in microbiology did physicians finally connect community sanitation, PERSONAL HYGIENE, and public health. In the millennia between, unsanitary and crowded living conditions fostered ravaging epidemics of CHOLERA (from contaminated water); bubonic plague (from flea-infested rats); yellow FEVER (from mosquitoes); and infectious diseases such as TUBERCULOSIS, SMALLPOX, and FOOD-BORNE ILLNESSES. In such times and circumstances personal bathing was more likely to spread disease than result in cleanliness.

By the start of the 20th century most industrialized countries incorporated public sanitation practices to separate sewage from drinking water supplies and to promote community as well as personal hygiene. Throughout the United States today strict regulations govern community sanitation, establishing processes for disposing of garbage and sewage as well as for maintaining the purity of drinking water and controlling living conditions. However, inadequate sanitation remains a key cause of disease and death in developing parts of the world that lack appropriate mechanisms for community and personal hygiene.

See also HAND WASHING; HEALTH EDUCATION; HEALTH RISK FACTORS; WATERBORNE ILLNESSES.

diabetes prevention DIABETES is emerging as one of the most significant health concerns facing the United States in the 21st century. Approximately 18 million Americans have diabetes and 16 million have prediabetes, a condition of INSULIN RESISTANCE that has a high risk for progressing to diabetes. Prevention efforts target type 2 diabetes, which primarily appears in adults as a manifestation of converging lifestyle factors. About 95 percent of diabetes in the United States is type 2, which many researchers and doctors believe appropriate preventive measures that focus on EATING HABITS and physical exercise can eliminate. Type 1 diabetes, which typically features sudden onset in childhood or ADOLESCENCE, is an autoimmune disorder. Most researchers do not consider type 1 diabetes preventable through lifestyle modifications although lifestyle measures can significantly influence insulin EFFICACY and the development of complications related to diabetes.

The discovery of INSULIN replacement therapy in the early 20th century provided the first viable treatment for diabetes, which until that time had been a diagnosis of death. Nearly 100 years later insulin replacement therapy remains the only treatment for type 1 diabetes. In the 1980s oral ANTIDIABETES MEDICATIONS became available to treat type 2 diabetes. Many of these medications work by increasing cellular sensitivity to insulin. Most type 2 diabetes develops over years to decades and manifests after age 40 years, though doctors are diagnosing the condition in an increasing number of adolescents. Doctors and researchers attribute the increase in young-onset type 2 diabetes to the rise in OBESITY among younger people.

Diet and exercise are the major lifestyle factors that contribute to type 2 diabetes. Improvements in both can delay or prevent the disease's development. In particular, exercise improves cell sensitivity to insulin. Numerous clinical studies have shown that 30 minutes a day of moderate physical activity such as walking, coupled with weight loss of 5 to 10 percent, improves insulin resistance more effectively than do antidiabetes medication. Diabetes is a leading cause of CARDIOVASCULAR DISEASE (CVD), KIDNEY disease, blindness, PERIPHERAL VASCULAR DISEASE (PVD), and limb AMPUTATION.

KEY MEASURES FOR PREVENTING DIABETES

- 30 to 45 minutes of physical exercise daily
- weight loss if necessary to achieve a BODY MASS INDEX (BMI) below 25
- diet that features fruits, vegetables, and whole grain products with fewer processed and fried foods
- annual blood GLUCOSE (sugar) test beginning at age 40 years (sooner in women who have had GESTATIONAL DIABETES)

See also AUTOIMMUNE DISORDERS; DIET AND CARDIOVASCULAR HEALTH; PHYSICAL EXERCISE AND CARDIOVASCULAR HEALTH.

drinking water standards Clean water is fundamental to health. In 1974 the US Congress passed into legislation the Safe Drinking Water Act (SDWA), which the Environmental Protection Agency (EPA) administers and enforces. Amended in 1986 and 1996, the SDWA regulates all public drinking water systems in the United States as well as the sources for drinking water supplies. Regulations define the operational parameters for maintaining safe drinking water systems. Though the SDWA does not apply to private wells that serve fewer than 25 people, the US Food and Drug Administration (FDA) encourages those who obtain their drinking water from private wells to maintain similar clean water standards.

HEALTH RISKS OF DRINKING WATER CONTAMINANTS

Contaminant	Potential Health Risks
disinfectants and disinfectant by-products	**localized irritation, CANCER, neurologic, LIVER, KIDNEY**
chlorine, chloramine, chlorite	EYE/NOSE irritation, ANEMIA
bromate, haloacetic acid	increased cancer risk
trihalomethane	increased cancer risk, liver disease, kidney disease, NERVOUS SYSTEM dysfunction
metals and minerals	**neurologic, SKIN, kidney, liver, thyroid, circulatory**
asbestos	INTESTINAL POLYP
arsenic	skin and circulatory problems, increased cancer risk
copper	liver and kidney damage
cyanide	nervous system damage, thyroid dysfunction
lead	developmental delays, kidney damage
mercury	kidney damage
selenium	circulatory damage, HAIR loss
pathogenic microorganisms	**GASTROENTERITIS (NAUSEA, vomiting, DIARRHEA)**
Giardia lamblia (PARASITE)	GIARDIASIS
Cryptosporidium (parasite)	CRYPTOSPORIDIOSIS
Fecal coliform (BACTERIA)	generalized gastroenteritis
Escherichia coli (bacteria)	*E. coli* gastroenteritis
legionella	LEGIONNAIRES' DISEASE (PNEUMONIA)
organic chemicals	**fertilizers, herbicides, industrial chemical**
altrazine, carbofuran, 1,2-dibromo-3-chloropropane	reproductive dysfunction
(DBCP), dioxin, ethylene dibromide, methoxychlor	increased cancer risk
dichloromethane, dichloropropane, heptachlor,	liver dysfunction
hexachlorobenzene, pentachlorophenol,	anemia and other blood disorders
tetrachloroethylene, trichloroethylene, vinyl chloride	immune dysfunction, neurologic disturbances, increased cancer
alachlor, carbon tetrachloride, chlordane, chlorobenzene,	risk, reproductive dysfunction
dichloroethylene, endrin, ethylbenzene, lindane	neurologic disturbances
benzene, simazine, styrene	
polychlorinated biphenyls (PCBs)	
acrylamide, toluene, xylene	
radionuclides	**increased cancer risk**
radium 226/228, uranium	increase in overall lifetime risk for developing cancer
viruses	**gastroenteritis**
enteroviruses, noroviruses, rotavirus	nausea, vomiting, cramping, diarrhea

Drinking water supplies contain numerous natural and manmade substances that are harmful to health. Under the SDWA, the FDA researches the effects of such contaminants and establishes standards that keep contaminants either out of drinking water supplies or at levels not expected to cause health problems in people with a healthy IMMUNE SYSTEM. These standards may be inadequate to protect people who are IMMUNOCOMPROMISED, such as people who have HIV/AIDS. Local health departments can provide information about contaminant levels in specific water supplies as well as recommendations for further purifying drinking water. Because it is not always possible to prevent contaminants from entering drinking water sources, water systems typically filter and treat (such as by chlorination) drinking water supplies to reduce contaminants to nonpathogenic levels.

FDA regulations currently address approximately 80 contaminants capable of causing acute (immediate and short term) or chronic (cumulative with exposure over time) health conditions. Among them are

- microorganisms such as BACTERIA (notably fecal coliform and *Escherichia coli*) and parasites

- enteric viruses (viruses that cause gastrointestinal INFECTION)
- disinfectants and disinfectant by-products
- organic and nonorganic chemicals (metals, minerals, and industrial chemicals)
- radionuclides (radioactive particles)

Because scientific knowledge continuously evolves, detecting and eliminating drinking water contaminants is a dynamic process. Generally, state and local water jurisdictions develop the procedures they follow to comply with FDA safe drinking water standards, with input from local health authorities as well as the general public.

See also COMMUNITY SANITATION; ENVIRONMENTAL HAZARD EXPOSURE; FLUORIDATION; WATERBORNE ILLNESSES.

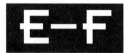

environmental hazard exposure Numerous substances in the environment create risk for a variety of health problems and conditions. They include pesticides, herbicides, industrial pollutants, minerals and metals, molds and fungi, BACTERIA, viruses, radiation, sewage, garbage, biological waste, and electromagnetic fields. These substances may be naturally occurring or the consequence of human actions, such as manufacturing and agricultural processes. They may cause a wide spectrum of health conditions ranging from hypersensitivity reactions to CANCER.

HEALTH CONDITIONS THAT MAY ARISE
FROM ENVIRONMENTAL HAZARD EXPOSURE

ALLERGIC RHINITIS	ALZHEIMER DISEASE
ASTHMA	AUTISM
brain cancer	chronic BRONCHITIS
CHRONIC OBSTRUCTIVE PULMONARY	DERMATITIS
DISEASE (COPD)	EMPHYSEMA
FIBROMYALGIA	GASTROENTERITIS
HEARING LOSS	HEAVY-METAL POISONING
INFECTION	LIVER CANCER
LUNG CANCER	MALIGNANT MELANOMA
METHEMOGLOBINEMIA	MULTIPLE SCLEROSIS
PNEUMONIA	poisoning
thyroid disease	

Often, environmental hazards may not directly cause disease but rather become added risk factors that, in aggregate with other factors or circumstances relevant to certain individuals or population groups, increase the likelihood of disease. For example, environmental chemicals may present little risk to the public overall yet confer significant risk on pregnant women. Young children are more likely than adults to experience lead poisoning due to water contamination, not only because of their smaller size but also because their bodies are still developing and cannot yet efficiently clear toxins. People who are IMMUNOCOMPROMISED are highly vulnerable to INFECTION resulting from foodborne or waterborne viruses and bacteria, whereas infection fails to gain a stronghold in people whose immune systems are healthy.

Federal, state, and local agencies oversee administration and enforcement of environmental health laws, regulations, and standards in the United States. Key among them are the US Centers for Disease Control and Prevention (CDC), the National Center for Environmental Health, the US Department of Agriculture (USDA), and the US Environmental Protection Agency (EPA). Collectively, these agencies operate programs to prevent, detect, mitigate, and remedy health conditions arising from exposure to environmental hazards.

See also BUILDING-RELATED ILLNESS; DRINKING WATER STANDARDS; FOODBORNE ILLNESSES; INDOOR AIR QUALITY; RADIATION EXPOSURE; SICK BUILDING SYNDROME; WATERBORNE ILLNESSES.

environmental cigarette smoke People who do not smoke but who live or work among people who smoke in their presence are at risk for the same health conditions that affect smokers, including LUNG CANCER, CHRONIC OBSTRUCTIVE PULMONARY DISEASE (COPD), EMPHYSEMA, CARDIOVASCULAR DISEASE (CVD), and chronic BRONCHITIS. Children who regularly breathe cigarette smoke from smokers in the home, also called secondhand smoke or passive smoking, have a much higher rate of chronic OTITIS media (middle EAR INFECTION), ASTHMA, allergies, and chronic bronchitis. Most schools, workplaces, government offices, and indoor public facilities ban cigarette smoking as a means to reduce exposure to environmental cigarette smoke. Some municipalities in the United States have banned all indoor smoking in locations open to the public.

One measure of cigarette smoke exposure is the blood cotinine level. The body produces cotinine when it breaks down (metabolizes) NICOTINE, the active chemical ingredient of TOBACCO. Researchers believe that while cotinine itself presents no health risk, it provides an accurate measure of exposure to other chemicals, many of which are carcinogenic (cancer-causing), that are present in cigarette smoke. Cotinine is among the chemical federal agencies monitor to assess the health risks of ENVIRONMENTAL HAZARD EXPOSURE.

See also ANTISMOKING EFFORTS; INDOOR AIR QUALITY; LIFESTYLE AND HEALTH; RADON EXPOSURE; SMOKING AND CANCER; SMOKING AND CARDIOVASCULAR DISEASE; SMOKING AND HEALTH.

ergonomics The interactions between people and their physical environments can support or challenge health. The primary role of ergonomics in health is to prevent injuries, particularly musculoskeletal injuries that result from repetitive motions, by identifying interactions that present a risk for injury and implementing interventions to mitigate the risk. Ergonomic interventions may be as simple as rearranging the work area to put commonly used items within easy reach or may require specialized devices and equipment such as telephone headsets, curved handles on tools, nonglare screens for computers, and implements designed specifically for left-handed use.

Ergonomics also evaluates the movements and actions of commonly performed tasks to minimize the risk of overuse to recommend improved methods and techniques. Many job tasks have evolved without formalized attention to the movements they require, with the consequence that employees develop habits for performing the tasks that may not be ergonomically sound. Actions that cause continual reaching across the body, for example, create repetitive stress for the shoulders, back, and neck. Changing the pattern of movement to use the other hand or rearranging the work area to eliminate cross-reaching can signifi-

ERGONOMICS-RELATED HEALTH CONDITIONS		
Health Condition	**Common Tasks**	**Remedies**
CARPAL TUNNEL SYNDROME	typing, keyboarding, production line, retail scanner	proper technique, ergonomically designed keyboard, frequent movement to stretch fingers and rotate wrists
EYE STRAIN	computer work, watching security monitors, reading, inadequate or inappropriate lighting	eyeglasses to accommodate midrange vision, frequent looking away from task to change focal distance, proper lighting
HEADACHE	noise exposure, bright lights	improved ventilation and airflow
low BACK PAIN	twisting, bending, lifting, extensive walking, prolonged standing	frequent stretching and position changes, proper lift and carry techniques, supportive shoes, shock-absorbent flooring
neck PAIN	holding telephone between chin and shoulder, looking at computer or video monitor, frequently turning head	headset, correct height and distance placement for monitor, rearrange workspace to minimize turning
ROTATOR CUFF IMPINGEMENT SYNDROME	reaching, production line, throwing	reorganize work area to minimize turning, frequent stretching and resting

cantly reduce this stress and its corresponding injuries. An improved method might be as simple as using a footstool or sliding ladder instead of reaching for items on shelves, or could require retraining employees in proper use of equipment and machinery.

Ergonomic factors account for about 4 million injuries among Americans each year, about half of which are serious enough to require medical care or limit participation in daily activities. Ergonomic injuries further account for a third of lost work time. Most of these injuries are musculoskeletal. The US Occupational Health and Safety Agency (OSHA) develops and administers guidelines for ergonomic standards and improvements in the workplace. Though implemented changes to improve the ergonomics of job tasks can prevent future injuries, people who have already experienced ergonomic-related injuries may have long-term or permanent health consequences.

See also ACCIDENTAL INJURIES; OCCUPATIONAL HEALTH AND SAFETY; REPETITIVE MOTION INJURIES.

food safety   FOODBORNE ILLNESSES sicken 76 million Americans each year, 5,000 of whom die as a result. Public health efforts target food safety on a community as well as an individual level. At the public safety level, the US Department of Agriculture (USDA) and the US Food and Drug Administration (FDA) oversee numerous programs that regulate food safety in the United States. These programs cover the gamut of food production and include pesticide and herbicide use, animal feed and use of supplements, food additives, product packaging and labeling, and safe food handling practices among wholesalers and retailers (including grocery stores and restaurants). These agencies inspect production facilities and test produce, grains, dairy products, meats, and other foods for biological and chemical contaminants.

The US Centers for Disease Control and Prevention (CDC) monitors foodborne illness outbreaks, in coordination with state and local health departments. These agencies investigate illnesses and recommend corrective procedures to prevent future outbreaks. They also provide education and training for people who work in food services industries. Though the public tends to fear outbreaks of foodborne illnesses that originate from

settings such as cruise ships or restaurants, most foodborne illness occurs as a result of contamination in home-prepared foods.

Summertime picnics, holiday parties, and other events where people entertain large groups in their homes or other private venues are common sources of "food poisoning." Nearly always, these events can be traced to improper food preparation, handling, serving, and storage. Using the same surfaces and implements to prepare meat or poultry and then vegetables and fruits allows cross-contamination of BACTERIA that may be present on countertops and cutting boards, in the air, or on foods.

Proper cooking kills the bacteria in the meat or poultry, but raw vegetables and fruits can carry bacteria and the potential for illness to those who eat them. The tendency to leave food out so people may help themselves or while other festivities take place can allow bacteria to flourish. Salads made with mayonnaise, cooked turkey, and pies left out too long at warm temperatures are commonly to blame for foodborne illness. More often than not, contaminated foods look and taste fine.

KEY INDIVIDUAL MEASURES
FOR PREVENTING FOODBORNE ILLNESSES

- Wash hands frequently with soap and warm water, especially before and after preparing food.
- Use separate surfaces for preparing meats and other foods.
- Thoroughly cook meats.
- Keep hot foods heated and cold foods chilled when serving them buffet-style.
- Promptly refrigerate leftovers and throw away most leftovers after five days.

See also HAND WASHING; WATERBORNE ILLNESSES.

fluoridation   Fluoride is a naturally occurring element that enhances a tooth's ability to retain hardening minerals such as calcium. US federal regulations began requiring communities to add fluoride to their water supplies, when naturally occurring levels of fluoride fall below 0.7 parts per million (ppm), in 1945 as a means of reducing DENTAL CARIES (cavities). Fluoride offers the greatest protection when it is in the bloodstream as the TEETH are forming, so it becomes part of the enamel. Even after the teeth have fully developed, fluoride continues to interact with the enamel through its presence in the saliva. Dentists also may apply topical fluoride to the surfaces of the teeth for added protection.

The American Dental Association and numerous other health organizations advocate fluoridation, though some groups question the safety of the practice. In the decades since fluoridation became public policy, numerous claims about adverse health effects have surfaced. Investigations of those concerns have failed to produce conclusive evidence to validate them, when fluoride levels are within the established therapeutic ranges. Excessive fluoride consumption can cause dental fluoridosis, in which dark stains appear on the teeth. Though harmless, the tooth stains are permanent. Children should use fluoridated toothpaste in small amounts and with close parental supervision.

See also ORAL HYGIENE.

hand washing Frequent hand washing with soap and warm water is one of the most effective means of preventing the spread of infectious diseases. Hand contact is a primary method of transmitting bacterial and viral infections. Hand washing kills or removes most pathogenic agents. To wash the hands:

- Turn on tap to dispense water that is warm but not too hot to hold the hands under its flow.
- Get hands wet.
- Apply soap, preferably liquid soap from a dispenser.
- Work the soap into a lather that covers all surfaces of the hands, taking a full minute.
- Rinse hands under running water.
- If it is not possible to turn off the water without touching the faucet handles, leave the water temporarily running.
- Dry hands thoroughly using disposable towels or a heated air dispenser.
- Use a paper towel to cover the faucet handle, then turn off the water.

WHEN TO WASH THE HANDS

after changing a diaper	after cleaning dirty dishes
after handling raw meat or poultry	after holding an infant
	after petting or handling
after sneezing or coughing into the hand	animals
	after sneezing, coughing, or
after using the bathroom	BLOWING THE NOSE
before eating	before holding an infant
before preparing food	before serving food

It is particularly important to wash the hands after going to the bathroom. Fecal-to-oral trans-mission spreads many gastrointestinal infections. Some studies suggest that many people wash their hands only when they believe someone is observing them. Though hand washing sounds like a simple solution to a complex problem, health experts project it could significantly reduce infectious diseases.

See also BACTERIA; ENTERITIS; FOODBORNE ILLNESSES; GASTROENTERITIS; PERSONAL HYGIENE; TRANSMISSION MODES; VIRUS.

health education Health experts consider instruction about health and disease to be a fundamental dimension of preventive medicine. Health education formalizes such instruction within structured settings such as schools, workshops, and classes. At its most basic level, health education the form of the fundamental instruction children receive in school about the functions of the human body. All states in the United States have governmentally mandated health education requirements, typically for kindergarten (K) through grade 8 or grades K through 12. Other health education curricula may target college-level students. Some health education programs focus on the needs of specific populations, such as childbirth education classes for pregnant women and their partners or DIABETES education classes for people who have diabetes. Businesses may offer health education programs for their employees and their families with the dual goals of improving personal health and reducing time lost to illness or injury.

See also LIFESTYLE AND HEALTH.

health insurance Health insurance is the financial platform for health care in the United States. As such, it plays a significant role in access to health-care services and in health-care treatment decisions. In 2004, about 250 million Americans had health insurance, just over two thirds through private coverage and the remainder through public programs such as Medicaid and state low-cost health plans.

Nearly all health insurance plans require participants to pay a portion of their medical expenses, typically in the form of annual deductibles and service co-payments. A deductible is payment at the front end, for example, the first $2,500.00 of medical costs each year. A co-payment shares the cost of each health-care service between the person and the insurer, either as a dollar amount or a percentage of the charge. Most plans have a cap on out-of-pocket medical expenses, after which the insurer pays the full amount for covered services. Nonetheless, people who experience serious illnesses or injuries can accumulate significant additional medical expenses for services the insurance plan does not cover. As well, most people pay a portion or all of their health insurance premiums.

Because the US health-care system intricately intertwines health-care services and health insurance, conflicts arise between care needs and insurance coverage. Doctors and hospitals coordinate with insurers to obtain approval for most non-emergency treatments before engaging in them. Most insurers have lists of approved procedures and medications to facilitate the administrative processes and issue payments directly to providers. Each state has laws and rules that regulate how these processes take place and establish procedures for handling disagreements with insurer decisions, and a state insurance commissioner oversees their enforcement.

Though 85 percent of the US population has health insurance and thus access to health-care services, 15 percent does not—about 42 million people. Those who do not have health insurance have great difficulty receiving needed health-care services. The federal government mandates that providers may not deny care to anyone for life-threatening illness or injury and for a pregnant woman's delivery of her child. All states have programs to provide basic health-care services for children and pregnant women. State and local programs attempt to fill in the gaps in providing

other care, though the need far exceeds available services.

The intertwining of health insurance and health services that can be an advantage for people who have health insurance becomes a barrier for the 42 million Americans who do not. They frequently go without medical care for conditions that prompt treatment would remedy but that without early intervention become serious and even life-threatening. Preemptive treatment, such as medications to lower blood cholesterol levels or control BLOOD PRESSURE, as well as preventive health measures such as ROUTINE PHYSICAL EXAMINATION, often are out of reach. Many health experts and public health policy planners view the lack of health insurance as one of the most significant challenges facing the health of Americans and the stability of the US health-care system.

See also HEALTH RISK FACTORS; HEALTHY PEOPLE 2010; QUALITY OF LIFE.

health risk factors The variables that create increased vulnerability to illness and injury are numerous and varied. Some health risks are fixed (immutable), such as those related to heredity, gender, and age. Many health risk factors are modifiable (mutable) and correlate to lifestyle and habit. The combination of fixed and modifiable risk factors helps one assess an individual's overall likelihood of developing health conditions such as CARDIOVASCULAR DISEASE (CVD), DIABETES, LIVER disease, KIDNEY disease, COLORECTAL CANCER, LUNG CANCER, PROSTATE CANCER, CERVICAL CANCER, and BREAST CANCER. Though researchers separate fixed and modifiable risk factors from the perspective of health prevention opportunities, within the body the effects of all health risk factors intertwine and affect each other in immeasurable ways.

Fixed (Immutable) Health Risk Factors
Age and gender are the primary fixed risk factors for health. Other fixed health risk factors include personal and family health history (heredity). Though it is not possible to change fixed risk factors, it is possible to influence and somewhat mitigate them through lifestyle and by controlling modifiable risk factors.

Age The risk for many health conditions increases with age as body systems and structures begin to deteriorate. Age further carries with it the specter of lifestyle choices and their health consequences, often compounding health risk. With increasing age, for example, the body becomes less efficient in its ability to use INSULIN. This increases the risk for type 2 diabetes. Physical inactivity and EATING HABITS may further challenge the body's insulin efficiency, as well as contribute to OBESITY, an independent risk factor for diabetes. In combination, these circumstances significantly boost the likelihood of developing diabetes in older age. Cardiovascular function also becomes less efficient with age, as blood vessels lose elasticity (often as a result of ATHEROSCLEROSIS).

Gender Some health conditions, of course, affect only men (prostate and testicular disorders) or only women (cervical, ovarian, and uterine disorders as well as PREGNANCY-related conditions). Other health conditions may predominantly affect one over the other gender, such as breast cancer. Popular perception erroneously holds that some health problems, such as cardiovascular disease and colorectal cancer, are primarily health risks for men. Though men are more likely than women to develop cardiovascular disease earlier in life, cardiovascular disease is the leading cause of death and disability among men and women alike. Doctors diagnose more women than men with colorectal cancer each year.

Health history PERSONAL HEALTH HISTORY significantly influences future health circumstances and often integrates with lifestyle (modifiable risk factors). Some health conditions are purely of hereditary origin, such as CYSTIC FIBROSIS, HEMOPHILIA, or congenital heart malformations. Some acquired conditions may result in residual health effects, such as chronic OTITIS media (middle ear INFECTION) that may have consequential HEARING LOSS. Other conditions may reflect a genetic predisposition as well as lifestyle choices, such as DIABETES AND CARDIOVASCULAR DISEASE.

Advances in genetics and molecular medicine are making it possible to determine whether a person has a hereditary health condition. Though such knowledge does not change the risk for developing the condition, it does allow the person and his or her doctor to establish a plan for managing the condition. Making changes in lifestyle

may delay the condition's development or further mitigate its the adverse effects.

Modifiable (Mutable) Health Risk Factors

Cigarette smoking, eating habits, and physical activity are the primary modifiable risk factors for health. Other health risk factors include occupation, recreational activities, ALCOHOL use, substance abuse, seat belt use, helmet use, and preventive health measures such as vaccination and safer sex practices. Modifiable health risk factors may directly cause disease, such as cigarette smoking, or contribute to the circumstances that allow health conditions to develop, as with diabetes.

Cigarette smoking Since the 1950s, research has linked cigarette smoking with a growing list of health conditions. There are no known health benefits of cigarette smoking. The leading health consequences of smoking are cardiovascular disease and lung cancer. Smoking also causes or contributes to dozens of other health conditions along the entire continuum of life: it influences CONCEPTION, pregnancy, childhood health (ENVIRONMENTAL CIGARETTE SMOKE), nutrition, chronic diseases, numerous cancers, and LIFE EXPECTANCY.

Eating habits The advent of fast food and processed food in the 1960s forever changed eating habits in the United States. Three decades later two thirds of the American population was overweight, a significant general health risk. Most fast foods and processed foods combine low nutritional content and excessive portion sizes.

Fast-food meals often feature "deals" that offer more food for a small increase in price, giving the impression of value. Processed foods, such as quick-prepare meals and snack items, come in packaging often implies the product is a single serving when instead the package contains two, three, or even four servings. When fast foods and processed foods are the mainstay of a person's eating habits, CALORIE consumption often is two to four times what it should be.

Fewer than 20 percent of Americans eat the American Cancer Society's recommended 9 to 12 daily servings of fruits and vegetables, yet more than a third exceed the American Heart Association's guideline limiting dietary fat consumption to 30 percent of total calories. Most Americans need to eat fewer processed and fried foods and more fruits, vegetables, and whole grain products to meet the nutritional needs of their bodies.

Physical activity Despite the proliferation of gyms, health clubs, and fitness centers over the past few decades, fewer than 20 percent of American adults get the daily physical exercise their bodies need to maintain cardiovascular health and overall metabolic efficiency. Lack of regular physical activity may be more of a factor than eating habits for health maintenance as well as development of health conditions. An adult needs a minimum 30 minutes of sustained, moderately intense, physical activity (such as walking) every day and one to two hours of sustained, moderate to high intensity, exercise (such as swimming, running, bicycling, or basketball) three or four times a week to maintain optimal health.

Obesity Obesity, a combination of factors with eating habits and physical activity at the hub, emerged in the 1990s as an independent health risk factor for numerous health conditions. Key among them are HYPERTENSION (high BLOOD PRESSURE), HEART FAILURE, OBSTRUCTIVE SLEEP APNEA, type 2 diabetes, OSTEOARTHRITIS, infertility, and GALLBLADDER DISEASE. The current clinical standard for assessing health risk associated with body weight is the BODY MASS INDEX (BMI), a mathematical calculation that converts height-and-weight ratio to an aggregate measure of body mass. Researchers have been able to correlate such measures with health conditions and know that lowering BMI, which only occurs through weight loss, correspondingly lowers health risk.

Reducing Personal Health Risk

Health risk factors tend to converge in patterns of increased susceptibility. A person who develops diabetes, for example, acquires an increased risk for cardiovascular disease, kidney disease, and cataracts. As well, the risks for these conditions further increase with age, and family history may also play a role. The key to mitigating health risks is sustained modifications in lifestyle habits that allow a person to maintain optimal health.

Sometimes these modifications are in response to the emergence of health conditions such as cardiovascular disease, diabetes, or cancer. Though the health condition becomes a risk factor as well, changes that improve modifiable risk factors provide cumulative health benefits. For example, a person who has a heart attack may begin walking every day as part of a cardiac rehabilitation program. The regular physical exercise improves cardiovascular health, and over time the person loses 10 or 20 pounds. Blood pressure, blood GLUCOSE (sugar), and blood cholesterol levels also come down.

Nearly everyone can benefit from doing as much as is possible to reduce health risk factors. Seldom is it too late to make changes that improve health and QUALITY OF LIFE.

See also ACCIDENTAL INJURIES; CONGENITAL ANOMALY; DIET AND HEALTH; INHERITANCE PATTERNS; LIFESTYLE AND HEALTH; EXERCISE AND HEALTH; RISK FACTORS FOR CARDIOVASCULAR DISEASE; SEXUAL HEALTH; SEXUALLY TRANSMITTED DISEASE (STD) PREVENTION; YOUTH HIGH-RISK BEHAVIOR.

Healthy People 2010 A program of health initiatives that numerous US health agencies jointly sponsor, the goals of which are to improve overall public health in key areas called leading health indicators. The first Healthy People program, Healthy People 2000, evolved from the 1979 US surgeon general's report of the same name. It established criteria for health monitoring and improvement. Various federal and state health organizations structured their objectives and programs to dovetail with Healthy People 2000. Though Healthy People 2000 did not achieve all of its goals, it resulted in measurable improvements in many areas of public health. Healthy People 2010 updates and expands the goals of its predecessor, with annual reports that identify accomplishments and challenges. Healthy People 2010 draws data from existing sources and mechanisms.

Among the participating US federal agencies are the Agency for Healthcare Research and Quality (AHRQ), Centers for Disease Control and Prevention (CDC), US Food and Drug Administration (FDA), Indian Health Service, National Institutes of Health (NIH), Office of Population Affairs, and President's Council on Physical Fitness and Sports. As well, more than 400 state and community health organizations form the Healthy People Consortium.

See also HEALTH RISK FACTORS; LIFESTYLE AND HEALTH.

heavy-metal poisoning Toxicity due to metals such as lead, mercury, copper, and iron can have serious and even lethal health consequences, especially among children. Heavy metals occur naturally in the environment. They are present in soil and in plants that grow underground, and in water. Heavy metals are also the by-products of manufacturing processes. They can quickly accumulate to hazardous levels when they leach into drinking water supplies or enter the food chain when farmers irrigate crops using contaminated water. Some metal pollutants are also present in the air. Numerous environmental laws enacted over the past 30 years have significantly reduced the presence of heavy metals as pollutants; and various standards, such as those for drinking water, require monitoring of metal and mineral levels. The US Environmental Protection Agency (EPA) monitors and enforces these laws.

Lead Federal regulations have banned lead in paints, inks, and gasoline for several decades. Nonetheless lead poisoning continues to be a problem, particularly among children, who are vulnerable to damage at much lower levels of ingestion. Houses built before 1977 may still have leaded paint on the walls and especially wood trim, which young children may peel off and eat. Lead also can enter water supplies when the pipes that carry it are made of lead. As the pipes deteriorate they release lead into the water they carry. Though many larger municipalities have replaced old lead pipes, many smaller ones have not. The smaller body size of children makes them especially vulnerable to toxic accumulations of lead. When the body stops receiving fresh supplies of lead, it can slowly process the lead that has accu-

mulated, and eventually most body systems return to normal.

Mercury The natural forms of mercury are liquid or gas. It forms different chemicals when it combines with other substances. Manufacturing processes combine mercury with oxygen or chlorine to form inorganic combinations, called salts, used in industrial applications such as caustic soda and batteries. Dentists use inorganic mercury compounds in fillings for TEETH. In nature mercury combines with carbon (methylmercury), usually in water, to form organic compounds. These organic mercury compounds accumulate in fish and shellfish.

> **The liquid nature of mercury has given rise to perceptions that it has mystical or supernatural abilities. Some spiritual and ritualistic practices use mercury, also called quicksilver or azogue, in baths, burned in candles, and sprinkled on surfaces. Like any other form of mercury, however, quicksilver is toxic. Many people who handle, breathe, or ingest quicksilver suffer mercury poisoning.**

Excessive amounts of mercury in the body can result in permanent damage to the BRAIN and kidneys. Studies link two forms of mercury—mercury chloride and methylmercury—with an increased risk for developing CANCER. Many people are concerned about the health risks possibly associated with mercury dental fillings (also called dental amalgam). The American Dental Association and the US Food and Drug Administration (FDA), among other health agencies, have issued position statements supporting the continued use of mercury fillings because there are no conclusive studies that correlate its use to mercury poisoning. However, most dentists offer alternative materials for people who are concerned about mercury fillings.

By far the most significant source of mercury among Americans is seafood. In 2004 the FDA issued a health advisory regarding mercury levels in four kinds of fish: swordfish, king mackerel, shark, and tilefish. These fish are at the top of the food chain; they live for many years, subsisting on a diet of other fish. Methylmercury levels in the flesh of these kinds of fish are higher than in other kinds of fish. The advisory recommends that pregnant women and women who are BREASTFEEDING avoid eating these kinds of fish. Salmon, cod, albacore tuna, pollock, haddock, ocean perch, tilapia, and fresh-water trout have the lowest levels of mercury.

Thimerosal, a common preservative in vaccines and some other biologic agents, contains mercury. Though pharmaceutical manufacturers are moving away from its use, thimerosal remains a concern especially with childhood vaccinations. Individuals should ask for thimerosal-free vaccines and other biologic agents for themselves and for their children. US health agencies have called for the complete eradication of thimerosal as a medicinal preservative.

Copper Though copper occurs in nature, the most common source of human exposure to copper is through water supplies that travel through copper pipes. Water that is highly acidic corrodes the pipes, drawing copper into the water. Excessive copper accumulations in the body can cause irreversible LIVER and KIDNEY damage. Copper also can accumulate in the brain, causing cognitive dysfunction. People who have WILSON'S DISEASE, a hereditary disorder in which the body cannot metabolize copper, are especially vulnerable to copper in the food supply and the environment because copper accumulates in their bodies. The body needs only a very small amount of copper, which it uses to make certain enzymes and to facilitate iron METABOLISM for HEMOGLOBIN production.

Iron The body needs iron to produce hemoglobin, the protein in the blood that binds with oxygen. Iron deficiency is fairly common, and many people take iron supplements. These supplements are the most frequent source for iron poisoning, especially among young children. Excessive amounts of iron in the body slow the HEART RATE and force of contractions, reducing the flow of blood. Other chemical changes that take place at the molecular level affect the ability of cells throughout the body to function. People who have the hereditary condition HEMOCHROMATOSIS cannot properly metabolize iron, resulting in toxic accumulations over years to decades. Iron is also highly toxic to the liver, resulting in hepatonecrosis (death of hepatocytes, the primary functional cells in the liver).

See also DRINKING WATER STANDARDS; POISON PREVENTION.

hepatitis prevention Although acute (sudden and limited) HEPATITIS infections are on the decline in the United States, chronic hepatitis infections (long-term) have reached epidemic proportions. Nearly a third of the US population has had hepatitis A INFECTION, an acute form of the disease that is sudden and limited. While the numbers of new cases are dropping each year because of vaccination and education efforts, hepatitis A remains a significant health threat because it can so easily be transmitted from one person to another. Hepatitis A spreads via oral–fecal contamination as a consequence of failing to wash the hands after using the bathroom. This spreads the VIRUS to items the infected person touches. A significant source of infection is contaminated uncooked foods such as salads. Hepatitis A outbreaks can sweep through schools, day care centers, cruise ships, prisons, and other environments in which large groups of people are in close contact.

Another 7 percent of Americans have chronic forms of hepatitis, either hepatitis B or hepatitis C. The rate of infection for chronic hepatitis is highest among injectable DRUG users and homosexual men (because of bodily fluid contact). Health-care and public safety workers are also at high risk for infection as a result of occupational exposures. However, hepatitis is so pervasive that anyone can become infected without being aware they have been exposed. Some people can carry hepatitis without themselves being sick and usually do not know they are carriers. Yet they can spread the hepatitis virus to others.

Of the five most common hepatitis viruses, fecal–oral contact is the primary infectious route for two: hepatitis A and hepatitis E. These forms of hepatitis are generally acute (sudden and limited). Blood and body fluid contact, such as via sexual intercourse and shared needles among injectable drug users, spread hepatitis B and hepatitis C. Hepatitis D is a risk only for people infected with hepatitis B, as it can replicate only by "hijacking" the hepatitis B virus's genetic material.

Hepatitis C is particularly insidious because the infection can take 20 to 30 years to progress enough to generate symptoms. A blood test can detect antibodies after the virus has been in the body for about six weeks, however, and health experts recommend that people who are at risk for hepatitis C be tested. People at highest risk for having hepatitis C infection are those who may have engaged in high-risk behaviors as long as 20 or 30 years ago. About 4 million Americans have chronic hepatitis C infection, nearly 2 percent of the U.S. population, and epidemiologists believe they may reflect only about 30 to 40 percent of those who are actually infected.

Hepatitis is a significant public health issue. Acute hepatitis sickens thousands of people each year and can be particularly serious, even fatal, in children and in people who are IMMUNOCOMPROMISED. Chronic hepatitis is the leading cause of LIVER FAILURE and leading reason for LIVER TRANSPLANTATION in the United States. A secondary public health concern is that a person who has had hepatitis, or who has chronic hepatitis, cannot donate blood. This has the potential to severely limit the availability of blood and blood products for transfusion.

KEY MEASURES FOR PREVENTING HEPATITIS

- Wash hands frequently with soap and warm water.
- Do not share food, drinks, or eating utensils.
- Receive the hepatitis A and hepatitis B vaccinations.
- Do not use injectable drugs.
- Use condoms during sexual intercourse, and limit sexual partners.
- Use barrier precautions (masks and gloves) to protect against INFECTION from occupational exposure.
- Receive prophylactic treatment (immunoglobulin injection) after suspected exposure.

See also SEXUALLY TRANSMITTED DISEASE (STD) PREVENTION.

HIV/AIDS prevention Researchers first detected the human immunodeficiency VIRUS (HIV) that causes acquired immunodeficiency syndrome (AIDS) in the early 1980s. New HIV/AIDS infections peaked about a decade later and have since slowly but steadily declined to reach a point over the past decade of holding relatively steady in the United States at about 40,000 a year. Advances in treatment, however, have resulted in increasing numbers of people living with HIV. Though this marks an exciting milestone in the fight against HIV/AIDS, it also means the risk for INFECTION is growing because more people are already infected. As well, health experts worry that improved treatment regimens that can forestall the transition from an HIV-positive status to AIDS may encourage complacency about HIV protection. AIDS remains ultimately fatal, and preventing infection remains the only cure. Though medical treatments can delay the disease's progression, there are as yet no treatments that can eradicate the virus. Research continues to search for both a cure and a VACCINE.

Prevention efforts target two dimensions of HIV/AIDS infection, halting the spread of infection and early diagnosis and treatment for those who become infected. Because of the long period of time during which a person can be infected and not know it, health experts view early diagnosis as a preventive measure; because most people, once diagnosed as HIV-positive, will take the recommended precautions to prevent spreading the virus to others. People who do not know they have HIV often do not feel the need to take significant precautions. A special focus area is preventing perinatal infection, in which an HIV-positive woman passes the virus to her unborn child.

Preventing New Infections
A person gets HIV/AIDS from close and regular contact with the body fluids, such as BLOOD and SEMEN, of another person who already has the virus. Abstinence is the only certain way to prevent infection via sexual activity with a partner. Barrier methods to prevent the body fluids of one person from contact with the mucous tissues of the other person during sex are the most effective approaches to reduce the risk for transmitting HIV. Consistent use of latex condoms during sex (anal, vaginal, and oral intercourse) significantly reduces the risk of passing HIV from the infected partner to the noninfected partner. People who inject drugs and share needles and paraphernalia can spread HIV through blood-to-blood contact. Breast milk can also transmit the virus from mother to infant. The average length of time from infection

to symptoms is about 10 years, during which time the person may not know he or she has HIV and can spread the infection to others.

In 1994 HIV/AIDS experts issued a recommendation to test high-risk pregnant women for HIV and to offer those with positive tests treatment with zidovudine (AZT), which slows the rate at which the virus replicates. This allows the infant's IMMUNE SYSTEM to develop sufficiently to produce resistance against HIV and stave off infection. The result was a two thirds reduction in the number of infants born with HIV between 1994 and 1997. Since then, HIV/AIDS programs have made a concerted effort to extend HIV testing and AZT treatment to all pregnant women with the hope that congenital HIV infections will decline even further. Many health-care providers believe HIV testing should be among the routine screenings pregnant women undergo.

Early Diagnosis and Prevention

Nearly a million Americans live with HIV/AIDS yet about 250,000 of them—one in four—do not know they do. The virus can exist in the body for decades without progressing to the disease condition of AIDS. During this time, however, the virus remains active and can spread to other people. By the time symptoms begin to manifest, an important window of therapeutic opportunity has closed. Treatment can still contain the progression of disease for years, but symptoms progress and will increasingly diminish QUALITY OF LIFE.

In 2004 the US Food and Drug Administration (FDA) approved the first rapid test to detect HIV-1 antibodies in a fingerstick blood sample. HIV-1 is the form of the virus that causes nearly all AIDS infections in the United States. More extensive and precise blood tests then confirm positive results. The US Centers for Disease Control and Prevention (CDC) and other health organizations recommend HIV testing become part of the ROUTINE MEDICAL EXAMINATION to facilitate early diagnosis.

KEY MEASURES FOR PREVENTING HIV/AIDS

- sexual abstinence
- when sexually active, latex condom use during every act of sexual intercourse unless in a longstanding monogamous relationship in which both partners have tested negative for HIV
- avoiding injectable drugs
- regular testing for all people who are sexually active
- frequent testing for people who engage in high-risk sexual behaviors (multiple sex partners, unprotected sex) or who use injectable drugs
- early intervention and monitoring for people who are HIV-positive, to start treatment at the most opportune times and to encourage preventive behaviors

---

See also OCCUPATIONAL HEALTH AND SAFETY; SEXUALLY TRANSMITTED DISEASES (STDS).

indoor air quality The average American spends 20 hours or more of each day in various indoor environments such as work, school, and home. Because the air they breathe recirculates, it accumulates pollutants. Indoor air may contain two to five times as much pollution as outdoor air. Health experts believe this contributes to the rise over recent decades in ASTHMA and other respiratory diseases. Indoor air pollutants may be visible, linger as odors, or remain undetected. The risk to health does not necessarily correlate with the ability to detect the pollutant; some of the most hazardous substances (such as carbon monoxide) have no smell or visible presence.

COMMON INDOOR AIR POLLUTANTS	
aerosol products	animal dander
asbestos in older structures	BACTERIA
body fragrances	CARBON DIOXIDE
carbon monoxide	cleaning solutions
dust	dust mites
formaldehyde	glues, paints, and solvents
lead	mercury
molds, mildew, and fungi	ozone
particulates	pesticides
radon	TOBACCO smoke
viruses	volatile organic compounds

Ventilation and outdoor air exchange are important for bringing fresh air into the building or home and releasing indoor pollutants so they can disperse. This helps reduce exposure to harmful substances and lower the risk of resulting health conditions. Federal regulations establish ventilation and air exchange rates for commercial buildings. Indoor air also may be too dry or too moist (humid), requiring humidification or dehumidification to make it more comfortable to breathe. Humid air supports the growth of molds and fungi, which can cause hypersensitivity response, ALLERGIC RHINITIS, chronic BRONCHITIS, and other upper respiratory tract conditions. Improperly cleaned humidifiers also can become pathogenic reservoirs, harboring and dispersing colonies of molds and bacteria. Central home heating systems have filters that homeowners or residents must periodically change.

The US Environmental Protection Agency (EPA) administers regulations and standards for indoor air quality, and recommends a three-prong approach:

1. Control pollutants at their sources: This may include no smoking indoors and installing carpets that do not contain VOCs,

2. Ventilate: Open windows and circulating fans move air containing pollutants outside and bring in fresh air.

3. Clean the air: Air cleaners and filters use various methods to extract specific kinds of pollutants from the air. The EPA cautions that air cleaners cannot substitute for proper ventilation and source control as the primary maintenance measures for clean air. Some air cleaners may add different pollutants to the air, such as particulates or ozone.

See also BUILDING-RELATED ILLNESS; ENVIRONMENTAL CIGARETTE SMOKE; LEGIONNAIRES' DISEASE; RADON EXPOSURE; SICK BUILDING SYNDROME.

influenza prevention INFLUENZA, commonly called the flu, is an upper respiratory INFECTION that causes epidemics (widespread outbreaks of disease) every year. In the United States each year about 20 percent of the population becomes ill with influenza (about 60 million people), and 30,000 to 40,000 people die as a result. Occasionally influenza occurs in a pandemic, in which people worldwide become ill. The most significant influenza pandemic in modern times was the Spanish influenza pandemic of 1918, which sickened 40 percent of the world population and caused more than 20 million deaths. Other pandemics occurred in 1957 (Asian influenza) and 1968 (Hong Kong influenza). Outbreaks of Avian flu created concern among public health officials in the early 2000s but containment efforts prevailed and limited the numbers of people who became ill.

Influenza Virus Strains: Moving Targets

Viruses cause influenza. There are three types of influenza viruses: influenza A, influenza B, and influenza C. Influenza A and B are responsible for most cases of illness; influenza C infections are generally mild and not so easily spread from one person to another as are A and B influenza viruses. Every year the strains of the influenza VIRUS responsible for causing illness are slightly different from the strains that caused infection the previous year (epidemiologists call this "drift"). These changes help the virus survive. Having an influenza infection confers IMMUNITY against the strain of virus that caused it. Because the strains vary each year, however, this immunity has value only for the duration of the flu season in which the virus strain is active (though a small amount of resistance may carry over to similar strains). Epidemiologists and researchers attempt to predict which strains will emerge each year, and base annual influenza vaccines on those strains.

Occasionally the influenza virus makes a dramatic alteration, a phenomenon epidemiologists call "shift." These are the influenza viruses capable of causing pandemic, or worldwide, infection because no immunity exists against them. Health organizations around the world have monitoring systems in place to detect these viruses and respond before pandemic infection develops. Because bird populations serve as reservoirs for influenza viruses that can also infect humans, health officials closely monitor avian influenza infections among birds. Avian influenza outbreaks among domesticated birds in parts of Asia in the late 1990s and early 2000s caused alarm for the potential of a pandemic, though containment responses were effective in confining the outbreaks. The ease with which people travel around the world creates considerable challenge for containing outbreaks.

Influenza Vaccination

Vaccines provide immunity by stimulating the IMMUNE SYSTEM enough to produce antibodies to fight the virus at its next attempt to enter the body but not enough to cause illness. The resulting immunity is effective against only the specific strain of virus. Two kinds of influenza vaccines are available in the United States:

- The conventional flu shot contains inactivated (killed) influenza virus, which, when injected into the body, cause the immune system to respond. The first killed-virus influenza VACCINE became available in the United States in 1945. Anyone older than six months of age can receive the flu shot.

- The live attenuated vaccine, which comes in the form of a nasal spray, contains live but weakened influenza virus genetically altered so it cannot cause illness (it is unable to survive at body temperature). The weakened virus enters the bloodstream via the mucous membranes of the nasal passages. Like the inactivated influenza injected vaccine, the live attenuated vaccine activates an immune system response to produce antibodies. The live attenuated influenza vaccine became available in the United States in 2003. Only people between the ages of 5 and 49 who are healthy can receive the live attenuated virus.

Health experts recommend getting the influenza vaccine in October or November, as the flu season in the United States typically runs December to March each year. Though everyone can benefit from vaccination, certain groups of people are at high risk for infection. They include

- children between the ages of six months and 2 years as well as their household members

- people age 50 and older

- people who live in extended-care facilities and other group settings

- people who work in health-care and public safety positions

- people over age six months who have chronic health conditions

Occasionally there are shortages of vaccine, as occurred in 2004, which is a significant public health issue. When this occurs, public health agencies such as the US Centers for Disease Control and Prevention (CDC) and the US Department of Health and Human Services (HHS) issue revised guidelines to protect those who are most vulnerable to complications.

Antiviral Medications

Because influenza is a viral infection, most treatment measures are supportive and target symptoms. From a prevention standpoint, ANTIVIRAL MEDICATIONS that can reduce the severity of symptoms can also reduce the spread of influenza infection. A doctor must prescribe an antiviral medication within 48 hours of the onset of symptoms; the more quickly after exposure, the more effective the medication. Antiviral medications available in the United States include amantadine (Symmetrel), rimantadine (Flumadine), zanamivir (Relenza), and oseltamivir (Tamiflu).

Frequent HAND WASHING and sneezing or coughing into a tissue or the sleeve rather than the hands are among the most effective measures for preventing the spread of the influenza virus from person to person.

See also INCUBATION PERIOD; TRANSMISSION MODES.

life expectancy A statistical calculation representing how many years a person might expect to live. Simple life expectancy calculates projected years of life from birth. Age-adjusted life expectancy projects how many more years a person of a certain age might expect to live. It is important to remember that such calculations are projections, not factual assertions of how long an individual will live. Any individual may live longer or less than his or her life expectancy as a result of numerous variables.

Life expectancy at birth has steadily increased in the United States, climbing by 60 percent overall between 1900 and 2000. A child born in 1900 could expect to live about 48 years, whereas a child born in 2000 could expect to live about 77 years. Though life expectancy for men remains less than that for women, the gap is slowly closing. Some health experts believe discoveries in genetics and molecular medicine in the early years of the 21st century have the potential to extend life expectancy 15 to 25 percent within the next decade.

Increases in life expectancy have historically reflected improvements in numerous areas of public health, ranging from sanitation to vaccinations. Current increases reflect health and healthcare improvements primarily in areas such as pharmaceuticals, diagnostic procedures that allow early detection of potentially fatal health conditions, and therapeutic technologies. Individual variables such as family and PERSONAL HEALTH HISTORY also influence life expectancy, as do behaviors that affect health such as cigarette smoking. Numerous government agencies publish life expectancy data, updated annually.

See also HEALTH RISK FACTORS; LIFESTYLE AND HEALTH; IMMUNIZATION; YOUTH HIGH-RISK BEHAVIORS.

lifestyle and health Many aspects of lifestyle influence health. Among the most significant are

- cigarette smoking and other tobacco use
- diet and nutrition
- physical activity and exercise
- occupational health risks
- WEIGHT LOSS AND WEIGHT MANAGEMENT and OBESITY
- seat belt and helmet use
- SAFER SEX PRACTICES

The correlations between lifestyle behaviors and health conditions are both direct and indirect and often intertwined. Numerous research studies show conclusively, for example, that cigarette smoking is a direct cause of CARDIOVASCULAR DISEASE (CVD), LUNG CANCER, CHRONIC OBSTRUCTIVE PULMONARY DISEASE (COPD), laryngeal CANCER, and STOMACH CANCER and a contributing cause to numerous other cancers and diseases. Scientists and researchers know, too, that OBESITY is a clear factor in health conditions such as cardiovascular disease and DIABETES. Furthermore, diabetes is one of the leading causes (along with cigarette smoking and obesity) of cardiovascular diseases such as HYPERTENSION (high BLOOD PRESSURE), PERIPHERAL VASCULAR DISEASE (PVD), and CORONARY ARTERY DISEASE (CAD).

Researchers also know that diet and nutrition are key factors in healthy body function as well as in disease states. Some diseases result directly from nutritional deficiencies, such as pernicious ANEMIA (vitamin B_{12} deficiency, which can occur from dietary insufficiency or due to MALABSORPTION disorders, PEPTIC ULCER DISEASE, or GASTRECTOMY). Researchers continue to investigate the ways in which nutritional and dietary factors contribute indirectly to health conditions, particularly with respect to the disease-fighting potential of antioxidants. Cancer researchers have made connections between the body's ability to fight off cancer and dietary habits such as eating 9 to 12 servings a day of fruits and vegetables.

Health conditions may also affect EATING HABITS, with further consequence for health and wellbeing. People who have LACTOSE INTOLERANCE, for example, cannot consume dairy products, the most common source of calcium and vitamin D. It is important for them to obtain these nutrients through other foods and through supplements. Some medications may require dietary restrictions. For example, people who take monoamine oxidase inhibitor (MAOI) medications, prescribed to treat DEPRESSION and occasionally to treat PARKINSON'S DISEASE, cannot eat foods such as cheeses and smoked meats that contain the amino acid tyramine. Health conditions may also limit what a person can eat; for example, a person who has CELIAC DISEASE (sprue) cannot eat foods that contain gluten.

Physical inactivity has come under intense scrutiny from health experts in recent years as more evidence emerges to connect physical activity with health and sedentary habits with disease. Though scientists do not fully understand the myriad ways in which exercise affects cell activity, they know that it increases INSULIN sensitivity and results in overall improved metabolic efficiency. In a sense, regular physical activity seems for the body like a tune-up is for a car—it keeps it running as smoothly as possible. Health experts urge people to get a minimum of 30 minutes of physical exercise, such as walking, every day.

The correlations between lifestyle and health take on particular relevance in the context of the aging of the American population. As people are living longer, QUALITY OF LIFE becomes an increasingly significant focus. Advances in medical technology now allow routine treatments for conditions that only a few decades ago were deadly. Thrombolytic medications can halt and even reverse HEART ATTACK and STROKE due to blood clots. ORGAN TRANSPLANTATION extends the promise of normal life to thousands of Americans. Prosthetic joints restore movement when arthritis or injury destroys joints and bones. Yet within the framework of these advances remains the reality that individual health is an individual responsibility. Medical science can fix quite a lot but the way in which a person chooses to protect the functions and structures of his or her body plays a significant role in health.

See also COENZYME Q10; OBESITY, HEALTH CONSEQUENCES OF; OCCUPATIONAL HEALTH AND SAFETY; SEXUALLY TRANSMITTED DISEASE (STD) PREVENTION; SMOKING AND HEALTH.

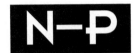

neural tube defects   BIRTH DEFECTS in which the neural tube, the precursor to the SPINAL CORD and BRAIN, fails to develop properly. The neural tube develops in the first few weeks of gestational life and may be complete by the time a woman knows she is pregnant. An open neural tube defect exposes the brain and spinal cord outside the body. SKIN and spinal structure abnormally encase a closed neural tube defect, typically involving only the spine (and usually the lower spine). Though there are associations between neural tube defects and CHROMOSOMAL DISORDERS such as DOWN SYNDROME, most researchers believe neural tube defects occur as a combination of random GENE MUTATION and environmental circumstances.

The most serious neural tube defect is anencephaly, in which the brain does not form. Anencephaly is always fatal. SPINA BIFIDA, in which the spinal column does not close properly, can result in mild to debilitating deformity and disability. The mildest form of spina bifida is myelomeningocele, in which the defect affects only a small portion of the lower spinal cord. Reconstructive surgery can improve protection of the spinal cord, though a degree of PARALYSIS affecting bowel, BLADDER, and lower body function typically remains. Occasionally a neural tube defect is so minor that it does not become apparent until later in life, even adulthood.

Folic acid supplementation, ideally beginning before CONCEPTION, can prevent most neural tube defects. Health experts recommend all sexually active women of childbearing age take folic acid supplements whether or not they plan PREGNANCY. (Folic acid supplementation also helps stabilize blood glucose levels in pregnant women who have DIABETES.) ALPHA FETOPROTEIN (AFP), CHORIONIC VILLI SAMPLING (CVS), and prenatal ULTRASOUND can detect most neural tube defects before birth, allowing women and their doctors to make decisions about the course of the pregnancy and care needs following birth. Doctors often recommend terminating the pregnancy when the neural tube defect is so severe that death of the infant would be certain and immediate after birth.

See also ABORTION; CONGENITAL ANOMALY; KYPHOSIS; SCOLIOSIS.

occupational health and safety   Work-related injuries account for about 6,000 deaths and 16 million health-care visits each year in the United States. There are literally thousands of hazards in the workplace, some common to nearly all jobs and others unique to specific occupations. In the United States, the Department of Labor, the Occupational and Health Safety Agency (OSHA), the Centers for Disease Control and Prevention (CDC), and the National Institute for Occupational Safety and Health (NIOSH) oversee workplace safety regulations, standards, and procedures. OSHA further has enforcement authority for compliance issues. Other federal and state organizations also participate in workplace safety.

MOST COMMON CAUSES OF WORKPLACE FATALITIES IN THE UNITED STATES	
drowning	ELECTROCUTION
falls from roofs and ladders	fires and explosions
MOTOR VEHICLE ACCIDENTS	overturned equipment
struck by falling objects	substance exposure
suicide	VIOLENCE

Employers are responsible for providing a working environment free from unreasonable risk to workers. Such an environment varies according to occupation. To the extent possible, federal and state laws mandate appropriate protective measures for workers in high-risk occupations. Occupational and industry standards often result in further measures to protect people from the hazards of their jobs. Individuals are responsible for following appropriate safety procedures.

MOTOR VEHICLE ACCIDENTS account for about 25 percent of workplace deaths. VIOLENCE also claims a significant number of deaths, particularly among retail cashiers and cab drivers who are at risk for death by homicide during robberies. Other occupations with high risk for injury and death are logging, commercial fishing, roofing, construction, and mining.

KEY INDIVIDUAL MEASURES
FOR PREVENTING WORKPLACE INJURIES

- Obtain proper training for operating devices and equipment.
- Integrate ergonomic standards and practices into work stations and job tasks.
- Use appropriate protective devices, clothing, and gear.
- Follow employer risk-management policies and procedures.
- Remain DRUG-free and ALCOHOL-free in the workplace.

See also ACCIDENTAL INJURIES; BUILDING-RELATED ILLNESS; OCCUPATIONAL HEALTH AND SAFETY; REPETITIVE MOTION INJURIES; SICK BUILDING SYNDROME; TRAUMA PREVENTION; WORKPLACE STRESS.

personal health history An ongoing record of an individual's health conditions including vaccinations, illnesses, injuries, operations, pregnancies and births, medications, and other information that might be relevant in the context of providing health-care services. A personal health history also helps determine future health risks and appropriate treatment options.

A personal health history might include these events (including dates)

- vaccinations, routine medical examinations, and routine diagnostic procedures such as MAMMOGRAM, PAP TEST, blood cholesterol test, tuberculin SKIN test, COLONOSCOPY
- common childhood diseases such as MEASLES, MUMPS, RUBELLA, CHICKENPOX
- uncommon childhood diseases such as SCARLET FEVER, rheumatic FEVER

- congenital anomalies, BIRTH DEFECTS, and congenital disorders (such as CEREBRAL PALSY), or GENETIC DISORDERS (such as SICKLE CELL ANEMIA or HEMOPHILIA)
- serious injuries such as BONE FRACTURE, CONCUSSION, major trauma
- serious illnesses such as ENCEPHALITIS, MENINGITIS, ENDOCARDITIS, HEPATITIS, PANCREATITIS
- surgeries (including TUBAL LIGATION or VASECTOMY)
- pregnancies, miscarriages, abortions, deliveries
- CONTRACEPTION, SEXUALLY TRANSMITTED DISEASES (STDS)
- DIABETES
- CARDIOVASCULAR DISEASE (CVD)
  - HEART ATTACK or STROKE
  - HYPERTENSION (high BLOOD PRESSURE)
  - ANGINA PECTORIS
  - ARRHYTHMIA
  - PERIPHERAL VASCULAR DISEASE (PVD), CORONARY ARTERY DISEASE (CAD), or CORONARY ARTERY BYPASS GRAFT (CABG)
  - HEART FAILURE or CARDIOMYOPATHY
  - VALVULAR HEART DISEASE or valve replacement
- pulmonary disease such as CHRONIC OBSTRUCTIVE PULMONARY DISEASE (COPD) or EMPHYSEMA
- gastrointestinal disorders such as INFLAMMATORY BOWEL DISEASE (IBD), GASTROESOPHAGEAL REFLUX DISORDER (GERD), PEPTIC ULCER DISEASE
- CANCER (including SKIN CANCER)
- neurologic conditions such as PARKINSON'S DISEASE or psychiatric conditions such as SCHIZOPHRENIA or BIPOLAR DISORDER
- chronic health conditions
  - infections such as OTITIS media, SINUSITIS, BRONCHITIS, CYSTITIS
  - OSTEOARTHRITIS, ANKYLOSING SPONDYLITIS, GOUT
  - thyroid disease such as HYPOTHYROIDISM, GOITER, or HYPERTHYROIDISM
  - DEPRESSION or GENERALIZED ANXIETY DISORDER (GAD)
- medications (including OVER-THE-COUNTER [OTC] DRUGS and herbal remedies)

- lifestyle factors such as smoking, EATING HABITS, physical exercise, and occupational health risks

It also is helpful to know about the general health histories of immediate family members (parents, siblings, and children), particularly in regard to health conditions that can have familial tendencies such as diabetes, cancer, and cardiovascular disease.

See also HEALTH RISK FACTORS.

personal hygiene Until researchers discovered BACTERIA and connected them with INFECTION, doctors went from one patient to another without washing their hands, and people did not bathe or otherwise manage personal hygiene. Before the 20th century most people believed bathing caused rather than prevented illness. Because sewage and garbage often contaminated water supplies, this all too frequently turned out the case. Doctors now know that cleanliness prevents the spread of many kinds of infection and disease. COMMUNITY SANITATION measures provide strict procedures for managing wastes, and clean DRINKING WATER STANDARDS help maintain the purity of water that flows from the tap.

Personal hygiene—regular bathing and cleansing of the body—helps control body odor, the result of bacterial growth on the SKIN (especially the underarms) in interaction with perspiration the body releases. It also can help prevent conditions such as athlete's foot and jock itch (types of yeast infections) and reduce the risk for bacterial infection following skin wounds such as cuts and scrapes.

See also HAND WASHING; HYPERHIDROSIS; NOSOCOMIAL INFECTIONS.

poison prevention Poisoning is the third-leading cause of ACCIDENTAL INJURIES, often affecting children who ingest toxic plants, cleaning products, and medications (over-the-counter as well as prescription). Poisoning also may affect adults when they consume more of a medication than is safe or plants and other substances that are toxic.

National poison control hotline:
1-800-222-1222
Available 24 hours a day, 7 days a week, from anywhere in the United States

---

Children especially are attracted to medications that are brightly colored and that may have a sweetened coating intended to make them more palatable to swallow. Medications designed for children are sweetened, chewable, or in other ways made enticing. Careful storage of potentially poisonous products could prevent many accidental poisonings. Older adults who are not accustomed to having children around or who have difficulty managing child-resistant closures often keep their medications in other containers or dispensers. This practice is a tragically frequent source of poisoning in children who find the containers and think they hold candy.

COMMON POISONOUS YARD AND HOUSE PLANTS

acorns	azalea
buckeyes	buttercups
castor bean seeds	crocus bulbs
daffodil bulbs	daphne berries
deadly nightshade	dieffenbachia
elderberry	foxglove
hyacinth bulbs	jack in the pulpit
jasmine berries	larkspur seeds
lily of the valley	mayapple
mistletoe berries	moonseed berries
mushrooms and toadstools	narcissus bulbs
oleander leaves and branches	poison hemlock
red sage berries	rhododendron
rhubarb leaves	thorn apple
wisteria	yew

Many decorative indoor and outdoor plants are poisonous, presenting a hazard especially for children young enough to put everything in their mouths and older children who may use leaves, berries, and branches as "play" food. Some common plants, such as oleander, are so toxic that plant juice on the hands can cause serious and sometimes fatal illness. Adults should teach children to never pick and eat any kinds of berries, fruit, leaves, mushrooms, nuts, or even sticks to use for campfire cooking without a knowledgeable adult's supervision and approval.

Do *not* give anything to, or induce vomiting in, a person who may have consumed a toxic substance, unless the substance is known and its original package or product label contains specific instructions for poisoning. Otherwise, contact emergency medical assistance (911, a hospital emergency room, or the national poison control hotline at 1-800-222-1222) and follow the recommended actions.

KEY MEASURES FOR PREVENTING POISONING

- Store all medications in their original labeled containers, with child-resistant lids or caps, in a locked cabinet or drawer out of the reach of children.
- Accurately measure medication doses, especially those given to children.
- Clear yards and play areas of toxic plants.
- Store cleaning products in locked cabinets out of the reach of children.

See also CONTACT TOXINS; INGESTED TOXINS; INHALED TOXINS; INJECTED TOXINS; OVERDOSE.

preventive health care and immunization Prevention measures are the mainstay of preventive medicine. Many such measures relate to lifestyle, such as smoking, EATING HABITS, and physical exercise. Others involve vaccinations to prevent disease and ROUTINE MEDICAL EXAMINATION and screening procedures to detect health conditions for early intervention and treatment. Key self-care measures are BREAST SELF-EXAMINATION (BSE) for women and for men, TESTICULAR SELF-EXAMINATION (TSE) for men, and SKIN self-examination for men and women. Immunizations provide protection against numerous potentially serious or life-threatening illnesses.

Recommendations for doctor examinations and screening tests vary according to gender and age. Appendix X, "Immunization and Routine Examination Scheldules," provides comprehensive information for infants and children, adolescents, men, and women.

See also HEALTH RISK FACTORS; LIFESTYLE AND HEALTH; TRAVEL IMMUNIZATIONS; VACCINE.

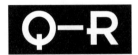

quality of life   The extent to which health supports, and disease or injury prevents, a person's ability to participate in and enjoy daily living activities is highly subjective though nonetheless a crucial measure of health care. Health experts use various tools, such as questionnaires, and methodologies to assess health-related quality of life (HRQOL). The findings become integral in determining the overall effectiveness of intervention and treatment approaches for all kinds of health circumstances from surgical operations to degenerative diseases.

Numerous factors influence quality of life for people living with chronic health conditions or disabilities, ranging from personal satisfaction with the process and outcome of medical treatment to the removal of barriers to participation in activities of interest. Removing barriers might include measures such as adaptive devices for HEARING LOSS and VISION IMPAIRMENT, voice-activated telephones and other electronics, prosthetic limbs, and mobility devices. Each person has activities that he or she considers essential for enjoying life.

Individual satisfaction with of quality of life correlates closely to expectations for outcomes, which vary among cultures and generations. Younger people tend to have higher expectations for treatments that return them to "normal" in relatively short order. Medical technology often makes such expectations reality. However, technology has its limitations and sometimes expectations exceed them. Doctors may be excited about the potential of new treatments, and individuals may be less than fully informed about potential benefits and risks. Taking the time to thoroughly investigate proposed treatments, including medications and surgeries, and obtaining second opinions from other doctors are key measures that can

help put those treatments in proper perspective and frame realistic expectations.

Quality of life is a particular concern for people who have severely debilitating or terminal health conditions. Issues such as independence, mobility, PAIN management, and dignity often arise. Most people are more accepting of chronic and even terminal conditions when they are able to discuss their concerns and fears openly and honestly with their doctors, and to establish treatment plans that are consistent with their wishes.

See also ADVANCE DIRECTIVES; CULTURAL AND ETHNIC HEALTH-CARE PERSPECTIVES; END OF LIFE CONCERNS.

radon exposure   Radon is a naturally occurring radioactive element, present as a gas in rocks and soil. Radon is also a CARCINOGEN (cancer-causing substance) that is the second-leading cause of LUNG CANCER in the United States. The highest rate of radon-induced LUNG cancer occurs among miners who work underground and breathe concentrated levels of radon over years to decades. Cigarette smoking, in addition to itself being the leading cause of lung cancer, greatly increases the risk for radon-induced lung cancer. Radon becomes a general health hazard when its levels rise inside houses and workplaces such as offices and stores. It seeps inside through cracks in foundations and floors, often drawn indoors by pressure inequalities (the air inside is generally lower pressure than the air outside).

The US Environmental Protection Agency (EPA) has established an "action level" for indoor radon concentrations of 4 picocuries per liter (pCi/L). The typical house has a radon concentration of about 25 percent of the maximum, 1.0 to 1.25 pCi/L; the air in an underground mine may contain four times the maximum, 20 pCi/L, or even more. Outdoor air typically contains about 0.4 pCi/L of radon. There is no determined safe level of radon. The public health goal is to lower all indoor radon levels to 2 pCi/L or less, with the eventual goal of lowering indoor radon levels to those of outdoor radon levels.

Home test kits, available through state radon offices and radon mitigation contractors, can measure radon levels. Among the most common methods for lowering indoor radon levels are beneath-ground ventilation systems that collect radon from under a house and release it via ventilation tubing into the outdoor air. These systems often can accommodate any kind of foundation (basement, slab, or slab with crawl space). Health experts recommend initial radon testing with regular follow-up testing regardless of the level.

See also ENVIRONMENTAL HAZARD EXPOSURE; HEALTH RISK FACTORS.

routine medical examination The examination a doctor conducts to assess an individual's health status typically includes certain procedures and tests that vary according to age and gender. A routine medical examination for adults consists of a physical examination, PERSONAL HEALTH HISTORY, general BLOOD tests (complete blood count [CBC], blood GLUCOSE, blood cholesterol), and URINALYSIS. Depending on the person's age, the doctor may order other diagnostic procedures such as blood tests for thyroid hormones, chest X-RAY, tuberculin skin test, COLONOSCOPY, MAMMOGRAPHY, and BONE DENSITY testing.

Some of the devices the doctor may use to assess physical health include

- ophthalmoscope to visualize the structures of the EYE

- otoscope to look at the structures of the outer EAR and the eardrum (TYMPANIC MEMBRANE)

- STETHOSCOPE to listen to the HEART and LUNGS (AUSCULTATION)

- sphygmomanometer to measure the BLOOD PRESSURE

- thermometer to take the temperature

- REFLEX hammer to test reflexes and other neurologic responses

- tuning fork to screen hearing and to assess sensory perception (neurologic function) in other parts of the body

Each doctor has his or her pattern for conducting a physical examination. A common pattern is to begin with vital signs and then go from head to foot.

Vital signs The typical vital signs are PULSE, RESPIRATION RATE, temperature, blood pressure, height, and weight. Temperature identifies whether there is a FEVER. Height and weight help the doctor to assess BODY MASS INDEX (BMI) and the likelihood of certain health conditions that correlate to body weight. Many doctors will take blood pressure readings at the start and end of the examination, because a person's anxiety about the examination may cause blood pressure to be artificially elevated. The doctor will typically take the pulse at each wrist and ankle, pressing against the pulse point with two fingers, and may check the pulses in the neck and groin as well. Respiration rate includes a count of how many breaths the person takes in a minute as well as an assessment of how deep or shallow the breaths are.

Head, face, and neck The doctor looks in the ears and the eyes, and may hold a tuning fork near each ear as a basic hearing screen. Many doctors use a SNELLEN CHART to assess basic visual acuity. When the doctor says, "Say ah," the sound causes the soft palate and related tissues at the back of the MOUTH to elevate. This allows the doctor to visualize the top of the THROAT. Sometimes the doctor presses a tongue depressor against the back of the mouth for a better view, which can unintentionally activate the GAG REFLEX. The doctor also looks at the structures of the mouth including the tongue. Palpating the neck helps identify thyroid nodules and enlargement; the doctor usually will feel the neck twice, first with the person sitting quietly and then when having the person swallow.

Chest The doctor listens to the heart and lungs with a stethoscope, and may tap on the chest and the back. The stethoscope allows the doctor to hear the heart valves open and close and the rhythm of the heart as it beats. It also lets the doctor hear the sounds of air entering and leaving the

lungs (breath sounds). The tapping helps to identify areas of unusual density that might suggest
enlargement of the heart, accumulated fluids, or
other circumstances that need further examination. The chest examination should also include
breast examination for men as well as women, to
detect lumps or other abnormalities.

Back The doctor may look at the back from the
back and each side when the person is standing, as
a general screen for SCOLIOSIS, KYPHOSIS, and other
back conditions. The doctor may palpate the spine
and have the person raise and lower the arms to
examine the shoulders and shoulder blades. The
back also is a common site for ACNE, ACTINIC KER-
ATOSIS, and other SKIN conditions.

Abdomen The doctor palpates the abdomen
from the base of the ribs to the pelvis, feeling for
any usual masses or tenderness. Abdominal palpa-
tion helps detect signs of ASCITES (collected fluid in
the abdominal cavity) abdominal ANEURYSM (weakening and ballooning of the major ARTERY in the
abdomen, the AORTA), LIVER or SPLEEN enlargement,
and tenderness of organs such as the GALLBLADDER,
STOMACH, and pancreas. The doctor will also listen
to the abdomen with a stethoscope, further checking for abdominal aneurysm as well as assessing
BOWEL SOUNDS. The doctor may also tap on the
belly, listening for differences in tones that might
suggest changes in density.

Arms and legs The doctor may move the arms
and legs to examine the joints, MUSCLE tone, and
range of motion. Small taps with the reflex hammer test TENDON responses as well as neurologic
reflexes. The doctor looks for unusual bruising,
swelling or edema, discolorations, and disparities
between sides of the body. The doctor may
observe as the person walks across the room and
back to assess gait and balance. Pulses in the feet
are good indicators of peripheral circulation.

Genitalia The doctor will palpate a man's testicles to check for lumps or swellings, and examine
the PENIS for structural anomalies or discharge. The
familiar "turn your head and cough" instruction
increases pressure in the lower abdomen to reveal
any HERNIA. A woman's physical examination typically includes a PELVIC EXAMINATION and PAP TEST.
Depending on age, the doctor may include a DIGI-
TAL RECTAL EXAMINATION (DRE) for men and women.

Job positions with highly physical demands
such as firefighter or police officer, school sports
and athletic programs, return-to-work following
injury, and certifications such as for aviation and
nautical pilots are among the special circumstances that may require routine medical examinations. The physical examination and diagnostic
procedures will include any additional tests to
meet the requirements. Appendix X, "Immunization and Routine Examination Schedules," provides information about how frequently a person
should have a routine medical examination and
what components the examination should
include.

See also HEALTH RISK FACTORS; LIFESTYLE AND
HEALTH; OCCUPATIONAL HEALTH AND SAFETY.

sexually transmitted disease (STD) prevention
Doctors diagnose and treat about 12 million new STD infections annually in the United States, and more than 70 million Americans live with incurable STDs. Nearly all STD infections are preventable through sexual abstinence, which is a certain though often undesirable preventive measure, or through safer sex practices, which include using latex condoms with every sexual act and regular screening tests for STDs.

SEXUALLY TRANSMITTED DISEASES (STDs)	
Curative Treatment	**Treatment but No Cure**
chancroid	GENITAL HERPES
CHLAMYDIA	HEPATITIS B
GONORRHEA	HIV/AIDS
lymphogranuloma venereum	HUMAN PAPILLOMAVIRUS (HPV)
nongonococcal URETHRITIS	
SYPHILIS	
TRICHOMONIASIS	

HEPATITIS C and TUBERCULOSIS also are often contracted through sexual contact though are not traditionally considered STDs. Untreated STDs can have significant health consequences including INFERTILITY, CENTRAL NERVOUS SYSTEM damage, generalized organ damage, and death. STDs can affect anyone who is sexually active. However, certain groups of people are more vulnerable to STD INFECTION and to the consequences of untreated STDs. Health experts classify these groups as special focus populations

- men who have sex with other men (MSM)
- injectable DRUG users
- men and women who have unprotected sex with multiple partners

- men and women entering correctional facilities
- adolescents and young adults
- women and infants

STDs may not cause symptoms, especially in women. A person who is unaware that he or she has an STD continues to spread the infection. The infection also has long-term personal consequences. For women, the key complication of untreated or repeated STD infection is PELVIC INFLAMMATORY DISEASE (PID), a leading cause of infertility. PID also can cause chronic PAIN and contribute to ECTOPIC PREGNANCY (also called tubal pregnancy), a life-threatening circumstance in which a pregnancy takes root in the fallopian tube or elsewhere in the abdominal cavity instead of the UTERUS.

Oral contraceptives (birth control pills), diaphragms, intrauterine devices (IUDs), and spermicides do not protect women from contracting STD infections.

Men may also have STDs without symptoms, though often develop urethritis (INFLAMMATION of the URETHRA) with discharge that leads to examination and diagnosis. In men and women alike, untreated SYPHILIS goes into stages of REMISSION. In most STDs, the infection remains contagious whether or not symptoms are present. The male latex condom is the most effective barrier against transmitting STDs. The pathogens that cause STDs cannot pass through the latex. However, contact between body fluids and mucous membranes can occur around the condom, so its protection is not foolproof. It is essential to use condoms properly (putting them on immediately upon erection and before pre-ejaculate appears) and consistently for maximum preventive benefit.

Infants whose mothers have active STDs, particularly GONORRHEA and CHLAMYDIA, during delivery are at great risk for blindness. Hospitals routinely put antibiotic drops in the eyes of all newborns as a prophylactic measure. Infants born to HIV-positive mothers are also at risk for acquiring the VIRUS during birth; prophylactic medications such as azidothymidine (AZT) can help thwart infection.

The US Centers for Disease Control and Prevention (CDC) has a national STD/HIV hotline available 24 hours a day, 7 days a week, for questions and information: 800-227-8922

Prevention efforts focus on education about STDs and their potential health consequences in combination with appropriate methods to reduce the likelihood of infection. The most effective prevention method is abstinence from sexual activity, or, when sexually active, sex exclusively within a monogamous relationship. Because some STDs may be present without symptoms in up to 70 percent of people infected, health experts recommend routine screening for all sexually active individuals as a preventive measure to help contain the spread of infection.

KEY MEASURES FOR PREVENTING STDS

- Use a latex condom for every sexual act.
- Restrict sexual activity to a monogamous relationship.
- Receive regular screening tests for STD infection.

See also CONTRACEPTION; HEALTH RISK FACTORS; LIFESTYLE AND HEALTH; YOUTH HIGH-RISK BEHAVIOR.

sick building syndrome A set of symptoms that appear when in a particular building and go away upon leaving the building. The US Environmental Protection Agency (EPA) defines sick building syndrome as symptoms that

- include HEADACHE, NAUSEA, itchy eyes and NOSE, and dry COUGH
- doctors cannot diagnose as any specific health condition

- are present only when within the building

Symptoms may affect a few people in a particular area or numerous people throughout the building. Because symptoms often are general and are present only when the person is in the building, obtaining a diagnosis of illness is challenging. Sometimes symptoms improve with ANTIHISTAMINE MEDICATIONS to combat allergic response, though most people do not want to take medications for symptoms they can relieve by being in a different location.

The causes of sick building syndrome are unclear though scientists believe they may relate to INDOOR AIR QUALITY, chemicals in the air from indoor or outdoor sources such as exhaust fumes or glues, contaminants such as molds or fungi that cause allergy-like reactions, and inadequate ventilation. Increased ventilation (higher turnover of air volume) and air-filtration systems may improve indoor air quality sufficiently to mitigate symptoms for most people. Some individuals may have heightened sensitivity to airborne substances.

See also ALLERGIC RHINITIS; BUILDING-RELATED ILLNESS; ENVIRONMENTAL CIGARETTE SMOKE; OCCUPATIONAL HEALTH AND SAFETY.

substance abuse prevention SUBSTANCE ABUSE is a complex health and social problem with public health as well as personal health consequences. Accordingly, substance abuse prevention efforts require coordinated efforts that align individuals, parents, schools, employers, and health-care providers toward common goals. Though education is the cornerstone of substance abuse prevention, it is naive to believe education alone is sufficient to stop a person from trying or using TOBACCO, ALCOHOL, drugs, and illicit substances. Many knowledgeable people have substance abuse problems.

Parents, teachers, sports figures, and other adults significantly influence the attitudes and actions of children. Adults who do not smoke or use illicit drugs and who use alcohol and medications appropriately and responsibly help model attitudes and behaviors that discourage substance abuse. Focused prevention efforts target underage smoking and drinking, emphasizing abstaining from both. Other efforts attempt to address issues of ADDICTION through treatment programs.

KEY MEASURES FOR PREVENTING SUBSTANCE ABUSE

- education through schools and community outreach regarding the health risks of substance abuse
- effective and appropriate modeling by adults
- access to treatment programs
- take medications, over-the-counter or prescription, only as needed and directed
- restrict underage access to TOBACCO, ALCOHOL, and medications of abuse

---

See also ALCOHOLISM; OVERDOSE; SMOKING CESSATION; TOLERANCE.

sudden infant death syndrome (SIDS) The unexpected and unexplainable death of an infant under age one year, most commonly between the ages of two and four months. Researchers do not know what causes SIDS, though believe a malfunction occurs in the infant's basic metabolic regulatory mechanisms that allows BLOOD PRESSURE, BREATHING, and body temperature to fluctuate. Also for reasons researchers do not understand, SIDS is three times more frequent among African American and Native American infants. SIDS is also more likely to occur among infants whose mothers are under age 20 years, smoke, gain inadequate weight during PREGNANCY, or have pregnancies less than a year apart.

Infants who sleep on their backs have a significantly lower rate of SIDS than infants who sleep on their sides or stomachs, prompting the national "Back to Sleep" campaign in 1994 to lower the risk for SIDS. Deaths due to SIDS dropped almost in half in subsequent years. Because researchers do not know why SIDS occurs, however, they are not certain how, or whether it is possible, to prevent it.

Because the infant's death is sudden and unexplained, local authorities must investigate. This adds to the emotional trauma for families because it is a difficult experience to undergo and even when SIDS is the conclusion, the question of why often remains unanswered. Inasmuch as the causes of SIDS remain unclear, health and law-enforcement experts do know that SIDS is *not* the result of parental neglect or CHILD ABUSE. Infants born pre-

maturely and those whose mothers smoked during pregnancy appear to have higher risk for SIDS. Pediatricians may recommend special monitors for especially vulnerable infants that sound an alarm when the infant's breathing rate or body temperature becomes higher or lower than normal.

KEY MEASURES FOR PREVENTING SIDS

- Place infant on his or her back to sleep, not on the side or STOMACH.
- Place infant to sleep in his or her own crib.
- Maintain the infant's room at a temperature warm enough to allow sleeping without blankets but not hot.
- Keep heavy blankets, quilts, and stuffed animals out of the infant's crib.
- Maintain a smoke-free living environment and prevent exposure to cigarette smoke in general.

See also NERVOUS SYSTEM; PRENATAL CARE.

trauma prevention Firearms, MOTOR VEHICLE ACCIDENTS, SEXUAL ASSAULT, DOMESTIC VIOLENCE, CHILD ABUSE, workplace and school VIOLENCE, animal bites, and major falls account for the majority of traumatic injuries. As is the case with other kinds of ACCIDENTAL INJURIES, most traumatic injuries are preventable. Traumatic injuries have a high likelihood of death within the first several hours after the events responsible for them, and require emergency medical treatment. Traumatic injuries

---

KEY MEASURES FOR PREVENTING TRAUMA

- Use trigger locks and gun safes to store guns, and separate guns from ammunition.
- Take firearms safety classes before hunting or target shooting, and always handle a gun as though it were loaded.
- Wear seat belts at all times when traveling in a motor vehicle and helmets when riding on a motorcycle, whether the driver or a passenger.
- Wear or use appropriate safety gear when using power tools and performing home repairs, and for recreational activities such as rock climbing.
- Stabilize ladders and do not step higher than recommended onto a stepladder or ladder.
- Keep dogs leashed or fenced, and do not approach wild animals.
- Seek professional help for anger management and DOMESTIC VIOLENCE issues

---

also account for a significant percentage of long-term recovery and permanent disability due to injury. Prevention efforts focus on increasing public awareness and reducing exposure to risks.

See also ANGER AND ANGER MANAGEMENT; BLUNT TRAUMA; GUNSHOT WOUNDS; MULTIPLE TRAUMA; OCCUPATIONAL HEALTH AND SAFETY.

tuberculosis prevention Until researcher Selman Waksman (1888–1973) discovered the powerful antibiotic streptomycin in 1944, TUBERCULOSIS (called "consumption" because its sufferers literally wasted away as the INFECTION consumed lung and other tissue) killed more people than any other disease. Antibiotic regimens developed in the ensuing decade significantly reduced tuberculosis infections in the United States by the mid-1960s. By the mid-1980s, however, strains of tuberculosis began appearing that were resistant to the conventional antibiotic therapy (now called multidrug-resistant tuberculosis or MDR-TB). Concurrently HIV/AIDS proliferated, making those who became infected highly susceptible to other infections such as tuberculosis. People who have DIABETES, kidney disease, LEUKEMIA, or LYMPHOMA or who receive IMMUNOSUPPRESSIVE THERAPY such as following ORGAN TRANSPLANTATION are also more susceptible to tuberculosis infection. Tuberculosis tends to develop more frequently among confined populations such as in prisons and crowded living conditions.

Doctors diagnose about 15,000 people with tuberculosis in the United States each year, about half of whom are immigrants who likely became infected in their native countries. Tuberculosis spreads by BREATHING droplets a person already infected with the disease breathes or coughs out into the air. Most people who have healthy immune systems can fight off infection, though the causative microorganism (*Mycobacterium tuberculosis*) may remain inactive in their bodies (called latent tuberculosis). Only people who have active tuberculosis can spread the infection to others. A SKIN test can detect the presence of *M. tuberculosis*. Public health policy in the United States requires skin testing, called a tuberculin skin test, in numerous occupations including public safety (police, fire, and emergency aid response), teaching, food handling and preparation, and health

care. The typical course of treatment for diagnosed active tuberculosis is a regimen of two or more ANTIBIOTIC MEDICATIONS taken for 6 to 10 months.

Prevention efforts focus on screening susceptible populations for early diagnosis and treatment, and on encouraging people who show symptoms of tuberculosis to receive medical treatment. Anyone who has had close contact with a person diagnosed with tuberculosis, as well as those who have HIV/AIDS and a marginal tuberculin skin test result should receive more frequent screening tests and discuss prophylactic antibiotic therapy with their doctors. Research continues the quest for a tuberculosis VACCINE. The BCG vaccine currently available provides very limited protection. Doctors administer it primarily to young children exposed to non-lung forms of tuberculosis infection.

KEY MEASURES FOR PREVENTING TUBERCULOSIS

- Receive periodic tuberculin SKIN tests to screen for the presence of *M. tuberculosis*.
- Receive prophylactic antibiotic therapy when at high risk for INFECTION.
- Take protective measures such as wearing a surgical mask when in close contact with someone diagnosed with tuberculosis.
- If being treated for tuberculosis, take the full course of antibiotic therapy as prescribed.

See also KIDNEYS; LUNGS; OCCUPATIONAL HEALTH AND SAFETY.

water safety More than 4,000 people drown in the United States each year, and as many as 12,000 experience near-drowning (also called submersion injury). The HYPOXIA (lack of oxygen) that occurs with submersion results in residual complications in about 40 percent of people who are revived, ranging from mild memory impairment and disturbances of cognitive function to PERSISTENT VEGETATIVE STATE. Virtually all water accidents are preventable.

The common scenarios for water-related injuries correlate with age:

- Children under age 1 year are most likely to drown in toilets, bathtubs, and buckets or other containers of water.

- Children between the ages of 1 and 4 years are most likely to drown in residential swimming pools.

- Young people between the ages of 15 and 19 are most likely to drown in lakes and rivers, and ALCOHOL consumption contributes up to half of their water-related injuries and deaths.

- Boating accidents are the most common cause of submersion injuries among adults. Alcohol consumption is a factor in nearly half of such accidents.

- Among adolescents and adults, diving into shallow water accounts for numerous HEAD AND SPINAL CORD INJURIES.

Three of four people who drown are adults. Even capable swimmers can experience exhaustion, MUSCLE cramps, and other challenges. Many people who die in boating accidents are not wearing personal flotation devices (PFDs) or lack other water safety devices that could have prevented their deaths. Alcohol consumption and swimming or boating factors in about 40 percent of water-related injuries among adolescents and adults.

KEY MEASURES FOR PREVENTING DROWNING
- Learn to swim.
- Learn CARDIOPULMONARY RESUSCITATION (CPR).
- Wear or use appropriate flotation devices when engaged in water activities such as boating.
- Closely supervise children in and near water, including pools, lakes, and rivers.
- Do not drink ALCOHOL when participating in activities on or in the water.

See also COLD WATER DROWNING; HYPOTHERMIA; SPINAL CORD INJURY; TRAUMATIC BRAIN INJURY (TBI); WARM WATER DROWNING.

youth high-risk behavior The US Centers for Disease Control and Prevention's (CDC's) Youth Risk Behavior Surveillance System (YRBSS) monitors behaviors among young people that can adversely affect their health. Key areas of focus include TOBACCO use, substance abuse, sexual activity, PREGNANCY, violent behavior, ACCIDENTAL INJURIES, physical inactivity, EATING HABITS, and attempted suicide. YRBSS data help public health organizations develop intervention strategies and programs to reduce adverse health consequences among youth. The CDC surveys students in middle schools and high schools throughout the United States to collect YRBSS data.

HIGH-RISK HEALTH BEHAVIORS AMONG YOUTH

anabolic steroid use	binge drinking
carrying a weapon	cigarette smoking
does not drink milk	does not eat fruit, vegetables
drinking and driving	failure to wear bike helmet
fast food consumption	fighting
ILLICIT DRUG USE	lack of seat belt use
laxatives or diet aids to lose weight	multiple sex partners
nonsmoking TOBACCO use	no regular physical exercise
overweight or obese	regular ALCOHOL consumption
riding with intoxicated driver	sexual activity without a condom
suicide ideation or attempts	

See also LIFESTYLE AND HEALTH; HEALTHY PEOPLE 2010.

ALTERNATIVE AND COMPLEMENTARY APPROACHES

The current time is one of a paradigm shift in the nature and delivery of health care that affects everyone—researchers, patients, doctors, and insurers—alike. Tremendous discoveries in medicine are leading to a reexamination of attitudes and practices across the spectrums of health and of disease. As conventional medicine intensifies its focus on lifestyle management and preventive measures and on viewing the patient as a "whole" person (the holistic view common to many alternative and complementary health systems), both doctors and individuals are finding therapeutic value in incorporating many alternative and complementary therapies within integrative treatment plans.

This section, "Alternative and Complementary Approaches," presents an overview discussion of treatment approaches that are beyond the boundaries of conventional medicine yet still within the realm of which conventional doctors may responsibly include them as elements of integrative treatment plans. The entries that follow represent the range of the alternative and complementary therapies available from ancient healing systems, such as TRADITIONAL CHINESE MEDICINE (TCM) and AYURVEDA, to MEDICINAL HERBS AND BOTANICALS. As well, several entries present methods that are controversial and potentially hazardous from the conventional medicine perspective, such as CHELATION THERAPY. Such entries are included not to give them credibility but because widespread misperceptions about them persist despite a clinically valid body of knowledge that supports concerns about their risks.

Context and Perspective

This section presents the discussion of alternative and complementary approaches within the context and perspective of conventional medicine as practiced in the United States, as this is the orientation of *The Facts On File Encyclopedia of Health and Medicine*. Some conventional doctors share the interest and enthusiasm of patients who want to incorporate alternative and complementary therapies, and some conventional doctors are less willing to entertain such inclusions. Much depends on the convergence of the patient's interests and condition with the doctor's knowledge and trust in specific alternative and complementary therapies. The efficacy of some ancient healing systems and methods is perhaps more trustworthy than that of isolated or obscure practices. The challenge for doctors and patients alike is to evaluate what bodies of knowledge exists about popular therapies, to understand which of them may have therapeutic value.

Most alternative therapies derive from healing systems deeply rooted in philosophical frameworks that differ dramatically from those of conventional Western medicine. A conventional physician's training does not include most of these methods, even the most studied or popular ones. Doctors must instead rely on evaluating the available research to determine whether, how, and when alternative and complementary approaches are appropriate in conjunction with conventional care. For some methods, not much data are available. As knowledge about these approaches increases, many conventional doctors may be more confident about incorporating them. Indeed, some conventional doctors seek additional education and certification in alternative and complementary therapies such as ACUPUNCTURE and herbalism so they can offer their patients a broader spectrum of therapeutic and preventive options.

The conventional framework that guides the practice of medicine in the United States is physician centered and based in measurable evidence and reliably repeatable results through controlled clinical studies. Though the true measure of a treatment's success is whether people improve or worsen with its use, evidence-based standards give conventional physicians a sense of reasonable expectation when making treatment decisions and recommendations. Many conventional doctors are increasingly interested and willing to add responsible alternative and complementary therapies to integrative treatment plans when they have reasonable expectations for how such therapies may benefit the patient's condition or QUALITY OF LIFE.

When looking at the broad range of alternative and complementary approaches from acupuncture to PRAYER AND SPIRITUALITY to VISUALIZATION it is also important to understand how patients look to these methods in preventive and lifestyle contexts. MEDITATION and YOGA, for example, have become fairly mainstream as practices to reduce stress and are gaining acceptance for their abilities to influence health conditions such as HYPERTENSION (high BLOOD PRESSURE). As researchers and doctors learn more about the pathways and mechanisms of MIND–BODY INTERACTIONS, they understand more fully how lifestyle and preventive health measures, with a holistic view of the individual, are important. Within such a context, yoga and exercise become comparable complements to good health. Whether one or the other is "alternative" or "conventional" has little relevance; each benefits health in similar ways.

COMMON ALTERNATIVE AND COMPLEMENTARY THERAPIES

ACUPUNCTURE	AROMATHERAPY
ART THERAPY	BIOFEEDBACK
Chinese herbal remedies	CRANIOSACRAL MASSAGE
FLOWER ESSENCES	HYPNOSIS
MAGNET THERAPY	MASSAGE THERAPY
MEDICINAL HERBS AND BOTANICALS	NUTRITIONAL THERAPY
OSTEOPATHIC MANIPULATIVE	PRAYER AND SPIRITUALITY
TREATMENT (OMT)	TAI CHI
VISUALIZATION	VITAMIN AND MINERAL
YOGA	THERAPY

Historical Traditions in Alternative Healing Systems

The oldest known healing systems still in practice today, traditional Chinese medicine (TCM) and Ayurveda, date to perhaps 3000 B.C.E., well before the advent of written language. NATIVE AMERICAN HEALING originating among the indigenous cultures of the North American continent melds spirituality and health in much the same fashion as does India's Ayurveda and, archaeological evidence suggests, could have origins that are nearly as ancient. In these systems, healers passed their knowledge from one to another, generation to generation, through tradition and experience. In some cultures each successive generation developed improvements on the methods of healing their ancestors used, and in other cultures each generation of healers practiced in precise compliance with the traditions they learned from the generations before them.

Some alternative healing systems are relatively modern, emerging within the past 100 or 200 years as outgrowths of what were the medical practices of their times. Though common perception views alternative and complementary therapies as Eastern in their philosophies and practices, these newer systems—notably HOMEOPATHY, NATUROPATHY, and OSTEOPATHY—are Western in origin and orientation. One alternative healing method, CHIROPRACTIC, is uniquely American.

ALTERNATIVE HEALING SYSTEMS

AYURVEDA	HOMEOPATHY
NATIVE AMERICAN HEALING	NATUROPATHY
OSTEOPATHY	TRADITIONAL CHINESE MEDICINE (TCM)

Interest in, and use of, alternative therapies is a growing phenomenon in the United States. According to a 2002 survey by the US National Center for Complementary and Alternative Medicine (NCCAM) and the US Centers for Disease Control and Prevention (CDC) National Center for Health Statistics (NCHS), nearly two thirds of Americans use some form of alternative health practice, most of them to complement their conventional medical care.

Surveys show that half choose alternative therapies on their own to complement conventional therapies, a quarter use alternative therapies their conventional physicians recommend, and a quarter use alternative therapies on their own because they believe conventional medicine will not help their conditions. Nearly 12 million Americans seek relief from BACK PAIN alone through alternative and complementary therapies (excluding prayer). Other common uses of alternative and complementary therapies (excluding prayer) include arthritis and JOINT PAIN, chronic HEADACHE, FIBROMYALGIA, anxiety and DEPRESSION, chronic gastrointestinal conditions, hypertension, and MENOPAUSE discomfort. Many people use alternative and complementary therapies to provide relief during cancer treatment and from cancer symptoms.

NCCAM/NCHS 2002 SURVEY'S TOP 10

Alternative/Complementary Practice	Percentage of Americans Who Use
prayer specifically for one's own health	43.0 percent
prayer by others for one's health	24.4 percent
natural products	18.9 percent
deep BREATHING EXERCISES	11.6 percent
participation in prayer group for one's own health	9.6 percent
MEDITATION	7.6 percent
CHIROPRACTIC care	7.5 percent
YOGA	5.1 percent
massage	5.0 percent
diet-based therapies	3.5 percent

Source: Barnes, P; Powell-Griner, E; McFann, K; and Nahin, R. CDC Advance Data Report #343. Complementary and Alternative Medicine Use Among Adults: United States, 2002. *May 27, 2004.*

"First, Do No Harm"

Alternative and complementary approaches often draw people to try them on their own, without consulting their conventional doctors. People may be curious about certain methods, frustrated or disappointed with the results of conventional treatments, or have limited access to conventional health care. In choosing from alternative and complementary therapies, it is prudent to learn as much as possible about the method so as to "first, do no harm" as the time-honored medical dictum cautions. And, when possible, seek the advice of a conventional doctor to gain perspective to what often is confusing or conflicting information.

Though it is seldom harmful to drink GREEN TEA, do yoga, or have REIKI, some alternative and complementary methods may be hazardous as may be some conventional methods—for people who have certain health conditions. For example, people who have RHEUMATOID ARTHRITIS or other degenerative musculoskeletal disorders may risk serious injury with craniosacral therapy, OSTEOPATHIC MANIPULATIVE TREATMENT (OMT), or chiropractic manipulation. NUTRITIONAL THERAPY may alter medication needs for people who have DIABETES, MALABSORPTION disorders, or conditions affecting the LIVER or KIDNEYS. It is important to choose the most reliable and credible methods and practitioners, and to coordinate care among all the providers involved in its delivery, conventional and complementary.

Using alternative and complementary approaches in coordination with conventional treatments may alleviate some symptoms but cannot effectively substitute for conventional medical care for many health conditions ranging from HYPOTHYROIDISM to CANCER.

For people who are undergoing conventional medical treatment such as CHEMOTHERAPY or RADIATION THERAPY, it is worthy to ask doctors what to eat, how and when to exercise, and what measures can support health; the environment of the body changes dramatically during such therapies, and sometimes approaches that are supportive and complementary to the conventional treatment can lessen the harshness of the experience. For many circumstances, however, available information fails to provide clear answers and it becomes a matter of trusting the doctor and making common sense decisions.

Science Meets Tradition: Evidence and Standards

Scientific evidence is scarce for many alternative and complementary therapies. Many therapies have evolved over centuries of use and produce reliable results even though contemporary clinical science cannot yet explain the mechanisms of the method. Acupuncture, for example, has been an integral component of TCM, as well as other healing systems, for several thousand years. At acupuncture's foundation, within these systems, is the presence of an extensive network of energy channels, called meridians, in the body. Though these meridians are not tangible, perceptible structures in the conventional sense, they are nonetheless a centuries-old map of energy pathways in the body. That contemporary researchers have yet to quantify them does not necessarily invalidate their existence. Indeed, not until the invention of devices such as the microscope in the eighteenth century, and really not until its application in exploring the structure of the human body in the nineteenth century, did scientists discover the networks of nerves that convey information and instructions from the BRAIN to each cell in the body. Medical science is ever-evolving, and new technologies continually reveal new and paradigm-shifting discoveries (such as mapping the human genome).

Herbal remedies and medicinal foods contain numerous potentially active ingredients. Conventional clinical studies of the intact substance, such as the soybean, may yield different results than studies of the substance's known active ingredients, such as SOY isoflavones. A substance may appear to be a "heal-all," raising questions about PLACEBO effect. And yet the substance may simply have such broad-reaching actions in the body, such as stimulating the immune system, that it truly does have healing effects for numerous health conditions.

Evidence of effectiveness and mechanism of action may be in short supply simply because the clinical research studies that are today the foundation of conventional medicine may not have investigated a particular therapy or may have produced inconclusive findings. Sometimes multiple studies generate conflicting data. Some methods have been copiously studied, though according to standards other than those common in the United States. And, of course, numerous "therapies" are available that have dubious therapeutic value (and may appear clearly ineffective or even harmful) and have no foundation within the context of any healing system.

As a result of these mixed circumstances, there is considerable disagreement among conventional doctors and clinical scientists about the effectiveness and potential risks of many alternative and complementary therapies. These possibilities apply as well to conventional therapies. Researchers do not fully understand the mechanisms of many drugs, such as levodopa to treat PARKINSON'S DISEASE, the tricyclic ANTIDEPRESSANT MEDICATIONS, and many of the medications doctors prescribe to treat HEART conditions. However, empirical evidence (observable, reproducible effects) support their effectiveness to the extent that conventional doctors are comfortable using them. Such is becoming the case with some alternative and complementary approaches that lend themselves to empirical study, such as acupuncture.

As the current health-care paradigm continues to change, it is natural to expect conflicting viewpoints about the best standard of care to emerge. Until there is a truly integrated approach, there will be a higher level of responsibility on the individual to participate in health-care decisions and to choose care that is wise and effective. This applies as much to the choice to use acupuncture as to enroll in a clinical study for an experimental drug or treatment.

Breakthrough Research and Treatment Advances

Advances in medical technology, particularly imaging procedures, have made possible the study of alternative and complementary therapies in ways that allow researchers to explore how they alter physiologic functions. POSITRON EMISSION TOMOGRAPHY (PET) SCAN and MAGNETIC RESONANCE IMAGING (MRI), for example, allow researchers to observe, in real time, the changes that take place in the brain and other parts of the body with therapies such as HYPNOSIS, acupuncture, MEDITATION, visualization, and even prayer. Numerous studies underway are investigating alternative therapies such as botanical and herbal remedies to relieve the discomforts of menopause, CANCER and CARDIOVASCULAR DISEASE PREVENTION and treatment claims, methods for pain management, and mind–body interventions to mitigate the symptoms of chronic health conditions.

The current health-care culture is reaching for new understanding that can unify technology, conventional techniques, and complementary methods in a single, amazing paradigm for treatment of the human being in health and in illness. Within this paradigm is the potential for many of the complementary approaches to be as "conventional" in their use and application as advances in technology such as GENE THERAPY, molecular medicine, diagnostic imaging, ORGAN TRANSPLANTATION, BIOLOGICAL RESPONSE MODIFIER, and PHARMACOGENOMICS.

Even today, hospitals are quietly becoming models of such an integrative paradigm. Neonatal intensive care units employ MASSAGE THERAPY and music therapy to soothe the fragile premature infants born before their bodies and systems developed fully. Patients waiting for organ transplants or undergoing high-tech cancer treatments receive instruction in meditation and visualization. Reflection gardens, labyrinths, Native American prayer wheels, meditation rooms, and chapels provide quiet, calming environments for prayer and contemplation.

This is a time of record breakthroughs in medical discoveries. Researchers are exploring more and more experimental treatments, conventional as well as alternative and complementary. Keeping up with the incredible pace of new knowledge challenges doctors and individuals alike. What is clear already is that as knowledge increases, the best care will be that which presents an informed integrative approach guided by progressive conventional doctors based on individual patient needs, using the simplest, most effective methods for restoring and maintaining health.

acupuncture A HEALING method in which the acupuncturist inserts hair-thin needles into the body at various locations along energy channels called meridians. The underlying premise is that disease represents imbalances of the flow of energy (chi), and the needles redirect the flow to restore balance and thus health. The practice of acupuncture dates back at least 2,500 years to the origins of TRADITIONAL CHINESE MEDICINE (TCM), and today remains an integral component of TCM.

The Western adaptation of acupuncture views the practice primarily from the perspective of PAIN relief and shifts the underlying mechanism to one in which the needles stimulate NERVE endings, eliciting biochemical and electromagnetic responses that interrupt the flow of pain messages to the BRAIN. Another Westernization of acupuncture is electrostimulation of the acupuncture needles after inserting them, which intensifies the effect.

COMMON THERAPEUTIC APPLICATIONS OF ACUPUNCTURE

ADDICTION	ASTHMA
BACK PAIN	CARPAL TUNNEL SYNDROME
CHEMOTHERAPY nausea	CHRONIC FATIGUE SYNDROME
CONVERT BREECH PRESENTATION IN PREGNANCY	dental PAIN
	ENDOMETRIOSIS
FIBROMYALGIA	HEADACHE
INDUCE LABOR IN PREGNANCY	IRRITABLE BOWEL SYNDROME (IBS)
menopausal HOT FLASHES	
menstrual cramps	motion sickness
OSTEOARTHRITIS	POLYCYSTIC OVARY SYNDROME (PCOS)
postoperative NAUSEA	
PREMENSTRUAL SYNDROME (PMS)	RELIEVE NAUSEA AND VOMITING
ROTATOR CUFF IMPINGEMENT SYNDROME	
	SMOKING CESSATION
sports injuries	tennis elbow (EPICONDYLITIS)

Numerous clinical studies of acupuncture have provided evidence that acupuncture does indeed relieve pain. However, no study has yet been able to identify the precise mechanisms by which relief takes place. In 1997 the US National Institutes of Health (NIH) issued a consensus statement acknowledging the primary therapeutic value of acupuncture for a variety of health situations and conditions such as NAUSEA, HEADACHE, dental pain, OSTEOARTHRITIS, and ADDICTION. This marked the turning point for acceptance of acupuncture as a mainstream treatment option for numerous health conditions.

The Acupuncture Experience

Most people find the experience of acupuncture relaxing, calming, and even somewhat euphoric. The hair-thin needles are so fine that they are difficult to see; most people do not feel them when the acupuncturist inserts them. The acupuncturist first directs the person to lie on a padded table or sit in a recliner-style chair, depending on the location of the acupuncture points and reason for treatment, and then inserts the needles. After insertion, the needles stay in place for 20 to 30 minutes. Occasionally a needle falls out; this is okay and does not affect the treatment.

Some conditions need only 2 or 3 treatments, usually about a week apart. Other conditions may require up to 10 or 12 weekly treatments for relief and occasional follow-up treatments for maintenance. For aural, or earlobe, acupuncture to treat addiction or for SMOKING CESSATION, the acupuncturist may place a small needle, like a button, leaving it in place until it falls out on its own hours to days later.

In the United States acupuncturists must use single-use, disposable needles to prevent the spread of bloodborne infections such as HEPATITIS and HIV/AIDS. Though adverse effects are rare, they can occur. Some people experience continued tingling at the site of a needle insertion, and occasionally there is very minor bleeding at a needle site. People who are uncomfortable with the thought or sight of needles may choose to close their eyes when the acupuncturist is handling and inserting needles. One of the most common side effects of acupuncture, typically among people who are new to the procedure, is fainting at the sight of a needle or when the acupuncturist inserts the first few needles. Such a response relates to the person's fear or concern about the procedure, not the acupuncturist's technique.

Choosing an Acupuncturist

Most acupuncturists in the United States are health-care practitioners such as conventional doctors (MDs and DOs), naturopathic doctors (NDs), chiropractors (DCs), and dentists (DDSs or DMDs). Most states have some level of certification or licensing, though standards are inconsistent among states. The minimum education and training required for MDs and DOs to become a licensed acupuncturist in the United States is 200 hours. Some states extend this requirement to NDs and DCs. States that will license an acupuncturist who is not a trained health professional typically require completion of an accredited acupuncture program that is about 3,000 hours of classroom education and experiential training. A licensed acupuncturist uses the designation L.Ac. after his or her name.

Because standards vary among states, health experts recommend obtaining recommendations and referrals for acupuncturists, especially for people who are new to acupuncture. As with any health-care practitioner, it is important to feel comfortable with, and to trust, the acupuncturist.

See also ALTERNATIVE METHODS FOR PAIN RELIEF; BIOFEEDBACK; MIND–BODY INTERACTIONS; OSTEOPATHIC MANIPULATIVE TREATMENT; REFLEXOLOGY; TRANSCUTANEOUS ELECTRICAL NERVE STIMULATION.

anti-aging approaches It is a common observation that people who fully engage in the activities of living from when they wake in the morning until they go to bed at night seem to be much younger than their chronological ages. They look younger, they act younger, they feel younger. With longevity continuing to increase, many people are searching for ways to be among those who seem young. It is enticing to think such efforts might be as simple as taking a pill every morning. While some methods to maintain the health and vigor of youth show intriguing promise, many are ineffective or potentially harmful.

Aging Interventions

Products marketed to slow the aging process seldom can substantiate their claims through clinical studies and objective measures. Nonetheless, they are appealing because everyone wants to believe they can work. And some may be helpful, though researchers do not yet know. Some products commonly marketed as anti-aging substances include

- Hormones such as DEHYDROEPIANDROSTERONE (DHEA) (a TESTOSTERONE/estrogen precursor the adrenal glands produce) and human GROWTH HORMONE (hGH), which marketers claim reverse aging effects such as lost MUSCLE mass and BONE DENSITY. Some clinical studies show these hormones can indeed have such effect. However, health experts caution that there are as yet no studies that evaluate the effects and consequences of these products over the long term.

- Antioxidants such as vitamins and COENZYME Q10, marketed as substances that can clean up the molecular waste that otherwise accumulates to cause disease. Indeed, antioxidants do bind with free radicals, molecular particles that remain in cells as byproducts of energy generation. What is much less clear is the precise role free radicals have in causing diseases such as DIABETES, CANCER, CARDIOVASCULAR DISEASE (CVD), OSTEOARTHRITIS, PARKINSON'S DISEASE, and other health conditions typically associated with aging.

Conventional health experts believe there is little value to claims about any products that say they can stop or reverse the aging process. Though such claims remain out there, the bigger truth also remains: None of these products ever kept anyone from growing older or from eventually reaching the end of his or her lifetime.

Healthy Aging

In the mid-1990s researchers at the Tufts University Center for Aging compared two groups of women ages 50 to 70. At the start of the study, the women in both groups were all sedentary. One group stayed that way. The other group participated in progressively intense physical STRENGTH training. At the end of 1 year the women in the strength training group looked, felt, and acted 20 years younger than the women in the sedentary group. Other studies involving other groups have shown, too, that people who stay physically and mentally active experience fewer illnesses and injuries, and maintain cognitive ability and memory function.

Many health experts believe the true "fountain of youth" is within each individual and the lifestyle choices he or she makes. Of course no one chooses to be sick. In fact, illness 40 years down the road is not what most people think about when making choices about eating, exercise, and smoking. Yet many of the choices people make lead to the chronic health conditions that have come to characterize growing older in America. Though not as glamorous as pills that promise to turn back the calendar, doing what is possible to contain the risks for these conditions, many health experts say, is the one anti-aging approach in which anyone and everyone can participate.

See also ESTROGENS; HEALTH RISK FACTORS; HORMONE; HUMAN GROWTH HORMONE (HGH) SUPPLEMENT; LIFESTYLE AND HEALTH; QUALITY OF LIFE.

aromatherapy The therapeutic use of essential oils of plants delivered via the sense of smell. Essential oils are highly concentrated liquid extracts from the stems, leaves, flowers, and other parts of plants that contain the energy essence of the plant. Aromatherapy is a form of energy HEALING always done to complement or accompany other therapeutic forms. A qualified aromatherapist can mix personalized blends as recipes to meet a person's individual needs. In the United States essential oils are available in health food stores, and many major grocery stores and drugstores carry common oils that anyone can buy.

COMMON ESSENTIAL OILS FOR AROMATHERAPY

Essential Oil	Therapeutic Use
anise	upper respiratory INFECTION
basil	focus and concentration
cedarwood	arthritis
citrus	mental clarity and alertness
eucalyptus	congestion
jasmine	DEPRESSION
lavender	anxiety, insomnia
peppermint	NAUSEA relief
rose	relaxation, gastrointestinal upset, dry SKIN
rosemary	MUSCLE relaxation
sandalwood	stress
thyme	circulation
vanilla	confidence, relaxation
ylang-ylang	anxiety, PALPITATIONS, stress

The most common method for dispensing an essential oil is diffusion, in which a heat source such as a candle or low-watt light bulb warms a solution of water and the essential oil. Often the essential oil also carries the fragrance of the plant, giving off a pleasant smell. However, according to the principles of aromatherapy, it is the energy nature of the essential oil, not necessarily its fragrance, that provides therapeutic benefit. Fragranced solutions that are not essential oils may smell no different but aromatherapists contend they have no therapeutic value.

Many alternative and complementary practices integrate aromatherapy, which health experts consider to be mostly safe. Some essential oils can stimulate physiologic changes in the body that may be hazardous during PREGNANCY; pregnant women should discuss using aromatherapy with their obstetricians or midwives. The essential oils for aromatherapy are for external use only. Most are harmful, and some can be fatal, if ingested. Many essential oils are irritating to the SKIN unless significantly diluted with neutral carrier oils (such as almond oil) before application.

See also FLOWER ESSENCES; HOMEOPATHY; MEDITATION; PRAYER AND SPIRITUALITY; VISUALIZATION.

art therapy A HEALING approach that uses the creative arts to help people, especially children, express suppressed emotions. Art therapy may employ drawing, writing, dancing, singing, drama, painting, storytelling, sculpting with clay, and other forms that allow free and creative expression. The underlying philosophy of art therapy is that the processes of creativity are also pathways of insight and understanding. With focused exploration of the art a person creates, he or she can gain new perspectives and learn to solve problems or reconcile situations that cause stress, anxiety, or DEPRESSION.

Art therapists typically have either a graduate degree in art therapy or dual graduate degrees in art and psychology (or related fields). A registered art therapist meets the education and experience requirements of the Art Therapy Credentials Board. In the United States, each state regulates the licensing requirements for art therapists. Art therapists may work in hospitals, health-care clinics, rehabilitation centers, and private practice.

See also COGNITIVE THERAPY; GENERALIZED ANXIETY DISORDER (GAD); MIND–BODY INTERACTIONS.

Ayurveda A philosophy of HEALING based in ancient Hinduism that dates perhaps to 4500 B.C.E. or earlier. Ayurveda considers all of existence in the context of energy, including human beings. Each person represents the essential elements of universal energy (fire, air, water, earth, and ether), which manifest in three states of physical existence called *doshas: vata, pitta,* and *kapha.* Health exists when there is balance among the *doshas,* and illness (or ailment) represents imbalance. The *dosha's* association indicates the general nature of the ailment. BACK PAIN, for example, represents a *vata* imbalance (movement) and indigestion is a *kapha* imbalance (structure).

Ayurvedic Diagnosis and Treatment
Key to the Ayurvedic diagnostic process is careful assessment of the tongue and the six pulses of each arm, three superficial and three deep. The pulses provide information about the balances and imbalances in the *doshas.* The Ayurvedic practitioner asks many questions about the individual's health, health concerns, family, lifestyle, and life in general. Ayurvedic therapies attempt to restore *dosha* balance through herbal remedies, YOGA poses, dietary changes, and lifestyle measures.

AYURVEDIC DOSHAS		
Dosha	**Elemental Energy**	**Association**
vata	ether (space) and air	movement
pitta	fire	transformation
kapha	earth and water	structure

Ayurvedic Practitioners
In India, Ayurvedic practitioners train for five to six years before going into practice on their own. A US-trained Ayurvedic practitioner completes a one-year program of study and then can practice. There are no licensing education or requirements for Ayurvedic practitioners in the United States. Some alternative health practitioners such as naturopathic physicians or chiropractors may complete additional training to practice Ayurvedic methods.

Benefits and Risks of Ayurveda
Ayurveda represents a lifestyle orientation to health and health care. All aspects of an individual's life and circumstances influence health and illness, and Ayurvedic therapies target bringing all back into balance. Some herbal remedies may interact with other substances including prescription medications. A conventional doctor should provide clinical oversight for people who have health conditions that require conventional treatment, such as DIABETES, CANCER, and CARDIOVASCULAR DISEASE (CVD).

See also MEDICINAL HERBS AND BOTANICALS; NATIVE AMERICAN HEALING; TRADITIONAL CHINESE MEDICINE (TCM).

B

bilberry A plant (*Vaccinium myrtillus*) whose berries, stems, and leaves are rich in antioxidants (notably anthocyanosides) and tannins. Even preserves made from the blue-colored berries of this bush contain high enough levels of these substances to have noticeable effect. Anthocyanosides have particular affinity for the walls of arteries, especially arterioles, the tiny, almost microscopic arteries deep within body tissues where nutrient/waste exchanges takes place. Anthocyanosides appear to keep the cells of these arterial walls healthy and structurally intact. This action has pronounced effects on the tiny blood vessels that supply the RETINA, CORNEA, and other structures of the EYE, protecting them from age-related damage such as AGE-RELATED MACULAR DEGENERATION (ARMD) and CATARACT. The tannins in bilberry seem to help INFLAMMATION and INFECTION affecting the MOUTH and THROAT, plus gastrointestinal upset.

Many ophthalmologists recommend that people over age 50, who are entering the high-risk period of life for conditions such as ARMD, night blindness, and cataracts, take bilberry to help protect their eyes and vision. Bilberry seems most effective in combination with the amino acids LUTEIN and ZEAXANTHIN, which also protect the retina and cornea. There are no known side effects or interactions with bilberry, and doctors consider it safe for most people to take long-term.

BILBERRY (Vaccinium myrtillus)

Uses	Risks/Side Effects	Interactions
improve night vision	none known	none known
prevent or slow ARMD		
prevent or slow growth of cataracts		
RETINOPATHY of DIABETES		

See also ARTERY; CATARACT EXTRACTION AND LENS REPLACEMENT; RETINOPATHY; VISION IMPAIRMENT.

biofeedback A method in which a person learns to influence certain body responses, such as to PAIN or stress. Biofeedback begins with learning sessions that use electronic measuring devices to report physiologic signs such as PULSE, BREATHING rate, or SKIN temperature. The device sends a visual or sound signal to help focus concentration on the particular sign, for example the pulse. The person then concentrates on slowing the rate of the sound or visual cue, indicating that the body is relaxing and the HEART RATE is slowing. Over the course of 5 to 10 biofeedback sessions, the person learns to "tune in" to the physiologic signs and no longer needs the device. Once the person masters the method of biofeedback, he or she can use it at will.

CONDITIONS BIOFEEDBACK MAY HELP

ASTHMA	chronic PAIN syndromes
HYPERTENSION	migraine HEADACHE
MUSCLE tension headache	PALPITATIONS
RAYNAUD'S SYNDROME	RETINOPATHY of DIABETES
SEIZURE DISORDERS	stress
STROKE recovery	URINARY INCONTINENCE

Though the most common application of biofeedback is stress relief, people who have chronic health conditions also can use it to manage pain and other symptoms. Numerous clinical studies over the past 25 years have supported the effectiveness of biofeedback, especially for relieving pain and stress. There are few risks with biofeedback, as it is noninvasive. Because biofeedback can alter body chemistry, it can change medication needs for chronic conditions such as

DIABETES (INSULIN or oral ANTIDIABETES MEDICATIONS) and HYPERTENSION (high BLOOD PRESSURE).

See also HYPNOSIS; MEDITATION; MIND–BODY INTERACTIONS; STRESS AND STRESS MANAGEMENT; VISUALIZATION.

black cohosh An herbal remedy women may take to treat HOT FLASHES at MENOPAUSE. The medicinal extract comes from the dark roots and rhizomes of the wildflower black cohosh (*Actaea racemosa* or *Cimicifuga racemosa*), a member of the buttercup family indigenous to North America. Medicinal uses of black cohosh derive from NATIVE AMERICAN HEALING traditions. In 2001 the American College of Obstetricians and Gynecologists (ACOG) issued a statement of support endorsing black cohosh as a short-term treatment (up to six months) for relief of menopausal discomforts. Sold without a doctor's prescription as a dietary supplement in the United States, black cohosh is an ingredient in numerous women's health products.

The apparent active ingredients of black cohosh are deoxyactein, triterpenes glycosides (also called triterpenes saponins), and fukinolic acid, phytoestrogenic chemicals that produce a weak estrogen effect in the human body. Clinical studies of black cohosh generally support its effectiveness for relieving hot flashes, though results for other menopausal discomforts are less consistent. Studies also have failed to demonstrate any benefit for OSTEOPOROSIS.

As hot flashes are the major symptom for about 80 percent of women who have discomfort when going through menopause, many gynecologists recommend an initial trial of black cohosh in lieu of conventional estrogen/progesterone or estrogen hormone replacement therapy (HRT) for menopause. Many women find that a combination of botanicals in addition to black cohosh (such as flaxseed, soy, and chasteberry) seems to more effectively relieve symptoms, though these clinical research studies so far have not generated supportive evidence. Black cohosh does not seem very effective for menstrual discomforts such as cramps and excessive flow, though women have used it as a premenstrual/ menstrual remedy for several centuries. It typically takes 8 to 10 weeks to experience benefits after starting black cohosh.

Herbalists recommend black cohosh products that contain freeze-dried root, which appears to have the most potent and consistent action. Women who are pregnant should not take black cohosh because its estrogen-like actions may interfere with the body's hormonal balance. Some women experience gastrointestinal upset or dizziness; reducing the DOSE and taking the remedy with meals can minimize these side effects. Women who are taking oral contraceptives (birth control pills) should check with their doctors or pharmacists about possible interactions.

BLACK COHOSH (*Actaea racemosa, Cimicifuga racemosa*)

Uses	Risks/Side Effects	Interactions
relieve menopausal HOT FLASHES	uterine contractions in PREGNANCY	oral contraceptives

See also DONG QUAI; GINSENG; PHYTOESTROGENS; SOY.

boswellia Medicinal preparations that derive from the resin of the *Boswellia serrata* tree native to the desert areas of India. Boswellia has strong anti-inflammatory characteristics and provides relief from OSTEOARTHRITIS and RHEUMATOID ARTHRITIS. It also provides relief from symptoms of INFLAMMATORY BOWEL DISEASE (IBD), especially in people who have Crohn's disease. In the United States boswellia is a dietary supplement available without a doctor's prescription. The typical course of treatment with oral forms of boswellia is 8 to 12 weeks. People who are taking prescription medications should check with their doctors before taking boswellia, though there are no known interactions between boswellia and other substances.

BOSWELLIA

Uses	Risks/Side Effects	Interactions
OSTEOARTHRITIS	none known	none known
RHEUMATOID ARTHRITIS		
INFLAMMATORY BOWEL DISEASE (IBD)		

See also NONSTEROIDAL ANTI-INFLAMMATORY DRUGS (NSAIDS).

chamomile An herb, *Matricaria recutita,* used for its abilities to calm anxiety, soothe gastrointestinal irritation, relieve menstrual cramps, and aid in sleep. Chamomile contains volatile acids and flavonoids, chemical substances that ease spasms of smooth muscles, such as in the intestinal tract and the UTERUS, and that have mild anti-inflammatory qualities. The most active of these is the flavonoid apigenin, which has antiseptic properties as well.

Chamomile tea is a common preparation for stress relief and relaxation. In oral forms chamomile is a dietary supplement in the United States, available without a doctor's prescription. Topical forms of chamomile, also available over-the-counter, relieve itching and other SKIN discomforts, including those of dermatitis, and mild to moderate SUNBURN. Some preparations of chamomile dissolve or mix in bath water, such as powders and oils, providing full body relief.

Though there are few clinical studies that affirm the effects of chamomile, health experts consider it a generally safe medicinal herb. There are no known interactions or side effects. People who have allergies to ragweed, daisies, chrysanthemums, and other plants in the *Aster* family may have cross-over sensitivity to chamomile.

CHAMOMILE *(Matricaria recutita)*		
Uses	**Risks/Side Effects**	**Interactions**
gastrointestinal upset	none known	none known
sleep aid		
general relaxant		

See also VALERIAN.

chelation therapy The therapeutic process of injecting or otherwise introducing a chemical agent, typically ethylenediaminetetraacetic acid (EDTA), into the body that binds with specific substances. The body then excretes the bound substances in the urine, safely eliminating them from the body. Doctors first used chelation therapy in the 1940s to treat poisoning with lead and other heavy metals, and that remains chelation therapy's accepted application in conventional medicine today.

Many of the first people to undergo chelation therapy were middle-aged men who had worked all their adult lives in factories where lead contamination was common. They also had the usual health conditions for men of their age, typically CARDIOVASCULAR DISEASE (CVD). As they completed the chelation therapy, many of the men also noticed they no longer had ANGINA PECTORIS (cardiac CHEST PAIN). The doctors conducting the chelation therapy treatments concluded the EDTA was also drawing calcium and other minerals from the ATHEROSCLEROTIC PLAQUE lining the CORONARY ARTERIES. The plaque narrowed the passageway for blood, causing the men to experience pain and shortness of breath particularly with exertion—the classic symptoms of CORONARY ARTERY DISEASE (CAD).

Though further testing and X-ray fluoroscopy of the men who experienced cardiovascular improvement failed to substantiate the theory, it has remained popular. However, there still are no clinical studies that support it. Another theory holds that chelation therapy removes from the body free radicals, particles of molecular waste that bind with any available molecule. This theory also remains unproven. Researchers believe free radicals that bind prevent bonded molecules from performing their intended functions, a process that over time results in degenerative diseases.

Though doctors in other countries may use chelation therapy before turning to surgical interventions to treat CAD, most conventional physicians in the United States feel the risks outweigh the benefits when it comes to chelation therapy as a treatment for atherosclerotic heart disease.

See also CORONARY ARTERY BYPASS GRAFT; HEAVY METAL POISONING; KIDNEY; LIFESTYLE AND CARDIOVASCULAR HEALTH; LIFESTYLE AND HEALTH.

Chinese herbal remedies See TRADITIONAL CHINESE MEDICINE (TCM).

chiropractic A system of health care that emphasizes manipulation of the spine and back to align the musculoskeletal system for optimal function and support of the rest of the body. Chiropractic originated in the United States with the work of Daniel David Palmer in the late 1890s. Palmer had a keen interest in magnetic HEALING and in what he perceived to be the body's natural tendency to keep itself in balance and thus in health. From his observations he began head and neck manipulations.

Chiropractic Diagnosis and Treatment

Chiropractic views the body as a system of balance, physical as well as emotional. When the spine is out of alignment, the rest of the body attempts to rebalance itself. When it cannot, one result is PAIN. Injuries and chronic health conditions may pull the spine out of alignment as well. The leading reason people seek chiropractic care is for treatment of musculoskeletal injuries and pain, particularly lower back pain. Chiropractic often is an effective approach for treating repetitious motion injuries as well as for teaching methods to avoid further injury. Chiropractic may incorporate ACUPUNCTURE, MASSAGE THERAPY, NUTRITIONAL THERAPY, or CRANIOSACRAL MASSAGE in addition to chiropractic manipulations.

The chiropractor begins an examination by asking questions about why the person has come for care and may take X-rays as well as look at the back. Observing posture and movement help the chiropractor assess overall musculoskeletal health, and the chiropractor will palpate the neck and spine. Most chiropractors also ask about diet and nutrition, physical activity and exercise, and occu-pation and recreational interests. The chiropractor should then explain his or her findings and the treatment options to correct them.

Chiropractic manipulations should not cause pain. Often the back makes popping sounds as the chiropractor uses pressure to correct subluxations (out of position vertebrae). Some chiropractors use devices, whereas others use only their hands. Most people feel relaxed after a chiropractic treatment. Chiropractic manipulation may correct one set of problems, which then reveals other problems. Some conditions require only a few visits and treatments, though others may require up to 10 visits over several weeks or occasionally more extensive therapy. No chiropractic therapy should continue indefinitely, though many people need to return periodically.

Chiropractic manipulation can restore the spine's correct alignment, but circumstances such as structural asymmetries, longstanding injury, and postural or function-oriented habits that remain unchanged may cause the spine to eventually return to misalignments. Many people have one leg slightly different length from the other, for example, or may sit at a computer all day leaning forward with shoulders hunched. These chronic sorts of circumstances account for about a third of chiropractic visits.

Chiropractic Practitioners

Over the decades since Palmer introduced his methods for manipulating the neck, chiropractic has evolved into a comprehensive and structured health-care discipline. Doctors of chiropractic (DCs) attend eight or more years of college and chiropractic medical school, completing extensive education and training in a broad spectrum of health-care areas. Many chiropractors have further training, certification, or licensure in acupuncture, nutrition, and specialized care such as sports injuries. All states in the United States require chiropractors to pass a national proficiency examination and meet the state's licensing requirements.

Benefits and Risks of Chiropractic

At one time in its evolution, chiropractic involved approaches and methods, arising from inconsistencies in practice and education, that sometimes did harm to people. Standardizations in philosophy, education, and licensing in the latter half of the twentieth century solidified chiropractic as a beneficial, reputable health-care profession and practice. In 1994 the US Agency for Health Care Policy and Research (AHCPR) endorsed chiropractic as a safe and appropriate first-line treatment for low back pain. Most insurers in the United States pay for limited chiropractic care.

Chiropractors may not prescribe medications, diagnose health conditions, provide medical treatments outside those necessary for spinal manipulations, or perform surgery. People who have health conditions that affect the spine such as ANKYLOSING SPONDYLITIS or RHEUMATOID ARTHRITIS should talk with their orthopedists before undergoing chiropractic treatment. A conventional doctor should evaluate back pain with FEVER, as this may be an indication of MENINGITIS or other potentially life-threatening infection.

See also NATUROPATHY; OSTEOPATHIC MANIPULATIVE TREATMENT (OMT).

chondroitin A chemical compound that occurs naturally in the CARTILAGE and other tissues in the joints, chondroitin appears to protect JOINT tissues from damage and deterioration by blocking the actions of certain destructive enzymes. There is substantial evidence, through clinical studies, that this blocking action can arrest and even reverse OSTEOARTHRITIS. In some studies, chondroitin was at least as effective as the commonly prescribed NON-STERIODAL ANTI-INFLAMMATORY DRUGS (NSAIDS) that are the standard treatment for osteoarthritis in the United States. Combining chondroitin with another natural compound, GLUCOSAMINE, intensifies the benefit.

Though researchers and practitioners have known of glucosamine and have recommended it to relieve joint INFLAMMATION and PAIN for decades, researchers discovered chondroitin only in the 1960s. A number of clinical studies conducted in the 1980s and 1990s began to make clear chondroitin's effects and benefits. Chondroitin seems most effective for osteoarthritis affecting the hips and knees and does not have any effect on RHEUMATOID ARTHRITIS, a deformative autoimmune disorder.

There seem to be few side effects or interactions with chondroitin. People who are taking anticoag-

ulant medications should check with their doctors before taking chondroitin. Though chondroitin does not directly affect clotting, many substances that affect inflammation have the potential for interfering with blood chemistry. It typically takes two to four months to notice appreciable results after starting chondroitin.

CHONDROITIN		
Uses	Risks/Side Effects	Interactions
OSTEOARTHRITIS	none known	possibly anticoagulants

See also ANTICOAGULANT THERAPY; AUTOIMMUNE DISORDERS; SAMe.

coenzyme Q10 An ANTIOXIDANT found in every nucleated cell in the body. It has numerous functions related to cell activity and repair. As a coenzyme, coenzyme Q10 facilitates or works in collaboration with enzymes in the cells. Enzymes carry out the genetic instructions of the cell. The more active the cell, the more coenzyme Q10 the cell contains. A HEART cell has considerably more coenzyme Q10 than does a SKIN cell, for example. Researchers discovered coenzyme Q10 in 1957 and continue to investigate how it works and what it does in the body.

People who have certain forms of heart disease, such as HYPERTENSION (high BLOOD PRESSURE) and HEART FAILURE, have lower than normal levels of coenzyme Q10. In some studies, giving them coenzyme Q10 improved heart function, most notably hypertension. Though researchers do not fully understand its mechanisms, boosting coenzyme Q10 levels in cardiac cells seems to improve their efficiency. This effect is less conclusive in people recovering from HEART ATTACK or who have other forms of heart disease.

There is some evidence that coenzyme Q10 supplementation has numerous beneficial effects on health. Researchers are exploring its role in preventing BREAST CANCER, periodontitis (INFLAMMATION and INFECTION of the gums), and ALZHEIMER'S DISEASE. Some health experts believe coenzyme Q10 may improve symptoms and QUALITY OF LIFE for people with MITOCHONDRIAL DISORDERS, MUSCULAR DYSTROPHY, and degenerative neurologic conditions such as PARKINSON'S DISEASE. Studies investigating the ability of coenzyme Q10 supplementation to prevent the onset of type 2 DIABETES have so far yielded no evidence that it can do so. Nor is there any conclusive evidence that coenzyme Q10 has any ability to enhance IMMUNE SYSTEM function, though all of these effects have theoretical potential. Across the spectrum of health knowledge, coenzyme Q10 is a relatively new discovery and much remains for researchers and doctors to learn and understand about its natural functions in the body as well as the benefits and possible risks of supplements.

Coenzyme Q10 is available in the United States as a dietary supplement that does not require a doctor's prescription to obtain. It does not appear to have side effects or interactions with other substances, though health experts encourage people to talk with their doctors about taking it if they are taking medications to treat health conditions, especially hypertension and heart failure. Pregnant or BREASTFEEDING mothers probably should not take coenzyme Q10 as researchers know little about how it might affect infants. Coenzyme Q10 is fat soluble; the body best absorbs it with foods that contain some dietary fat.

COENZYME Q10		
uses	Risks/Side Effects	Interactions
HYPERTENSION	none known	none known
HEART FAILURE		
recovery after		
HEART ATTACK		
periodontitis		

See also LIFESTYLE AND CARDIOVASCULAR HEALTH; PERIODONTAL DISEASE.

craniosacral massage   A form of bodywork, also called craniosacral therapy, in which the practitioner gently manipulates the head, neck, and spine to balance the fluids around the head and SPINAL CORD. The movement of this fluid, in the context of craniosacral massage, is the cranial rhythmic impulse. The intended goal is somatoemotional release, the discharge of physical and emotional tension the head and spine hold as a result of stress and daily experiences. Injuries may also contribute to the tension.

For many people the experience evokes the sensation of floating or dreaming and is profoundly relaxing. Though the craniosacral therapist's movements are gentle and touch is very light, there is a sensation of movement throughout the body. Sometimes the craniosacral therapist will also manipulate the spine, though also very gently and not at all in the way a chiropractor performs spinal manipulation.

A craniosacral therapist is usually trained and licensed (in compliance with relevant state requirements) as a massage therapist or physical therapist, though some naturopathic physicians, chiropractors, and osteopathic physicians also have training in craniosacral techniques. As with all touch therapy, it is important to feel comfortable with, and trust, the practitioner. The manipulations of the body release stored physical and emotional energy that can result in unexpected surges of feelings and even discomfort. But nearly everyone feels deeply relaxed following a craniosacral massage.

See also CHIROPRACTIC; MASSAGE THERAPY; MIND–BODY INTERACTIONS; PHYSICAL THERAPY.

D–F

dehydroepiandrosterone (DHEA) A steroid HORMONE that occurs naturally in the body. It serves as a precursor primarily to estrogen in women and TESTOSTERONE in men, though women also convert small amounts to testosterone and men convert small amounts to estrogen. Levels of endogenous DHEA gradually diminish with aging. As a supplement, DHEA provides a similar source to the body for these hormones. DHEA is available without a doctor's prescription in the United States, marketed as a dietary supplement sold mostly in health food stores.

People take DHEA supplement for numerous and diverse uses such as to increase libido, reduce the effects of aging, boost immune function, prevent OSTEOPOROSIS, relieve symptoms associated with FIBROMYALGIA and SYSTEMIC LUPUS ERYTHEMATOSUS (SLE), and prevent degenerative diseases related to aging such as CARDIOVASCULAR DISEASE (CVD). There is scant clinical evidence to support any of these uses, and doctors worry that increasing the body's levels of sex hormones may increase the risk for hormone-driven BREAST CANCER and PROSTATE CANCER. There is some evidence that long-term DHEA use damages the LIVER.

Though DHEA is an over-the-counter dietary supplement in the United States, doctors encourage people to obtain blood tests to measure their levels of estrogen or testosterone before taking DHEA. The greatest risk for adverse health circumstances occurs when products such as DHEA increase estrogen or testosterone blood levels to higher than normal. Researchers believe this make increase the risk for some cancers, although again clinical evidence is lacking. Health experts recommend that people under age 50 do not take DHEA unless a doctor prescribes it to treat conditions in which endogenous DHEA levels are low.

DEHYDROEPIANDROSTERONE (DHEA)

Uses	Risks/Side Effects	Interactions
FIBROMYALGIA	acne flareups	none known
SYSTEMIC LUPUS ERYTHEMATOSUS (SLE)	mood swings	
	LIVER damage	
mental alertness in aging		
slow OSTEOPOROSIS		

See also ADRENAL INSUFFICIENCY; ANABOLIC STEROIDS AND STEROID PRECURSORS; HUMAN GROWTH HORMONE (HGH) SUPPLEMENT; MELATONIN.

dong quai An ancient remedy for relieving menstrual and menopausal discomforts. It contains phytoestrogens, which are estrogen-like chemicals that are much weaker than those the human body produces though are nonetheless capable of binding with estrogen receptors. Researchers do not know the extent to which dong quai's phytoestrogens have any effect in the body, however, because dong quai contains other active ingredients and often appears in combination with other herbs. Dong quai (*Angelica sinensis*) also contains coumarins, chemicals that cause smooth MUSCLE tissue to relax. This effect dilates blood vessels, increasing blood flow. It also acts to relax the UTERUS, which is also smooth muscle tissue. Many health experts believe coumarins are responsible for most of dong quai's effects. Dong quai is sold as an over-the-counter dietary supplement in the United States.

Dong quai also contains psoralens, chemicals that interact in the SKIN when exposed to sunlight. Psoralens intensify the effects of ultraviolet light with the result of unusually rapid and severe SUNBURN. Women should limit sun exposure when taking dong quai. Dong quai also may interact with NONSTEROIDAL ANTI-INFLAMMATORY DRUGS (NSAIDS), causing stomach upset, irritation, and bleeding. Because dong quai affects blood flow, it may also alter the intended effects of anticoagulant medications. And because of its actions to relax smooth muscle including the UTERUS, women should not take dong quai when they are pregnant.

DONG QUAI *(Angelica sinensis)*		
Uses	Risks/Side Effects	Interactions
menstrual cramps	excessive bleeding	anticoagulants
menopausal discomforts	stomach irritation	NSAIDs
ENDOMETRIOSIS		

See also BLACK COHOSH; DYSMENORRHEA; MENOPAUSE; MENSTRUATION; PREMENSTRUAL SYNDROME; SOY.

echinacea An herb with immune-supportive properties. Echinacea remedies incorporate stems, leaves, and seeds or their extracts from three of the nine species of echinacea (*Echinacea angustifolia, E. pallida, E. purpurea*). Though herbalists typically use certain of the species according to the desired immune effect, commercially produced echinacea products typically contain a mix. The most common use of echinacea is to lessen the severity of COLDS, INFLUENZA, and other upper respiratory infections. Echinacea seems most effective when taken at the first indication of symptoms and can shorten the length of illness by 20 to 60 percent.

Echinacea seems less effective in protecting against upper respiratory infections when taken as a general prophylactic measure, though regular use may prevent canker sores. Health experts caution people to take echinacea for no longer than three weeks to give their immune systems a break from the echinacea's stimulation and to wait one week before taking another course of echinacea. Some herbalists recommend using echinacea in rotation with other immune-boosting herbs. There is no clinical evidence to support a role for echinacea in preventing infections such as HIV/AIDS or HEPATITIS. Though echinacea may additionally support the IMMUNE SYSTEM when taken in conjunction with ANTIBIOTIC MEDICATIONS to treat bacterial infections, it cannot replace antibiotics.

Some studies have shown echinacea to have adverse effects in people who are IMMUNOCOMPROMISED, although this finding has been inconsistent. Doctors generally recommend against echinacea for people who have chronic immune system disorders such as RHEUMATOID ARTHRITIS, MULTIPLE SCLEROSIS, and SYSTEMIC LUPUS ERYTHEMATOSUS (SLE), because echinacea can overstimulate the immune system and make symptoms worse. Some people who have CHRONIC FATIGUE SYNDROME have experienced improvement with echinacea and other immune-enhancing herbs, however. People who have immune system disorders should discuss echinacea with their regular doctors before taking echinacea. Echinacea is available as a dietary supplement in the United States. People who are allergic to plants in the daisy (*Aster*) family may also be allergic to echinacea.

ECHINACEA *(E. angustifolia, E. pallida, E. purpurea)*		
Uses	Risks/Side Effects	Interactions
prevent COLDS and INFLUENZAnone	none known	none known
reduce cold/flu duration		
general IMMUNE SYSTEM support		

See also CANKER SORE; GOLDENSEAL; INFECTION.

feverfew An herb once popular for, as its name implies, lowering FEVER. However, current use focuses on its ability to prevent migraine headaches from developing and to minimize the symptoms of migraines when they do occur. The primary active ingredients researchers have isolated in feverfew (*Tanacetum parthenium*) are parthenolides, a group of mild prostaglandin suppressants. PROSTAGLANDINS are chemicals the body releases that are associated with PAIN. Aspirin and other NONSTEROIDAL ANTI-INFLAMMATORY DRUGS (NSAIDS) achieve much of their pain-relieving effects through prostaglandin suppression. Prostaglandins also are factors in the inflammatory processes associated with fever.

The form of feverfew that appears most effective in preventing migraine headaches is the freeze-dried herb. However, the level of parthenolides in feverfew plants varies widely. Capsules and tablets appear to have little or no effect for migraines, though may provide a level of relief for menstrual discomforts. Results become evident after taking feverfew for eight weeks or longer. Feverfew inhibits PLATELET AGGREGATION, slowing the initiation of COAGULATION (the formation of blood clots). People who take feverfew should let their surgeons know of this, if they are planning surgery, and stop taking the herb for the time period the surgeon recommends. People should not take feverfew with prescribed anticoagulant medications such as warfarin or enoxaparin.

FEVERFEW *(Tanacetum parthenium)*		
Uses	Risks/Side Effects	Interactions
migraine HEADACHE	excessive bleeding	anticoagulants
menstrual discomfort		aspirin, NSAIDs

See also ANALGESIC MEDICATIONS; BIOFEEDBACK; BIOFEEDBACK AND PAIN RELIEF.

flower essences Remedies that capture the energy and HEALING qualities of plants and flowers and impart them to alter emotional responses that might be causing physical disease. The most widely use flower essence formulas are the Bach flower essences, named for the Dr. Edward Bach, who developed and popularized flower essence therapy in the 1930s. Bach, a homeopathic physician, observed the correlations between emotion and physical illness. He surmised that plants and flowers could alter emotional responses, freeing the body to return to a state of health. In the tradition of HOMEOPATHY, Bach created mixtures that started with parts of plants in solutions of water and ALCOHOL. He repeatedly diluted the solutions until virtually no plant particle remained. The residual solution retained the energy of the flower, however, which could influence the emotions of people who used the solution.

No clinical studies support the effectiveness of flower essences, though people who use them typically report improvement in their symptoms. From the homeopathic perspective the flower essences influence health in the fashion of "like cures like," the underlying philosophy of homeopathy. From the conventional medicine perspective, flower essences may improve the emotional well-being of people who take them through the PLACEBO effect. Most health experts agree that with remedies, such as flower essences, that have no potential side effects, there is no harm in using the remedies. It is important to remember, however, that some emotional states may reflect potentially serious conditions such as GENERALIZED ANXIETY DISORDER (GAD) and DEPRESSION. There are conventional medicine therapies for these conditions that are likely to provide more rapid and effective intervention. Flower essences are widely used in an integrative manner in many European countries.

See also ANTIANXIETY MEDICATIONS; ANTIDEPRESSANT MEDICATIONS; AROMATHERAPY.

garlic In ancient times people used garlic to ward off the evil vapors and spirits they believed responsible for illness. In modern times doctors know more about what really causes many of the health circumstances that result in disease. People use garlic and garlic supplements to improve BLOOD circulation, lower BLOOD PRESSURE, and reduce blood cholesterol, the key factors that contribute to CARDIOVASCULAR DISEASE (CVD). The active ingredients in garlic (*Allium sativum*) are allium compounds (also found in onions and leeks), sulfur-based substances that give garlic its distinctive odor and flavor as well as its medicinal benefits.

More than 100 clinical research studies point to allium compounds as the substances responsible for these benefits. Allium compounds contain two dozen or so chemicals that

- reduce PLATELET AGGREGATION, making it more difficult for the blood cells that initiate the clotting process to stick together
- help maintain the FLEXIBILITY of ARTERY walls
- may block cholesterol production in the LIVER, reducing the blood levels in particular of the low density lipoprotein (LDL) and very low density lipoprotein (VLDL) cholesterols associated with ATHEROSCLEROSIS and CORONARY ARTERY DISEASE (CAD)
- have mild anti-inflammatory effects, helping reduce irritation and INFLAMMATION of the inner walls of the arteries that researchers believe sets the stage for arterial plaque accumulations that form the basis of atherosclerosis and CAD
- have mild antibacterial effects that improve resistance to infections affecting the MOUTH and THROAT

These effects seem the same whether the source of the garlic is the natural bulb or supplements. Some studies show as much as a 6 to 10 milligram per deciliter (mg/dL) reduction in total blood cholesterol levels after taking garlic supplements for three months, about the same result doctors expect to see with lipid-lowering medication therapy. The combined effect of garlic's actions on the cardiovascular system help lower blood pressure by decreasing the resistance blood encounters as it flows through the arteries. Though the preventive benefit for HEART ATTACK and STROKE is difficult to measure, many health experts agree that the many effects of garlic, however small, add up to reduced risk for cardiovascular disease, especially in combination with other lifestyle factors such as regular daily exercise, weight loss, and SMOKING CESSATION. Some health experts believe garlic and garlic supplements also lower the risk for DIABETES type 2 by improving INSULIN sensitivity, though clinical studies so far have failed to bear this out. Nor is there much evidence supporting garlic's ability to reduce CANCER risk.

Garlic and garlic supplements are relatively safe for most people to take, though may intensify the effect of many common antihypertensive medications. People who are taking medications to treat high blood pressure should first talk with their doctors before beginning a garlic regimen. The amounts of garlic a person might use in seasoning foods are not enough to cause this interference, though the amounts of garlic in therapeutic products can interact with numerous medications. Because garlic affects clotting, surgeons generally request people stop taking it before any scheduled operations.

GARLIC (Allium sativum)

Uses	Risks/Side Effects	Interactions
lower blood cholesterol	gastrointestinal upset strong body and	antihypertensives
lower risk for ATHEROSCLEROSIS	breath odor excessive bleeding	
reduce BLOOD PRESSURE	with surgery	

See also ANTICOAGULATION THERAPY; COAGULATION; INFECTION; LIFESTYLE AND CARDIOVASCULAR HEALTH.

ginger An herb that soothes gastrointestinal upset. More likely to be in the kitchen spice cabinet than the medicine cabinet, ginger (*Zingiber officinale*) is one of the most popular spices. Herbalists and cooks alike use the gnarly root fresh or dried, sliced or powdered, in natural form or prepared as an extract. TRADITIONAL CHINESE MEDICINE (TCM) considers ginger a hot, yang energy that brings warmth to the HEART, LUNGS, and especially the STOMACH to improve their functions. Folk medicine advises pregnant women to suck on thin slices of fresh gingerroot to alleviate symptoms of MORNING SICKNESS. A popular home remedy for stomach upset is sipping on a flat gingerale. Ginger also contains substances that act as mild antihistamines, helping relieve allergy symptoms such as ALLERGIC RHINITIS.

Clinical research studies provide supporting evidence of ginger's abilities to relieve

- NAUSEA, particularly that related to PREGNANCY (morning sickness), motion sickness, and CHEMOTHERAPY

- nausea and VOMITING due to gastrointestinal viruses

- dizziness related to motion sickness

- digestive upset, particularly FLATULENCE (intestinal gas)

- congestion due to COLDS, INFLUENZA, and seasonal allergies

Though some people experience mild gastric irritation when taking ginger supplements or drinking ginger tea, ginger causes very few side effects and health experts consider it safe for nearly everyone to take. Ginger may affect

PLATELET AGGREGATION, and thus BLOOD clotting (COAGULATION), in some people so surgeons generally ask people to stop taking ginger a few days before any planned surgery.

GINGER (Zingiber officinale)

Uses	Risks/Side Effects	Interactions
general NAUSEA	excessive bleeding	anticoagulants
MORNING SICKNESS		ASPIRIN THERAPY
motion sickness		
nausea of CHEMOTHERAPY		
digestive upset		

See also ANTIEMETIC MEDICATIONS; ANTIHISTAMINE MEDICATIONS; HISTAMINE.

ginkgo biloba An herbal product with many uses. The ginkgo biloba tree is the oldest living species of tree on Earth, believed to have first appeared more than 200 million years ago in the area that is now China. Individual trees typically live hundreds of years, with some documented to be nearly 1,000 years old, and now grow in many parts of the world. Herbal remedies made from the leaves and seeds of this ancient tree have been popular for centuries for increasing longevity and improving mental focus. It contains numerous antioxidants (notably quercetin), collectively identified as ginkgo biloba extract (GBE) on supplement product labels. In the United States ginkgo biloba is a dietary supplement available without a doctor's prescription.

Clinical research studies conducted in the 1990s and early 2000s demonstrated ginkgo's ability to improve BLOOD circulation in the BRAIN and the smallest of arteries, the arterioles, throughout the body. Studies among people with ALZHEIMER'S DISEASE and other forms of DEMENTIA (diminished thought capacity and memory) showed significant improvement after taking ginkgo biloba supplements for eight weeks or longer, especially in combination with *Panax* GINSENG. Many people of all ages who take ginkgo biloba do so for these cerebrovascular benefits. The effect seems to arise from ginkgo's mild anticoagulant action in combination with its ANTIOXIDANT activity. Ginkgo's ability to open up peripheral circulation also improves conditions such as PERIPHERAL VASCULAR DISEASE (PVD), NEUROPATHY of DIABETES, and ERECTILE DYS-

FUNCTION related to ATHEROSCLEROSIS (as is most erectile dysfunction in men age 60 and older). There is also likely a preventive effect against embolytic STROKE and HEART ATTACK.

For most people, health experts consider ginkgo biloba safe at recommended doses. Because ginkgo biloba affects blood clotting, people who are having surgery should let their surgeons and anesthesiologists know they are taking it. The doctor may ask the person to stop taking the supplement for a week or two before the surgery and for a period of time after the surgery, until HEALING is adequate to end the risk for postoperative bleeding. People who take ANTICOAGULANT THERAPY (including ASPIRIN THERAPY) should talk with their doctors before taking ginkgo, as it may intensify the anticlotting effect. Gingko biloba also affects INSULIN production and sensitivity, which may improve prediabetes and noninsulin-dependent type 2 diabetes though can interfere with ANTIDIABETES MEDICATIONS and INSULIN THERAPY in people who have insulin-dependent diabetes (type 1 or type 2).

GINKGO BILOBA		
Uses	**Risks/Side Effects**	**Interactions**
RAYNAUD'S SYNDROME	excessive bleeding	anticoagulants
	elevated BLOOD PRESSURE	antihypertensives
INTERMITTENT CLAUDICATION		thiazide diuretics
		trazodone
PERIPHERAL VASCULAR DISEASE (PVD)		prochlorperazine
		ASPIRIN THERAPY
ATHEROSCLEROSIS		
CORONARY ARTERY DISEASE (CAD)		
ALZHEIMER'S DISEASE		

See also ANTI-AGING APPROACHES; ARTERY; INSULIN RESISTANCE; LIFESTYLE AND HEALTH.

ginseng A botanical product prepared from the root of the ginseng plant. There are two major varieties of ginseng, Asian ginseng (*Panax ginseng*) and American ginseng (*Panax quinquefolius*). As well, there are dozens of subvarieties within each. Asian ginseng, also called Chinese or Korean ginseng, is indigenous to the Asian continent. American ginseng, also called North American ginseng, grows naturally on the North American continent. The designation "*Panax* ginseng" refers to the major varieties and their subvarieties collectively; "*Panax ginseng*" with both words italicized refers to Asian ginseng. The herb commonly called Siberian ginseng (*Eleutherococcus senticosus* or *Acanthopanax senticosus*) is not true ginseng but rather a "look-alike" botanical cousin that has a different chemical composition and different effects as an herbal remedy. Ginseng is sold as a dietary supplement in the United States and available in various forms without a doctor's prescription.

Panax Ginseng

The varieties of *Panax* ginseng include differing amounts of three major kinds of chemicals

- ginsenosides, which function as mild stimulants to sharpen mental focus and possibly improve cognitive function and memory

- panaxans, which may improve INSULIN sensitivity

- polysaccharides, complex sugar molecules that aid IMMUNE SYSTEM functions

PANAX GINSENG		
Uses	**Risks/Side Effects**	**Interactions**
mental clarity and focus	insomnia	loop diuretics
	excitability	CAFFEINE
memory improvement		
IMMUNE SYSTEM support		
aphrodisiac		
INSULIN RESISTANCE		
type 2 DIABETES		

The color of ginseng, red or white, reflects the kind of processing method used in its preparation. Medicinal preparations use only the ginseng root. Red ginseng is steam processed, which preserves more of the natural ginsenosides. White ginseng is sun dried. Herbalists consider red ginseng more potent than white ginseng. Most people take ginseng for improved mental alertness, and for its IMMUNE RESPONSE properties. Ginseng also has gained popularity as an aphrodisiac, likely as a result of its mild STIMULANT effect. Some research studies support the claimed benefits of sharpened mental focus and improved cognitive function, especially when taken in combination with GINKGO

BILOBA, though any effects on LIBIDO beyond heightened alertness remain unclear. A number of energy drinks and similar products contain ginseng, though not in amounts likely to produce any effects.

Acanthopanax (Siberian Ginseng)

Herbalists call this ginseng cousin by the common name Acanthopanax. The plants of Acanthopanax look similar to true ginseng and are indigenous to northern China and the region of southern Russia once called Siberia, hence the misnomer Siberian ginseng. However, Acanthopanax contains eleutherosides, which have strong STIMULANT characteristics, rather than ginsenosides. Both eleutherosides and ginsenosides belong to the same chemical family, saponins, which have a range of actions including CENTRAL NERVOUS SYSTEM stimulation, antibiotic properties, and immune response. Asparagus root, onion, and GARLIC also contain saponins. The stimulant effect of Acanthopanax is strong enough that this ginseng relative is on the list of banned substances for Olympic athletes. Herbalists value Acanthopanax as a tonic (preparation that increases STRENGTH and ENDURANCE) rather than a medicinal herb.

People who have HYPERTENSION (high BLOOD PRESSURE) and women who are pregnant should not take Acanthopanax. Women should temporarily stop taking Acanthopanax during their menstrual periods as it may cause excessive bleeding. Most herbalists recommend taking Acanthopanax no longer than 90 days, then taking a three- to six-week break before taking it again.

ACANTHOPANAX GINSENG		
Uses	**Risks/Side Effects**	**Interactions**
alertness	elevated BLOOD	antihypertensive
athletic	PRESSURE	medications
enhancement	excitability,	furosemide (Lasix)
	irritability	
	insomnia	
	excessive menstrual	
	bleeding	

See also TRADITIONAL CHINESE MEDICINE (TCM).

glucosamine A GLUCOSE compound the body uses to produce the chemical substances it needs to repair and maintain JOINT CARTILAGE, ligaments, and tendons. In health, the body generates sufficient quantities of endogenous glucosamine through a complex series of metabolic interactions. When damage through wear and tear occurs to the joints, the body may have difficulty keeping pace with its glucosamine needs. The older the person, the more quickly the body reaches the point at which it cannot produce enough glucosamine to produce the substances to repair joint tissues. The result is OSTEOARTHRITIS—INFLAMMATION and degeneration of the cartilage and related tissues in the joint.

Doctors in Europe and numerous countries around the world prescribe glucosamine supplementation to replenish the body's supply and allow the natural HEALING processes to take place. Veterinarians in the United States similarly use glucosamine to treat osteoarthritis in domestic pets as well as large animals such as horses. However, doctors in the United States do not often consider glucosamine as a possible treatment for osteoarthritis, in part because NONSTEROIDAL ANTI-INFLAMMATORY DRUGS (NSAIDS), which became popular in the late 1970s and early 1980s, are so effective at controlling both the PAIN and the inflammation characteristic of osteoarthritis and in part because there were few clinical research studies to support glucosamine's effectiveness.

Clinical studies in the 1980s and 1990s began to show objective evidence that glucosamine supplements (exogenous glucosamine) seemed able to at least partially restore the body's ability to heal osteoarthritis damage, and some doctors started recommending it for people who could not tolerate the gastrointestinal irritation of NSAIDs. About half of the people in the studies experienced moderate to significant relieve from pain, stiffness, and limited range of motion in arthritic knees and hips. The effect seems even more profound when taking glucosamine in combination with CHONDROITIN, another glucose-based structure (called a complex polysaccharide).

However, researchers continue to debate whether glucosamine taken as a supplement has the same action in the body as endogenous glucosamine. So far clinical research studies have failed to reveal the actions of exogenous glucosamine once it enters the body. Because glucosamine is a dietary supplement in the United States, it is available without a doctor's prescription, so people who have osteoarthritis can sidestep the controversy and take the substance if they choose. Glucosamine seems to have little effect on RHEUMATOID ARTHRITIS, an autoimmune disorder that not only destroys but also deforms the joints.

Glucosamine partially blocks the absorption of many diuretic medications such as furosemide (Lasix) and the thiazides. Though people can take both products at the same time, doctors may increase the diuretic DOSE for as long as the person is also taking glucosamine. Among the minor side effects are NAUSEA and gastrointestinal upset.

GLUCOSAMINE		
Uses	Risks/Side Effects	Interactions
OSTEOARTHRITIS	gastrointestinal upset	loop diuretics
chronic BACK PAIN		

See also AUTOIMMUNE DISORDERS; LIGAMENT; SAMe; TENDON.

goldenseal An herb (*Hydrastis canadensis*) with anti-inflammatory and possibly anti-INFECTION properties. Indigenous to the North American continent (and in particular to the Pacific Northwest), goldenseal is a mainstay of NATIVE AMERICAN HEALING. Early tribes ground the roots into a mushy paste to use as a poultice to treat insect bites, LACERATIONS, and rashes. They also brewed the roots into tea, which though bitter to the taste was an effective remedy for digestive upset. Today products containing goldenseal extract come in topical, oral, and dried forms.

Researchers have isolated goldenseal's active ingredients as berberine and hydrastine, substances that now manufacturers extract and produce as prescription medications for use as in a number of European countries. Berberine in particular has strong antibiotic action and acts to stimulate IMMUNE RESPONSE in the body. Goldenseal taken in combination with ECHINACEA, another herb that boosts immune function, appears to increase resistance to many infections from COLDS and INFLUENZA to HEPATITIS.

Goldenseal is often an ingredient in herbal preparations to relieve the adverse effects of CHEMOTHERAPY and to support the IMMUNE SYSTEM in

fighting the cancer. As with other immunosupportive therapies, health experts recommend using goldenseal for no longer than three weeks consecutively, with two to four weeks between treatments. This allows the immune system to rest and restore itself. There are no known side effects or interactions with goldenseal.

GOLDENSEAL (*Hydrastis canadensis*)		
Uses	Risks/Side Effects	Interactions
topical and systemic antibioticnone	none known	none known
stimulate IMMUNE RESPONSE		
soothe digestive upset		
calm and help heal canker sores		
increase resistance to urinary tract infections		

See also CANKER SORE; GASTROENTERITIS; GREEN TEA; RASH; SAMe; URINARY TRACT INFECTION (UTI).

green tea The unfermented, dried leaves of the tea plant (*Camellia sinensis*), brewed into a drink. Black tea and green tea come from the same plant. The difference between them is that processing and drying of green tea leaves takes place immediately after harvesting them and black tea leaves undergo a processing that includes fermentation before drying. Though both kinds of tea leaves contain the same chemical compounds, green tea contains them in far greater concentrations. Green tea is also available in the United States as a dietary supplement, packaged in capsules or as tablets that contain the dried leaves ground into powder. Green tea contains a number of antioxidants, called polyphenol catechins. They include gallocatechin (GC), epigallocatechin (EGC), epicatechin (EC), and the especially potent epigallocatechin gallate (EGCG). Red grapes and red wine also contain high amounts of these catechins.

EGCG appears to interfere with enzyme processes necessary to allow healthy cells to mutate into cancerous cells, thus thwarting the development of CANCER. It also seems to initiate apoptosis, a sequence of natural events leading to cell death, in cancer cells that are already present. In addition to its cancer-fighting actions, EGCG has the ability to kill certain BACTERIA including *Helicobacter pylori*, the bacteria responsible for much PEPTIC ULCER DISEASE, and *Escherichia coli*, the bacteria that causes serious GASTROENTERITIS. Researchers continue to study all of these actions to further understand how they occur and what they might bode for cancer prevention efforts.

The other catechins have ANTIOXIDANT actions that appear to help the body resist changes in the cells of the ARTERY walls that allow ATHEROSCLEROSIS to establish itself. Other ingredients in green tea include tannins, which act to soothe mild to moderate digestive upset, and fluoride, which strengthens the TEETH. Green tea and green tea extract products naturally contain CAFFEINE. Green tea also contains theanine, a substance with anti-anxiety effects that somewhat counter the effect of the caffeine. Though there are no known health risks or interactions with green tea, people who ingest high quantities may experience sleep disturbances and irritability as a consequence of too much caffeine. Because of green tea's caffeine content, health experts recommend pregnant and nursing mothers limit consumption.

GREEN TEA *(Camellia sinensis)*		
Uses	**Risks/Side Effects**	**Interactions**
prevent development of cancer	excessive CAFFEINE consumption	none known
prevent spread of cancer		
eliminate existing cancer cells		
soothe digestive upset		
decrease low-density lipoprotein cholesterol (LDL-C)		
improve circulation		
strengthen the TEETH		
fight bacterial MOUTH infections		

See also COENZYME Q10.

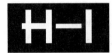

homeopathy A system of medicine based on the philosophy that symptoms represent the body's efforts to heal. Homeopathic treatment attempts to further stimulate those efforts through the premise that "like cures like," as homeopathy founder Samuel Hahnemann expressed it. Treatment employs homeopathic remedies that are extremely diluted solutions of substances such as herbs, plants, and minerals; some may contain chemicals and even toxins. In the United States, the US Food and Drug Administration (FDA) regulates homeopathic remedies. Manufacturers must comply with the standards and procedures of the *Homeopathic Pharmacopoeia of the United States*.

Homeopathic Diagnosis and Remedies

The homeopathic practitioner makes a diagnosis of symptoms rather than disease. He or she does so by listening to what the person describes and conducts an examination appropriate for the practitioner's scope of practice. The practitioner then prescribes homeopathic remedies that support the symptoms to help the body use those symptoms to rid itself of whatever ailment is present. The premise is that the body uses its own resources and energy to heal itself. There are more than 3,000 homeopathic remedies, each of which applies to a certain symptom or constitution. A person takes the remedies that apply to his or her circumstances, making homeopathic treatment entirely individualized.

The essential principle of homeopathic remedy preparation is that the vigorous shaking, called succession, that follows each step of dilution intensifies the potency of the solution by dispersing the energy of its molecules into the molecules of the water and ALCOHOL in the solution. Even when the solution has become so dilute that there

are no detectable molecules of the original ingredient remaining, homeopathy asserts the remedy still holds the "molecular memory" of the active ingredient. The concentrations of homeopathic remedies reflect sequential dilutions. Mixing the solution with powdered lactose creates product forms other than liquids.

HOMEOPATHIC REMEDY DILUTIONS		
Dilution	**Sequential Ratios**	**Designation**
decimal	1:10	C (1C, 2C, 3C, etc.)
centesimal	1:100	X (1X, 2X, 3X, etc.)
millesimal	1:1000	M (1M, 2M, 3M, etc.)

Homeopathic remedies carry the Latin names of their original ingredients, along with the designations for their dilutions. Many also include common names as well. The higher the dilution ratio, the more dilute the remedy. Homeopathic remedies come in tablets, granules, liquids, ointments, creams, and suppositories.

Homeopathic Practitioners

Homeopathy originated in Europe in the 1700s with the work of Samuel Hahnemann, a German chemist. Hahnemann embarked on a quest to find better ways to treat illness than the harsh and often damaging methods, such as bloodletting (the practice of bleeding a person who was ill to rid the body of toxins), popular at the time. His approach was, for its time, highly scientific and the mildness of homeopathic remedies quickly acquired a loyal following. A Boston physician, Hans Burch Gram, studied homeopathy in Europe and opened a homeopathic practice when he returned to the United States in 1825. The philosophy gained popularity over the ensuing decades, peaking at the start of the 20th century with two dozen colleges of homeopathy and over 100 homeopathic hospitals throughout the United States. Scientific discoveries in bacteriology and disease processes that accompanied the turn of the century marked a turning point in the practice of medicine, however, and homeopathy soon went the way of bloodletting.

In the United States today practitioners of homeopathy typically learn the philosophy and methods through graduate classes during the course of their conventional education or through supplemental courses and programs they enroll in after completing their conventional education (though homeopathy is part of the regular curriculum for NATUROPATHY). However, because federal guidelines classify most homeopathic remedies as OVER-THE-COUNTER (OTC) DRUGS, they are available for anyone to purchase and use. Some remedies do contain ingredients that require a medical doctor's prescription. Surveys show that most of the 6 million Americans who use homeopathic remedies treat themselves without consulting a health-care practitioner.

Each state regulates the practice of homeopathy. In most states physicians (MD and DO), chiropractors (DC), naturopathic physicians (ND), and dentists (DDS and DMD) can make homeopathic diagnoses and prescribe homeopathic remedies. A few states have specific licensing requirements for MDs and DOs who also practice homeopathy. In Europe homeopathy remains a distinct discipline in health care, and homeopathic physicians receive specific training and credentialing.

Benefits and Risks of Homeopathy

Homeopathic remedies are so dilute, some as much as one part per million, that by conventional clinical standards they do not contain active ingredients. Because of this, they do not interact with other medications or cause side effects. Aside from the risks of improper manufacturing and potential contamination, health experts generally regard homeopathic remedies as safe, though some remedies contain significant quantities of alcohol. FDA regulations require homeopathic remedy labels to list the ingredients as well as the instructions for use (including conditions the remedy treats).

Health experts caution people to seek conventional medical care for symptoms that do not improve after five to seven days of treatment with homeopathic remedies, the same caution they extend for self-treatment with any over-the-counter product. Clinical studies of homeopathic remedies have produced mixed results, with some studies showing no greater effect than PLACEBO (an inactive substance) and others showing measurable improvement beyond placebo effect.

See also AROMATHERAPY; FLOWER ESSENCES.

human growth hormone (hGH) supplement A controversial anti-aging approach of injecting synthetic hGH to raise the body's natural levels of this HORMONE, known as growth hormone (GH) in its endogenous form (the form the body naturally produces). The PITUITARY GLAND produces endogenous GH. GH levels are highest in childhood and ADOLESCENCE, when the body is growing. GH stimulates this growth through various biochemical actions. GH levels stay fairly high through early to middle adulthood, during which time GH shifts its role to maintaining MUSCLE mass, BONE density, and cardiac STRENGTH (the HEART's ability to pump forcefully and efficiently). By about age 50, the pituitary gland produces less GH and levels in the bloodstream begin to decline. The characteristic physical changes of aging, such as increased body fat and decreased muscle mass, begin to manifest. OBESITY also slows hGH release.

Some children have deficiencies of GH, usually due to a tumor, endocrine disorder, or other dysfunction of the pituitary gland. GH deficiency in childhood and adolescence causes stunted growth and blocks many of the body's normal maturation processes. Some adults also have GH deficiencies; hGH supplementation similarly restores body levels to those needed for healthy muscles, bones, and cardiac function. Doctors have prescribed hGH supplementation to treat such deficiencies since the 1970s.

Many people who support hGH supplementation as an anti-aging measure point to the success of such treatments as evidence that hGH is safe. Some doctors agree that there is no difference between therapeutic hGH given to adults whose GH levels fall before age-related declines naturally take place; symptoms and response are the same. Other doctors question the therapeutic value of giving hGH to counter a process that seems purely the result of the aging process rather than of a disease process. Proponents of hGH supplementation counter that reversing some of the effects of aging prevents age-related diseases, such as ATHEROSCLEROSIS and OSTEOARTHRITIS, from developing. This, they argue, is clearly a therapeutic effect. Those who question the safety of hGH supplementation note that researchers do not know the functions of GH in adults, or how GH influences factors such as body fat distribution and muscle mass. They further observe that though muscle mass increases with hGH supplementation in adults, muscle strength does not, raising more questions about the role of GH in the adult body. The debate touches on a number of key ethical issues that are not easy to resolve.

At present the US Food and Drug Administration (FDA) approves hGH supplementation only for people who have clinical GH deficiencies—that is, GH deficiencies resulting from pituitary dysfunction rather than aging. hGH supplement is available only with a doctor's prescription. Treatment with hGH supplement can cause HYPERTENSION, edema (fluid retention), and HEART FAILURE, and hGH supplement may interact with other hormone supplements such as thyroid and hydrocortisone. A rare but serious complication arising from too much GH is ACROMEGALY, in which the bones of the jaw, hands, and feet grow disproportionately large. Though the excessive growth stops when GH levels drop, changes that have already occurred are permanent.

HUMAN GROWTH HORMONE (HGH) SUPPLEMENT		
Uses	Risks/Side Effects	Interactions
increase MUSCLE mass	ACROMEGALY edema	CORTISOL, hydrocortisone
decrease body fat	HEART FAILURE	thyroid supplement
improve cardiovascular function		
prevent OSTEOPOROSIS		

See also ANTI-AGING APPROACHES; HORMONE THERAPY; POLYGLANDULAR DEFICIENCY SYNDROME.

hypnosis A method of induced deep relaxation, sometimes perceived as an altered state of CONSCIOUSNESS, in which a person often is more responsive to suggestion than during normal consciousness. Studies show changes in the patterns of electrical activity in the BRAIN when a person is under hypnosis, suggesting some parts of the brain become more active and others less active. Many people are able to recall details when hypnotized that they cannot otherwise remember. Though a person may not be able to recall a suggestion the hypnotherapist gives during hypnosis, he or she may act on the suggestion during full consciousness, often without full awareness.

FACTS ABOUT HYPNOSIS

- A person retains full control of his or her thoughts, emotions, and actions when under hypnosis.
- Hypnosis is fully voluntary. A person cannot be hypnotized against his or her will or without knowledge and participation.
- A person will not say or do anything, under hypnosis or as the result of hypnotic suggestion, that violates his or her values and sense of what is right and wrong.
- Some people do not respond to hypnosis or hypnotherapeutic suggestions, regardless of their willingness to do so.
- Most people fully remember everything that occurs under hypnosis.

Hypnotherapy may help people who are trying to make lifestyle changes such as in EATING HABITS or SMOKING CESSATION. It is also a clinically accepted method for managing chronic PAIN and stress. Sometimes people use hypnosis to help them visualize a state of health they desire to achieve, with the residual effect supporting them while they work toward their health goals. Such goals may include restoration of function after serious injury, weight loss, fitness level, and even REMISSION from CANCER. Hypnosis should always be an adjunct, not a primary, treatment; it accompanies and supports other therapies and treatments.

A typical hypnotherapy session takes place in a professional setting and may last 30 to 45 minutes. A person should emerge from hypnosis feeling refreshed and invigorated, fully capable of returning to the day's regular activities. Some circumstances may need several hypnotherapy sessions, though many require only a session or two. In addition to performing hypnosis, a hypnotherapist can teach self-hypnosis. Self-hypnosis may be helpful for reinforcing suggestions the hypnotherapist provides during a hypnotherapy session. Self-hypnosis is also an effective stress relief method, particularly for people who have chronic health conditions that cause discomfort or pain. Often the hypnotherapist will make a recording of the first session for the person to replay at home.

A person who practices hypnosis may be a doctor, nurse, psychologist, psychotherapist, dentist, naturopathic physician, or certified hypnotist. Most states do not regulate hypnotherapy, so it is important to fully understand the hypnotherapist's education, credentials, and experience even when the hypnotherapist is a certified or licensed health practitioner. It is important to feel a high level of trust in the hypnotherapist. Hypnosis itself is generally a safe practice, though it can allow people to recall circumstances that are emotionally painful. Once those emotions surface, the person may need professional guidance to address them.

See also BIOFEEDBACK; MIND–BODY INTERACTIONS.

integrative medicine An approach to the practice of medicine that uses conventional and complementary therapies in conjunction with one another. In the United States integrative medicine typically refers to physicians (MDs and DOs) who practice conventional medicine that incorporates complementary therapies, such as ACUPUNCTURE and herbal remedies, or who work in close association with complementary practitioners such as massage therapists and chiropractors.

Doctors in the United States who practice integrative medicine typically use complementary methods that clinical studies have shown to provide therapeutic benefit or at the least have not shown to cause harm. Hospitals often use integrative methods such as MEDITATION and VISUALIZATION with people who are undergoing major surgery or CANCER treatment. The ORNISH PROGRAM for CARDIO-VASCULAR DISEASE (CVD) presents an integrative approach that has obtained Medicare approval, a step that speaks to the effectiveness and acceptability of its methods.

See also HOMEOPATHY; MEDICINAL HERBS AND BOTANICALS; NATUROPATHY; TRADITIONAL CHINESE MEDICINE (TCM).

L

labyrinth A spirituality-based approach that features a geometric, symmetrical pattern that a person walks in prayer, MEDITATION, VISUALIZATION, or quiet contemplation. Many hospitals have labyrinths, which may be small or large, indoors or outdoors, permanent or temporary. The tradition of the labyrinth dates to medieval times and has integrated with a number of religious and spiritual practices through the centuries. The winding, convoluted path of the labyrinth physically and symbolically draws the person into the center. Once at the center, the person turns and follows the path back out. Many people experience profound calm and inner peace as they complete their labyrinth journeys. People who have chronic or terminal conditions often find the labyrinth gives them respite from their symptoms while within the labyrinth and often for hours to days afterward.

See also NATIVE AMERICAN HEALING; PRAYER AND SPIRITUALITY; REIKI; TRADITIONAL CHINESE MEDICINE (TCM).

lutein An ANTIOXIDANT belonging to the carotenoid family. Lutein, along with another carotenoid, ZEAXANTHIN, helps protect against AGE-RELATED MACULAR DEGENERATION (ARMD) and other retinal disorders. ARMD is the leading cause of progressive vision loss among adults. Some studies suggest lutein may also help lower the risk for LUNG CANCER. Ophthalmologists often recommend lutein in combination with ZEAXANTHIN, an antioxidant that occurs in many of the same foods as lutein, for people in middle age and older. There is limited evidence that lutein and other carotenoids may also help prevent cataracts from forming.

Lutein occurs naturally in the dark yellow pigments found in red bell peppers, pumpkin, and in dark green vegetables such as spinach and broccoli. It is also available as a dietary supplement, usually in combination with other carotenoids. Too much lutein or other carotenoids, which typically occurs only when taking high doses of carotenoid supplements, can cause the palms of the hands and soles of the feet to turn orange or dark yellow. This is a temporary effect that goes away when the amount of consumed carotenoids decreases. Penicillin-based ANTIBIOTIC MEDICATIONS may decrease lutein absorption.

LUTEIN		
Uses	Risks/Side Effects	Interactions
prevent cataracts	excessive amounts may turn the palms and	none known
reserve macular function	soles of the feet orange or dark yellow	
possibly protect against LUNG CANCER		

See also BILBERRY; CATARACT; CATARACT EXTRACTION AND LENS REPLACEMENT; LYCOPENE; RETINOPATHY; VITAMIN AND MINERAL THERAPY.

lycopene An ANTIOXIDANT that is one of the carotenoids. Lycopene emerged in the 1990s as an adjunct (secondary) therapy for PROSTATE CANCER because of its ability to slow the growth of prostate CANCER cells. It may also help to slow the growth of cancer cells in other locations, notably the LUNG and LIVER. In combination with LUTEIN and ZEAXANTHIN (other carotenoids), lycopene helps protect the RETINA and vision.

Lycopene occurs naturally in fruits and vegetables that have red flesh, such as tomatoes, guava, and watermelon. The highest levels of lycopene occur in cooked tomatoes and tomato products such as tomato soup, tomato sauce, and ketchup. Most studies investigating the effects of lycopene involved consuming high amounts of foods containing lycopene, notably cooked tomato products. The findings seem to substantiate lycopene's role in inhibiting the growth of cancer cells, particularly prostate cancer cells. However, few research studies have evaluated lycopene supplements. Because tomatoes contain numerous nutrients, it is difficult to assess the effects of only one.

Most doctors agree that while there is likely little harm to come of taking lycopene supplements, there is not enough evidence to recommend doing so except as an adjunctive therapy (in addition to other therapeutic approaches). Men who have prostate disease or PROSTATE CANCER may benefit from increasing their consumption of foods containing cooked tomatoes. Excessive ingestion of lycopene and other carotenoids can cause the palms of the hands and the soles of the feet to turn dark yellow or orange, a temporary circum-

stance that returns to normal when carotenoid levels drop after stopping or reducing the supplement. There are no other known risks or side effects when using lycopene, though taking penicillin-based ANTIBIOTIC MEDICATIONS may decrease the amount of lycopene absorbed into the bloodstream from the gastrointestinal tract.

LYCOPENE		
Uses	**Risks/Side Effects**	**Interactions**
prevent or slow PROSTATE CANCER	excessive amounts may turn the palms and	none known
possibly protect against LUNG CANCER	soles of the feet orange or dark yellow	
preserve retinal function		

See also AGE-RELATED MACULAR DEGENERATION (ARMD); BILBERRY; CATARACT EXTRACTION AND REPLACEMENT; RETINOPATHY; SAW PALMETTO; VISION IMPAIRMENT; YOHIMBE/YOHIMBINE.

magnet therapy The use of static magnets to create magnetic energy fields, which are alignments of the atoms within them. The most common use of magnet therapy is to treat chronic PAIN such as from OSTEOARTHRITIS, RHEUMATOID ARTHRITIS, FIBROMYALGIA, and CARPAL TUNNEL SYNDROME.

People who have implanted medical devices such as pacemakers, defibrillators, and INSULIN pumps should not use therapeutic magnets because they may interfere with the electrical functions of the devices.

Therapeutic magnets come in many strengths and configurations, from adhesive-backed strips to items of jewelry such as necklaces and bracelets to magnets designed for placement under the mattress. The only aspects of magnet therapy that fall within regulatory reach are labeling and marketing. Because there are no clinical studies to support the therapeutic qualities of static magnets, the US Food and Drug Administration (FDA) prohibits therapeutic magnet manufacturers from claiming health benefits from their products. Magnet STRENGTH varies widely among manufacturers and products, and often varies from the stated strength on the product packaging.

MAGNETIC ENERGY MEASURES

Earth's magnetic field	0.5 gauss
refrigerator magnets	35 to 200 gauss
therapeutic magnets	300 to 5,000 gauss
MAGNETIC RESONANCE IMAGING (MRI) magnet	200,000 gauss

Source: National Center for Complementary and Alternative Medicine (NCCAM)

The earliest documented use of magnets for HEALING comes from medieval times, when surgeons used lodestones and magnets made from them to locate and remove iron fragments and arrowheads from soldiers on the battlefield. With understanding of the body's functions in health or disease considerably limited until the start of the twentieth century, magnets remained among the most popular tools in the doctor's medicine bag.

Though several theories for how magnets may exert therapeutic influence seem plausible, particularly because neurologic and other cellular functions generate electromagnetic fields. so far clinical studies have not produced findings that support them. A number of studies have shown therapeutic benefit with pulsed electromagnetic therapy, in which a rapidly pulsating electrical current creates a temporary, powerful magnetic field. Only health-care professionals may use electromagnetic therapeutic devices under current regulations in the United States.

Most health experts believe static magnets have very limited therapeutic effect though are not likely to cause harm in most people. Pregnant women (because effects of magnetic energy fields on a developing fetus remain unknown) and people who have implanted electronic devices (because the magnet may interfere with the device's electromagnetic field) should not use magnet therapy. Magnets cannot treat or cure diseases such as CANCER, DIABETES, and CARDIOVASCULAR DISEASE (CVD), though some disreputable vendors may represent them as being able to do so. A doctor should evaluate any condition that does not improve within 7 to 10 days.

See also ALTERNATIVE METHODS FOR PAIN RELIEF; BIOFEEDBACK FOR PAIN RELIEF; TRANSCUTANEOUS ELECTRICAL NERVE STIMULATION (TENS).

massage therapy   A touch therapy, also called therapeutic massage or bodywork, that acts on the body as well as the mind and the emotions. About 25 percent of people who seek massage therapy do so to relieve PAIN and stiffness related to musculoskeletal injuries, and a third are interested in stress relief. There are dozens of therapeutic massage techniques and methods, though all share the common intent of stimulating the flow of BLOOD through the muscles and soft tissues to cleanse metabolic toxins, tone MUSCLE tissues, and release tension.

Though a doctor may recommend massage therapy in conjunction with PHYSICAL THERAPY, the two have distinctly different approaches. Physical therapy is fix-oriented: there is a problem and massage can help make it better. Therapeutic massage in the context of physical therapy is one component of a treatment plan that might also include therapies such as hydrotherapy (whirlpool or soaking bath), ULTRASOUND, and electrotherapy (gentle stimulation of the muscles with mild electrical current). The treatment plan focuses on the injured body part, and the massage therapist or physical therapist does not usually massage other parts of the body.

INFANT MASSAGE

Many neonatal care units use massage therapy with premature infants. The gentle touch of the massage therapist seems to calm and relax these babies born before their bodies are quite ready to process the stress of external stimulation. Studies show that infants who receive massage therapy gain weight and grow faster, and go home earlier from the hospital.

Massage therapy independent of physical therapy has a holistic orientation, approaching manipulation of the body within the context that the body holds physical, emotional, and spiritual tension. The massage therapist may focus on a particular area of the body that he or she detects is holding more tension than other parts of the body. Though the intent is not necessarily one of HEALING a musculoskeletal injury, massage therapy typically results in improvement of FLEXIBILITY and mobility. When the muscles release stored physical tension, they often also release stored emo-

tional tension. The result of this release can be quite profound. Many people begin to cry during massage therapy or find themselves recalling past experiences that caused them pain or grief. From a holistic perspective, this release is essential to healing in a broad context.

Massage therapy also facilitates the flow of lymph, helping the body to clear metabolic toxins stored in the muscles. Particularly in people who are sedentary, lymph flow may be sluggish. Chronic health conditions also may impair lymph circulation. People who have had lymph nodes surgically removed (lymphectomy) to treat cancer may have gaps in the lymph circulatory structures; massage therapy helps LYMPH to work around those areas to restore its movement (lymphatic drainage). As the LYMPHATIC SYSTEM is key to immune function, stimulating lymph circulation improves resistance to illness and INFECTION.

In the United States, each state regulates the practice of massage therapy. Thirty states have specific education, training, and certification requirements. Health experts recommend that regardless of state standards, massage therapists should have passed the certification requirements of the National Certification Board for Therapeutic Massage and Bodywork (NCTBMB) and belong to the American Massage Therapy Association (AMTA). Naturopathic (NDs), CHIROPRACTIC (DCs), and osteopathic physicians (DOs) are among the practitioners who most often also have formal training in massage therapy. In addition to an individual's credentials, however, the most important factors in selecting a massage therapist are trust and comfort.

See also LYMPHEDEMA; REFLEXOLOGY; REIKI.

medicinal herbs and botanicals   Plants have been the source of HEALING therapies for all of known history and among all societies. The earliest written records across cultures make reference to teas, berries, salves pounded and mixed from leaves and barks, seeds, roots, and other plant parts as remedies for ailments ranging from HEADACHE to digestive upset to GOUT. The ubiquitous aspirin, whose chemical basis is salicylic acid, derives from the bark of the willow tree. For centuries Native Americans chewed this bark to relieve TOOTHACHE, headache, and other pains, yet it was not until 1899 that researchers isolated and synthesized this key ingredient. About 30 percent of the drugs and medicines in use today derive from plant sources—the HEART medication digoxin from foxglove, for example, and the anticancer DRUG tamoxifen from the yew tree. Complementary and alternative therapies employ hundreds of plant-based remedies.

Effectiveness

Until the 1980s, there were few US clinical research studies to evaluate the benefits, risks, and effectiveness of botanical therapies, though European countries have conducted countless clinical studies. Germany's *Commission E Monographs*, a document that extensively documents the effectiveness and safety of more than 300 herbs and botanicals, stands as one of the definitive treatises on botanical remedies, analogous to Western medicine's pharmacopoeias. The Commission E updates the *Monographs* every few years as it completes investigation of additional products. Many practitioners around the world rely on the *Monographs* for information about benefits, risks, dosages, and forms of botanical therapies.

As interest has surged among Americans in using these therapies, US researchers have expanded their studies of them. Plant-based therapies in the research spotlight are PHYTOESTROGENS, for their effects in relieving hormonal discomforts related to MENOPAUSE and their potential ability to head off PROSTATE CANCER and BREAST CANCER, and SOY for its role in preserving cardiovascular health. Recent clinical studies have demonstrated the value of the herb BILBERRY to improve night vision and prevent cataracts, the herb MILK THISTLE to protect the LIVER's ability to restore itself, the herb ST. JOHN'S WORT to treat mild to moderate DEPRESSION, and the extract SAW PALMETTO to treat BENIGN PROSTATIC HYPERPLASIA (BPH).

Other remedies have failed to produce clinical evidence of their effectiveness, such as the herb DONG QUAI to treat HOT FLASHES and other discomforts of menopause. This does not mean the remedy is ineffective; it means only that so far researchers do not understand how the remedy functions in the body and cannot consistently reproduce the claimed beneficial results. Much research continues in the areas of botanicals and herbal remedies.

Forms and Preparations

The part of the plant from which the botanical product derives also affects its potency. Seeds and roots generally contain the highest concentrations of plant chemicals, while leaves or stems contain weaker concentrations. Common preparations of botanicals include the following:

- Extracts are made by soaking the plant in water to draw out its active ingredients, and the liquid becomes the product. Extracts also are evaporated out to leave the product in a powder form that manufacturers may package as loose powder or in capsules, or form into tablets.

- Tinctures are made by soaking the plant in ALCOHOL or a mixture of alcohol. The water draws out the active ingredients, and tinctures remain in liquid form.

- Teas are made from fresh, dried, or freeze-dried parts of the plant. Manufacturers may package them loose or in tea bags.

- Capsules contain powdered plant parts (usually extracts).

- Tablets are compressed powders containing the plant ingredients as well as inert binders and fillers.

- Liquids are usually extracts or decoctions in bottled form.

Most herbalists recommend staying as "close to the earth" as possible, using actual plant parts (fresh, dried, or extracted) rather than supplements manufactured from isolated ingredients.

Standardization

Medicinal botanicals have been in use in Europe for millennia, and strict standards now govern their manufacture and use in most European countries. Many require a doctor's prescription. In the United States, most medicinal botanicals and herbal preparations fall under minimal regulatory oversight as dietary supplements. The US Congress passed the Dietary Supplement Health and Education Act in 1994, allowing dietary supplement classification for any substance other than TOBACCO that, according to the US National Institutes of Health (NIH) Office of Dietary Supplements

- has the intention to supplement dietary intake
- contains dietary ingredients such as vitamins, minerals, amino acids, or botanical substances, including herbs
- is taken in some form by MOUTH (such as liquid, tablet, capsule, gel, tea, freeze-dried, or powder) either by itself or mixed with food or water
- carries clear labeling on the front of the package that identifies the product as a dietary supplement

Further, dietary supplements may not make health claims unless the US Food and Drug Administration (FDA) approves them. Dietary supplements are thus exempt from the rigorous standards that medications must meet.

In the United States, there are no standards for product ingredients or consistency for dietary supplements, other than the product may not contain substances that the law prohibits or claim to contain ingredients that it does not. The term *standardized* on a dietary supplement label can mean anything the manufacturer desires, from consistency in following the same recipe and balance of ingredients in making every batch of the supplement to all tablets in the same bottle are the same color. Many manufacturers strive to produce supplements that have consistent ingredients and potency across batches though some do not. Though reading product labels for the percentages or measurements of included ingredients is helpful, health experts point out that because there are no standards to control those measurements, there is no way to know how accurate they are.

THE USP QUALITY STANDARD

The United States Pharmacopeia (USP) maintains a verification program of stringent guidelines to assure the quality of dietary supplements. Manufacturers whose products meet the quality guidelines may place the designation "USP" on product labels. The organization's Web site (www.usp.org) maintains a current list of USP-verified products.

Another factor affecting the consistency of botanical supplements manufactured from harvested plants (as opposed to synthesized ingredients) is the wide variation possible among the source plants. Soil conditions, mineral content of the water, the amounts of water and sunshine, the part of the world where the plant grows, and numerous other environmental factors influence the plant's growth and the potency of its active ingredients. The time and method of harvest also affects potency. As well, there may be different species of the plant, such as GINSENG (Siberian, Korean, Red, *Panax*), that have differing potencies and characteristics. Manufacturers may blend several species or use whatever species is available or less expensive.

Safety
There is a tendency to view herbs and botanicals as "safe" because they are natural. However, any substance that alters the functions of the body has the capacity to be both helpful and harmful. Foxglove provides digoxin, a medication that maintains heart rhythm and STRENGTH in millions of people. Foxglove also is one of the most potent poisons; the sap residue left on the fingers after picking its beautiful purple and white bell-like flowers is enough to cause life-threatening ARRHYTHMIA (disturbance of the heart's rate and rhythm) especially in children.

Herbal remedies, like conventional medications, can interact with each other as well as with conventional medications. Most herbal products available over-the-counter are mild formulas that generally are safe when people take them according to recommended guidelines or package instructions. Some herbal formulas are potent enough, or carry sufficient risk for harmful effects, that the FDA regulates them as drugs. An example is the "herbal Viagra" remedy YOHIMBE/YOHIMBINE, derived from the bark of the African yohimbe tree, which is available in the United States only with a doctor's prescription. It is important for doctors to know, when considering prescription medications, all of the remedies, including vitamin and mineral supplements, people are taking.

See also ALTERNATIVE AND COMPLEMENTARY REMEDIES FOR CANCER; TRADITIONAL CHINESE MEDICINE.

THERAPEUTIC BOTANICALS, HERBS, AND SUPPLEMENTS

Name	Common Uses/Benefits	Risks/Side Effects
BILBERRY (*Vaccinium myrtillus*)	improve night vision, prevent AGE-RELATED MACULAR DEGENERATION (ARMD), prevent cataracts, prevent RETINOPATHY of DIABETES	none known
BLACK COHOSH (*Actaea racemosa, Cimicifuga racemosa*)	relieve menopausal HOT FLASHES	can cause uterine contractions and interfere with oral contraceptives
BOSWELLIA (*Boswellia serrata*)	relieve pain of OSTEOARTHRITIS, RHEUMATOID ARTHRITIS, IRRITABLE BOWEL DISEASE (IBD), and other AUTOIMMUNE DISORDERS	none known
CHAMOMILE (*Matricaria recutita*)	relieve gastrointestinal upset, sleep aid, general relaxation	none known
CHONDROITIN	reduce INFLAMMATION and relieve PAIN of osteoarthritis may prevent or reverse damage to JOINT tissues	may interfere with actions of anticoagulant medications
COENZYME Q10	lower BLOOD PRESSURE, strengthen force of HEART'S contractions, help heart to recover after HEART ATTACK, prevent PERIODONTITIS may prevent cancers and chronic health conditions related to oxidation	none known
DONG QUAI (*Angelica sinensis*)	relieve menstrual cramps, menopausal discomforts, and ENDOMETRIOSIS symptoms	may cause STOMACH irritation and excessive menstrual bleeding may interfere with actions of anticoagulant medications and NONSTEROIDAL ANTI-INFLAMMATORY DRUGS (NSAIDS)
ECHINACEA (*Echinacea angustifolia, Echinacea pallida, Echinacea purpurea*)	prevent or reduce symptoms of upper respiratory infections such as COLDS and INFLUENZA (flu) general IMMUNE SYSTEM support	none known
FEVERFEW (*Tanacetum parthenium*)	relieve migraine HEADACHE and menstrual discomfort	may cause excessive bleeding may interfere with anticoagulant medications, aspirin, and NSAIDs
GARLIC (*Allium sativum*)	lower BLOOD cholesterol and risk for ATHEROSCLEROSIS, CORONARY ARTERY DISEASE (CAD), and PERIPHERAL VASCULAR DISEASE (PVD)	interferes with many antihypertensive medications may cause excessive bleeding with surgery

Name	Common Uses/Benefits	Risks/Side Effects
GINGER *(Zingiber officinale)*	relieve general NAUSEA, nausea of CHEMOTHERAPY, MORNING SICKNESS, motion sickness, and digestive upset	may interfere with anticoagulant medications and ASPIRIN THERAPY may cause excessive bleeding
GINKGO BILOBA	relieve symptoms of RAYNAUD'S SYNDROME, INTERMITTENT CLAUDICATION, and ALZHEIMER'S DISEASE may improve PVD, CAD, and atherosclerosis	interferes with numerous medications including anticoagulants, antihypertensives, thiazide diuretics, prochlorperazine, trazodone interferes with aspirin therapy
GINSENG *(Panax ginseng, Panax quinquefolius)*	improved mental clarity and focus, memory general immune system support improved INSULIN sensitivity aphrodisiac	interferes with loop diuretics can result in excitability and insomnia when combined with CAFFEINE
GLUCOSAMINE	reduce inflammation and relieve pain of osteoarthritis relieve chronic BACK PAIN may prevent or reverse damage to joint tissues	may cause gastrointestinal upset interferes with loop diuretics
GOLDENSEAL *(Hydrastis canadensis)*	topical and systemic antibiotic general immune system support relieve digestive upset relieve and help heal canker sores increase resistance to URINARY TRACT INFECTION (UTI)	none known
GREEN TEA *(Camellia sinensis)*	prevent development and spread of CANCER lower low-density lipoprotein (LDL) cholesterol improve circulation strengthen TEETH and resist bacterial MOUTH infections	contains significant amount of caffeine
LUTEIN	preserve macular structure and function, protect vision, prevent cataracts	none known
LYCOPENE	prevent development and spread of PROSTATE CANCER preserve retinal function and protect vision	none known
MELATONIN	relieve insomnia prevent jet lag alter sleep patterns to accommodate shift work	causes strong drowsiness numerous medication interactions may raise blood pressure should not take with diabetes, CARDIOVASCULAR DISEASE (CVD), kidney disease

Name	Common Uses/Benefits	Risks/Side Effects
MILK THISTLE *(Silybum marianum)*	protect the LIVER from damage due to CIRRHOSIS, chronic HEPATITIS, mushroom poisoning, and DRUG poisoning	interferes with insulin therapy for diabetes
PHYTOESTROGENS	relieve menopausal discomforts and PREMENSTRUAL SYNDROME (PMS) symptoms lower blood cholesterol enhance BONE DENSITY and STRENGTH to prevent osteoporosis possibly prevent prostate cancer and some kinds of BREAST CANCER	may diminish fertility may increase risk of certain kinds of breast cancer
SAME (S-adenosylmethionine)	relieve mild to moderate DEPRESSION relieve symptoms of osteoarthritis, back pain, and CHRONIC FATIGUE SYNDROME	may cause insomnia and gastrointestinal upset interferes with monoamine oxidase inhibitor (MAOI) antidepressants
SAW PALMETTO *(Sabal serrulata)*	stop PROSTATE GLAND from enlarging relieve symptoms of benign PROSTATIC HYPERPLASIA (BPH)	may interfere with some treatment for prostate cancer
soy	lower LDL cholesterol, reduce risk for CAD reduce risk for osteoporosis, prostate cancer, and certain breast cancers relieve menopausal discomforts, especially hot flashes	may cause gastrointestinal upset may increase risk for certain estrogen-driven breast cancers
ST. JOHN'S WORT *(hypericum perforatum)*	relieve mild to moderate depression	increases sensitivity to the sun and ultraviolet light interferes with some chemotherapy agents, HIV/AIDS medications, immunosuppressive drugs, and selective serotonin reuptake inhibitor (SSRI) and MAOI antidepressants
SUN'S SOUP	slow metastasis of non-small cell LUNG CANCER (NSCLC) reduce HIV/AIDS symptoms and progression	none known
VALERIAN *(Valeriana officinalis)*	sleep aid relieves anxiety	may cause excessive drowsiness in combination with other substances and medications that also cause drowsiness
YOHIMBE/YOHIMBINE *(Pausinystalia yohimbe)*	treat ERECTILE DYSFUNCTION aphrodisiac	may cause elevated blood pressure interferes with MAOI antidepressants interacts with foods containing tyramine

Name	Common Uses/Benefits	Risks/Side Effects
ZEAXANTHIN	prevent cataracts	none known
	preserve macular function and protect vision	
	possibly protect against LUNG CANCER and	
	OVARIAN CANCER	

meditation A method of focusing the mind for HEALING VISUALIZATION, relaxation, stress relief, and contemplation. Though meditation can have a spiritual dimension for people who desire it, meditation is not a religious practice. Clinical studies show that daily meditation has the ability to

- reduce EPINEPHRINE production, thereby lowering BLOOD PRESSURE and the frequency of ANGINA PECTORIS
- relax BLOOD vessels, which also lowers blood pressure
- relax musculoskeletal structures
- instill a sense of inner calm and peacefulness
- decrease the frequency, duration, and severity of menopausal HOT FLASHES

When meditation becomes a routine of daily life, these effects can help lower blood pressure by reducing the resistance blood encounters as it flows through the arteries. They also increase the flow of blood to muscles, helping muscle cells to more efficiently clear lactic acid accumulations and other metabolic wastes that cause cramping and discomfort. Some people use meditation as a platform to "go within" their bodies and visualize healthy, strong cells, tissues, organs, and functions. Such visualization may aid in healing during illness or injury as well as in maintaining health.

There are many methods of meditation. Meditation centers, YOGA centers, community centers, and health organizations often teach classes in meditation techniques. Meditation may take place while sitting quietly, while walking, or while engaged in mind–body practices such as yoga and TAI CHI. Some people chant when meditating, to focus their meditations with specific sounds or intents. Though a quiet location best facilitates meditation, a person can meditate anywhere.

Many people take five-minute meditation breaks while at work to help dissipate job stress. Children also can learn to meditate. Meditation has no known health risks.

See also MIND–BODY INTERACTIONS; PRAYER AND SPIRITUALITY; STRESS AND STRESS MANAGEMENT.

melatonin An endogenous (naturally occurring within the body) HORMONE the PINEAL GLAND produces that maintains the body's circadian rhythms (cycles of waking and sleeping). Melatonin may also have ANTIOXIDANT functions, helping protect cells from damage. Researchers first discovered melatonin in the late 1950s, and early studies suggested endogenous melatonin (melatonin the body manufactures) production diminished with increasing age. This gave rise to speculation that melatonin played a role in the aging process. Subsequent studies have been unable to substantiate such involvement, however, and most doctors do not believe melatonin can halt, prevent, or reverse aging.

The daily level of melatonin in the body cycles a pattern of peaking between 2 o'clock and 4 o'clock in the morning (which is the middle of the night for most people) and reaching its lowest point around midday. Researchers believe the HYPOTHALAMUS, a structure deep within the BRAIN that regulates vital body functions such as BREATHING and BLOOD PRESSURE, receives signals from the RETINA via the OPTIC NERVE that indicate whether it is light or dark. When it is dark, the hypothalamus signals the pineal gland to begin releasing melatonin and when it is light, to stop releasing melatonin. This may in part explain why people feel drowsy when spending several hours in dark settings such as movie theaters, or want to go to sleep earlier in the winter when daylight is short and have trouble falling asleep in summer when daylight is much longer.

Raising the level of melatonin in the bloodstream increases drowsiness, which has led to the use of melatonin supplement as a sleep aid. In the United States melatonin is available as an over-the-counter dietary supplement. In most European countries, however, melatonin is available only with a doctor's prescription. This is because researchers do not fully understand the functions of melatonin in the body though they do know that as a hormone, melatonin has numerous effects within the body in addition to the roles it plays in sleep cycles and the circadian rhythm. Some studies have found that melatonin causes blood vessels to constrict, perhaps by stimulating the release of CORTISOL, raising blood pressure. Though this finding is not conclusive, health experts advise people who have HYPERTENSION (as well as people who have other forms of CARDIOVASCULAR DISEASE (CVD), DIABETES, and KIDNEY disease) not to take melatonin to avoid this risk.

A number of studies support melatonin's ability to relieve jet lag and help people adjust to sleeping during the day when they work during the night. However, there are no studies that conclusively identify supplemental melatonin's benefits or risks. Melatonin interacts with numerous prescription medications and should be taken only after a doctor's examination determines there are no neurologic or other physiologic causes for insomnia. Even people taking melatonin for jet lag or to restructure their sleep patterns to accommodate shift work should first consult with their doctors to make sure they have no health conditions that make it unsafe for them to take melatonin supplements.

Melatonin causes drowsiness within 20 to 30 minutes of taking a DOSE, an effect that lasts four to six hours. Some people experience a "hangover" effect when they wake up, feeling groggy and disoriented for as long as several hours. People must not drive or operate machinery after taking a melatonin dose, as the onset of sleepiness can be sudden and irresistible. Some people also experience increased insomnia or have vivid dreams and nightmares as well as fatigue after taking melatonin. Melatonin taken in combination with other medications that cause drowsiness can result in an intensified effect (excessive sleepiness).

MELATONIN

Uses	Risks/Side Effects	Interactions
sleep aid	drowsiness	CORTICOSTEROID MEDICATIONS
	possible fertility problems	prescription sleep aids
		ASTHMA medications
	may elevate BLOOD PRESSURE	ANTIHISTAMINE MEDICATIONS
		narcotic ANALGESIC MEDICATIONS
	insomnia	
	fatigue	ANTIANXIETY MEDICATIONS
		MUSCLE RELAXANT MEDICATIONS
		ANTIDEPRESSANT MEDICATIONS

See also ANTI-AGING APPROACHES; SLEEP DISORDERS; VALERIAN.

milk thistle A medicinal herb, also called holy thistle, that helps protect the LIVER from INFECTION and improves the liver's ability to regenerate from damage. Numerous clinical studies support this benefit. The active ingredient in milk thistle is silymarin, a composite of five flavonoids (siliandrin, silibinin, silydianin, silymonin, and silychristin), which is in highest concentrations in the milk thistle seeds. Silymarin strengthens the structure of hepatocytes, the cells in the liver that metabolize toxins. It may also influence aminotransferases, the enzymes the liver produces to break down chemical substances the liver extracts from the blood.

Doctors often recommend milk thistle for people who have LIVER DISEASE OF ALCOHOLISM, CIRRHOSIS, or chronic HEPATITIS, or who have ingested toxic mushrooms or toxic doses of medications such as acetaminophen. Some people who have HIV/AIDS take milk thistle or silymarin extract to protect their livers from the potentially damaging effects of some of the medications used to treat HIV/AIDS. There also is limited evidence that milk thistle has a similarly protective function in the kidneys though researchers continue to explore this possible effect. A folk medicine use for milk thistle, likely the origin of the plant's name, is to stimulate BREAST milk production in nursing mothers. Of the few studies that have investigated this use, there have been no conclusive findings about benefits or risks. Because the effects are unknown, health experts recommend BREASTFEEDING mothers do *not* use milk thistle or silymarin extract.

Milk thistle is available in dried plant form in teas, and also in preparations of silymarin extract in tablet form. People who are allergic to common thistle, daisies, artichokes, or kiwi (all of which are in the same plant family as milk thistle) should not take milk thistle or silymarin in any form. Milk thistle or silymarin extract may cause digestive upset including NAUSEA and DIARRHEA. Because of its enzymatic inhibitory actions, milk thistle may interfere with INSULIN–GLUCOSE processes. People who have DIABETES should consult with their doctors before using milk thistle or silymarin.

MILK THISTLE *(Silybum marianum)*		
Uses	**Risks/Side Effects**	**Interactions**
CIRRHOSIS	allergic reaction	INSULIN therapy
chronic HEPATITIS	digestive upset	
mushroom poisoning		
DRUG poisoning		

See also HEPATOTOXINS.

mind–body interactions   Approaches of care that engage the interrelationships between the mind and the body for HEALING and health. Healers have known for centuries that the state of the mind influences the condition of the body. Contemporary physicians will not hesitate to say that the patient's attitude and outlook are at least as important as any technology modern medicine has to offer. Though the mind alone cannot pre-

vent or heal significant physical conditions such as CANCER or CARDIOVASCULAR DISEASE (CVD), an individual's mindset shapes the determination with which he or she approaches treatment and treatment's ultimate success or failure.

MIND–BODY THERAPIES	
AROMATHERAPY	ART THERAPY
BIOFEEDBACK	CRANIOSACRAL MASSAGE
HYPNOSIS	MASSAGE THERAPY
MEDITATION	PRAYER AND SPIRITUALITY
REIKI	TAI CHI
VISUALIZATION	YOGA

At the most basic level, perceptions about health, illness, and the success or failure of treatment influence a person's compliance with the doctor's recommendations from the taking of prescription medications to lifestyle modifications such as weight loss or SMOKING CESSATION. At a more sophisticated level, clinical studies demonstrate the ability of some people to consciously alter body functions such as HEART RATE and BLOOD PRESSURE through methods such as BIOFEEDBACK and MEDITATION. Cancer treatment programs use healing visualization, in which the person in treatment meditates to visualize his or her cancer gone and the body strong and healthy. Surgeons and anesthesiologists often recommend visualization before and after surgery, encouraging people to "see" the surgery succeed and the body restore itself to health.

See also BEHAVIOR MODIFICATION THERAPY; LIFESTYLE AND HEALTH; ORNISH PROGRAM.

Native American healing A spirituality-based approach, also called traditional North American medicine, that incorporates ceremony, ritual, and symbolism. In the Native American tradition, intent is as important as action and there are no distinctions between body, mind, and spirit. The illness or health of one affects the well-being of the whole. As well, traditional Native American medicine holds that HEALING takes place within the body's sense of time and timing, and efforts to rush or otherwise influence this timing extend rather than shorten the healing process.

Traditional Native American healing practices made use of the sweat lodge, a small enclosed structure in which a fire burned hot. The heat would flush the cause of the ailment to the surface, where it would manifest in the form of a vision. People stayed in the sweat lodge until the heat initiated within them the vision necessary for healing. The person might then go into the forest, desert, or mountains to be with the vision and allow the natural environment to reveal its meanings. The experience also restores the balance between the individual and the natural environment, an essential component of the healing process from the traditional perspective.

Some hospitals in areas where there are Native American populations are beginning to incorporate Native American healers among the complementary providers available to patients, notably in the American Southwest. Drumming, chanting, smudging, and dancing may be among the elements of healing rituals. One of the most common ceremonies is the medicine wheel, a form of ritual MEDITATION or prayer similar to a LABYRINTH. The circle of the wheel represents the continuous harmony of the universe, with the four spokes representing the four directions and their correlations to body (north), spirit (south), mind (east), and inner peace (west).

See also AYURVEDA; MIND–BODY INTERACTIONS; PRAYER AND SPIRITUALITY; TRADITIONAL CHINESE MEDICINE (TCM).

naturopathy A system of medicine that uses methods and substances found in nature to maintain and restore health. The philosophical foundation of naturopathy rejects interventions such as major surgery, RADIATION THERAPY, and drugs other than elements, minerals, and other natural compounds. Naturopathy incorporates or supports therapeutic approaches such as ACUPUNCTURE, energy medicine, NUTRITIONAL THERAPY using diagnostic testing through functional medicine, hydrotherapy, physiotherapy, MEDICINAL HERBS AND BOTANICALS, HOMEOPATHY, and manipulative therapies (such as CHIROPRACTIC, MASSAGE THERAPY, and OSTEOPATHIC MANIPULATIVE TREATMENT [OMT]).

Naturopathic Diagnosis and Treatment

The naturopathic physician assesses symptoms and examines patients in much the same fashion as a conventional doctor, though spends considerably more time addressing lifestyle factors such as nutrition, activity, relationships, stress, and emotional well-being. The naturopathic physician may function as a consultant for botanical or nutritional therapies, or as a primary-care provider who works collaboratively with other health-care professionals and refers people for specialty care as needed, as would a conventional doctor (MD or DO). The naturopathic approach considers the person holistically and incorporates therapeutic methods that both treat symptoms and restore overall health and well-being. Naturopathic physicians spend much time educating people about how to better manage their health to prevent illness.

Naturopathic Practitioners

Naturopathy traces its origins to ancient HEALING methods based entirely on natural methods, the only approach available for centuries. Today in the United States, naturopathic physicians complete comprehensive education and training programs and must pass licensing examinations in the states in which they practice. A naturopathic physician receives a doctor of naturopathy degree and puts the initials "ND" or "NMD" after his or her name. Many naturopaths have additional training and certification in ACUPUNCTURE and TRADITIONAL CHINESE MEDICINE (TCM), broadening the scope of their perspectives and abilities to accommodate diverse interests in health care among the people who come to them for care.

Benefits and Risks of Naturopathy

Naturopathy as practiced in the United States today functions synergistically with conventional therapies. The risks of naturopathic remedies vary according to the person's primary and secondary health conditions and with the therapeutic approach. Within such a context, and because naturopathy does not use medications or major surgery, naturopathy is overall less risky than conventional medicine. It is important for people to receive appropriate conventional medical treatments for conditions that require it, such as type 1 DIABETES. Herbal remedies can interact with each other as well as with conventional medications. A person who receives care from conventional as well as naturopathic doctors should be sure all practitioners know they are collectively participating in that care.

See also OSTEOPATHY; REFLEXOLOGY.

nutritional therapy   A therapeutic approach that uses nutraceuticals, foods, vitamins, minerals, and special diets to fight disease and maintain health. Nutritional therapy as a complementary method is not the same as the NUTRITIONAL ASSESSMENT a registered dietitian (RD) might provide for compliance with conventional nutrition requirements. Nutritional therapy instead blends holistic concepts with dietary modifications.

From a conventional medicine perspective, the premise that nutrition and diet influence health and disease is not new or unique. Foods may contribute to numerous health conditions. Some foods energize and others relax the body. Foods also can be harmful to people who have certain medical conditions. For example, people who have HEMOCHROMATOSIS, a metabolic disorder that allows iron to accumulate in various organs, worsen the condition when they eat foods high in iron such as spinach. Food allergies, such as to peanuts, can have lethal consequences.

HEALTH CONDITIONS FOODS INFLUENCE	
ANEMIA	ATHEROSCLEROSIS
ATTENTION DEFICIT HYPERACTIVITY	AUTISM
DISORDER (ADHD)	CARDIOVASCULAR DISEASE
CELIAC DISEASE (sprue)	(CVD)
chronic OTITIS media	ECZEMA
GASTROESOPHAGEAL REFLUX	GOUT
DISORDER (GERD)	HEMOCHROMATOSIS
INFLAMMATORY BOWEL DISEASE	IRRITABLE BOWEL SYNDROME
(IBD)	(IBS)
migraine HEADACHE	multiple metabolic
OBESITY	syndrome
OSTEOARTHRITIS	OSTEOPOROSIS
PREMENSTRUAL SYNDROME (PMS)	PSORIASIS
RECURRENT YEAST INFECTIONS	RHINITIS
type 2 DIABETES	WILSON'S DISEASE

Many of the most significant health conditions facing Americans today in some way relate to EATING HABITS. Many people eat too much in general, too much of foods that do not support health, or not enough foods that provide the body with the nutritional foundation it needs to meet its energy and maintenance requirements. The most compelling evidence of this is the OBESITY rate in the United States; more than two thirds of Americans are overweight (5 to 20 percent above healthy weight) and nearly a third have obesity (20 percent or higher above healthy weight). Of special concern is the significant rise in the number of children who have obesity, particularly children under 10 years old. Some studies also link dietary habits with health conditions such as COLORECTAL CANCER.

Because many people do not eat nutritiously, dietary changes to improve nutrition nearly always

result in health improvements. However, the scientific connections between nutrition and health or disease are not entirely clear and sometimes appear even conflicting. As yet, there are very few circumstances (other than those that are the direct result of nutritional deficiencies) in which consuming or not consuming certain foods can prevent health conditions. Foods, and the nutrients they contain, certainly can support wellness or contribute to disease. But nutritional therapy that restricts or emphasizes certain nutrients may create nutritional deficiencies and imbalances.

See also ALTERNATIVE AND COMPLEMENTARY REMEDIES FOR CANCER; DRUG INTERACTIONS; LIFESTYLE AND HEALTH; MALNUTRITION; NUTRITIONAL NEEDS; NUTRITIONAL SUPPLEMENTS.

osteopathic manipulative treatment (OMT) A touch therapy that uses pressure, stretching, and manipulation of the muscles and joints to relieve musculoskeletal discomfort. The goal of OMT is to release restrictions within musculoskeletal structures to restore FLEXIBILITY and mobility. OMT may improve chronic BACK PAIN, FIBROMYALGIA, CHRONIC FATIGUE SYNDROME (CFS), and REPETITIVE MOTION INJURIES such as CARPAL TUNNEL SYNDROME, and ROTATOR CUFF IMPINGEMENT SYNDROME. OMT represents one of the founding principles of OSTEOPATHY, that the structure of the body supports the body's health. Often, a doctor of osteopathy (DO) has the training and expertise to perform OMT.

See also ALTERNATIVE METHODS FOR PAIN RELIEF; CHIROPRACTIC; JOINT; MASSAGE THERAPY; MUSCLE; REFLEXOLOGY.

osteopathy A philosophy of health care that emphasizes preventive approaches and self-care to manage lifestyle choices in ways that encourage wellness. Osteopathy strives to support the structures of the body to maintain health. In the United States, a doctor of osteopathy (DO) has the same practicing privileges and licensing requirements as a medical doctor (MD) and is considered a conventional physician. The osteopathic medicine curriculum is comparable to the curriculum at a conventional medical school, typically a four-year graduate program with a subsequent internship and residency though with more opportunity to learn manipulations such as OSTEOPATHIC MANIPULATIVE TREATMENT (OMT) and craniosacral massage. Though many osteopathic physicians choose to practice in primary care, they may become specialists in any area of medicine.

See also AYURVEDA; HOMEOPATHY; NATUROPATHY; OSTEOPATHIC MANIPULATIVE TREATMENT; REFLEXOLOGY; TRADITIONAL CHINESE MEDICINE (TCM).

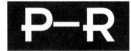

phytoestrogens   Plant-based ESTROGENS, many of which are similar in chemical structure to the estrogens the human body produces. In plants, phytoestrogens are part of the botanical IMMUNE SYSTEM, helping protect the plant from fungal and bacterial INFECTION. In humans, phytoestrogens exert a weak estrogenic effect relative to that of endogenous (produced within the body) or supplemental estrogen. Though an abundance of research supports numerous health benefits from eating foods high in phytoestrogens, questions remain about the effectiveness of phytoestrogens in supplement forms as well as the precise mechanisms and consequences of them in the human body.

DIETARY SOURCES OF PHYTOESTROGENS

Isoflavones	Lignans	Coumestans
soybeans	flaxseed	red clover
SOY-based foods	flaxseed oil	pinto beans
red clover	lentils	lima beans
textured vegetable protein	carrots	split peas
soy protein isolate	oat bran	alfalfa sprouts
soy milk	oatmeal	red clover sprouts
licorice	asparagus	

There are two main classifications of phytoestrogens: isoflavonoids (isoflavones) and lignans. Soybeans are the primary source of isoflavones such as genistein and daidzien, and nuts and flax are the primary sources of lignans. A third classification of phytoestrogens, coumestans, appears to have an even stronger estrogen effect in the body though research has not focused on them. Red clover and alfalfa, especially sprouts, contain coumestans. Most plants have combinations of phytoestrogens with one that is dominant. Supplements prepared from extracts of these substances often combine the various phytoestrogens into formulas for specific uses, such as MENOPAUSE symptoms or DYSMENORRHEA (difficult menstrual periods or menstrual cramps).

The primary therapeutic uses for phytoestrogens are to improve the discomforts of PREMENSTRUAL SYNDROME (PMS) and menopause. Some studies support the value of some phytoestrogens, notably isoflavones, in preventing or limiting PROSTATE CANCER and BREAST CANCER though health experts do not agree on the extent to which these actions result from the isoflavones. Studies using isoflavone extracts in supplement form produce less conclusive findings than those studies that use isoflavone-containing (SOY-based) foods. Isoflavones may also help reduce the risk for CARDIOVASCULAR DISEASE (CVD) by lowering blood cholesterol levels and for OSTEOPOROSIS by aiding the bones in retaining calcium. Some studies show soy has limited ability to slow osteoclastic activity (bone destruction) and promote osteoblastic activity (bone construction).

Because their chemical structures are similar to those of endogenous estrogens, phytoestrogens are able to bind with estrogen receptors (specialized molecular "switches" in cells) in the body. However, the bond is an incomplete fit and more fragile than the bond of endogenous or supplemental estrogen, and produces a weaker estrogen response. Health experts disagree on the role this weaker bond and response may play in reducing the risk for breast cancer in women. Some believe phytoestrogens, because they occupy estrogen receptors, prevent more potent endogenous estrogen from binding and thus suppress estrogen availability. Less estrogen means less fuel for potential CANCER cells, theoretically inhibiting their ability to manifest as breast cancer.

Other health experts worry that by only partially blocking estrogen effect in the body, phytoestrogens allow other chemical communications to take place that could actually increase the risk for estrogen-driven breast cancers in some women who have previously had estrogen-driven breast cancer. However, it remains unclear whether endogenous estrogen binding creates a greater risk. Some studies show a stronger preventive effect in premenopausal women and a less conclusive preventive effect in postmenopausal women, which researchers correlate to the differences in the kinds of breast cancers likely to affect each age group. Research continues to explore these issues, and doctors remain divided in their recommendations. Many health experts recommend obtaining phytoestrogens through natural food sources rather than supplements, to receive the additional benefits of other nutrients in the foods.

PHYTOESTROGENS

Uses	Risks/Side Effects	Interactions
relieve MENOPAUSE discomforts	fertility disturbances	none known
relieve PREMENSTRUAL SYNDROME	possible increased risk of breast cancer in certain women	
lower blood cholesterol		
enhance BONE calcium		
possibly prevent BREAST CANCER		
possibly prevent PROSTATE CANCER		

See also BLACK COHOSH; DONG QUAI; SOY AND CARDIOVASCULAR HEALTH.

prayer and spirituality Faith-based approaches to HEALING. Numerous anecdotal reports as well as clinical studies support a connection between healing and belief practices such as prayer and spiritual MEDITATION. Researchers at Duke University's Center for Spirituality, Theology, and Health have conducted a number of studies measuring different immune function indicators in people who regularly attend religious services and in people who do not. Over time, researchers found, the immune systems of people who regularly participate in religious or spiritual activities (regardless of belief system) have higher levels of INTERLEUKINS and other immune factors.

Two thirds of American medical schools now teach courses in prayer and spirituality, and all hospitals have chaplains on staff or clergy on call. Most hospitals have chapels or meditation rooms for where patients can go privately, as well as locations where family members and friends may gather to pray or meditate. Many people participate in prayer circles, through churches or through other common structures, in which they pray specifically for others who are injured or ill. A number of studies suggest that the beneficiaries of these prayers, called intercessory prayers, tend to improve more quickly. In degenerative conditions such as ALZHEIMER'S DISEASE, the ritual of shared spiritual or religious practices often provides comfort and a sense of stability. Spiritual practices also help provide a sense of meaning and acceptance when health conditions are terminal.

See also END OF LIFE CONCERNS; NATIVE AMERICAN HEALING; SPIRITUAL BELIEFS AND HEALTH CARE.

qigong See TRADITIONAL CHINESE MEDICINE (TCM).

reflexology A therapeutic approach that uses massage and pressure on the feet and hands. The philosophy of reflexology holds that the soles of the feet (and to lesser extent, the palms of the hands) contain reflex points that correlate to body structures and functions. Activating these points affects the correlating structure or function, relieving energy blockages that might be causing symptoms or disease. People receiving reflexology treatments often experience the pressure of the reflexologist's touch as well as tingling or other sensations in the area of the body that correlates with the reflex point.

The sole of each foot contains more than 7,000 NERVE endings. Nerve pathways branch through various regions of the body on their way to or from the SPINAL CORD and BRAIN. One theory for how reflexology might work is that activating a nerve ending such as on the bottom of the foot could result in a nerve response elsewhere along the path of the nerve structure. Other theories correlate reflexology to energy channels and networks similar to those of ACUPUNCTURE (though acupuncture and reflexology are not related in philosophy or practice). However, there are no clinical studies to substantiate any of these theories, or that reflexology produces objective results. Most conventional doctors are skeptical that reflexology has therapeutic value beyond that which one might expect from a thorough foot massage.

See also MASSAGE THERAPY; REIKI.

Reiki   A 3,000 year-old system of energy HEALING that originated with Tibetan monks. The word *Reiki* means "universal life force." Reiki practitioners use their hands, without touching the person, to focus energy. The energy might come from the person's body, identifying the location of illness or injury. Sometimes the Reiki practitioner experiences these locations as feeling hot or cold. The energy also comes through the Reiki practitioner to the person, focusing healing where the body needs it. Many people feel profound relaxation and release during a Reiki session and often relief from PAIN. It is common for both the person receiving Reiki and the Reiki practitioner to emerge from a Reiki session feeling a heightened sense of awareness.

Because there is no clinical substantiation for the effects of Reiki, many doctors tend to be skeptical. However, there are no known risks associated with Reiki when it is a complementary component of overall care and treatment. Unlike MASSAGE THERAPY, with Reiki there is no, or only very light, touching. The primary concern of conventional doctors is that people continue to receive conventional medical care when necessary.

A number of hospitals make Reiki practitioners available to people who are waiting for transplant organs or undergoing strenuous CANCER treatment. Some conventional health-care practitioners, such as nurses, become Reiki practitioners. Some researchers believe the deep relaxation that people experience with Reiki sessions causes the body to release natural PAIN-relieving chemicals (endorphins and enkephalins), accounting for effects such as pain relief and stress reduction. Reiki may be especially helpful for people who have conditions, such as BURNS or major trauma, that make touch therapies difficult or unfeasible.

Reiki practitioners designate their levels of expertise according to degrees. A first-degree Reiki practitioner has received basic Reiki training, typically a two-day session. A second-degree Reiki practitioner has been practicing Reiki for a minimum of three months and has completed an additional Reiki training session, typically a two-day workshop, to learn more advanced techniques including mental healing and distance healing. A third-degree Reiki practitioner is a Reiki master. A Reiki master has practiced Reiki for at least a year and then has completed a year-long training program. Reiki masters also teach Reiki. As with other forms of bodywork and energy healing, it is essential to trust in, and feel comfortable with, the Reiki practitioner.

See also ACUPUNCTURE; REFLEXOLOGY.

SAMe A chemical that occurs naturally in the BRAIN. SAMe, which is short for S-adenosylmethionine, participates in the brain's synthesis of DOPAMINE and serotonin, neurotransmitters that have key functions in brain communication regarding emotions and mood. SAMe is available in the United States as a dietary supplement and as a prescription medication in most European countries. People commonly take SAMe to relieve symptoms of DEPRESSION, OSTEOARTHRITIS, chronic BACK PAIN, and CHRONIC FATIGUE SYNDROME (CFS). Clinical studies support SAMe's effectiveness in treating depression and osteoarthritis, though are not entirely conclusive. So far research findings have failed to support a conclusive benefit from SAMe for chronic back pain and CFS.

Depression

In a number of clinical studies SAMe appears as effective as prescription tricyclic ANTIDEPRESSANT MEDICATIONS for treating mild to moderate depression and without the side effects, such as drowsiness and dry mouth, common to them. However, depression can be a serious medical condition. Doctors worry that people who use over-the-counter remedies to self-treat depression may put themselves at risk. Conventional medical approaches to treating depression may incorporate antidepressant medications with PSYCHOTHERAPY to resolve the underlying causes of the depression.

As well, any substance that alters the production and ratio of brain neurotransmitters has the potential to create imbalances in those vital brain chemicals that cause further problems. One such consequence is serotonin syndrome, a serious and potentially fatal accumulation of serotonin in the brain. SAMe appears to suppress monoamine oxidase, the same NEUROTRANSMITTER that tricyclic

antidepressants target. While doctors monitor people taking tricyclics for evidence of serotonin syndrome, a person who is self-medicating with SAMe may not recognize the symptoms of serotonin toxicity (HEADACHE, dizziness, vomiting, disorientation and confusion, unconsciousness) as related to SAMe. Also because of SAMe's monoamine oxidase inhibition ability, people who are taking monoamine oxidase inhibitor (MAOI) antidepressants should not take SAMe.

Serotonin syndrome is a serious and potentially fatal SIDE EFFECT of ANTIDEPRESSANT MEDICATIONS. It requires immediate medical attention.

Osteoarthritis

A number of clinical research studies show that osteoarthritis improves after taking SAMe for four to six weeks. However, researchers have yet to identify the actions of SAMe responsible for this improvement. The METABOLISM of endogenous (naturally occurring) SAMe produces various chemical substances (notably amino acids) that the body can use to repair JOINT tissues and produce the synovial fluid that lubricates joints. Some researchers believe SAMe as a supplement provides more of these amino acids. Because of the length of time it takes to see improvement, however, other researchers question whether it is the SAMe supplement or the natural processes of the body that result in reduced PAIN and INFLAMMATION.

Chronic Back Pain and CFS

Chronic back pain and CFS can be debilitating conditions that defy attempts to improve symptoms. The mechanisms of both are poorly understood, though theories abound. Most doctors feel that low doses of SAMe do no harm and thus are worth trying if they might bring improvement. The precautions that apply to other uses of SAMe remain pertinent. People taking SAMe for chronic back pain or CFS should do so only with the knowledge of their doctors, to avoid any possible interactions with prescription medications and to monitor for adverse effects or further deterioration of the underlying condition.

SAMe		
Uses	**Risks/Side Effects**	**Interactions**
DEPRESSION	serotonin syndrome	MAOI antidepressants
OSTEOARTHRITIS	gastrointestinal upset	
chronic BACK	insomnia	
PAIN		
CHRONIC FATIGUE		
SYNDROME		

See also CHONDROITIN; GLUCOSAMINE; ST. JOHN'S WORT.

saw palmetto   A botanical preparation made from the berries of the saw palmetto tree (*Sabal serrulata*) native to the American coastal southwest. Saw palmetto prevents the PROSTATE GLAND from enlarging, though it does not appear to reduce enlargement that has already occurred. Though many people believe saw palmetto can prevent PROSTATE CANCER, so far there is no conclusive evidence to support this effect.

Researchers do not know for certain what ingredients in saw palmetto have an active effect, though believe its fatty acids contain substances that mildly suppress TESTOSTERONE and its precursors (chemicals the body converts to testosterone). This action reduces testosterone levels enough to inhibit the growth of prostate cells but not so much as to cause other symptoms related to low testosterone such as diminished LIBIDO or ERECTILE DYSFUNCTION. Such symptoms are common with conventional medications such as finasteride (Proscar) to treat BENIGN PROSTATIC HYPERPLASIA (BPH), a condition affecting about half of men over age 60. Many doctors recommend a trial of saw palmetto before moving to finasteride, as saw palmetto is significantly less expensive as well as less likely to cause undesired side effects.

Men who take saw palmetto for BPH should have an annual prostate examination to check for early signs of prostate cancer. Saw palmetto is available in numerous formulations as dietary supplements, many of which include other ingredients. Health experts recommend choosing products that contain 90 to 95 percent saw palmetto sterol oils or fatty acids. Combination products may not contain enough saw palmetto to be effective. Saw palmetto can cause gastrointestinal distress; doctors recommend taking it with meals. Men who have prostate cancer should take saw palmetto only if their doctors approve; saw palmetto may interfere with some hormone-based prostate cancer treatments.

SAW PALMETTO (*Sabal serrulata*)		
Uses	**Risks/Side Effects**	**Interactions**
stop PROSTATE	stomach upset	some PROSTATE
gland enlargement		CANCER
relieve BPH		treatments
symptoms		

See also AGING, URINARY SYSTEM CHANGES THAT OCCUR WITH; LYCOPENE; PROSTATE HEALTH; PROSTATITIS.

soy   Researchers have noticed since the 1970s that people whose diets include soybeans and soy-based foods such as tofu have lower blood cholesterol levels and lower rates of CARDIOVASCULAR DISEASE (CVD). Numerous research studies have isolated various soy proteins such as genistein and daidzein that have demonstrated their ability to decrease low-density lipoprotein (LDL) cholesterol. The US Food and Drug Administration (FDA), which regulates the health claims manufacturers may make about their products, allows manufacturers to tout this effect on products that contain 25 grams or more of soy protein.

FOOD SOURCES OF SOY	
immature soybeans (edemame)	mature soybeans
roasted soy nuts	textured vegetable
tofu	protein (TVP)
miso	dried soybeans
tempeh	soymilk
soy protein isolate	soy flakes
soy cheese	

The primary active ingredients in soybeans are PHYTOESTROGENS, chemicals that function in the human body like weak ESTROGENS. Researchers have connected estrogen with numerous health conditions including BREAST CANCER, PROSTATE CANCER, cardiovascular disease, and OSTEOPOROSIS. Though soy and phytoestrogens appear to improve these conditions, researchers remain uncertain as to the mechanisms of phytoestrogens in the human body and the potential risks that they present. Estrogen can both prevent and cause BREAST cancer, for example. Much research continues to explore these issues. In the meantime, health experts recommend most people substitute soy products for meats to reduce dietary saturated fats as a measure for reducing the risk of heart disease. Soybeans are the only plant-based source of complete protein, providing all of the essential proteins the body requires.

SOY		
Uses	Risks/Side Effects	Interactions
lower LDL cholesterol	may increase risk for estrogen-driven breast cancers	none known
reduce risk for HEART disease	gastrointestinal upset	
reduce risk for OSTEOPOROSIS		
relieve menopausal discomforts		
reduce risk for PROSTATE CANCER		
reduce risk for some BREAST CANCERS		

See also GREEN TEA; HORMONE-DRIVEN CANCERS; HORMONE THERAPY; SOY AND CARDIOVASCULAR HEALTH.

St. John's wort An herb, *Hypericum perforatum,* that healers have used for centuries to treat DEPRESSION. The actions of St. John's wort appear similar to those of the serotonin reuptake inhibitor (SSRI) antidepressants. St. John's wort is available in teas, extracts, and capsules as a dietary supplement in the United States, and as a medication that requires a doctor's prescription in most of Europe. In Europe, St. John's wort is the most widely prescribed of the ANTIDEPRESSANT MEDICATIONS. Researchers believe the active ingredients are hypericin and hyperforin, though in isolation

these substances do not produce the same results as the intact herb. These are the substances most commonly available in extract products.

Most health experts agree that while St. John's wort may help mild to moderate depression as well as mild to moderate anxiety, it is not effective in major depression or in BIPOLAR DISORDER, a combination of depressive and manic symptoms. St. John's wort interacts with a number of medications, including some HIV/AIDS medications, certain CHEMOTHERAPY agents, and IMMUNOSUPPRESSIVE MEDICATIONS such as cyclosporine taken following ORGAN TRANSPLANTATION. Because St. John's wort extends the presence and action of serotonin, people who take SSRI or monoamine oxidase inhibitor (MAOI) antidepressants should not take St. John's wort. A serious and sometimes fatal complication, serotonin syndrome, may result.

Serotonin syndrome is a serious and potentially fatal SIDE EFFECT of ANTIDEPRESSANT MEDICATIONS. It requires immediate medical attention.

Because depression can be a serious medical condition, most doctors prefer that people receive conventional medical treatment. That treatment may include St. John's wort, after a thorough evaluation of the person's physical and mental health status. But health experts caution that self-diagnosis and self-treatment can be risky.

ST. JOHN'S WORT *(Hypericum perforatum)*		
Uses	Risks/Side Effects	Interactions
mild to moderate DEPRESSION	serotonin syndrome sun sensitivity	CHEMOTHERAPY agents HIV/AIDS medications immunosuppressive drugs SSRIs and MAOIs

See also SAMe; VALERIAN.

Sun's Soup A formula of herbs and vegetables, formally called Sun Farms Vegetable Soup (SFVS) and sometimes referred to as Selected Vegetables, developed to treat non-small cell LUNG CANCER (NSCLC) and HIV/AIDS. The formula's developer,

Alexander Sun, a biochemist and former researcher at Yale and Mount Sinai schools of medicine, selected ingredients that appear to have cancer-fighting properties.

Though the actual formula is proprietary, published reports identify the original ingredients as shiitake mushrooms, mung beans, hawthorn fruit, onion, GINGER, American GINSENG, lentils, leeks, and the Chinese herbs bai hua she she cao and ban zhi lian. Sun's Soup comes in freeze-dried packages that the person mixes with hot water or hot soup once daily. In several small clinical studies with people who had moderate to advanced NSCLC, Sun's Soup produced measurable improvements. However, the small study size limited the value of the findings. Researchers are continuing to evaluate Sun's Soup in its various formulations.

There appear to be few side effects with Sun's Soup, with the primary complaints being dissatisfaction with the taste and gastrointestinal upset. As with other complementary therapies, it is important to continue appropriate conventional treatments. The conditions Sun's Soup targets, NSCLC and AIDS, are very serious diseases. Though there are few cures with NSCLC and there is no known cure for AIDS, there are treatments that prolong life and improve QUALITY OF LIFE.

See also NUTRITIONAL THERAPY; TRADITIONAL CHINESE MEDICINE (TCM).

tai chi A gentle form of martial art that features slow, fluid movements (called forms) combined with MEDITATION. Tai chi forms represent imagery found in nature. Tai chi improves balance, STRENGTH, FLEXIBILITY, and breath control. Most people participate in tai chi in groups with a leader (master) who guides the session's movements and length, though some choose to do tai chi as a solitary practice. Many community centers, health clubs, programs for seniors, and sometimes colleges offer tai chi classes.

A typical tai chi session may take 10 minutes to an hour, depending on the form. Most people begin a tai chi session with a few minutes of meditation and BREATHING EXERCISES to help cleanse the body and focus the thoughts. Sometimes the focus on performing the motions of the form is its own meditation, and sometimes the person has a specific meditative focus that he or she holds for the duration of the session. Though tai chi is not typically aerobic because its movements are so slow, it does stretch and exercise the entire body. Often tai chi groups meet outdoors, and some people like to do tai chi barefoot to symbolically and tangibly connect themselves with the Earth and nature.

Anyone of any age can benefit from tai chi as a meditation practice and for improved balance and coordination. Doctors often recommend tai chi for people who

- are older and have increased risk for age-related falls, to help prevent injuries such as fractured hip
- have chronic health conditions such as OSTEOARTHRITIS or RHEUMATOID ARTHRITIS that threaten to restrict mobility
- have degenerative conditions such as PARKINSON'S DISEASE or MULTIPLE SCLEROSIS, to maintain

as much mobility as possible for as long as possible

- have ALZHEIMER'S DISEASE, to encourage social engagement and for the sense of comfort that the routine of tai chi imparts
- have CARDIOVASCULAR DISEASE (CVD) such as HYPERTENSION (high BLOOD PRESSURE), ATHEROSCLEROSIS, mild to moderate HEART FAILURE, or PERIPHERAL VASCULAR DISEASE (PVD), to improve blood flow and strengthen the HEART
- have OBESITY or are overweight and need a mild method to ease back into physical activity
- have CEREBRAL PALSY or other congenital disorders that affect coordination and movement

Because tai chi's movements are slow and gentle, there are few risks for most people. A tai chi master can help individuals modify tai chi forms to accommodate specific limitations and needs. People who have significantly impaired balance should do tai chi only in a group or with a partner, in case they do stumble or fall. Medications that cause drowsiness may decrease stability and balance. Most people feel relaxed yet invigorated following a tai chi session.

See also HIP FRACTURE IN OLDER ADULTS; TRADITIONAL CHINESE MEDICINE (TCM); YOGA.

therapeutic massage See MASSAGE THERAPY.

traditional Chinese medicine (TCM) A philosophy of holistic HEALING that dates to about 100 B.C.E., anchored in the premise that the energy that sustains the universe also sustains the body. Energy in balance is health; energy in imbalance is illness. Disease reflects blockages of energy that TCM therapies attempt to clear. The primary

101

energy balances are yin and yang, reflecting dual qualities of hot and cold, dark and light, male and female, and so on. TCM also draws from the five elements of nature—fire, earth, water, metal, and wood—and symbolic representations of organ systems. TCM's primary therapeutic approaches are herbal remedies and ACUPUNCTURE.

TCM physicians, also called doctors of Oriental medicine (OMDs), complete experience-based programs of study in which they serve in an apprentice fashion with a practicing TCM physician. Many of the written guidelines TCM physicians follow today derive from texts nearly as old as the practice of TCM itself, updated to accommodate modern knowledge and methods. Some states in the United States require specific licensing for TCM physicians and others for acupuncturists. A few states limit the practice of acupuncture to conventional health-care practitioners.

The TCM Physician's Examination

The TCM physician's examination differs from a conventional physician's examination in that there is considerable focus on factors such as posture, SKIN texture and tone, and how a person handles or carries his or her body. These factors often reveal to the TCM physician where and how the body's energy channels are blocked. The TCM physician also closely examines the tongue, from which TCM derives information about the state of the body's energy balances and blockages. The TCM physician also checks the PULSE at numerous points, some of which are not conventional pulse points. The TCM physician also asks many questions about the symptoms, how the person feels (physically and emotionally), the person's life experiences and circumstances, and in general listens closely to what the person describes and explains. TCM diagnoses blend symptoms, energy balance and imbalance, and the elements with perceptions of the affected organ systems and their functions. Treatments then undertake to release energy blockages to restore the flow of energy to organ systems and throughout the body.

Acupuncture

Acupuncture is a key therapeutic form in TCM. In traditional acupuncture, the TCM physician inserts hair-thin needles into specific points along energy channels called meridians. In the United States, TCM physicians and other acupuncturists use sterile, single-use needles. The needles, according to TCM, redirect the flow of energy. Contemporary Western medicine, which also incorporates acupuncture for treating chronic PAIN, ADDICTION, and other conditions, views the placement of needles as stimulating electrochemical responses in the NERVE endings. The process is painless, though some people feel a tingling sensation.

The TCM physician may place the needles in locations considerably distanced from the affected organs. For example, numerous acupuncture points on the outer EAR correlate to structures throughout the body. The outer ear is also the primary location for acupuncture points related to addiction. The needles typically stay in place for 20 to 30 minutes. Simple or acute conditions may require one to three treatment sessions; chronic or complex conditions may require a number of sessions over a period of weeks. Seldom does a condition require more than 12 treatments in total.

Chinese Herbal Remedies

Chinese herbal remedies derive from ancient recipes handed down through generations and generations of practitioners. They are precise measures of specific herbs, in specific preparations and intended for use exactly as the TCM physician prescribes, and there are thousands of different formulas as well as custom preparations that blend specific herbs into a combination to meet an individual's health needs. The remedies typically have Chinese names that reflect either the herbs they contain or the effects they are intended to achieve. Major remedies have four groups of herbs to treat four levels of the condition. The order in which the herbalist mixes the herbs together has symbolic significance that is as important as the herbs themselves. Major remedies have an emperor, minister, assistant, and envoy.

Most Chinese herbal remedies, when experienced and knowledgeable herbalists prepare them, are safe to take as the physician prescribes. Many herbal combinations contain potent ingredients and can evoke strong responses. It is important to know the source of the herbs as some herbs that come from directly from China may contain heavy metal contamination. Some herbs interact with medications, so the person always should tell the TCM physician of any medications he or she is taking. Similarly, a person taking conventional medications should first discuss Chinese herbal remedies with his or her doctor before taking the remedies.

Moxibustion

Moxibustion is a technique for heating an herbal remedy, which the TCM physician often rolls into a wicklike structure and holds just above the skin while the herbs burn. The heat further stimulates the acupuncture point below the herb, drawing the herb's healing qualities into the body's meridians (energy channels) to release stubborn energy blockages. The TCM physician may combine moxibustion with cupping, in which the physician places a small glass cup over the skin while it is still warm. The cup contains the heat, which sucks the skin surface into the cup. This also intensifies the herb's actions.

Qigong

Qigong is a form of energy work that employs structured breathing, meditation, and physical movements, similar to TAI CHI or YOGA. Qigong is an integral aspect of nearly all TCM treatment approaches because it emphasizes balancing the flow of energy. The movements and BREATHING stimulate the flow of blood as well as the LYMPH circulation, helping clear toxins and metabolic wastes more quickly from the body. Many people practice qigong privately as they would MEDITATION. The movements are more simple than those of tai chi or yoga, and easier to learn from videotapes or books. Conventional doctors may recommend qigong separate from TCM as a means of improving balance, FLEXIBILITY, and mobility in people who are elderly or who have chronic health conditions that make movement difficult.

Many communities have classes in qigong, and some hospitals use it as part of their rehabilitation programs or for stress relief. Qigong is gentle and rhythmic, providing a sense of calm and relaxation at the same time that it tones and stretches the muscles and joints. Qigong is especially helpful for people who have conditions that restrict mobility, because its regular practice improves flexibility and range of motion.

Benefits and Risks of TCM

When practiced as a complementary approach, TCM offers considerable benefits without many risks. As with all alternative and complementary methods, conventional doctors become concerned when people forgo proven conventional treatments in lieu of alternative practices. TCM methods are not proven to cure HEART disease, CANCER, DIABETES, and other such conditions. Most TCM physicians in the United States are accustomed to working in close coordination with conventional practitioners, and refer people for conventional care for conditions that require it.

See also AYURVEDA; NATIVE AMERICAN HEALING.

valerian A medicinal herb (*Valeriana officinalis*) that causes drowsiness and relaxation, commonly taken as a sleep aid. Until the twentieth century physicians also used valerian for seizures, to relieve anxiety, for mild sedation, and as a diuretic. The valerian root, or rhizome, contains the highest concentration of active ingredients and is the source of medicinal preparations. Though valerian has an unpleasant taste and smell, herbalists recommend the tea, brewed from freshly harvested or freeze-dried rhizomes, for optimal benefit. Other forms, including capsules and tablets containing ground valerian root, are also available as dietary supplements in the United States.

VALERIAN (*Valeriana officinalis*)		
Uses	Risks/Side Effects	Interactions
insomnia	excessive drowsiness	other sleep aids or
relieve		medications
anxiety		narcotic ANALGESIC
		MEDICATIONS
		ANTIANXIETY MEDICATIONS
		ANTIDEPRESSANT
		MEDICATIONS
		ANTIHISTAMINE MEDICATIONS
		MUSCLE RELAXANT
		MEDICATIONS

Efforts to isolate valerian's active ingredients have so far eluded researchers, though a number of clinical studies affirm its effectiveness as a mild sedative and sleep aid. Health experts recommend using valerian, like any other sleep aid, for no longer than two weeks. A doctor should evaluate sleep disturbances that continue longer. People who are taking other medications that cause drowsiness should not take valerian. ALCOHOL consumption also intensifies the drowsiness effect. There are no known health risks associated with valerian, though women who are pregnant or BREASTFEEDING should not take it because doctors and researchers do not know what effects, if any, it might have on the developing fetus or newborn infant.

See also GENERAL ANXIETY DISORDER (GAD); MELATONIN; SLEEP DISORDERS.

visualization A form of MEDITATION in which the person envisions his or her desired state of health or a treatment outcome such as surgery. Hospital surgery programs, CANCER recovery programs, and hospice programs began to integrate visualization methods in the 1990s. Many people find it calming and comforting to visualize themselves as healthy and whole, and many practitioners believe such visualization improves recovery rates and levels. Some people prefer guided imagery, in which a practitioner offers suggested visualizations and guides the person through the visualization process. Other people prefer to establish their own visualizations, and may integrate them with PRAYER AND SPIRITUALITY practices.

See also BIOFEEDBACK; LABYRINTH; MIND–BODY INTERACTIONS; NATIVE AMERICAN HEALING.

vitamin and mineral therapy Doses of vitamins and minerals that are higher than those typically recommended for health maintenance. Vitamin and mineral therapy derives from the perspective that depletions of vital nutrients are the primary cause of disease and that preventing these depletions can prevent the health concerns. Vitamin and mineral therapy in this context differs from routine vitamin supplementation and treatments that target specific nutritional deficiencies.

Vitamins and minerals are important nutrients the body needs to carry out its many functions. All such nutrients the body needs exist in nature and typically enter the body through foods and drinks. Even drinking water contains numerous minerals. Most people in the United States obtain adequate amounts of vitamins and minerals through appropriate dietary choices, despite concerns that the American diet on the whole is less than ideal to support health. People who live in areas where certain essential nutrients are lacking, such as selenium, which occurs in specific kinds of soil and the foods grown in them, may need to take supplements to acquire adequate amounts of those nutrients. Women who menstruate monthly may need supplemental iron to replace that lost to menstrual bleeding, and health recommendations call for supplementation of calcium and other key minerals at age 50 and older to maintain BONE density.

Conventional health experts are divided about whether healthy adults need or benefit from additional vitamins and nutrients. Some believe the ANTIOXIDANT actions of vitamins helps to prevent chronic diseases that result from cumulative damage to cells from free radicals, molecular particles that are the waste products of OXYGENATION functions (the ways in which cells metabolize nutrients to produce energy). Clinical research studies have produced conflicting results about antioxidants, however, and there remains little scientific evidence that they prevent disease or the degeneration associated with aging.

The body requires fairly small amounts of many minerals and vitamins to meet its functional needs, and excretes or stores any excess. Accumulations of certain vitamins, such as the fat-soluble vitamins A and E, may become toxic and cause health problems. Excessive mineral consumption (sodium, potassium, calcium, magnesium) can affect the body's electrolyte balance, consequentially altering KIDNEY function, cardiovascular function, and NERVOUS SYSTEM function with potentially harmful or life-threatening outcomes. The body excretes excess water-soluble vitamins (the B vitamins and vitamin C), so ingesting more than the body needs has no value. Researchers have established nutritional value ranges for most identified nutrients.

Nonetheless, many complementary approaches incorporate moderate to high doses of certain vitamins and minerals, depending on the person's symptoms. Health experts urge caution, and suggest a comprehensive NUTRITIONAL ASSESSMENT before beginning any intensive vitamin and mineral therapy. Pregnant or BREASTFEEDING women and people receiving treatment for chronic or degenerative health conditions who take regular medications should consult with their doctors, as some medications and vitamins interact to alter the action of one or the other or both. Practitioners such as naturopathic physicians and chiropractors often incorporate vitamin and mineral therapy in their practices.

See also DRUG INTERACTIONS; NUTRITIONAL THERAPY.

Y-Z

yoga A 5,000-year old practice originating in China that blends exercise and MEDITATION. Yoga incorporates specific configurations of the body called poses. Many poses are gentle and easy for most people to perform regardless of fitness level or expertise with yoga, and some poses are complex and difficult for the novice or the unconditioned to perform. Some poses are static (the person moves into and holds the pose) and some are dynamic (moving). There are several kinds of yoga. The yoga most Americans practice is Hatha yoga and its derivations. Astanga yoga, also called power yoga, is highly aerobic and requires a good FITNESS LEVEL. Some people chant during yoga, while others meditate quietly.

The essence of yoga is breath control, which ancient practitioners believed was the connection among body, mind, and spirit. Every yoga pose incorporates patterned, structured BREATHING. There are dozens of such breathing patterns, which a person also can perform independent of the yoga postures that employ them. Pulmonary care specialists often recommend yogic breathing for people who have chronic LUNG diseases or who are recovering from extensive injuries or surgery. Yogic breathing emphasizes opening the full body to the breath, and uses methods that help the body to extract more oxygen from each breath.

People who have musculoskeletal conditions such as chronic BACK PAIN or REPETITIVE MOTION INJURIES often experience pronounced benefits from yoga. Yoga can help such conditions heal by increasing blood flow to the area and by gently stretching, toning, and strengthening the involved musculoskeletal structures. Athletes may use specific yoga poses to stretch and warm up before practices, events, and competitions. Pregnant women, particularly those in the third trimester of pregnancy, often find yoga an effective way to stay fit and relieve stress. A yoga instructor can help an individual select poses specifically for his or her condition as well as modify poses to accommodate any limitations.

Health clubs, community centers, and private yoga instructors offer classes and sessions in yoga in many communities throughout the United States. Numerous books and videotapes also can teach yoga poses, though most people benefit from having a qualified yoga instructor observe their poses and help them get them right. Even the basic poses are precise in how they position and hold the body, and doing them incorrectly lessens the benefit and may cause discomfort or injury. There are no health risks associated with properly performed yoga poses.

See also TAI CHI.

yohimbe/yohimbine An herbal preparation from the bark of the African yohimbe tree (*Pausinystalia yohimbe*) taken to improve erectile function in men or as a treatment for ERECTILE DYSFUNCTION. Yohimbe may also produce a mild sense of euphoria, resulting in its reputation as an aphrodisiac. In the United States yohimbe is marketed as a dietary supplement and available without a doctor's prescription. The active ingredient in yohimbe is yohimbine. Yohimbine is available as a concentrated extract, which is much more potent than herbal yohimbe, and requires a doctor's prescription.

People sometimes call yohimbe "herbal Viagra," a reference to the prescription medication (sildenafil) for erectile dysfunction. Yohimbine, yohimbe's active ingredient, works in somewhat similar fashion to sildenafil in that causes an increase in the body's production of NOREPHINE-PHRINE which in turn increases the flow of blood to the PENIS. Norepinephrine has numerous other effects on cardiovascular function, including BLOOD PRESSURE and HEART RATE, so the US Food and Drug Administration (FDA) restricts the amount of it that is permissible in over-the-counter products.

Most health experts feel the amount of yohimbine, and thus the amount of norepinephrine, in over-the-counter yohimbe herbal remedies is too low to have a physiologic effect. They recommend that men instead see their doctors when erectile dysfunction is a concern, to identify any physical problems that might be responsible as well as to discuss options for treatment. The doctor can write a prescription for the more potent yohimbine extract if that is an appropriate therapeutic approach. Common causes of erectile dysfunction include ATHEROSCLEROSIS and PERIPHERAL VASCULAR DISEASE (PVD) resulting from CARDIOVASCULAR DISEASE (CVD) or DIABETES. Treating these underlying conditions often improves erectile function at the same time that it improves overall health. Men who have these conditions, or who take antihypertensive medications to treat HYPERTENSION (high blood pressure) generally should not take yohimbe and yohimbine products.

Yohimbe and yohimbine also block the actions of the NEUROTRANSMITTER monoamine oxidase, which may account for the mild euphoria some people experience when taking yohimbe-derived products. Monoamine oxidase affects BRAIN activity related to mood and emotion. Men who are taking monoamine oxidase inhibitor (MAOI) medications, either as ANTIDEPRESSANT MEDICATIONS or as treatment for PARKINSON'S DISEASE, should not use yohimbe products. Men who do use yohimbe products should avoid foods containing the amino acid tyramine, which requires monoamine oxidase for METABOLISM. Excess tyramine can produce numerous unpleasant symptoms, including severe HEADACHE and possible extreme spikes in blood pressure that could result in STROKE. Foods that contain tyramine include red wines, smoked meats and fish, aged cheeses, and dark chocolate.

YOHIMBE (PAUSINYSTALIA YOHIMBE)

Uses	Risks/Side Effects	Interactions
aphrodisiac ERECTILE DYSFUNCTION	elevated BLOOD PRESSURE	MAOI medications tyramine in foods

See also AROMATHERAPY; GINKGO BILOBA; LIBIDO; SAW PALMETTO.

zeaxanthin An ANTIOXIDANT that is one of the carotenoids. Zeaxanthin helps protect the health of the RETINA and to prevent AGE-RELATED MACULAR DEGENERATION (ARMD). Ophthalmologists often recommend zeanthin in combination with another carotenoid, LUTEIN, for people who are middle-aged and older. These antioxidants are present in the cells of the retina, where they absorb blue light that can damage the retina. As an antioxidant, zeaxanthin helps the retinal cells rid themselves of metabolic waste. Some studies suggest zeaxanthin and lutein may also help prevent cataracts from forming in the EYE's LENS.

ZEAXANTHIN

Uses	Risks/Side Effects	Interactions
prevent CATARACT preserve macular function possibly protect against LUNG CANCER possibly protect against OVARIAN CANCER	excessive amounts may turn the palms and soles of the feet orange or dark yellow	none known

Foods that contain zeaxanthin include dark leafy vegetables such as spinach, collard greens, broccoli, and kale. Yellow fruits and vegetables such as peaches, mangoes, squash, and corn also contain zeaxanthin. Many of the foods that are rich in zeaxanthin also contain lutein and other carotenoids. As an antioxidant, zeaxanthin may also protect against certain cancers, notably LUNG CANCER and OVARIAN CANCER. In supplement form, zeaxanthin typically appears in products that are blended carotenoids. Carotenoids appear to have greater effect in combination rather than in isolation, which is how they occur in nature, despite their individual actions and benefits.

People who take excessive amounts of carotenoid supplements may find the palms of their hands and soles of their feet take on a yellowish orange discoloration. This is a temporary effect that wears off when stopping the supplement allows the amounts of carotenoids present in the body to decrease. Taking zeaxanthin with foods that contain some fat increases the amount of zeaxanthin that enters the bloodstream from the digestive tract. Taking penicillin-based ANTIBIOTIC MEDICATIONS may decrease zeaxanthin absorption.

See also BILBERRY; LYCOPENE; PHYTOESTROGENS; RETINOPATHY.

GENETICS AND MOLECULAR MEDICINE

Genetics and molecular medicine are the disciplines in health care that focus on genetic encoding and molecular function within the cell as the foundations for health and disease. Many medical researchers believe nearly every component of health—and correspondingly, every presentation of disease—has some degree of genetic involvement and an individual acquires whatever propensity toward health that his or her genes convey. The manifestations of health and disease in many situations then become a combination of genetics and environment (lifestyle factors). The specialists who diagnose and treat GENETIC DISORDERS are geneticists.

This section, "Genetics and Molecular Medicine," presents an overview discussion of the structures and functions of human genetics and entries about genetic health and disorders. The entries in this section focus on genetic consequences for health across the spectrum of the body as a whole, including disorders and diseases that affect multiple systems. Entries in other sections of *The Facts On File Encyclopedia of Health and Medicine* provide detailed content about conditions that result from genetic disorders that affect single body systems. Cross-references connect entries with one another.

Structures of Genetics

GENE/ALLELE	cell
CHROMOSOME	nucleus
DNA	cytoplasm
RNA	ribosome
	mitochondrion
	molecule

Functions of Genetics

Genetics determines every aspect of human existence, from appearance and structure to function. Each individual acquires one set of chromosomes, the molecular presentation of heredity, from each parent. Each complete complement of chromosomes (23 pairs) contains 25,000 to 30,000 genes, the smallest structural and functional units of heredity. Each GENE pair within the structure of a

CHROMOSOME has a single and specific task. It accomplishes this task by instructing the cell to make a particular protein, a process called protein encoding. Through protein encoding genes direct every action of every cell.

The genome: the book of life The complete complement of chromosomes is the human GENOME, quite literally the book of life. The genome contains all of the instructions the body requires to take shape and to function. Within a single individual, every one of the body's 100 trillion cells contains the same set of chromosomes, so all cells in the body read from the same book of life.

DNA (deoxyribonucleic acid) is the ink of the genome, the biochemical substance that allows the GENETIC CODE to express itself. DNA organizes itself in chemical presentations called nucleotides, which function somewhat like letters. Human DNA presents a surprisingly brief alphabet for the extensive range of genetic expression it permits, forming only four NUCLEOTIDE compounds that subsequently shape the 30,000 or so genes the human genome contains. One of the most intriguing discoveries of the HUMAN GENOME PROJECT is that there are vast amounts of "empty" DNA. Only 1 to 2 percent of DNA encodes. The remaining 98 to 99 percent of DNA is noncoding, much like white space on the printed page of a book. Researchers believe noncoding DNA somehow stabilizes or in other ways supports the structure of DNA within the chromosomes.

Each gene, like a word, contains patterns of nucleotides. Chromosomes, like sentences and paragraphs, present strings of genes that convey integrated and coordinated sets of instructions for specific structures and functions throughout the body. Collectively these genetic instructions are the pages, written in code, that form an individual's GENOTYPE. The outcome, the individual's outward presentation of his or her genetic code from appearance to health, is the PHENOTYPE.

Decoding the messages: the cells The cells decode, interpret, and implement an individual's genotype. Each gene carries an encoded message that it transcribes to RNA (ribonucleic acid), a carrier molecule within the cell. The RNA conveys the gene's message to the cell's ribosomes. Ribosomes are organelles (defined structures with specific functions) within the cell. The job of the ribosome is to translate the gene's message into a specific protein. The protein then carries the message to its target within the body, which is usually molecular.

Transmitting the code: inheritance patterns The function of conveying a genotype is as much one of mathematics as biology. INHERITANCE PATTERNS—the ways in which genes reorganize into new pairs at CONCEPTION—are the patterns of statistics. A geneticist can calculate with astonishing accuracy the likelihood of certain traits passing from parents to offspring. Such calculations accommodate the potential combinations that can arise from each parent's genotype.

Health and Disorders of Genetics

In some respects what is perhaps most remarkable about human genetics is the precision and consistency with which myriad, intricate, and complex biochemical actions take place not only to produce a new human being but also to choreograph its functions for eight decades or longer. Though everyone's genotype contains some mutations, researchers believe most mutations have no consequence for the body's structure or function. However, understanding of the complex interactions among genes continues to evolve as geneticists engage in further research.

It is a common misperception that there are genes that cause disease, such that there are specific genes for HEMOPHILIA or CYSTIC FIBROSIS in the same fashion as there are certain genes for brown HAIR or green eyes. There are not really "disease" genes, however. There are instead flaws and errors in the structures of certain genes (mutations) that cause them to give the wrong instructions for synthesizing their specific proteins. The consequence is a gap, expansion, or rearrangement in the information. In some situations a gene, or more commonly a segment of or an entire chromosome, is missing—as if pages or chapters are torn from the genetic book of life. In other situations the gene may have extra material or its material is rearranged—as if pages or chapters are inserted into the book. The resulting errors in structure or function can be quite significant.

IDENTIFIED GENETIC AND MOLECULAR DISORDERS

ALPORT SYNDROME	CLEFT PALATE/CLEFT PALATE AND
CONGENITAL HEART DISEASE	LIP
CYSTIC FIBROSIS	DOWN SYNDROME
EDWARDS SYNDROME	EPIDERMOLYSIS BULLOSA
FAMILIAL ADENOMATOUS	FAMILIAL MEDITERRANEAN FEVER
POLYPOSIS (FAP)	FANCONI'S SYNDROME
FRAGILE X SYNDROME	G6PD DEFICIENCY
HEMOCHROMATOSIS	HEMOPHILIA
HEREDITARY NONPOLYPOSIS	HUNTINGTON'S DISEASE
COLORECTAL CANCER (HNPCC)	hypertrophic
KERATOCONUS	CARDIOMYOPATHY
KLINEFELTER'S SYNDROME	LONG QT SYNDROME (LQTS)
MARFAN SYNDROME	MUSCULAR DYSTROPHY
MYOPATHY	myotonia congenita
NEURAL TUBE DEFECTS	PATAU SYNDROME
PHENYLKETONURIA (PKU)	POLYDACTYLY
PORPHYRIA	PROGERIA
RETINOBLASTOMA	SICKLE CELL DISEASE
SYNDACTYLY	TAY-SACHS DISEASE
THALASSEMIA	TRIPLE X SYNDROME
TURNER'S SYNDROME	VACTERL
WILSON'S DISEASE	VON WILLEBRAND'S DISEASE
WOLFF-PARKINSON-WHITE	
SYNDROME	

Researchers have identified more than 6,000 monogenic (single gene) mutations that result in health disorders, affecting 1 child in every 200 born. Among them are CYSTIC FIBROSIS, SICKLE CELL DISEASE, MARFAN SYNDROME, HUNTINGTON'S DISEASE, and HEMOCHROMATOSIS. Other disorders, such as CLEFT PALATE/CLEFT PALATE AND LIP, result from polygenic (multiple gene) mutations or CHROMOSOMAL

DISORDERS, such as DOWN SYNDROME. Though as yet there are few treatments to alter the course of genetic and chromosomal disorders, continuing research holds promise that doctors may in the foreseeable future have the ability to offer effective therapeutic interventions.

Traditions in Medical History

In the 1660s English scientist Robert Hooke (1635–1703) used his newest invention, the compound light microscope, to examine a thin slice of cork. The increased magnifying power of this new microscope's dual lenses was considerable compared to the standard single-lens microscope of the time; and with its improved light source of reflected and focused candlelight, it revealed a level of structure in living organisms scientists had not known existed: the tight clustering of tiny compartments. Hooke called these compartments cells because they reminded him of the living quarters of monks in monasteries. Hooke described his findings and explorations of cells in his 1665 manuscript *Micrografia,* which became an epochal publication in the field of biology during Hooke's lifetime—short order for such significant recognition.

Not for another 150 years, however, did biologists finally and fully comprehend the interrelationships and organizations of cells within organisms. British botanist Robert Brown (1773–1858) discovered the cell nucleus in 1831, establishing it as the foundation of cell division; 36 years later Swiss biologist and chemist (Johann) Friedrich Miescher (1844–1895) isolated and identified the active protein–acid structure in the cell nucleus responsible for cell division. Miescher called the structure nuclein, and speculated that it not only was the key player in cell reproduction but also was the decanter of heredity itself. Miescher would never know the prophecy of his speculation because the technology to further explore such a hypothesis was still three quarters of a century away.

The words might well have gone from the scientist's mouth to the monk's ear, however. Merely a country's border away Gregor Johann Mendel (1822–1884) spent his days nurturing sweet peas in his monastery's gardens. Mendel, an Augustinian monk, observed in nature what Miescher studied in the laboratory: the paths of heredity.

Mendel crossbred his sweet peas, detailing the patterns of their varieties and alternate characteristics. Mendel would later achieve full recognition for identifying the predictable variations that occurred as the consequence of what he called paired elements of heredity. Less than two years apart these two researchers, the chemist and the botanist, published their respective findings.

In 1933 Thomas Hunt Morgan (1866–1945) received the Nobel Prize in Physiology or Medicine for proving the existence of chromosomes. By the 1940s numerous scientists were trying to unravel the cryptogram of the chromosome. James Watson and Francis Crick, working in collaboration, and Maurice Wilkins, working independently, finally succeeded. In 1953 Watson and Crick unveiled their model of the double-helix structure of deoxyribonucleic acid. DNA, the master code of genetics, was no longer a secret. Watson, Crick, and Wilkins received the 1962 Nobel Prize in Physiology or Medicine "For their discoveries concerning the molecular structure of nucleic acids and its significance for information transfer in living material."

Increasingly sophisticated technology made it possible to study the activity of the cell at the level of the molecule. Following numerous affirming discoveries about genes and DNA sequencing in the 1960s, 1970s, and 1980s, scientists began to talk of sequencing the human genome—unraveling the molecule of heredity. The effort began formally in 1988 with James Watson at the helm of the planning process. Watson saw the Human Genome Project through its official launch in 1990. Only 13 years later, 2 years ahead of schedule and on the 50th anniversary of Watson and Crick's unveiling of the double helix, the Human Genome Project announced completion of the sequencing of the human genome. "Never would I have dreamed in 1953 that my scientific life would encompass the path from DNA's double helix to the three billion steps of the human genome," Watson said in comments to the media at the events celebrating the completion of the Human Genome Project.

Breakthrough Research and Treatment Advances

The high-tech world of genetics and molecular medicine continues to drive the direction of medicine. RECOMBINANT DNA technology debuted in the

1970s, representing a breakthrough in the ability to manipulate synthetic substances such as INSULIN to create products biologically identical to endogenous substances and launching what has become known as the biotech industry. Pharmacogenomics expands the intersection of genetics and pharmacology, with researchers in both disciplines developing customized medications that integrate with an individual's genotype to produce predictable, reliable, and effective results with minimal potential for adverse DRUG reactions. Many researchers believe aging itself is a function of genetics. Continued work to understand the details of the human genome makes it not only conceivable but likely that on the horizon are therapies to correct genetic mutations and chromosomal errors, and perhaps to overcome the dimensions of aging, that are deleterious to health.

Genetics and molecular medicine open new vistas in medical ethics as well. The line between life-altering treatments and altering life itself becomes increasingly blurred. GENETIC TESTING has the capability to tell not only what is already wrong with a person but what will go wrong in the future, and sometimes even with a timeline. Medical ethicists worry that such information is too much to know and that the risk is high for physicians and their patients (and other parties that have access to the information) to believe the book of life, as it were, is carved in stone rather than set in proteins. Many variables still remain within the control of individuals in regard to health and medical decisions. Environmental interactions—lifestyle factors—can modify most health conditions associated with genetic alterations. Even with all the knowledge arising from the science fiction–like world of genetics and molecular medicine, for many people lifestyle remains the critical turning point between health and disease.

allele Any of the variations of a GENE that may occupy the same position (locus) on a CHROMOSOME. The gene controlling a particular trait or function always occupies the same locus on the same chromosome. Genes occur as pairs, with one gene coming from each parent. The pairing determines how the gene's traits are expressed in the individual. For example, the gene for BLOOD TYPE occurs at region 34 on the long arm of chromosome 9, indicated as 9q34. This gene has three alleles, identified as 9q34IA, 9q34IB, and 9q34i (which geneticists sometimes abbreviate as IA, IB, and i, respectively). These alleles can occur in one of six pairings to produce the blood type A, B, O, or AB.

When the two alleles at the same locus are the same the individual is said to be homozygous for that gene; when the alleles are different the individual is heterozygous. In a heterozygous individual generally one allele is dominant and the other recessive. Occasionally each allele in a pairing has equal dominance, a circumstance called codominance. The 9q34i allele (type O) is recessive; the 9q34IA and 9q34IB alleles (type A and type B) are dominant. When the 9q34IA and 9q34IB alleles pair, their expression is codominant. The possible allele pairings for blood type can produce any of these expressions.

For further discussion of alleles within the context of the structures and functions of genetics, please see the overview section "Genetics and Molecular Medicine."

See also GENOTYPE; INHERITANCE PATTERNS; PHENOTYPE.

apoptosis The natural mechanism through which a cell engages in actions that lead to its death, often called programmed cell death or cell suicide. Apoptosis appears linked to SENESCENCE, an inherent limitation on the number of times a cell can divide. Both apoptosis and senescence play significant roles in the aging process. Once the cell initiates apoptosis there is no reversal; the process proceeds until the cell dies.

Apoptosis begins when the cell's DNA fragments, signaling or switching the rest of the process in motion. Once activated apoptosis sets in motion the subsequent events result in the cell's disman-

EXAMPLE ALLELE PAIRINGS AND EXPRESSION: BLOOD TYPE		
Allele Pairing	**Expression**	**Blood Type**
IaIa (A+A)	Homozygous dominant	Type A
Iai (A+O)	Heterozygous dominant	
IbIb (B+B)	Homozygous dominant	Type B
Ibi (B+O)	Heterozygous dominant	
ii (O+O)	Homozygous recessive	Type O
IaIb (A+B)	Heterozygous codominant	Type AB

tling, assimilation, and recycling. In some respects cells become endlessly renewable resources for the body. Specialized cells called phagocytes break down dying and dead cells into basic components such as amino acids that other the body can use to construct new cells.

Apoptosis is necessary for growth, development, and change in the body. The process of the death of cells that experience injury or damage is called necrosis and by definition occurs outside the natural order of cell life expectancy. Extrinsic, rather than intrinsic, factors initiate necrosis.

See also CELL STRUCTURE AND FUNCTION; METABOLISM; PHAGOCYTE; PHAGOCYTOSIS; STEM CELL.

autosomal trisomy   A chromosomal disorder in which there are three instead of the normal two copies of an AUTOSOME (nonsex chromosome). An autosomal trisomy may be complete (affect all cells) or mosaic (affect only some cells). The most commonly occurring complete autosomal trisomies that are survivable are those involving chromosomes 21, 18, and 13, which result in the chromosomal disorders DOWN SYNDROME (trisomy 21), EDWARDS SYNDROME (trisomy 18), and PATAU'S SYNDROME (trisomy 13). These trisomy disorders may also occur as a mosaic. Mosaic autosomal trisomies typically produce less severe, though still significant, physical and mental impairments. Complete autosomal trisomies affecting other chromosomes are often lethal, nearly always causing death early in development and well before birth.

Though the risk for autosomal trisomy disorders increases with a woman's age at the time she becomes pregnant, most autosomal trisomy disorders occur in pregnancies in younger women because the rate of CONCEPTION is significantly higher among younger women. The risk is highest for women who have previously given birth to a child with a trisomy disorder. Obstetricians can detect fetal trisomy disorders generally within the first and early part of the second trimesters of PREGNANCY with prenatal tests. The diagnostic path usually incorporates a combination procedures including

- BLOOD tests that look at the levels of proteins the FETUS and placenta are making

- ULTRASOUND, which shows physical anomalies that suggest a chromosomal disorder

- CHORIONIC   VILLI   SAMPLING   (CVS)   and AMNIOCENTESIS, which permit examination of fetal cells

See also BIRTH DEFECTS; CHROMOSOMAL DISORDERS; CONGENITAL ANOMALY; GENETIC COUNSELING; GENETIC TESTING; MOSAICISM; PREGNANCY.

autosome   A CHROMOSOME that appears as a pair in which both chromosomes are the same in either sex, also called a nonsex chromosome. In contrast, the sex chromosomes appear as a pair that is different in males and females. The human GENOME contains 22 autosomes and one pair of sex chromosomes for a total complement of 46 chromosomes as 23 pairs.

For further discussion of autosomes within the context of the structures and functions of genetics, please see the overview section "Genetics and Molecular Medicine."

See also GENE; GENOTYPE; KARYOTYPE; PHENOTYPE; SEX CHROMOSOME.

cell structure and function   The cell is the basic structural and functional unit of all living organisms. About 100 trillion cells make up one of the most complex of such organisms, the human.

Types of Cells in the Human Body
There are three basic types of cells in the body: stem cells, germ cells, and somatic cells.

The foundation of life: stem cells   Stem cells are the primal, undifferentiated cells that give rise to all other cells. They are primarily abundant and functional during early embryonic development (embryonic stem cells). These are the cells of the blastocyst, the earliest form of a new life, and at this stage are totipotent: They have the ability to become any other kind of cell. Genes instruct dividing stem cells how to differentiate or form specific kinds of cells that then develop into various organs and body structures.

UMBILICAL CORD BLOOD STEM CELLS

The BLOOD that remains in the UMBILICAL CORD and PLACENTA at birth is an abundant source of multipotent BLOOD STEM CELLS. Cord blood transplantation is an emerging treatment for LEUKEMIA and other cancers as well as SICKLE CELL DISEASE and other blood disorders. Many people now opt to collect and store or donate the cord blood of their newborns after birth.

As the body takes shape stem cells become increasingly diffuse and specialized, transitioning to pluripotent (able to become cells of distinct body systems such as cardiovascular or gastrointestinal) and finally multipotent (able to become cells of specific kinds, such as BLOOD or BONE). The most versatile stem cell that remains when development is complete is the blood stem cell, which has the ability to differentiate into various types of blood cells throughout life. Other adult stem cells (also called somatic stem cells to distinguish them from embryonic stem cells) exist in most body tissues though are interspersed among other cells. Their role remains unclear though they appear responsible for large-scale regeneration of tissue such as can occur in the LIVER.

The cells of reproduction: germ cells   Germ cells, also called gametes, are the cells of reproduction: the OVA or eggs (female) and the spermatozoa or SPERM (male). Gametes are haploid cells; each GAMETE contains one-half the complement of chromosomes. When two gametes merge in CONCEPTION, the resulting ZYGOTE acquires the full complement of genetic material.

The cells of the functioning body: somatic cells   All cells that are not stem cells or germ cells are somatic cells. Somatic cells make up more than 99 percent of the cells in the adult body. They are diploid cells; each somatic cell contains the full complement of chromosomes. Somatic cells make up the organs and structures of the body. They are the body's primary working units, responsible for carrying out the myriad functions of METABOLISM that support life. Though similar in structure and function, somatic cells are broadly diverse in their activities and specializations.

Cell Structure
Most cells have standard, key structural components in common. These include

- PLASMA membrane, the cell's outer wall made up of a protein layer and a lipid (fatty) layer, that separates the cell's contents from its external environment yet permits interaction between the cell and the external environment

- cytoskeleton, a dynamic construct of filaments and fibers that support the cell's shape and inner components
- cytoplasm, a watery fluid that suspends the inner structures of the cell, moves substances through the cell, and conducts electricity
- nucleus, the core of the cell, separated from the cytoplasm by a thin membrane called the nuclear envelope, which contains the cell's chromosomes and genetic material
- mitochondria, self-replicating structures called organelles that generate the energy, in the form of adenosine triphosphate (ATP), the cell needs to function
- ribosomes, another type of organelle, which synthesize proteins according to genetic directions the mitochondrial RNA brings to the ribosomes
- lysosomes and peroxisomes, also organelles, which contain enzymes to break down cellular wastes into component molecules the cell can recycle

Cell Function

The cell is responsible for all of the functions of metabolism that support the body. Most of the body's 100 trillion cells have specialized responsibilities. Blood cells transport oxygen, GLUCOSE, and other NUTRIENTS throughout the body and collect molecules of metabolic waste that cells in the liver and KIDNEYS dismantle, recycle, or eliminate from the body. NERVE cells conduct electrical impulses. MUSCLE cells contract the HEART and move the body. Other cells make hormones, absorb nutrients, fight INFECTION, and so on. Regardless of their specializations, however, the primary activity of all cells is the synthesis of the enzymes and proteins that carry out the biochemical tasks of living.

Cell Division

One of the most important functions of a cell is to replicate itself, as this is the activity that sustains life. Some cells, such as those that line the gastrointestinal tract, replicate every 12 hours. Other cells, such as those in the heart and the liver, divide perhaps once every 12 months or so. Though cells have vast ability to perpetrate themselves in such fashion, there appear to be gene-

mediated limits to the number of times cells may divide.

Cells replicate by dividing themselves, a process called mitosis (somatic cells) or meiosis (gametes). Mitosis is a multistage process during which the cell's chromosomes pull together and duplicate themselves. When this duplication is complete the cell then pulls apart into two new cells, called daughter cells, with one package of chromosomal content (called a CHROMATID) going with each daughter cell. In this way each daughter cell receives the full complement of chromosomes. Meiosis has two stages, meiosis 1 and meiosis 2. There is duplication of chromosomal material in meiosis 1 but not in meiosis 2, such that one cell ultimately produces four gametes.

For further discussion of cell structure and function within the context of genetics, please see the overview section "Genetics and Molecular Medicine."

See also APOPTOSIS; BLOOD TRANSFUSION; CENTROMERE; CHROMOSOME; HORMONE; INHERITANCE PATTERNS; PREGNANCY; SENESCENCE; SOMATIC CELL; STEM CELL; TELOMERE.

centromere   The position on a CHROMOSOME where the chromosome separates during cell division. The centromere is a structure of noncoding DNA (DNA that does not convey genetic information). When the cell divides the strands of the chromatids migrate in opposite directions (pull apart) at the centromere. In a photomicrograph, the centromere appears as an indented, waistlike area on the chromosome. Geneticists use the centromere's position, along with other characteristics of the chromosome, to match chromosomes into their pairs when creating KARYOTYPES.

For further discussion of centromeres within the context of the structures and functions of genetics, please see the overview section "Genetics and Molecular Medicine."

See also ALLELE; CELL STRUCTURE AND FUNCTION; CHROMATID; GAMETE; GENE; GENOTYPE; PHENOTYPE; SOMATIC CELL; TELOMERE.

chromatid   A replica of a CHROMOSOME that develops in preparation for cell division. Chromatids are "sister" pairs of each chromosome that contain identical genetic material. They remain attached to each other at the CENTROMERE until cell division. When the mother cell divides, the sister chromatids separate at the centromere and migrate into the new daughter cells, forming the chromosome pairs for the new cells. Though minor variations are normal and frequently occur without causing problems because they affect relatively few cells, errors in chromatid replication and separation affect many or all cells and can be responsible for CHROMOSOMAL DISORDERS such as DOWN SYNDROME.

For further discussion of chromatids within the context of the structures and functions of genetics, please see the overview section "Genetics and Molecular Medicine."

See also CELL STRUCTURE AND FUNCTION; DNA; GENETIC DISORDERS; MOSAICISM; MUTATION; NUCLEOTIDE; VARIATION.

chromosomal disorders Abnormalities affecting the chromosomes that result in syndromes (constellations of symptoms) having characteristic physical or functional anomalies. Most chromosomal disorders occur because of alterations in the number of chromosomes or the structure of chromosomes. Though an individual may inherit a chromosomal disorder, more commonly chromosomal disorders represent random occurrences. Typically all the cells in the body reflect the abnormality. Occasionally some but not all cells carry the chromosomal abnormality; this is a mosaic chromosomal disorder. A mosaic presentation tends to be milder than that observed when all cells carry the chromosomal abnormality

Disorders of Replication

Normally chromosomes exist in pairs. Replication errors can result in an incorrect number of chromosomes passing to new cells. Though such errors can occur in any cell with any episode of cell division, they are most harmful when they affect gametes (the sex cells, the ovum in the female and the spermatozoon in the male). Replication errors in gametes become chromosomal disorders in the new life created through their union. These errors may take the form of trisomy (an extra CHROMOSOME), monosomy (a missing chromosome), or uniparental disomy (both copies of a chromosome come from the same GAMETE or parent).

Trisomy Disorders of trisomy occurs when the ZYGOTE receives three instead of the normal two copies of a chromosome. Most trisomies are autosomal, and most autosomal trisomies are lethal very early in embryonic development. Most early losses due to trisomy thus likely escape detection. The survivable autosomal trisomies affect chromosome 13 (PATAU'S SYNDROME), chromosome 18 (EDWARDS SYNDROME), and chromosome 21 (DOWN SYNDROME). Trisomies can also involve the sex chromosomes. The most common such disorder is KLINEFELTER'S SYNDROME, in which the zygote receives two (and sometimes more) X chromosomes and one Y chromosome. Though the Y chromosome determines the gender as male, the additional X chromosome affects sexual development and FERTILITY. The zygote may also receive three X chromosomes (triple X syndrome) or one X chromosome and two Y chromosomes. These trisomies may not produce obvious symptoms, though often boys who have XYY syndrome have developmental delays and learning disabilities.

Monosomy Monosomy occurs when the zygote receives only one copy of a chromosome and overall occur far less frequently than trisomy because an entire missing autosome (nonsex chromosome) is nearly always lethal. The monosomy disorder Turner syndrome, in which the zygote receives only one X SEX CHROMOSOME, is one of the few survivable monosomy disorders. Because the single sex chromosome is X, the zygote is female although breast development at sexual maturity is diminished.

Uniparental disomy In uniparental disomy the zygote receives two copies of a chromosome from one gamete and none from the other gamete. Though in many cases this REPLICATION ERROR may result in no adverse symptoms or consequences, it can allow rare recessive disorders to manifest. Uniparental disomy also causes symptoms when the involved chromosome is one in which GENETIC IMPRINTING is essential. In such circumstances the chromosome pairing requires one chromosome from each parent to activate the chromosome's genetic functions.

Disorders of Structure

Chromosomal disorders of structure occur when there are physical changes to the chromosome that alter its configuration. In TRANSLOCATION, fragments of a chromosome break away and reattach to other chromosomes or are lost, potentially changing several chromosomes with unpredictable and random results. Inversions, rings, duplications, and deletions are other disorders of structure involving fragments of the chromosome that are fairly uncommon though tend to produce symptoms when they occur. The types of symptoms depend on the involved chromosome.

Inversions In a chromosomal inversion the chromosome breaks in two or more locations, then the segments rejoin with one or more segments inverted (upside-down). Some genetic material may be lost in the process, and the genes are out of position. Inversions may or may not cause symptoms, depending on the involved chromosome and the degree of inversion.

Rings Chromosomal rings occur when the ends of the chromosome are missing and the remaining chromosome reshapes itself into a ring. The extent and nature of symptoms depends on the involved chromosome and the amount of missing genetic material. A ring of chromosome 15, for example, tends to produce symptoms such as facial anomalies and growth deficiency.

Duplications and deletions In duplications and deletions, the chromosome acquires (duplication) or loses (deletion) fragments of its structure. The severity of the consequences depends on the chromosome involved and the extent of the altered genetic material.

Symptoms and Diagnostic Path
The symptoms of chromosomal disorders vary with the chromosome involved and the extent of damage present. Because chromosomal disorders tend to affect large segments of genetic material, the resulting symptoms and syndromes are often complex and affect multiple organs, structures, functions, and systems. The diagnostic path may include imaging procedures such as ULTRASOUND, COMPUTED TOMOGRAPHY (CT) SCAN, and MAGNETIC RESONANCE IMAGING (MRI) to evaluate structural anomalies of internal organs. A KARYOTYPE (picture of the chromosomes a in a cell) reveals overt chromosomal problems, and molecular studies may be necessary to unravel the circumstances of less obvious chromosomal disruptions.

Treatment Options and Outlook
For nearly all chromosomal disorders, treatment focuses on improving physical anomalies and maintaining function to the extent possible. Children born with chromosomal disorders often require ongoing medical care and other kinds of support. Outlook and QUALITY OF LIFE vary widely even within the same syndrome.

Risk Factors and Preventive Measures
Most chromosomal disorders are random events for which there are no preventive measures. Parental age and exposure to teratogenic substances (chemicals, drugs, or other materials that disrupt embryonic or fetal development) are risk factors for certain chromosomal disorders. Doctors recommend all women of childbearing age who could become pregnant, whether or not they are planning PREGNANCY, take folic acid supplementation, which appears to reduce the risk for numerous congenital anomalies and perhaps chromosomal damage.

See also CONGENITAL ANOMALY; GENETIC DISORDERS; INHERITANCE PATTERNS.

chromosome A coiled DNA molecule within the cell's nucleus that carries an individual's GENETIC CODE. Most of the time the chromosome's structure is loose and indistinguishable. Only in the stage of cell division immediately before the cell divides (the metaphase) does the chromosome draw itself into a compact, rodlike structure the geneticist can see under a microscope after applying a special dye to the cell that the chromosomes absorb. It is this ability to absorb a colored dye that gives the chromosome its name, which means "colored body."

Chromosome Complements
The nucleus of every diploid cell, also called a SOMATIC CELL, contains the full complement of 46 chromosomes arranged in 23 pairs. One pair contains the sex chromosomes that establish gender, paired either as XX (female) or XY (male). The other 22 pairs are autosomes. The haploid cells, the gametes (spermatozoa and OVA), contain one half the chromosome complement. When gametes merge in CONCEPTION the diploid cell they form, the ZYGOTE, acquires the full chromosomal comple-

ment. The only cells in the body that do not have chromosomes are the erythrocytes, which do not have nuclei.

Autosomes carry the bulk of genetic code. Thousands of genes line each autosome, each in its ordained position. The sex chromosomes carry several hundred genes. The GENE positions, called loci (in the singular, each position is a locus), are constant. For example, the gene loci for the ABO BLOOD TYPE are always on chromosome 9, those for the rhesus (Rh) blood type are on chromosome 1, and those for EYE color on chromosomes 15 and 19.

CHROMOSOME SIZE

The HUMAN GENOME PROJECT, completed in 2003, revealed the structure of chromosomes to be much larger and more complex than scientists previously had theorized. Chromosome 1, the largest CHROMOSOME, contains 2,968 genes. The smallest chromosome, the Y chromosome, contains 231 genes.

Nomenclature

Geneticists designate the normal female chromosome complement as 46,XX and the normal male chromosome complement as 46,XY. Deviations from the norm are CHROMOSOMAL DISORDERS geneticists designate according to the deviation, for example 47,XY,+21 denotes AUTOSOMAL TRISOMY 21 (DOWN SYNDROME) in a male. The designation 45,X denotes TURNER SYNDROME, a monosomy disorder (missing chromosome) affecting the SEX CHROMOSOME in a female. A comprehensive standard of nomenclature (naming) exists so all geneticists can use a common "language" when describing chromosomal and genetic configurations.

A chromosome's structure consists of two telomeres (end segments), a CENTROMERE (waistlike indentation), and two arms (the segments above and below the centromere). The centromere is somewhat off-center, such that each chromosome has a short arm (designated "p" for *petite*) and a long arm (designated "q" because scientific nomenclature is alphabetical). The regions of each arm are numbered. Geneticists identify a gene's locus relative to its placement on the chromosome. The gene responsible for CYSTIC FIBROSIS, for example, is identified as CFTR 7q31.2—cystic fibrosis transmembrane conductance regulator located in band 31, region 2, on the long arm of chromosome 7.

For further discussion of chromosomes within the context of the structures and functions of genetics, please see the overview section "Genetics and Molecular Medicine."

See also AUTOSOME; ERYTHROCYTE; GAMETE; GENETIC DISORDERS; GENOME; GENOTYPE; PHENOTYPE; SPERM; TELOMERE.

cloning The creation of exact copies of a GENE, cell, or entire organism. Such exact copies occur naturally when a ZYGOTE divides to become identical multiples such as twins or, less commonly, triplets. Manipulated cloning is primarily a research method at present, though scientists use cloning for therapeutic applications in creating RECOMBINANT DNA products such as INSULIN. Insulin was the first human gene cloned (1978) as well as the first genetically engineered product approved for use in the United States (1982). The cloning of entire organisms, such as Dolly the sheep in 1997, though sensational, is extraordinarily challenging. Currently, cloned organisms appear prone to numerous health problems and tend to die prematurely, which somewhat mystifies researchers because natural clones such as identical twins do not experience these challenges. Numerous ethical issues surround the use of entire organism cloning, particularly EMBRYO cloning.

Scientists create gene clones by removing the DNA from a vector such as a bacterium cell and replacing it with the DNA of choice. The bacterium rapidly replicates, creating multiple identical copies of the DNA. Similarly, this process can create identical replicas of cells. Researchers are hopeful that this technology will someday lead to the ability to generate replacement tissues and organs to treat various health conditions that currently rely on therapies such as ORGAN TRANSPLANTATION. This technology further holds promise for treating degenerative conditions such as PARKINSON'S DISEASE and HUNTINGTON'S DISEASE. Cloning is also one method of potential GENE THERAPY.

See also CELL STRUCTURE AND FUNCTION; ETHICAL ISSUES IN GENETICS AND MOLECULAR MEDICINE.

congenital anomaly A physical abnormality present at birth. Congenital anomalies, also called BIRTH DEFECTS, can affect nearly any structure in the body and may be hereditary or random. GENETIC DISORDERS and exposure to teratogens (substances, such as drugs, that alter the development of the embryo or fetus) account for the majority of congenital anomalies. The symptom constellations that characterize CHROMOSOMAL DISORDERS typically contain multiple congenital anomalies.

Some congenital anomalies are almost always treatable, such as atrial septal defect (an abnormal opening in the septum, or wall, between the two atria in the HEART) or CLEFT PALATE/CLEFT PALATE AND LIP (failure of the oral structures to properly close). Other congenital anomalies are life-altering or life-threatening, such as severe forms of SPINA BIFIDA (in which the spine fails to form properly) or transposition of the great arteries (incorrect alignment of the major BLOOD vessels in the heart).

Many congenital anomalies are physically apparent at birth or manifest symptoms that reveal their presence. An infant born with congenital anomalies of the heart, for example, may have a bluish hue to the SKIN (CYANOSIS) that indicates insufficient oxygen to the tissues. The diagnostic path may include imaging procedures such as ULTRASOUND, COMPUTED TOMOGRAPHY (CT) SCAN, and MAGNETIC RESONANCE IMAGING (MRI) that allow the neonatologist to visualize and identify the anomaly. GENETIC TESTING may also be appropriate, depending on the nature of the anomaly. Treatment depends on the type, extensiveness, and complexity of the anomaly. Surgeons often can easily repair isolated anomalies, such as cleft lip or atrial septal defect, with minimal or no residual consequences. Extensive or multisystem anomalies may not be treatable.

See also CONGENITAL HEART DISEASE; HORSESHOE KIDNEY; REPLICATION ERROR.

cystic fibrosis An inherited genetic disorder resulting from multiple mutations of the cystic fibrosis transmembrane conductance regulator (CFTR) GENE on CHROMOSOME 7, inherited as autosomal recessive mutations. Researchers believe as many as 10 million people may be cystic fibrosis carriers and unaware of it. Though researchers

know of approximately 600 CFTR mutations, one MUTATION, called the delta F508 mutation, accounts for about 70 percent of cystic fibrosis in the United States. About 30,000 Americans live with cystic fibrosis.

CFTR is a protein that, when functioning normally, facilitates the transport of chloride and other ions across cell membranes. In cystic fibrosis the presence of CFTR is greatly diminished and salts fail to properly cross the cell membranes. One result is very high concentrations of salts in the sweat, particularly chloride, giving the SKIN a salty taste. The effect of diminished CFTR is most pronounced on epithelial secretory cells—the cells that form mucous membranes and make up the linings of the intestinal tract, LUNGS, and urinary system, which rely on sodium chloride and other salts to draw fluid into their secretions. Without CFTR the normal watery secretions of these cells become thick and sticky.

Cystic fibrosis most seriously affects the pulmonary and gastrointestinal systems, and does so in all people who have the disorder, though the disorder involves all body systems to varying extents. Thickened secretions accumulate in the airways in the lungs, creating obstructions that interfere with BREATHING as well as establish breeding grounds for BACTERIA and other pathogens. Furthermore, the high chloride content on the surface of the epithelial cells that line the bronchial structures suppresses the body's natural bacterial-control mechanisms. People who have cystic fibrosis have frequent or chronic upper respiratory infections and pneumonias. About 85 percent of people who have cystic fibrosis also develop pancreatic insufficiency, in which the DIGESTIVE ENZYMES the PANCREAS normally secretes do not adequately support digestion.

Symptoms and Diagnostic Path

Infants who have cystic fibrosis may have MECONIUM ileus at birth, an obstruction of the bowel with meconium, a tarry substance that normally passes from the RECTUM within a few hours of birth. Other signs and symptoms of cystic fibrosis may emerge at any time and include

- large, foul-smelling, greasy-looking stools
- frequent bowel blockages

- thick SPUTUM
- coughing and wheezing
- clubbing of the fingers and toes
- INTUSSUSCEPTION (a segment of the bowel "telescopes" into another segment), a potentially life-threatening circumstance
- RECTAL PROLAPSE
- nasal polyps

Men who have cystic fibrosis nearly always have congenital bilateral absence of the vas deferens, which results in INFERTILITY, though the TESTES and other structures of the male sex organs function normally.

The diagnostic path begins with a skin salt test that measures the amount of chloride present on the surface of the skin. In cystic fibrosis these levels are five to six times normal; such a finding is generally conclusive of a diagnosis of cystic fibrosis, especially in combination with other characteristic symptoms. A BLOOD or saliva test also can confirm the presence of a cystic fibrosis mutation. Other blood tests help to assess the level of damage organ systems have experienced.

Treatment Options and Outlook

The most serious and common consequence of cystic fibrosis is lung damage. Doctors may prescribe ANTIBIOTIC MEDICATIONS to curtail infections, mucolytic agents and mechanical methods such as CHEST PERCUSSION AND POSTURAL DRAINAGE to help thin secretions, and bronchodilator medications to open the airways. An aerosol spray medication, dornase alpha, uses enzymes to break up secretions so the person can more easily COUGH them up. Other treatments may include pancreatic enzyme supplementation and high liquid consumption.

Cystic fibrosis is the leading reason for LUNG TRANSPLANTATION, which is a treatment that becomes necessary when the lungs can no longer function. Some people who have severe cystic fibrosis undergo simultaneous pancreas and lung transplantation. Such surgery is extensive and ORGAN TRANSPLANTATION requires lifelong IMMUNOSUPPRESSIVE THERAPY. These treatments are relatively new, so doctors do not know their long-term success. With appropriate medical management some people who have cystic fibrosis can live into at least midlife with relatively few significant complications.

Risk Factors and Preventive Measures

Cystic fibrosis is an autosomal recessive disorder acquired when each parent carries the gene mutation. Preconception GENETIC SCREENING is the only way to prevent parents from passing cystic fibrosis to their children. Because the projected number of cystic fibrosis carriers is so high (1 in 20 among Caucasians of northern European ancestry), many doctors offer cystic fibrosis screening to adults who are planning families. Though researchers hope GENE THERAPY may offer a cure for cystic fibrosis in the future, such approaches are only in the early stages of experimentation.

See also CARRIER; CYSTIC FIBROSIS AND THE LUNGS; FAMILY PLANNING; GENETIC COUNSELING; GENETIC DISORDERS; INFECTION; INHERITANCE PATTERNS; NASAL POLYP; PATHOGEN; PNEUMONIA.

D

DNA The abbreviation for deoxyribonucleic acid. DNA is the molecule of heredity; its sequences form the body's GENETIC CODE. Each cell in the body contains DNA within the chromosomes in its nucleus (except erythrocytes, which do not have nuclei). DNA has a characteristic double-helix structure that resembles a gently twisting ladder. The supporting rails of this structure are deoxyribose, a sugar-phosphate, and the cross-bands are nitrogen bases: adenine (A), thymine (T), guanine (G), and cytosine (C). These bases pair in precise, predictable patterns arranged in nearly endless combinations, more than three billion in all.

British scientists James Watson and Francis Crick unraveled the double-helix structure of DNA in 1953, identifying its two spiraling, sugar–phosphate (deoxyribose) supports and cross-bands of paired nucleic acids. Just 50 years later researchers involved with the HUMAN GENOME PROJECT concluded their mapping of the human GENOME, which included determining the entire biochemical sequence of human DNA. Chromosomes are structures of DNA, and genes are segments of chromosomes (also made up of DNA).

For further discussion of DNA within the context of the structures and functions of genetics, please see the overview section "Genetics and Molecular Medicine."

See also CELL STRUCTURE AND FUNCTION; CHROMOSOME; ERYTHROCYTE; GENOTYPE; RNA.

Down syndrome An AUTOSOMAL TRISOMY disorder that results from a REPLICATION ERROR during cell division in which a GAMETE (sex cell) ends up with two copies of CHROMOSOME 21 instead of the normal single copy (as haploid cells, gametes contain one half the complement of chromosomes). At CONCEPTION the ZYGOTE thus ends up with three instead of the normal two copies of chromosome 21, which ultimately produces multiple congenital anomalies. When all cells carry the extra chromosome, the resulting anomalies occasionally may be so severe that the disorder is lethal before birth. Sometimes Down syndrome occurs as a mosaic disorder in which some but not all cells contain the extra chromosome 21, which typically produces milder symptoms.

Down syndrome occurs in about 1 in 1,200 live births in the United States and about 350,000 Americans currently live with Down syndrome, many independently. Though the risk for Down syndrome increases dramatically with maternal age, most infants who have Down syndrome are born to younger mothers because the increased rate of CONCEPTION more than offsets the increase in age-related risk. Down syndrome is the most commonly occurring of the autosomal trisomy disorders.

Symptoms and Diagnostic Path
Children born with Down syndrome often have characteristic facial features, which include

- flat, upwardly slanting eyes with extra fatty tissue in the lids
- rounded face with a small NOSE and MOUTH
- small ears
- broad, short neck
- short stature with noticeably small hands and short fingers

Other findings of Down syndrome include congenital anomalies affecting the HEART, intestines, and other organs. About half of infants born with

Down syndrome have atrial or ventricular septal defects (openings or holes in the septum, or wall, between the chambers of the heart). About half also have impaired vision (notably, congenital cataracts and AMBLYOPIA) and partial to complete HEARING LOSS. About 10 percent have malformations of the intestines that require surgical correction. All individuals with Down syndrome have some intellectual impairment. Mild to moderate intellectual impairment is most common. Some children who have Down syndrome do well in regular classes in school and grow up to be capable of independent living.

Doctors often can diagnose Down syndrome and other autosomal trisomy disorders before birth using prenatal screening methods such as blood tests, ULTRASOUND, AMNIOCENTESIS, and CHORIONIC VILLI SAMPLING (CVS). These methods retrieve cells from the FETUS from which a geneticist can construct a KARYOTYPE, which presents photomicrographic images of the fetus's or infant's chromosomes. Advanced maternal age (mother's age over 40) and the previous conception of a child with Down syndrome or another autosomal trisomy disorder are the leading risks for Down syndrome. Whether done prenatally or after birth the karyotype provides definitive diagnosis.

Treatment Options and Outlook

There are no specific treatments for Down syndrome. Because children who have Down syndrome are more susceptible to INFECTION, they often need more medical care while growing up. There is a high correlation between early-onset ALZHEIMER'S DISEASE and adults who have Down syndrome. Typically men who have Down syndrome are sterile, though women who have Down syndrome may be fertile and can become pregnant. Their risk for conceiving a child with Down syndrome is very high, however, and doctors strongly recommend GENETIC COUNSELING.

About 350,000 Americans live with Down syndrome. Because Down syndrome is the mildest of the survivable trisomy disorders and because it can occur in a mosaic rather than a complete presentation, some people who have it are able to lead relatively independent and productive lives, living into their mid-50s or beyond. Early treatment for the anomalies common with Down syndrome, such as septal defects, and ongoing care for other health conditions, such as HYPOTHYROIDISM and VISION IMPAIRMENT, have greatly improved both health and QUALITY OF LIFE for people who have Down syndrome.

Risk Factors and Preventive Measures

Down syndrome occurs as a replication error that does not appear to be preventable, though recent research suggests that folic acid supplementation beginning before conception and extending through PREGNANCY, such as obstetricians recommend for preventing NEURAL TUBE DEFECTS, may reduce the risk for Down syndrome. Older women, who have a higher risk of conceiving a child with Down syndrome, may opt for genetic testing early in pregnancy to determine whether the fetus has the trisomy 21 GENOTYPE. Knowing allows the woman to make appropriate plans and decisions regarding the pregnancy and potential care needs of the child.

CONGENITAL ANOMALIES CHARACTERISTIC OF DOWN SYNDROME	
AMBLYOPIA	atrial septal defect
BOWEL ATRESIA	broad, short neck
congenital cataracts	developmental delays
flat, upwardly slanting eyes	HEARING LOSS
intellectual impairment	rounded face
short stature	small ears
small hands and short fingers	small NOSE and MOUTH
ventricular septal defect	

See also AUTOSOME; CATARACT; CONGENITAL ANOMALY; CHROMOSOME DISORDERS; CONGENITAL HEART DISEASE; EDWARDS SYNDROME; ETHICAL ISSUES IN GENETICS AND MOLECULAR MEDICINE; GENETIC SCREENING; INHERITANCE PATTERNS; MOSAICISM; PATAU'S SYNDROME; PRENATAL CARE.

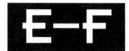

Edwards syndrome An AUTOSOMAL TRISOMY disorder that results from a REPLICATION ERROR during cell division in which a GAMETE (sex cell) ends up with two copies of CHROMOSOME 18 instead of the normal single copy (as haploid cells, gametes contain one half the complement of chromosomes). At fertilization the ZYGOTE thus ends up with three instead of the normal two copies of chromosome 18, which ultimately produces multiple and life-threatening congenital anomalies.

When all cells carry the extra chromosome 18), the anomalies are so severe that the defect often is lethal well before birth. Sometimes Edwards syndrome occurs as a mosaic trisomy disorder (some but not all cells contain the third chromosome 18), which tends to produce milder though nonetheless significant symptoms. Edwards syndrome occurs in about 1 in 5,000 live births in the United States, 80 percent of which are females. Researchers do not know whether Edwards syndrome affects females more often or if females are more likely to survive beyond birth.

Children born with Edwards syndrome have severe and complex physical deformities involving multiple organs and systems that require extensive medical care from the time of birth. Most also have profound intellectual impairment arising from malformations affecting the BRAIN and NERVOUS SYSTEM. A KARYOTYPE confirms the diagnosis. Fewer than 10 percent of infants born with Edwards syndrome survive the first year after birth; those who do require extensive, ongoing medical care and developmental support. Survival beyond five years is extremely rare.

Doctors often can diagnose Edwards syndrome and other autosomal trisomy disorders before birth, through prenatal screening methods such as AMNIOCENTESIS and CHORIONIC VILLI SAMPLING (CVS).

These methods retrieve cells from the FETUS from which a geneticist can construct a karyotype. Advanced maternal age (mother's age over 40) and the previous CONCEPTION of a child with Edwards syndrome or another autosomal trisomy disorder are the leading risks for Edwards syndrome. Whether done prenatally or after birth the karyotype, which presents photomicrographic images of the fetus's or infant's chromosomes, provides definitive diagnosis.

CONGENITAL ANOMALIES
CHARACTERISTIC OF EDWARDS SYNDROME

facial deformities
fingers curled over one another in clenched fists
heart defects
kidney abnormalities
low, small ears
microcephaly (small head and BRAIN)
small MOUTH and cleft deformities
spina bifida
SYNDACTYLY
TALI PEDES (club foot)

See also AUTOSOME; CHROMOSOME DISORDERS; CONGENITAL ANOMALY; CONGENITAL HEART DISEASE; DOWN SYNDROME; ETHICAL ISSUES IN GENETICS AND MOLECULAR MEDICINE; GENETIC SCREENING; INHERITANCE PATTERNS; MOSAICISM; PATAU'S SYNDROME; PRENATAL CARE.

ethical issues in genetics and molecular medicine The questions and concerns that arise for physicians and individuals in regard to the information GENETIC SCREENING, GENETIC TESTING, and genetic and molecular therapies. Though advances in genetics have produced significant breakthroughs in understanding, diagnosing, and sometimes treating health conditions that occur as a result of GENETIC

DISORDERS, doctors and their patients grapple with the ethics of both research and therapeutics. The issues touch many of what have long been the sacred tenets of the practice of medicine: privacy, access to care, autonomy in decision making, and protection against discrimination.

Privacy

Most health conditions, with the exception of infectious diseases, affect only the individuals who have them. Matters of diagnosis, treatment, and prognosis remain private between physician and patient (and, some would add, third-party insurers). Genetic issues affect families, current and prospective. Doctors, especially family practitioners who care for multiple members of the same family, may find themselves in conflict in regard to genetic information about one family member that affects the health or health prospects of other family members.

Access to Care

Diagnostic and therapeutic applications of genetic technology are both complex and expensive. Many procedures are available only in research facilities or are not covered by conventional HEALTH INSURANCE plans. People who participate in clinical studies may have access to technologies that people who choose not to participate in research cannot have. As well, questions arise in regard to the relative value of certain applications of genetic technology. What purpose does genetic testing serve when there is no treatment or cure for the genetic condition? This is a particular issue for adults who may carry GENE mutations for genetic disorders such as HUNTINGTON'S DISEASE, for whom the disease is inevitable if they have the MUTATION but for which at present there is no means to mitigate symptoms or the disease's unpleasant progression, although promising therapies may be available soon. Some health experts argue that resources provide greater benefit for the larger good when they go toward conditions for which prevention, treatment, or cure is possible.

Informed and Autonomous Decision Making

For as much as researchers have learned and now know about human genetics there remain vast unknowns about the potential benefits, risks, and complications of genetically based treatments. In 2003 the US Food and Drug Administration (FDA), which oversees clinical research and approves new treatments, suspended certain GENE THERAPY methods after people receiving apparently successful results suddenly acquired lethal leukemias. Informed consent, long the mainstay of treatment decision making, is increasingly difficult to apply. Other ethical issues arise in regard to making decisions about genetic conditions that affect the lives and circumstances of children or other family members. Further concerns involve legal and forensic applications of genetic information.

Discrimination

As technology provides ever-expanding knowledge, concerns also grow that what people learn about their health status could end up being used against them in settings ranging from health and life insurance coverage to job offers and even medical care opportunities. Though such concerns are not new, the inevitabilities of certain genetic outcomes put discrimination concerns in new perspective.

For further discussion of medical ethics within the context of the structures and functions of genetics, please see the overview section "Genetics and Molecular Medicine."

See also CLONING; LEUKEMIA; QUALITY OF LIFE.

familial Mediterranean fever An inherited genetic disorder that results in repeated episodes of arthritis (INFLAMMATION of the joints), PERITONITIS (inflammation of the membrane that lines the abdominal cavity), pleuritis (inflammation of the membrane that surrounds the LUNGS), and PERICARDITIS (inflammation of the membrane that contains the HEART). FEVER accompanies the outbreaks of inflammation, which occur without apparent precipitating factors and not in any particular pattern. In some people the disorder also includes AMYLOIDOSIS, in which deposits of amyloid (a waxlike substance) accumulate in organs such as the KIDNEYS.

Familial Mediterranean fever, as the name implies, occurs predominantly among people of Mediterranean descent and is an autosomal recessive disorder. The responsible mutated GENE is on the short arm of CHROMOSOME 16. At present there are no genetic tests or diagnostic procedures that conclusively diagnose familial Mediterranean fever; the doctor makes the diagnosis on the basis of family history and the pattern of symptoms.

See also AUTOSOME; GENETIC DISORDERS; INHERITANCE PATTERNS; MUTATION; RENAL FAILURE.

family medical pedigree A comprehensive listing of relatives and their medical conditions, including information about diseases that may have genetic foundations. A family medical pedigree looks somewhat like a genealogic family tree, with branched lineage to show family relationships (such as marriage, birth, half-siblings). The family medical pedigree should extend at least three generations and list each person's age at the time of death, the cause of death, and any known history of diseases or symptoms.

Many of the health conditions doctors know today are genetic in origin were not known, either as diseases or as GENETIC DISORDERS, even one or two generations ago, so documenting symptoms can help reveal undetected genetic conditions. Maintaining a record of personal health symptoms and conditions, and similar information for children, can further provide important clues about genetic factors in health and in illness.

See also GENOME; INHERITANCE PATTERNS; MUTATION; PERSONAL HEALTH HISTORY.

fragile X syndrome An inherited genetic disorder that results in significant intellectual impairment. Fragile X syndrome arises from a monogenic (single-GENE), increased repeat MUTATION affecting the FMR1 gene on the X CHROMOSOME and is the leading cause of inherited intellectual impairment in males. Fragile X syndrome more severely affects males because females have a second X chromosome that can somewhat override the mutated gene on the other X chromosome. Most females are unaffected carriers. Because males have one X chromosome and one Y chromosome, they lack this dampening affect. A male can also be an unaffected CARRIER of the mutated gene, though this is very rare, and will thus pass the mutation to all of his daughters though none of his sons.

The symptoms of fragile X syndrome vary in severity though typically include

- developmental delays
- speech impairments
- intellectual impairment (sometimes profound)
- seizures
- behavioral problems
- AUTISM-like characteristics
- physical features that may include overly flexible joints, flat feet, long facial configuration, and oversized ears

Diagnosis occurs through GENETIC TESTING, typically cytogenic analysis. Treatment may include supportive measures such as special education in school, speech and language pathology, and medications to moderate behaviors and control seizures. Children who are mildly affected may require little extra care and may attend regular classes and schools; those who are severely affected may require ongoing support and institutional care.

See also DOWN SYNDROME; GENETIC COUNSELING; GENETIC DISORDERS; INHERITANCE PATTERNS; PHENYLKETONURIA (PKU); SEIZURE DISORDERS.

gamete A spermatozoon (SPERM cell) or an ovum (egg cell). A gamete, also called a germ cell or sex cell, is a haploid cell; it contains half the complement of chromosomes and genetic material necessary to encode (result in creating) an individual. When two gametes merge they produce a single diploid cell, the ZYGOTE, which then contains the full complement of chromosomes needed for life.

For further discussion of gametes within the context of the structures and functions of genetics, please see the overview section "Genetics and Molecular Medicine."

See also CELL STRUCTURE AND FUNCTION; CHROMOSOME; CONCEPTION; OVULATION.

gene A segment of coding DNA (DNA that instructs the structure and function of cells throughout the body) composed of a specific sequence of nucleotides. The gene is the basic unit of inheritance that directs every facet of the body's appearance and functions. Genes align along chromosomes in pairs. Each CHROMOSOME (AUTOSOME) contains thousands of genes, except the sex chromosomes which contain only a few hundred genes.

Each gene has a specific location on the chromosome, called its locus, and encodes a specific function (either a protein or RNA transcription). The HUMAN GENOME PROJECT identified 19,599 confirmed genes and 2,188 probable genes at its conclusion in April 2003. GENETIC DISORDERS occur when there are disruptions of the ALLELE pairings or there is damage to the gene or the chromosome at or near the gene's locus.

Each gene has a specific task, which it carries out through a process called encoding. The gene instructs the cells to synthesize (produce) a specific protein. Ribosomes, specialized structures within each cell, synthesize the proteins. The protein then carries the gene's message to its target and initiates the appropriate sequence of biochemical events to implement the message.

For further discussion of genes within the context of the structures and functions of genetics, please see the overview section "Genetics and Molecular Medicine."

See also CHROMOSOMAL DISORDERS; GENOME; INHERITANCE PATTERNS; MUTATION; NUCLEOTIDE; SEX CHROMOSOME.

gene therapy Treatment methods, most of which remain experimental, that attempt to manipulate genetic structure or gene encoding. GENE therapy targets either germline (GAMETE) or somatic cells, using vectors to deliver genes within cells. Germline gene therapy aims to prevent a genetic disorder from passing to new generations, while somatic gene therapy targets genetic disorders that already exist in individuals. Most often the goal of gene therapy is to replace a defective gene with a healthy, functional gene. The vectors typically used are inactivated viruses into which scientists insert the replacement gene. The VIRUS enters the target cell and delivers the gene.

Applications of gene therapy have not been as successful as researchers have hoped was possible, however, and at present the US Food and Drug Administration (FDA) has not approved any gene therapy methods for use in the United States. The effects of gene therapy appear time-limited, and viral vectors often initiate immune responses. Researchers continue to investigate safe and effective mechanisms to therapeutically manipulate genes with the goal of treating or curing GENETIC DISORDERS.

See also ETHICAL ISSUES IN GENETICS AND MOLECULAR MEDICINE; MOLECULARLY TARGETED THERAPIES; RECOMBINANT DNA; SOMATIC CELL.

genetic carrier   An individual whose GENOTYPE contains a recessive GENE MUTATION capable of causing a genetic disorder though the individual does not have or show symptoms of the disorder the mutation causes. Typically a genetic CARRIER has one "good" gene and one mutated gene. A genetic carrier may pass on the mutated gene to his or her biological children, though typically two mutated genes are necessary for the child to acquire the genetic disorder.

See also CELL FUNCTION AND STRUCTURE; GENETIC DISORDERS; GENETIC SCREENING; GENETIC TESTING; INHERITANCE PATTERNS.

genetic code   The organizations of nucleotides (DNA sequences) within messenger RNA into triplet structures called trinucleotides or codons. The codons convey the order of amino acids for the structure of the protein for which a particular GENE encodes. The process of protein synthesis takes place in the ribosomes in the cell cytoplasm; the messenger RNA carries the encoding to the ribosomes.

See also CELL STRUCTURE AND FUNCTION; CHROMOSOME; GENOME; GENOTYPE; NUCLEOTIDE; PHENOTYPE.

genetic counseling   A multidisciplinary approach to evaluating the risk for specific genetic diseases or CHROMOSOMAL DISORDERS. Doctors often recommend genetic counseling for people who have strong family history for GENETIC DISORDERS such as TAY-SACHS DISEASE or HUNTINGTON'S DISEASE and older women who are or who are planning to become pregnant. Obstetricians also will recommend genetic counseling for couples who receive positive results from prenatal genetic tests so they may make informed decisions and conduct appropriate planning for pregnancies in which there are genetic or chromosomal abnormalities.

A genetic counseling team may include a clinical geneticist (physician specializing in genetics and molecular medicine), genetic psychologist, and a social worker. The intent of genetic counseling is to evaluate family history, results of genetic tests, and current health circumstances to provide individuals, couples, or families with as much information as possible about whatever genetic risks or situations they are facing and the options for addressing them.

The role of the genetic counseling team is to answer questions and provide support for the decisions individuals and couples make. Major healthcare centers and high-risk obstetrical practice groups generally have genetic counseling practitioners and services available.

See also ETHICAL ISSUES IN GENETICS AND MOLECULAR MEDICINE; FAMILY MEDICAL PEDIGREE; GENETIC SCREENING; GENETIC TESTING; PREGNANCY.

genetic disorders   A collective classification for syndromes, diseases, and congenital anomalies that result from alterations of the genes and chromosomes. There are four general categories of genetic disorders, each relating to the way in which the alterations manifest.

Chromosomal Disorders

The normal human GENOME contains 23 paired chromosomes. CHROMOSOMAL DISORDERS occur when there are disruptions in these pairings in which there is an extra CHROMOSOME (trisomy) or a missing chromosome (monosomy). Chromosomal disorders also occur when large segments of a chromosome are damaged or missing (deletion syndromes). Less often, a broken segment of a chromosome attaches itself to another chromosome (TRANSLOCATION). Common chromosomal disorders include DOWN SYNDROME, EDWARDS SYNDROME, PATAU'S SYNDROME, TURNER SYNDROME, and KLINEFELTER'S SYNDROME.

Single-Gene Disorders

Each GENE encodes, or directs, a specific action within the body. Single-gene disorders, in which a MUTATION of a gene or set of genes causes malfunctions of the proteins that carry out the gene's instructions, cause conditions of faulty encoding, either because the gene's protein messenger is missing or incomplete. The disorders that result often become more severe over time as the malfunction continues to repeat itself. CYSTIC FIBROSIS, SICKLE CELL DISEASE, Duchenne's MUSCULAR DYSTROPHY, HUNTINGTON'S DISEASE, and MARFAN SYNDROME are single-gene disorders.

Multifactorial Disorders

Researchers suspect many health conditions arise as a result of an interplay between genetic and environmental factors. Geneticists call such conditions multifactorial disorders because it appears a certain combination of events must take place for disease to result; doctors may refer to them as conditions of GENETIC PREDISPOSITION. These are the conditions that tend to run in families; some family members develop them and others do not. Health conditions in which genetics, lifestyle, and other variables participate in the development of disease are numerous. Some of those that are common include CORONARY ARTERY DISEASE (CAD), HYPERTENSION (high BLOOD PRESSURE), CANCER, DIABETES, GALLBLADDER DISEASE, and NEPHROLITHIASIS (kidney stones), and numerous other conditions.

Mitochondrial Disorders

Mitochondria are self-replicating structures within a cell (called organelles) that carry out the metabolic functions of the cell. Mitochondria have their own DNA that directs their specific functions, and have multiple copies; MITOCHONDRIAL DNA (MTDNA) is different from the cell's nuclear DNA. MITOCHONDRIAL DISORDERS, which are the rarest of the genetic disorders, occur when the genes that encode mitochondrial activity contain mutations or when there are defects in the mtDNA. Mitochondrial disorders tend to vary widely among individuals, causing different symptoms because they affect different, and usually multiple, organs or structures. Doctors define the disorder as a complex of symptoms. Some forms of ENCEPHALOPATHY, MYOPATHY, and CARDIOMYOPATHY are mitochondrial disorders.

See also CONGENITAL ANOMALY; INHERITANCE PATTERNS; MOSAICISM.

genetic imprinting The inactivation of certain genes, determined by whether the GENE is maternal (comes from the mother) or paternal (comes from the father). Genetic imprinting, also called genomic imprinting, appears to be another method of controlling genes by requiring one copy of each of certain chromosomes from each parent.

INHERITANCE PATTERNS, which establish gene expression through dominance, regulate most gene expression and normally present paired chromosomes that determine which traits are expressed in the PHENOTYPE. However, it is possible for mutations to occur that result in both sets of a particular chromosome coming from the same parent (uniparental disomy). Though such mutations likely occur with no noticeable effect and thus remain undetected, they can allow rare recessive abnormalities to be expressed.

Though rare, the CHROMOSOMAL DISORDERS Prader-Willi syndrome and Angelman syndrome represent the most common pathology of genetic imprinting. These syndromes reflect uniparental disomy of CHROMOSOME 15, one of the chromosomes known to incorporate genetic imprinting. Chromosome 15 regulates numerous neurologic and musculoskeletal structures and functions that affect intelligence, cognition (the ability to think, reason, and remember), behavior, emotion, physical appearance, MUSCLE tone, movement, and METABOLISM as well as reproductive health and capability.

Normal development requires one copy of chromosome 15 from each parent. When both copies of chromosome 15 are maternal (called paternal deletion), genetic imprinting produces a constellation of symptoms known as Prader-Willi syndrome. When both copies of chromosome 15 are paternal (called maternal deletion), genetic imprinting produces a constellation of symptoms known as Angelman syndrome. Each syndrome presents differing manifestations of neurologic dysfunction, musculoskeletal and other physical anomalies, and intellectual impairment.

Researchers believe genetic imprinting is a mechanism intended to prevent damaging mutations from propagating (extending themselves). Genetic imprinting appears to affect only certain chromosomes and, when it causes a disease state, results in related though differing symptoms, depending on the deletion.

See also CELL STRUCTURE AND FUNCTION.

genetic predisposition The tendency to develop a health condition as a consequence of the interaction between genetics and lifestyle factors. Doctors believe genetic influences underlie many if not all health conditions that develop over time, such as HYPERTENSION (high BLOOD PRESSURE), ATHEROSCLEROSIS, OSTEOARTHRITIS, RENAL FAILURE, LIVER disease, and type 2 DIABETES. An individual's GENOTYPE establishes genetic vulnerability through mechanisms researchers do not fully understand.

These genetic elements influence the effects of environmental factors such as cigarette smoking, physical activity and inactivity, exposure to chemical toxins, ALCOHOL consumption, and nutrition (lack of certain NUTRIENTS or excesses of other nutrients) in the development of disease processes. Once the disease becomes established, its genetic underpinnings may allow more rapid progression of damage or severity of symptoms.

Unlike GENETIC DISORDERS that encode for specific disturbances of structures and functions that inevitably produce a disease state (such as DOWN SYNDROME), genetic predisposition for a condition does not make that condition certain. Many doctors and researchers believe knowing of genetic predispositions gives an individual the opportunity to engage in lifestyle modifications to prevent health problems from developing.

See also LIFESTYLE AND HEALTH.

genetic screening Procedures that indicate whether an individual has the potential to have a genetic disorder. Among the most commonly performed genetic screening procedures in the United States are prenatal ULTRASOUND and maternal BLOOD levels of multiple biomarkers, such as ALPHA FETO-PROTEIN (AFP), during PREGNANCY. These procedures may present suspicious findings though are not precise enough to allow diagnosis. Other genetic screening procedures are those that test for conditions that occur in the general population and have significant consequences when undetected and untreated. For example, hospitals in the United States conduct routine newborn testing for PHENYLKETONURIA (PKU), an inherited metabolic disorder that results in severe intellectual impairment without treatment at the time of birth.

The findings of genetic screening, positive or negative, can have a margin of error for false-negative as well as false-positive results. However, doctors use genetic screening when factors of increased risk for GENETIC DISORDERS, such as maternal age in pregnancy or family history, exist. The doctor may conduct further GENETIC TESTING and diagnostic testing when the overall health picture points to an increased risk for genetic disorders,

even when the findings of genetic screening procedures appear normal. Genetic screening procedures are minimally invasive and typically present no risk to the mother or the fetus in prenatal screening or to the individual in screening conducted following birth or in adults.

See also AMNIOCENTESIS; AUTOSOMAL TRISOMY; CHORIONIC VILLI SAMPLING (CVS); CHROMOSOMAL DISORDERS; ETHICS IN GENETICS AND MOLECULAR MEDICINE; FAMILY PLANNING; FOLIC ACID SUPPLEMENTATION; GENETIC TESTING; NEURAL TUBE DEFECTS.

genetic testing Methods and procedures to determine the presence of a genetic disorder. The KARYOTYPE, which uses microphotographs to examine and depict an individual's chromosomes, is one of the more common methods of genetic testing. Other methods include cytogenic analysis, AMNIOCENTESIS, and CHORIONIC VILLI SAMPLING (CVS). Some genetic testing methods are highly sophisticated and require specialized equipment and knowledge available only in research centers. Other methods, such as CVS, have become fairly commonplace.

Diagnostic genetic testing can identify the cause of symptoms resulting from GENE mutations and CHROMOSOMAL DISORDERS. This knowledge can be helpful when there are treatments and treatment choices for the resulting conditions, and in FAMILY PLANNING decisions. The matter of genetic testing to screen for the presence of GENETIC DISORDERS, particularly in people who do not have symptoms or apparent increased risk for conditions of genetic origin, remains an issue of intense ethical debate. Some such practices, such as testing for PHENYLKE-TONURIA (PKU) in newborns, have become standard in the United States. Others, such as those for the so-called CANCER genes (BRCA-1, BRCA-2, CA-125, and others), often raise more questions than answers because the consequence of having such genes remains uncertain.

Even when the outcome is certain, the knowledge of the genetic disorder may have little therapeutic value yet create distress for the individual. This is currently a significant issue with genetic testing for HUNTINGTON'S DISEASE, for example, a fatal neurodegenerative disorder for which there is no treatment or cure. People who carry the gene MUTATION for Huntington's disease are certain to develop the disease in midlife. GENETIC COUNSELING is almost always a valuable and necessary component of genetic testing.

See also ETHICAL ISSUES IN GENETICS AND MOLECULAR MEDICINE; GENETIC PREDISPOSITION; LIFESTYLE AND HEALTH.

genome The total genetic material, including coding and noncoding sequences, a cell contains in its chromosomes. Each organism has a unique genome. Scientists define the size of a genome by the number of its base pairs. The human genome contains 3.2 billion base pairs, which make up that comprise about 23,000 genes.

See also CELL STRUCTURE AND FUNCTION; CHROMOSOME; GENE; GENOTYPE; HUMAN GENOME PROJECT; PHENOTYPE.

genotype The contents of an individual's GENETIC CODE. The genotype directs the structures and functions of the human body. A person's genotype is to the human body what an architect's blueprint is to a house: It provides the directions for the construction and operation of the human organism.

See also GENOME; KARYOTYPE; PHENOTYPE.

G6PD deficiency An inherited genetic disorder in which the body lacks the enzyme glucose-6-phosphate dehydrogenase (G6PD). Erythrocytes (red BLOOD cells) normally produce G6PD, which aids in metabolizing carbohydrates and also helps to protect erythrocytes from oxidation (damage resulting from metabolic waste). The absence of G6PD causes health problems when the body experiences unusual stress, such as illness, or with certain medications such as aspirin and sulfa antibiotics. These circumstances cause oxidants to accumulate in the blood. Without G6PD to neutralize these oxidants, they destroy erythrocytes, resulting in hemolytic ANEMIA.

The symptoms of hemolytic anemia resulting from G6PD deficiency include

- dark URINE
- pale SKIN
- weakness
- JAUNDICE (yellowish discoloration of the skin and sclera of the eyes)
- HEPATOMEGALY (enlarged LIVER) and SPLENOMEGALY (enlarged SPLEEN)
- tachycardia (rapid HEART RATE)
- FEVER

Symptoms and family history may cause the doctor to suspect G6PD deficiency. Blood tests will reveal the hemolytic anemia. Treatment generally consists of avoiding circumstances and substances that trigger oxidative stress. Many people are able to avoid symptoms entirely through such an approach. Because G6PD is an inherited condition, there are no methods for prevention. The inheritance pattern for G6PD is X-linked recessive; G6PD affects twice as many males as females and is more prominent in people of African American heritage and Mediterranean heritage.

See also ERYTHROCYTE; GENETIC DISORDERS; INHERITANCE PATTERNS; PHENYLKETONURIA (PKU); PORPHYRIA.

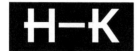

Human Genome Project   A collaborative undertaking among researchers around the world, organized under the joint auspices of the U.S. Department of Energy and the National Institutes of Health, to identify and map the human GENOME (genetic material that defines the human being). Altogether, more than 20 research centers in the United States, United Kingdom, China, France, Germany, and Japan participated in the DNA sequencing. The Human Genome Project began in 1990 and concluded with the full mapping of the human genome in April 2003, 50 years after Watson and Crick unveiled their double-helix model of DNA. Researchers expect data analysis and new findings to continue for the indefinite future. The Human Genome Project's Web site, (www.ornl.gov), regularly posts updates.

HUMAN GENOME PROJECT FINDINGS: HIGHLIGHTS

- The human GENOME consists of 3,164,700,000 NUCLEOTIDE bases.
- The largest GENE (dystrophin) contains 2.4 million nucleotide bases.
- 99.9 percent of the nucleotide bases are identical in all people.
- The human genome contains about 30,000 genes.
- CHROMOSOME 1 contains 2,968 genes and chromosome Y contains 231 genes, the most and the fewest, respectively.

Source: The Science behind the Human Genome Project, *www.ornl.gov/hgmis; updated October 27, 2004.*

See also CELL STRUCTURE AND FUNCTION; CLONING; ETHICAL ISSUES IN GENETICS AND MOLECULAR MEDICINE; GENOTYPE; PHENOTYPE; RECOMBINANT DNA.

inheritance patterns   The ways in which genotypes pass among individuals and generations. Many inherited traits are either autosomal or X-linked and either dominant or recessive. Such inheritance patterns reflect statistical calculations assessing the mathematical likelihood of certain traits or mutations passing from one generation to the next. Inheritance patterns consider the genotypes of each parent. Inheritance patterns vary according to whether the chromosomes responsible are autosomesal or sex-linked chromosomes. Geneticists often refer to these patterns as Mendelian, in reference to the foundational work of botanist Gregor Mendel (1822–1884), who was the first to delineate inheritance patterns.

Recent research, notably through the HUMAN GENOME PROJECT, has shown that much of human inheritance may not be quite so simple as the Mendelian model. Multiple genes and chromosomes share responsibility for traits ranging from EYE color to the development of diseases, such as DIABETES AND CARDIOVASCULAR DISEASE, that also have environmental (lifestyle) components. This circumstance of multiple factors makes it far more difficult to statistically represent a delineated pattern of inheritance. Multifactorial inheritance is not clearly dominant or recessive, though is commonly autosomal (derives from autosomes rather than sex chromosomes).

The least common pattern of inheritance is mitochondrial, which comes only from the mother and involves traits and mutations affecting mitochondrial, not nuclear, DNA. This pattern is exclusively maternal because only the ovum (female GAMETE or egg) contains mitochondria. Mitochondria affect functions rather than structures of the body, and thus, mitochondrial mutations cause numerous, nonspecific multisystem disturbances. Because mitochondria are the energy generators of the cells, mitochondrial mutations affect functions that require energy

INHERITANCE PATTERNS: AUTOSOMAL TRAITS AND MUTATIONS

Autosomal Recessive		Autosomal Dominant	
Both parents carriers	One parent carrier, one parent noncarrier	Both parents affected	One parent affected, one parent unaffected
Each child:	Each child:	Each child:	Each child:
25% condition	50% noncarrier	25% unaffected	50% unaffected
25% noncarrier	50% carrier	25% more severely affected than parents	50% affected
50% carrier		50% affected	

Percentages refer to the probability of occurrence.

INHERITANCE PATTERNS: X-LINKED TRAITS AND MUTATIONS

X-Linked Recessive		X-Linked Dominant	
Mother CARRIER, father noncarrier	Mother noncarrier, father affected	Mother affected, father noncarrier	Mother noncarrier, father affected
Each daughter:	Each daughter:	Each daughter or son:	Each daughter:
25% noncarrier	100% carrier	50% affected	100% affected
25% carrier	Each son:	50% nonaffected	Each son:
Each son:	100% noncarrier		100% nonaffected
25% noncarrier			
25% affected			

Percentages refer to the probability of occurrence.

rather than affect structures of the body. Though mitochondrial mutations may be single-GENE, they often have widespread effects across types of cells in which energy needs are high, such as NERVE cells and MUSCLE cells.

See also AUTOSOME; CHROMOSOME; FAMILY MEDICAL PEDIGREE; GENOTYPE; MITOCHONDRIAL DISORDERS; MITOCHONDRIAL DNA (MTDNA); MUTATION; SEX CHROMOSOME.

karyotype A pictorial presentation of an individual's chromosomes, taken from microphotographs (photographs taken through a microscope) and arranged in a numeric sequence that aligns the chromosomes from largest to smallest. This standardized presentation allows the geneticist to analyze an individual's chromosomal profile. A geneticist can structure a karyotype from any SOMATIC CELL (nonsex cell) in the body. The most common application of karyotyping is GENETIC SCREENING of a fetus. A geneticist constructs a karyotype to evaluate whether an individual has a GENETIC DISORDER. A karyotype requires DNA from a representative cell in the body, from which the geneticist extracts and prepares the DNA for examination under the microscope.

See also CHROMOSOME; GENETIC COUNSELING; GENETIC DISORDERS; GENETIC TESTING.

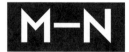

M–N

mitochondrial disorders Inherited mutations in mitochondrial genes that result in functional disturbances in various body systems. Mitochondria are structures within the cell that generate the energy, in the form of adenosine triphosphate (ATP), the cell requires to function. A cell may contain dozens of mitochondria. Each mitochondrion contains the specific genetic material (MITOCHONDRIAL DNA [MTDNA]) to encode the enzymes (specialized proteins) that regulate the biochemical reactions within the mitochondrion that generate ATP. The only function of mtDNA is to regulate these processes of energy production.

Each mitochondrion contains multiple copies of its DNA. Mutations typically affect some but not all DNA copies, so mitochondrial function continues though may be impaired whenever the mutated mitochondrial GENE sends incorrect code. Only the ovum contains mitochondria that pass on to the ZYGOTE at CONCEPTION. SPERM cells contain few mitochondria, and these are in the sperm cell's tail, which breaks away as soon as the sperm penetrates the ovum. As the zygote continues to divide, it may perpetuate errors in mtDNA that are widespread or pervasive.

Mitochondrial disorders include myositis, some types of CARDIOMYOPATHY, some types of MYOPATHY, and carnitine deficiency syndrome. Often, symptoms are multisystem and inconsistent with the conventional presentations of the health conditions they suggest. MUSCLE and NERVE cells have particularly high energy needs, so mitochondrial disorders often manifest symptoms such as weakness and poor muscle tone (hypotonia).

Because mitochondrial disorders are rare and their symptoms are confusing, the diagnostic path may lead to numerous dead ends. Though this process rules out other diagnoses, it is a frustrating experience for those patients looking for answers for their symptoms. There are no definitive diagnostic tests for mitochondrial disorders, though muscle biopsy often can provide strong evidence supporting diagnosis once doctors rule out other conditions and disorders. Treatment targets managing symptoms and preventing common complications such as DEHYDRATION. Some doctors advocate COENZYME Q10 supplementation for people who have mitochondrial disorders, which appears to improve the efficiency of cellular METABOLISM as well as protect cells from oxidative damage. People who have mitochondrial disorders should include GENETIC COUNSELING in their FAMILY PLANNING efforts.

See also CELL STRUCTURE AND FUNCTION; CHROMOSOME DISORDERS; GENETIC DISORDERS; MUTATION; REPLICATION ERROR.

mosaicism A chromosomal disorder in which some cells are normal and some cells contain the chromosomal abnormalities of the disorder, in contrast to a complete distribution of the abnormal chromosomes throughout all cells. The distribution of abnormal cells in mosaicism is usually random and unpredictable. Mosaicism most commonly occurs in AUTOSOMAL TRISOMY, in which there is an additional copy of one CHROMOSOME that appears in some cells and not in others. The result generally is a milder presentation of symptoms when only some cells express the abnormality (mosaic disorder) than occurs when all cells express the abnormality (complete disorder). People who have a mosaic expression of the autosomal trisomy disorder DOWN SYNDROME, for example, typically have milder symptoms than people who have a complete expression. Mosaicism may also affect genetic expressions other than health disorders.

See also CELL STRUCTURE AND FUNCTION; CHROMO-
SOMAL DISORDERS; EDWARDS SYNDROME; INHERITANCE
PATTERNS; MUTATION; PATAU'S SYNDROME; REPLICATION
ERROR.

mutation Permanent alterations in the ALLELE
pairings, or genes, on the chromosomes that pass
on to new cells and ultimately to offspring. Mutations are the process through which genetic
change takes place. Some mutations are beneficial, some are neutral, and some are harmful.
Mutations occur as changes in the GENE'S
NUCLEOTIDE sequences. These changes may take the
form of

- point mutations, also called base mutations,
  which are analogous to changing one letter in a
  word and occur when one nucleotide substitutes for another
- deletion mutations, which are analogous to
  removing a word from a sentence and occur
  when the gene drops a nucleotide sequence
- insertion mutations, which are analogous to
  adding a word to a sentence and occur when
  the gene adds a nucleotide sequence
- increased repeat mutations, which occur when
  a normally repeated nucleotide repeats extra
  times

A germline mutation affects a GAMETE (ovum or
spermatozoon) or ZYGOTE and is present from CON-
CEPTION, passing to the child. WILMS'S TUMOR and
HEMOPHILIA are examples of germline mutations
that cause disease. A monogenic MUTATION affects a
single gene. Duchenne's MUSCULAR DYSTROPHY and
SICKLE CELL DISEASE are among the conditions that
occur as a result of monogenic mutations. Polygenic mutations involve multiple alleles of numerous genes, often across chromosomes. Polygenic
mutations often do not clearly result in GENETIC
DISORDERS though establish GENETIC PREDISPOSITION.
Conditions such as CARDIOVASCULAR DISEASE (CVD),
DIABETES, and some types of cancer occur as a
result of polygenic mutations in combination with
lifestyle (environmental) factors.

See also AUTOSOMAL TRISOMY; CHROMOSOMAL DIS-
ORDERS; LIFESTYLE AND HEALTH.

nucleotide A structural component of DNA and
RNA. A DNA nucleotide contains deoxyribose and
a nitrogen base of adenine, guanine, thymine, or
cytosine, which form pairs called base pairs. An
RNA nucleotide contains ribose and a nitrogen
base of paired adenine, guanine, uracil, or cytosine. Each DNA or RNA molecule contains thousands of nucleotides. The order in which the
nucleotides appear is the base sequence and conveys the GENETIC CODE for the proteins the DNA or
RNA molecule encodes. Base sequences, arranged
in triplets (trinucleotides), make up GENES.

See also CELL STRUCTURE AND FUNCTION; CHROMO-
SOME; GENOME.

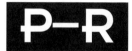

Patau's syndrome An AUTOSOMAL TRISOMY disorder that results from a REPLICATION ERROR during cell division in which a GAMETE (sex cell) ends up with two copies of CHROMOSOME 13 instead of the normal single copy (as haploid cells, gametes contain one-half the complement of chromosomes). At CONCEPTION the ZYGOTE thus ends up with three instead of the normal two copies of chromosome 13, which ultimately produces multiple and life-threatening congenital anomalies. When Patau's syndrome occurs as a complete trisomy disorder (all cells carry the extra chromosome), the anomalies are so severe that the disorder often is lethal well before birth. Occasionally Patau's syndrome occurs as a mosaic disorder (some but not all cells contain the extra chromosome 13), which typically produces milder though nonetheless significant symptoms. Patau's syndrome occurs in about 1 in 10,000 live births in the United States.

CONGENITAL ANOMALIES CHARACTERISTIC OF PATAU'S SYNDROME

atrial septal defect (ASD)	CLEFT PALATE/CLEFT PALATE
malformed KIDNEYS	AND LIP
malformed or absent eyes	malformed KIDNEYS
malformed or absent NOSE	microcephaly (small head
multiple hernia	and BRAIN)
patent ductus arteriosus	polycystic kidneys
(PDA)	POLYDACTYLY
ventricular septal defect (VSD)	vextrocardia (HEART on right
	side of chest)

Children born with Patau's syndrome have severe and complex physical deformities involving multiple organ systems that require extensive medical care from the time of birth. Most also have severe developmental delays and intellectual impairment arising from malformations affecting the BRAIN and NERVOUS SYSTEM. KARYOTYPE confirms the diagnosis. It is rare for a child who has Patau's syndrome to survive beyond early childhood; there are no documented survivals to adulthood. Ongoing medical care to accommodate physical anomalies and developmental support to achieve optimal learning potential provide the child who survives the best possible QUALITY OF LIFE.

See also AUTOSOME; CHROMOSOME DISORDERS; CONGENITAL ANOMALY; CONGENITAL HEART DISEASE; DOWN SYNDROME; EDWARDS SYNDROME; ETHICAL ISSUES IN GENETICS AND MOLECULAR MEDICINE; GENETIC SCREENING; INHERITANCE PATTERNS; MOSAICISM; POLYCYSTIC KIDNEY DISEASE.

phenotype The outward presentation, or features, of an individual's GENOTYPE (genetic composition). The phenotype is the construction and operation that results from implementation of the genotype, much as a house is the outcome of a building contractor's implementation of an architect's blueprints. A phenotype consists of such obvious characteristics as EYE color and HAIR patterns as well as less apparent traits such as BLOOD TYPE and proclivity for health or certain diseases. The genotype for lipid METABOLISM, for example, may support effective use of lipids within the body (supporting health) or the tendency for high levels of lipids to accumulate in the BLOOD (increasing the risk for CARDIOVASCULAR DISEASE [CVD]).

See also ALLELE; ALOPECIA; CELL STRUCTURE AND FUNCTION; FAMILY MEDICAL PEDIGREE; VARIATION.

phenylketonuria (PKU) An inherited genetic disorder in which the enzyme phenylalanine hydroxylase is missing or severely deficient, preventing the METABOLISM of the essential amino acid (one the body must acquire from dietary sources) phenylalanine. Phenylalanine is common in all foods that contain protein (such as meats, dairy products, fish, and legumes) and in artificial sweeteners such as aspartame. Avoiding foods that contain phenylalanine, which means following a strict low-protein diet, prevents phenylalanine accumulations and the resultant damage that affects primarily the NERVOUS SYSTEM. The most significant consequence of undiagnosed PKU is irreversible, and usually severe, intellectual impairment.

Symptoms and Diagnostic Path

Early symptoms of PKU appear soon after birth and include restlessness, irritability, stunted growth, and a characteristic musty smell to the breath. The appearance of symptoms means neurologic damage is already occurring, however. Newborn screening to identify PKU before symptoms appear is essential to prevent intellectual impairment. Hospitals in the United States routinely screen newborns, typically within two days of birth, to detect elevated levels of phenylalanine in the blood. Further testing can confirm the diagnosis, and immediate dietary restrictions can prevent the disorder from causing permanent damage.

Treatment Options and Outlook

Treatment is stringent restriction of dietary phenylalanine, which includes BREAST milk. Infants require special phenylalanine-free formulas. Dietary restrictions are lifelong. Many food products contain labeling information that states their phenylalanine content, and a number of food manufacturers produce low-phenylalanine versions of popular foods such as cereals as well as phenylalanine-free protein substitutes. Fruits, vegetables, breads, and pastas contain very low amounts of phenylalanine. In the United States foods that contain aspartame must state on the label that they contain phenylalanine.

Women who have PKU can safely carry a PREGNANCY to term though must be especially diligent to maintain a low phenylalanine diet because excessive phenylalanine in the mother's BLOOD circulation also affects the developing FETUS and can cause permanent neurologic and other damage before birth. Because the inheritance pattern for PKU is autosomal recessive, women who have PKU will pass the disorder to their children only if the father carries the mutated gene or also has PKU.

Risk Factors and Preventive Measures

PKU is an autosomal recessive, single-GENE mutation. Both parents must carry the PKU mutation for a child to have the disorder. However, PKU carriers often do not know they have the mutated gene because they do not show any indications of the disorder. People who know they are PKU carriers or who have PKU should consider GENETIC COUNSELING as an element of their FAMILY PLANNING.

See also CARRIER; GENETIC DISORDERS; INHERITANCE PATTERNS; NUTRITIONAL NEEDS; PORPHYRIA.

porphyria The collective term for a group of eight inherited GENETIC DISORDERS of METABOLISM in which deficiencies of certain enzymes block the production of heme and allow the accumulation of porphyrins. Heme is an iron-containing pigment normally present in nearly all tissues in the body, notably as a component of HEMOGLOBIN in the BLOOD and of electron transport proteins called cytochromes. The LIVER produces cytochromes, which are essential for metabolizing numerous drugs, hormones, NUTRIENTS, and other substances. Heme synthesis occurs in a sequence of eight steps, each occurring through the actions of a particular enzyme. Each of the eight forms of porphyria represents the absence of one of these enzymes.

Symptoms and Diagnostic Path

Symptoms vary with the type of porphyria and may be neurologic (affect the NERVOUS SYSTEM), dermatologic (affect the SKIN), hepatic (involve the liver), or erythropoietic (involve the BONE MARROW and blood). Typically symptoms are episodic, occurring as attacks that last for days to weeks and sometimes longer. Symptoms vary widely in appearance, severity, and duration and may include

- eruptive skin rashes (bullae)
- PHOTOSENSITIVITY
- severe ABDOMINAL PAIN
- NAUSEA, VOMITING, and DIARRHEA
- MUSCLE weakness and possibly PARALYSIS
- agitation and hallucinations

THE PORPHYRIAS

Porphyria	Deficient Enzyme	Inheritance Pattern
acute intermittent porphyria (AIP)	porphobilinogen deaminase (PBG-D)	autosomal dominant
ALAD-deficiency porphyria (ADP)	aminolevulinic acid dehydratase (ALAD)	autosomal recessive
congenital erythropoietic porphyria (CEP)	uroporphyrinogen III cosynthase	autosomal recessive
erythropoietic protoporphyria (EPP)	ferrochelatase	autosomal dominant
hepatoerythropoietic porphyria (HEP)	uroporphyrinogen decarboxylase	autosomal recessive
hereditary coproporphyria (HCP)	coproporphyrinogen oxidase	autosomal dominant
porphyria cutanea tarda (PCT)	uroporphyrinogen decarboxylase	autosomal dominant
variegate porphyria (VP)	protoporphyrinogen oxidase	autosomal dominant

- tachycardia (rapid HEART RATE)
- URINARY RETENTION and URINARY INCONTINENCE

The diagnostic path includes blood and urine tests to measure the presence of key porphyric enzymes. In people who know they have porphyria, exposure to identified precipitating factors —which include numerous drugs, hormones, and nutrients—will bring on an attack. HYPERTENSION (high BLOOD PRESSURE) can develop during an attack and persist after symptoms subside.

Treatment Options and Outlook
Severe symptoms, particularly neurologic, require hospitalization and aggressive treatment that may include intravenous heme administration (the only form in which heme is available). Medications safe to take to relieve and control symptoms include narcotic pain relievers and phenothiazines to relieve nausea and vomiting or neuropsychiatric symptoms. It is crucial to stop any substances that may have precipitated the attack. Most symptoms subside within two to three weeks, and most people fully recover within six weeks. Some people experience extended muscle weakness. Attacks may occur without provocation. Many people who have porphyria seldom experience attacks, however.

Risk Factors and Preventive Measures
The porphyrias are inherited genetic disorders. The risk of porphyria depends on the inheritance pattern. There are no measures to prevent porphyria. People who have porphyria, or who have family members who have porphyria, might consider GENETIC TESTING and GENETIC COUNSELING. It is possible to be a CARRIER for the autosomal recessive forms of porphyria.

See also BULLA; CYTOCHROME P450 (CYP450) ENZYMES; GENE; HALLUCINATION; HORMONE; MUTATION; RASH.

progeria   A very rare genetic disorder, commonly called severe premature aging, that arises from a MUTATION in a single GENE on CHROMOSOME 1 called lamin A (LMNA). The gene encodes a protein, also called lamin A, that is important for proper functioning of the membrane of the cell nucleus. In progeria this protein is abnormal, resulting in rapid deterioration of the nuclear membrane and destruction of the cell. The diagnostic path is primarily clinical, based on symptoms. Most children who have progeria die of cardiovascular problems such as HEART ATTACK or STROKE by the age of 12 or 13 years. As a consequence of research into the causes of progeria, scientists have discovered other mutations of the same gene that cause uncommon forms of MUSCULAR DYSTROPHY. At the present time there is no treatment, cure, or prevention for progeria.

See also CELL STRUCTURE AND FUNCTION; GENETIC DISORDERS.

recombinant DNA A biotechnology technique that replaces DNA to alter a cell's function. There are several methods for performing recombination, though all ultimately involve extracting the native DNA from a carrier (called a vector) and replacing it with the desired DNA. Modified BACTERIA and viruses are common vectors—bacteria because they replicate rapidly, and viruses because they can deliver modified DNA into the nucleus of cells within the body (GENE THERAPY).

One of the most significant uses of recombinant DNA technology is the production of substances such as human INSULIN supplementation to treat DIABETES, which recombinant technology can synthesize in vast quantities in the laboratory to meet strict quality and consistency standards. Because such recombinant products are biochemically indistinguishable from their endogenous (naturally produced in the body) counterparts, they are an exact replacement, and the body accepts them as though they were endogenous. Recombinant DNA technology produces other hormones, too, such as HUMAN GROWTH HORMONE (HGH) SUPPLEMENT.

See also CELL STRUCTURE AND FUNCTION; CLONING; HORMONE; VIRUS.

replication error A mistake that occurs when DNA sequences duplicate before cell division. Replication errors are accountable for CHROMOSOMAL DISORDERS such as AUTOSOMAL TRISOMY, in which a GAMETE (also called a sex cell or germ cell) receives two copies of a CHROMOSOME instead of the normal single copy. Gametes, which are haploid cells, each carry one-half the complement of chromosomes so when they unite to form the ZYGOTE that will become a new human being, the zygote contains the full complement of genetic material. With a replication error such as an autosomal trisomy, the zygote receives an extra chromosome—two copies from one gamete and one copy from the other gamete. The result is a chromosomal disorder such as DOWN SYNDROME. Replication errors also may have harmless consequences when they occur in DNA sequences that do not encode structural or regulatory sequences of gene activity.

See also MUTATION; VARIATION.

RNA The abbreviation for ribonucleic acid. RNA is a single-strand molecule consisting of ribose; a sugar; and nucleotides made up of the nitrogen bases adenine, uracil, guanine, and cytosine. RNA exists in a number of forms, all of which serve as biochemical messengers that carry the instructions of DNA to the ribosomes, structures in the cell's cytoplasm. Ribosomes synthesize (manufacture) the proteins the genes encode. RNA also may function as the carrier of GENETIC CODE within the mitochondria.

For further discussion of RNA within the context of the structures and functions of genetics, please see the overview section "Genetics and Molecular Medicine."

See also CELL STRUCTURE AND FUNCTION; GENE; NUCLEOTIDE.

S

senescence The gradual and progressive slowing of cellular activity, including cell division, that occurs with aging. Cells lose the ability to divide over time, a phenomenon researchers call Hayflick's limit. The limit relates to the number of times the cell divides. During cell division, fibers of DNA called telomeres attach to the chromatids, facilitating their separation from each other to enter the new daughter cells. The process destroys the segment of the TELOMERE attached to the CHROMATID, causing the telomere to shorten with each cell division. When the cell runs out of telomeres it can no longer divide and it dies.

The exceptions are cancer cells, which seem to be nonsenescent. Cancer cells produce increased levels of an enzyme called telomerase, which acts to restore the length of the telomeres and gives cancer cells the ability to endlessly divide. Normal cells also produce telomerase but not in quantities sufficient to regenerate telomeres. Researchers do not know what causes cancer cells to increase the amount of telomerase they produce. As well, other factors are at play in the processes of senescence, which researchers continue to study.

See also APOPTOSIS; CELL STRUCTURE AND FUNCTION; PROGERIA.

sex chromosome The structure of GENETIC CODE that determines gender (male or female). The male sex CHROMOSOME has the appearance of the letter *Y* and the female sex chromosome has the appearance of the letter *X*. A combination of XY results in male and a combination of XX results in female. The Y chromosome contains fewer than 100 genes, while the X chromosome carries several hundred genes. A number of GENETIC DISORDERS are X-linked—that is, they result from mutations that occur among genes the X chromo-

some carries. HEMOPHILIA and some forms of MUSCULAR DYSTROPHY (notably Duchenne's and Becker's) are X-linked genetic disorders.

See also AUTOSOME; GAMETE; GENE; MUTATION; SOMATIC CELL.

somatic cell A cell that is not a GAMETE (sex cell). More than 99 percent of the body's trillions of cells are somatic cells. Somatic cells are diploid; their nuclei contain the full complement of paired chromosomes and genetic material necessary to encode an organism. When somatic cells divide, their chromosomes replicate so the new daughter cells receive the full complement of paired chromosomes as well.

For further discussion of somatic cells within the context of the structures and functions of genetics, please see the overview section "Genetics and Molecular Medicine."

See also CELL STRUCTURE AND FUNCTION; CHROMOSOME; CONCEPTION; REPLICATION ERROR; ZYGOTE.

stem cell An undifferentiated, primal cell that has the capability to endlessly divide and develop into numerous types of cells. Totipotent stem cells exist primarily in the early EMBRYO (blastocyst) and can differentiate into (become) virtually any type of cell in the body. As the body becomes more complex and develops beyond the blastocyst stage, stem cells become specialized to produce certain kinds of cells, which they retain the ability to do endlessly. These stem cells, though found in tissues of all kinds throughout the body, are most highly concentrated in the BONE MARROW (BLOOD STEM CELLS). UMBILICAL CORD BLOOD is another source of highly concentrated blood stem cells. Blood stem cells can differentiate into any type of blood cell.

Researchers have had some success with stimulating blood stem cells, in the laboratory, to function as though they were other types of cells such as NERVE cells or MUSCLE cells, and are hopeful that stem cells will someday become a source of cultivated replacement tissues and organs. Multipotent stem cells that occur in other tissues are difficult to identify and extract from their source tissues though may also hold similar potential.

For further discussion of stem cells within the context of the structures and functions of genetics, please see the overview section "Genetics and Molecular Medicine."

See also ETHICAL ISSUES IN GENETICS AND MOLECULAR MEDICINE; GAMETE; HEMATOPOIESIS; STEM CELL THERAPY.

stem cell therapy   Implantation of STEM CELLS to become specialized cells for tissue and organ repair or replacement. Though most STEM CELL therapy applications remain experimental, BONE MARROW TRANSPLANTATION (also called BLOOD stem cell transplantation) has become a standard of treatment for many cancers affecting the blood and the lymphatic system (leukemias and lymphomas) as well as certain other cancers. Researchers have also been successful in cultivating stem cells into SKIN for skin grafting, to treat severe BURNS, and into pancreatic islet cells that produce INSULIN, to treat severe type 1 DIABETES. Though these applications of stem cell therapy remain experimental, they raise the potential for stem cell therapy to become viable in treating numerous health conditions.

Two significant concerns with stem cell therapy are the potential for cancer to develop and the rejection of the cultivated cells or tissue. A prime value of the stem cell is its unlimited ability to divide. However, a function called APOPTOSIS limits most division of the cells in the body. It appears that cells can divide only a certain number of times, then begin to shut down. The exceptions are stem cells and cancer cells, and researchers are not certain what will keep stem cells from becoming cancer cells. Apoptosis remains a focus of much research. And as is the case with organs donated for transplantation, the body can reject stem cell transplantations. When this occurs the body's IMMUNE SYSTEM attacks the transplanted stem cells, killing them.

See also BLOOD STEM CELLS; CELL STRUCTURE AND FUNCTION; GENE THERAPY; ISLETS OF LANGERHANS; LEUKEMIA; MOLECULARLY TARGETED THERAPY.

T–Z

Tay-Sachs disease An inherited genetic disorder that causes a progressive, fatal form of gangliosidosis (the accumulation of gangliosides within NERVE cells). Tay-Sachs disease involves mutations of a pair of genes on CHROMOSOME 15 that encode for the enzyme hexosaminidase-A (hex-A). The mutation blocks production of hex-A. The body requires hex-A to metabolize GM2 ganglioside, a fatty acid that nerve cells need to metabolize and produce energy. Without adequate hex-A this METABOLISM cannot take place, and the GM2 ganglioside that enters the cell accumulates. GM2 ganglioside concentrations are highest within the nerve cells in the BRAIN as these nerve cells have the highest energy needs among nerve cells. GM2 ganglioside accumulates in other nerve cells as well. The accumulation causes the nerve cell to swell and eventually rupture.

Though the accumulation of GM2 ganglioside begins before birth, symptoms do not become apparent until age four to six months. Around this age the damage to brain tissue reaches a critical level and begins to disrupt brain activity. The child appears to regress developmentally. Brain function continues to decline, affecting intellectual and thought processes as well as voluntary and involuntary functions throughout the body. Tay-Sachs disease is usually fatal before age five years. An uncommon variation, late-onset Tay-Sachs disease, allows slight amounts of hex-A, delaying the onset of symptoms until ADOLESCENCE or early adulthood. However, the progressive loss of neurological and cognitive function follows a similar timeline once symptoms start.

Symptoms and Diagnostic Path

The earliest indication of Tay-Sachs disease is a characteristic round, cherry-red spot on the macula at the back of the EYE, the point where the ocular nerve joins the RETINA. The spot represents the onset of gangliosidosis in the optic nerve. Other symptoms include

- flaccid MUSCLE tone (early)
- loss of voluntary muscle control and movement (late)
- irritability (early)
- intellectual impairment
- seizures (late)
- diminishing responsiveness and awareness (progressive)
- loss of vision (progressive)

The diagnostic path includes family history, ethnic heritage, BLOOD tests to measure the level of hex-A present in the circulation, and GENETIC TESTING such as cytogenetic analysis and DNA sequencing. The genetic tests provide the definitive diagnosis.

Treatment Options and Outlook

There is no treatment or cure for Tay-Sachs disease. Nearly all children who have Tay-Sachs disease die before the age of five years. Research exploring methods to replace hex-A so far have been unsuccessful. Currently the most effective efforts target prevention by identifying carriers, who do not themselves have Tay-Sachs disease and who may not know they carry the GENE MUTATION.

Risk Factors and Preventive Measures

Tay-Sachs disease is an autosomal recessive disorder, meaning both parents must have the mutated gene for them to have a child with the disease, a one in four chance with each CONCEPTION. People at highest risk for Tay-Sachs disease are those of Ashkenazi Jewish heritage. A blood test became available in 1985 to detect carriers of Tay-Sachs disease, who do not themselves have the disease but who have lower than normal amounts of hex-A in their blood. GENETIC COUNSELING can help couples who are carriers make informed decisions about whether to have children. Assisted reproductive technologies (ARTs) such as in vitro fertilization allow genetic testing before implantation so the couple knows the conceived child does not carry the mutated genes.

See also ASSISTED REPRODUCTIVE TECHNOLOGY (ART); ETHICAL ISSUES IN GENETICS AND MOLECULAR MEDICINE; GENETIC CARRIER; GENETIC DISORDERS; INHERITANCE PATTERNS.

telomere A structure of noncoding DNA (DNA that does not convey genetic instruction) at each end of a CHROMOSOME. Telomeres are essential for chromosome duplication during cell division. They function as handles to pull the chromatids (dividing chromosomes) apart as the mother cell divides into the two new daughter cells. The process of cell division permanently destroys a tiny fragment of the telomere, however. Eventually the telomere becomes too short to participate in chromosome duplication, and the cell stops dividing. Researchers believe the shortening of telomeres is key to APOPTOSIS, the apparently programmed death of cells. In cancer cells the telomeres regenerate after cell division, which researchers believe is one of the factors that allows cancer cells to grow uninhibited.

For further discussion of telomeres within the context of the structures and functions of genetics, please see the overview section "Genetics and Molecular Medicine."

See also CELL STRUCTURE AND FUNCTION; CENTROMERE; CHROMATID; SENESCENCE.

translocation A chromosomal disorder in which a fragment of a CHROMOSOME breaks from its original chromosome and attaches itself to a different chromosome. The fragment may exchange with another fragment, may add itself to another chromosome, or may become lost. Some translocations are random and others occur in predictable patterns. Translocations can be reciprocal, in which

chromosome fragments trade places with one another. Such balanced translocations are common and usually do not produce symptoms because all the normal genetic material remains within the GENOME.

A Robertsonian translocation occurs when the long arms of two acrocentric chromosomes, in which the CENTROMERE (waistlike indentation) is so high on the chromosome that the upper arms appear nonexistent and the upper arms contain almost no genetic material. Robertsonian translocations occur only among the five acrocentric chromosomes, which are chromosomes 13, 14, 15, 21 and 22. Like reciprocal translocations, Robertsonian translocations generally do not produce harmful consequences because the genetic material remains unadulterated despite the translocation. Robertsonian translocations are fairly common.

One reciprocal translocation that tends to produce harmful health effects is the Philadelphia chromosome, in which a segment of chromosome 9 and a segment of chromosome 22 exchange places. Geneticists commonly find this translocation in people who have chronic myeloid LEUKEMIA (CML).

See also CELL STRUCTURE AND FUNCTION; CHROMOSOMAL DISORDERS; DNA.

trisomy 13 See PATAU'S SYNDROME.

trisomy 18 See EDWARDS SYNDROME.

trisomy 21 See DOWN SYNDROME.

variation The genetic differences among individuals. There are trillions of possible GENE combinations within the human GENOME. Except for identical twins, no two people share exactly the same GENOTYPE (genetic constitution). Though any two individuals may have 99.9 percent of the same DNA sequences and gene pairings, the 0.1 percent of pairings that differ accounts for the endless details that make each individual unique.

The same genotype can have multiple expressions (phenotypes) among individuals. The genotype for EYE color, for example, can express itself as blue eyes in one person and brown eyes in another. Such variability exists for every gene pairing, with more or less obvious results. VARIA-TION also occurs through MUTATION, in which DNA sequences change during replication. Polymorphisms and mutations may have positive, neutral, or negative effects, which differ among individuals based on circumstance, lifestyle, and other factors.

See also ALLELE; CELL STRUCTURE AND FUNCTION; GENETIC PREDISPOSITION; INHERITANCE PATTERNS; PHENO-TYPE.

zygote   The fertilized ovum (egg) before it begins to divide. The spermatozoon (SPERM cell) and the ovum are each haploid cells (gametes); they con-tain half the complement of chromosomes neces-sary to create an organism. When two gametes join they form a single diploid cell that contains the full complement of chromosomes. The zygote then divides as a haploid cell, becoming a blasto-cyst and eventually forming an EMBRYO.

For further discussion of zygotes within the context of the structures and functions of genetics, please see the overview section "Genetics and Molecular Medicine."

See also ASSISTED REPRODUCTIVE TECHNOLOGY (ART); CELL STRUCTURE AND FUNCTION; CHROMOSOME; CONCEP-TION; GAMETE; OVULATION.

DRUGS

The area of health care concerned with drugs and medicinal therapies is pharmacology. Health-care professionals who dispense prescription drugs are pharmacists, who may be registered pharmacists (RPh) or doctors of pharmacy (PharmD).

This section, "Drugs," presents an overview discussion of pharmacologic concepts and entries about drugs and their use for the maintenance of health and the treatment of infection, injury, and disease.

Pharmaceutical Traditions in Medical History

The earliest written medical documents reference often elaborate preparations of botanicals used as medicines to treat a broad spectrum of ailments, ranging from HEADACHE and itching to weak PULSE and infected wounds. Healers in the times of ancient Babylonia, Mesopotamia, Egypt, and China relied on extensive collections of herbs, roots, barks, and seeds from which they concocted tinctures, teas, poultices, and other remedies. Ancient pharmacopeias outlined the formulations and uses of hundreds of plant forms for medicinal purposes.

ALCOHOL, too, was a major weapon in the early physician's pharmaceutical arsenal, serving as a topical antibacterial as well as an ingested analgesic (PAIN reliever) and quasi-anesthetic. Opium poppies and coca leaves yielded the first NARCOTICS, opium and COCAINE. Coffee beans and tea leaves yielded CAFFEINE, a potent stimulant. Tobacco leaves, chewed or smoked, were the source of another powerful stimulant, NICOTINE. Coca leaves and tobacco leaves acquired such high value in some early cultures that they served as currency.

Today medicinal herbs and botanicals remain the mainstay of TRADITIONAL CHINESE MEDICINE (TCM) and form the foundation of the modern pharmaceutical industry. As many as 5,000 medicinal plants grow in various regions around the world, many in the rain forests of South America. About 25 percent of modern medicines trace their derivations directly or indirectly to plants. Laboratories now produce synthetic forms of many drugs once extracted from plants, such as the antiarrhythmia DRUG digoxin (digitalis from the foxglove plant), the pain reliever aspirin (salicin from the bark of the willow tree), and the antimalarial drug quinine (quinaquina from the bark of the chinchona tree). Other drugs, such as the anticancer drug paclitaxel (Taxol), which is an extract from the bark of the Pacific yew tree, still derive from their botanical sources.

Drug Controls and Regulations

The regulation of drugs—from effectiveness and safety to production and availability—that is the foundation of today's pharmaceutical industry is a modern phenomenon. Until the early 20th century narcotics such as opium and HEROIN were freely available in the United States. Patent medicines (an odd assortment of liniments, elixirs, tinctures, nostrums, bitters, extracts, and compounds) dominated the druggist's apothecary. From Lydia E. Pinkham's Vegetable Compound, which contained far more alcohol than vegetable, to Mrs. Winslow's Soothing Syrup, a sedating preparation of morphine, patent medicines claimed to treat just about any ailment . . . and many claimed to treat just about *every* ailment.

The Pure Food and Drugs Act of 1906 was the beginning of the end for patent medicines; requiring medicine labels to list the product's ingredients and spawning the federal oversight agency that was to become the US Food and Drug Administration (FDA). In 1938 the Food, Drugs, and Cosmetics Act extended the authority of the FDA to regulate the safety and therapeutic effectiveness (and labeling claims thereof) of drugs, requiring manufacturers to prove a drug's safety before being allowed to market the drug. The regulations arose from the sometimes deleterious adulteration of drug products, brought to the forefront of public outrage when the use of poisonous wood alcohol in a sulfa preparation caused the deaths of more than 100 people. Shortly thereafter the FDA established separate classifications for prescription drugs and OVER-THE-COUNTER (OTC) DRUGS, prescription drugs being those whose safe use required a physician's oversight and guidance and OTC drugs being those that individuals could safely use without the guidance of a doctor or pharmacist.

Drug advertising remained under the jurisdiction of the Federal Trade Commission (FTC) until the Drug Amendments of 1962, the first of several key amendments to the Food, Drugs, and Cosmetics Act. The 1962 Drug Amendments also gave the FDA the regulatory authority to require evidence of a drug's safety as well as effectiveness before granting approval for the drug. The Dietary Supplements and Nutritional Labeling Act of 1994 drew back some authority from the FDA, however, reclassifying herbal and botanical products as dietary supplements and removing from FDA regulatory oversight.

Challenges in Pharmaceutical Therapy

Drugs have transformed health care over the past half century, relegating to insignificance many infections and diseases that in previous generations meant lifelong disability or early death. Drugs treat INFECTION, DIABETES, CARDIOVASCULAR DISEASE (CVD), kidney disease, LIVER disease, gastrointestinal disease, neurologic disorders, and cancer. Doctors in the United States write more than 14 billion prescriptions a year for nearly 3,000 different drugs, and another 2,000 medications are available in over-the-counter (OTC) products that are available without a doctor's prescription.

Indeed, there are few health conditions for which there are not pharmaceutical treatments. Nonetheless, significant challenges exist. Health experts worry that the expense of drugs puts them out of reach for many people who need them and that collectively people are developing habits in regard to drug therapies that ultimately put health at greater risk.

Drug costs and availability Pharmaceutical manufacturers spend millions of dollars every year to develop new drugs. Yet as many as 20 promising drug concepts may die in the laboratory for every one that makes it clinical testing. For the length of time a drug remains under patent after its approval, an average of 14 years, the drug's manufacturer has an exclusive piece of a multi-billion-dollar market. Though few dispute a pharmaceutical company's right to expect a financial return on its investment, the high cost of drugs still under patent makes the drugs unaffordable for many people. Older people take the hardest hit, caught in an intersection between increasing health-care needs and a fixed income.

One major effort to reduce drug costs is generic drugs, which are identical to their trade name counterparts (innovator drugs) in terms of active ingredients, DOSE, form, and efficacy (action in the body). The Government Accountability Office (GAO), the official expenditure watchdog of the federal government, estimates that generic drugs save Americans more than $10 million a year.

The high cost of drugs in the United States has fueled interest in purchasing drugs from countries in which they are not as expensive, such as Canada and Mexico. Although US law prohibits bringing imported drugs into the country, many people order them from Internet and mail-order sources nonetheless to save hundreds to thousands of dollars each year.

Patient compliance and lifestyle choices Treating or preventing a health condition can be as easy as taking a few pills a day. However, though precise statistics are difficult to determine health experts estimate that perhaps half of people for whom doctors prescribe regular medications do not take them as directed. They may miss doses, combine drugs to consolidate dosages, take a reduced dose to "stretch" the prescription, or take the drug only when they feel symptoms. In some situations, however, taking a drug improperly is more of a health hazard than not taking the drug at all. The problem is significant enough to support a thriving secondary market that sells various "medication minder" methods. Unfortunately thousands of Americans require additional medical care for circumstances, including unintentional OVERDOSE, that develop as a consequence of failing to follow label instructions.

Health experts also worry that medications are becoming substitutes for healthful changes in lifestyle habits. For example, people who take drugs such as lipid-lowering medications may become complacent about making lifestyle changes that would allow them to stop taking the medication while reducing their risk for cardiovascular disease. Often it is easier to take the pill rather than to change EATING HABITS and exercise habits, another method for lowering blood lipid levels.

Antibiotic resistance The first antibiotics, sulfa and penicillin, became lifesavers during and after World War II. Antibiotics put a rapid end to the often deadly infections rampant at the time, such as PNEUMONIA, TONSILLITIS, GONORRHEA, and TUBERCULOSIS. Within 25 years, however, infections began to appear that were resistant to penicillin, the most commonly used antibiotic, and doctors had to prescribe newly developed alternatives.

ANTIBIOTIC RESISTANCE emerged as a full-blown health issue in the latter decades of the 20th century with the appearance of multiple-drug-resistant infections of tuberculosis, gonorrhea, and pneumonia. By 2002 some strains of *Staphylococcus aureus*, a BACTERIA family accountable for a wide range of infection, including pneumonia and wound infections, had acquired resistance even to the most powerful antibiotic available, vancomycin. Of the most critical concern are NOSOCOMIAL INFECTIONS, infections that result from exposure to bacteria that thrive in environments such as hospitals and extended-care facilities. These bacteria have often evolved to a high level of multiple-drug resistance, making the infections they cause very difficult to treat.

Interactions among drugs An estimated 30 million Americans take multiple prescription medications. Though these drugs keep potentially disabling or deadly health conditions in check, the risk for serious drug interactions increases exponentially with each additional drug. Factor in OTC drugs and herbal remedies, and drug interactions become more likely than not to occur. Such interactions can result in reduced or potentiated effectiveness of any or all of the drugs the person is taking. Doctors and pharmacists urge people always to tell each doctor who provides care, whether or not the doctor writes a prescription, about all drugs they are taking because sometimes the health problems that send them to the doctor result from interactions among their medications.

Breakthrough Research and Treatment Advances

Pharmaceutical research began to focus on pharmacogenomics—the interactions between genetics and medications—in the 1990s. Doctors have known for quite some time that some people metabolize certain drugs more or less efficiently than do other people. This can result in altered efficacy. Researchers have been able to identify genes, some of which regulate CYTOCHROME P450 (CYP450) ENZYMES, the collective of enzymes that metabolize most drugs that enter the body. Subtle differences in protein encoding may slow or speed drug absorption, METABOLISM, or length of time in the BLOOD circulation. Particularly in areas such as cancer treatment, researchers are searching for ways to use pharmaceuticals to manipulate genetic encoding. Other research focuses on developing "smart" drugs, which specifically and narrowly target certain kinds of cells.

adverse drug reaction An undesired, negative, and often unpleasant response to a medication. People commonly refer to adverse DRUG reactions as side effects, which is not entirely accurate because a SIDE EFFECT may have therapeutic value whereas an adverse drug reaction is potentially harmful. Adverse drug reactions are common, affecting more than two million Americans each year. They can occur with any drug a person takes or uses, ranging in severity from upset STOMACH or HEADACHE, which often subside after taking the drug for several doses, to URTICARIA (hives) or ANAPHYLAXIS (life-threatening closure of the airways), which are usually allergic reactions. RASH and itching are also common adverse reactions. Adverse drug reactions may also affect the composition of the BLOOD or the function of organs such as the HEART, LIVER, and KIDNEYS.

Intentional misuse of a DRUG, including taking more than recommended or in combination with other drugs, increases the likelihood of adverse drug reaction.

All drugs have some identified potential adverse reactions. These are the events that usually surface during the human testing phase of clinical research studies. Some such reactions may be inherent to the properties of the drug—that is, result from the drug itself. Many ANTIBIOTIC MEDICATIONS, for example, kill BACTERIA in the intestines at the same time they kill bacteria that are causing INFECTION, resulting in DIARRHEA because intestinal bacteria are essential for proper digestion. NAUSEA, VOMITING, and HAIR loss are known adverse reactions with CHEMOTHERAPY drugs. Other such reactions may result from DRUG INTERACTIONS with other medications the person is using or from

the ways in which the body responds to the drug over the long term. Tardive DYSKINESIA is a known adverse reaction to long-term use of ANTIPSYCHOTIC MEDICATIONS, for example. Long-term use of CORTICOSTEROID MEDICATIONS, such as taken to treat INFLAMMATORY BOWEL DISEASE (IBD) or ADDISON'S DISEASE, have numerous adverse effects on the body.

Adverse drug reactions may be localized, such as DERMATITIS, or systemic (involve multiple body systems). Doctors generally classify adverse drug reactions as immunologic (those that involve an IMMUNE RESPONSE) or nonimmunologic (those that do not involve an immune response). People who are IMMUNOCOMPROMISED (such as those who have HIV/AIDS or take IMMUNOSUPPRESSIVE THERAPY), have an autoimmune disorder such as RHEUMATOID ARTHRITIS or SYSTEMIC LUPUS ERYTHEMATOSUS (SLE), have liver or kidney disease, take multiple medications (often called polypharmacy), or are age 60 or older have increased risk for adverse drug reactions. Most drug reactions occur within several days to three weeks of beginning the drug, though some long-term adverse reactions occur up to years after the drug's initiation.

COMMON ADVERSE DRUG REACTIONS		
allergic response	ANAPHYLAXIS	ANEMIA
ANGIOEDEMA	ARRHYTHMIA	arthralgia
CANDIDIASIS	DERMATITIS	DIARRHEA
GLOMERULONEPHRITIS	LYMPHADENOPATHY	NEUTROPENIA
PRURITUS	RASH on trunk	tardive DYSKINESIA
TINNITUS	URTICARIA	VOMITING

It is important, when beginning treatment with a new medication or adding a different drug to a treatment regimen, to know the expected results and possible adverse reactions. People who take multiple drugs, including OVER-THE-COUNTER (OTC)

DRUGS and MEDICINAL HERBS AND BOTANICALS, should make sure the prescribing physician and the dispensing pharmacist know all of them. Numerous products interact with one another in ways that alter their effects in the body, increasing the risk for adverse drug reactions.

Many countries have regulatory requirements for documenting and reporting adverse drug reactions. Such requirements help oversight agencies and health-care professionals monitor issues with drugs that may not have been apparent during preapproval testing. In the United States the US Food and Drug Administration (FDA) oversees compliance with these requirements and works with pharmaceutical manufacturers to resolve issues that arise.

See also ALCOHOL INTERACTIONS WITH MEDICATIONS; AUTOIMMUNE DISORDERS; CIRRHOSIS; DRUG INTERACTION; LIVER FAILURE; OFF-LABEL USE; RENAL FAILURE; TOXIC EPIDERMAL NECROLYSIS.

aging, effects on drug metabolism and drug response Many drugs have different therapeutic effects as well as potential adverse DRUG reactions, depending on a person's age. The very young and the very old often have limited LIVER function, which affects the ways in which the liver metabolizes drugs, resulting in lower thresholds for toxicity and unpredictable therapeutic effects. In the infant and young child, the liver has not yet fully developed and lacks the structural capacity to metabolize certain substances. The elderly may lose liver function due to CIRRHOSIS, fatty deposits accumulating within the liver (STEATOHEPATITIS), or the normal loss of cells that occurs with aging. Reduced kidney function may further affect drug response by slowing clearance of the drug from the body and thus maintaining higher than expected concentrations of the drug in the BLOOD circulation.

Drugs in Children

Two significant issues surround medication therapy in children. The first is the continually changing metabolic capability and status of the child's body as organ systems grow and mature. The liver remains relatively unsophisticated in its function until a child reaches age 10 or 12 years. Not only does this limit the liver's ability to metabolize drugs such as antibiotics and analgesics (pain relievers), the most common kinds of drugs children may need, but also it makes the liver vulnerable to damage from substances that enter the blood circulation. Incompletely metabolized drugs increase the risk for damage to other developing organ systems as well, notably the CENTRAL NERVOUS SYSTEM. These factors become of therapeutic concern when treating serious childhood diseases for which medications are the primary course of treatment, such as SEIZURE DISORDERS, CONGENITAL HEART DISEASE, and cancer.

The second issue in regard to medication therapy in children is that many drugs do not undergo testing or evaluation for their effectiveness or safety in pediatric use because children make up a very small percentage of the drug's intended patient population or because the potential risks of involving children in clinical research studies are too high. The consequence is that doctors rely on best practices standards and OFF-LABEL USE of drugs in prescribing medications, which are safe and effective in adults but untested in children, to treat health conditions in children.

Drugs in the Elderly

The body undergoes significant metabolic and functional changes by the seventh and eighth decades of life, a blend of the normal processes of aging and the cumulative effect of health conditions. The liver and KIDNEYS become less efficient, which affects the amount of a drug that enters the blood circulation and how long the drug remains in the body. Health conditions such as ATHEROSCLEROSIS (fatty deposits in the walls of the arteries) may alter the flow of blood through the body. Changes in NERVOUS SYSTEM function may alter the release of neurotransmitters. These kinds of changes in the body influence how, and how well, drugs work.

Often the very reasons elderly people need to take therapeutic drugs (such as to treat CARDIOVASCULAR DISEASE [CVD], DIABETES, kidney disease) have significant effects on the ways in which the body can handle the drugs and how those drugs affect the body. As well, older people are more likely to have complex or multiple health conditions and take multiple medications, increasing the risk for ADVERSE DRUG REACTION, DRUG INTERACTION, and OVERDOSE.

See also APOPTOSIS; NEUROTRANSMITTER; ORPHAN DRUG.

antibiotic resistance The adaptation of bacterial strains to certain of the ANTIBIOTIC MEDICATIONS doctors prescribe to treat infections the BACTERIA cause, rendering the antibiotic ineffective. Such adaptation is an evolutionary mechanism that allows the strain of bacteria to survive. Though in most situations the strain of bacteria remains sensitive to other antibiotics even as it develops resistance to a particular antibiotic, antibiotic resistance is a very serious concern in modern health care because the more common strains of bacteria are developing broad bases of resistance to multiple antibiotics. A few strains have mutated to resist all available antibiotics, presenting a worrisome challenge for fighting the infections they cause.

Bacteria, Infection, and Antibiotics

Bacteria are single-cell microorganisms that exist in broad families with numerous strains, or variations, within the same family. Under supportive circumstances each individual strain can cause unique and specific infections. Most bacteria that cause INFECTION in people are normally present in the body and the environment. Ordinarily these bacteria are harmless or even beneficial to body functions, such as the bacteria in the gastrointestinal tract that aid in digestion. NORMAL FLORA bacteria become pathogenic when there is a breach, such as a wound, in the body's protective mechanisms, or when something goes awry with the body's balance of microorganisms and the IMMUNE SYSTEM cannot keep bacterial growth in check.

Antibiotics kill bacteria, either by direct toxicity to the bacteria or by preventing the bacteria from reproducing. Antibiotics are effective for treating only *bacterial* infections; they cannot treat viral infections. Chronic conditions such as BRONCHITIS and OTITIS media (middle EAR infection) are often viral, yet are among the top ailments for which doctors prescribe antibiotics. It is not possible to determine the cause of an infection by evaluating the symptoms, though certain characteristics make it more likely that an infection is bacterial. Only a laboratory culture of cells from the infection, in which cells of a bacterial strain may or may not grow in the lab, can identify the cause of an infection as bacterial.

How Bacteria Acquire Resistance

Bacteria reproduce rapidly, which gives them the opportunity to change rapidly. Over multiple generations the bacteria's DNA—its GENETIC CODE—mutates to establish adaptations beneficial to the bacterial strain's survival. These adaptations include increased resistance to the antibiotics that people take to fight the infections the strain causes. Bacteria generally mutate through one of three processes:

- Spontaneous MUTATION is when changes occur within the DNA alter the bacteria's adaptive ability across the bacterial strain. Resistance due to spontaneous mutation, also called evolutionary mutation, develops over multiple generations of the bacterial strain.

- Transformation is when the DNA from resistant bacteria enter another bacteria that are not yet resistant. Also called DNA uptake, transformation expedites the mutation process to allow bacterial strains to become more rapidly resistant than they would through spontaneous mutation.

- Plasmid transfer is when plasmids (molecules that contain incomplete fragments of genetic material) move among different kinds of bacteria. Plasmids impart limited genetic encoding related primarily to the survivability of a bacterial strain and can result in rapid adaptation to produce antibiotic resistance. Because antibiotic resistance has become a key purpose of plasmid transfer, researchers designate such plasmids as R plasmids.

Resistance resulting from spontaneous, or evolutionary, mutation is the most common adaptation process and accounts for most of the resistant strains of GONORRHEA and *Staphylococcus aureus* infections. Transformation, or DNA uptake, is a more sophisticated, biologically intentional process than spontaneous mutation. Among the three mutation processes plasmid transfer is the most efficient and creates the greatest concern in regard to antibiotic resistance. Plasmids can transfer among different strains of bacteria within a bacterial family, sharing adaptive mutations for multiple resistance. Plasmid transfer accounts for resistance to entire classifications of drugs such as the quinolones, a family of antibiotics that attack enzymes that facilitate DNA cleavage (the division of DNA in preparation for cell reproduction) in bacteria.

Factors That Contribute to Antibiotic Resistance

Antibiotic use itself is the precipitating factor for the adaptive changes that occur in bacteria to result in antibiotic resistance, as these changes represent natural survival efforts. Key circumstances that further encourage survival adaptations include the following:

- Inappropriate prescribing of antibiotics for infections that are viral or of uncertain cause. The US Centers for Disease Control and Prevention (CDC) believes about half of the 100 million antibiotic prescriptions US doctors write each year are unnecessary because the conditions they are treating are not bacterial.

- Failing to complete the full course of antibiotic therapy, which allows some bacteria to escape eradication. It is important to take a therapeutic antibiotic long enough to kill all the bacteria, extending through their complete life cycle, that are causing infection. Bacteria that are exposed to the antibiotic but do not die have the opportunity to undergo adaptive mutation, which results in antibiotic resistance.

- Prophylactic antibiotics given to food animals such as cattle, pigs, and chickens to prevent them from getting infections that slow their growth. The constant exposure to the same antibiotics fosters adaptive mutation in bacteria that may then become infective agents in people. Humans become vulnerable to infection from resistant bacteria through eating meat from treated animals that is not thoroughly cooked, which allows the bacteria to enter the body. Exposure to the bacteria in environmental settings also is a source of infection.

Limiting Antibiotic Resistance

The most effective measure for reducing antibiotic resistance is to decrease the use of antibiotics. To this end, health experts offer these recommendations for individuals:

- Take antibiotics only for infections that laboratory tests prove are bacterial.

- Take all doses of the antibiotic for the full course of prescribed treatment.

- Wash hands frequently with soap and warm water to prevent the spread of infection-causing bacteria and other pathogens.

- Limit exposure to other people who are ill.

- Choose meat and poultry products that are labeled antibiotic free.

Health experts also are reexamining the practice of ANTIBIOTIC PROPHYLAXIS (administering antibiotics to prevent infection in people who are IMMUNOCOMPROMISED or exposed to risk for NOSOCOMIAL INFECTIONS). The US Food and Drug Administration (FDA), which oversees drug approval and prescribing practices in the United States, issued new regulations in 2003 that establish stringent criteria for doctors to follow in prescribing antibiotics and is spearheading public education efforts to improve public awareness of antibiotic resistance.

See also BACTEREMIA; FOOD SAFETY; HAND WASHING; OPPORTUNISTIC INFECTION; PATHOGEN; PERSONAL HYGIENE.

antitoxin   A serum product, cultivated from animal (usually horse) BLOOD, that counteracts the effects of toxins (poisons) certain strains of anaerobic BACTERIA produce when they enter the body. The antitoxin binds with the toxin that is circulating in the bloodstream, neutralizing it. Some antitoxins, such as those for *Clostridium tetani* (tetanus) and *Corynebacterium diphtheriae* (DIPHTHERIA), are effective prophylactically (administered to prevent illness); doctors administer these as vaccines. Others are effective therapeutically; doctors administer them when exposure triggers illness, such as to *Clostridium botulinum* (BOTULISM). Antitoxins for tetanus and diphtheria also have therapeutic action in people who develop these conditions. About 10 percent of people have allergic reactions to antitoxins. Giving smaller amounts of the antitoxin over a longer period of time, such as when treating disease, often mitigates the reaction.

See also ANTIVENIN; CHILDHOOD DISEASES; PREVENTIVE HEALTH CARE AND IMMUNIZATIONS; VACCINE.

antivenin A serum product, also called antivenom, cultivated from animal BLOOD and given therapeutically to neutralize the effects of poisonous venoms such as from BITES AND STINGS. Antivenin is specific to a particular venom and works by activating antibodies that enable the person's IMMUNE SYSTEM to fend off the effects of the venom.

> When possible, safely capture the snake or spider that renders the bite for positive identification and the correct antivenin.

A person generally must receive antivenin within about four to eight hours of the bite or sting for the antivenin to be effective. Antivenin is commonly available in the United States for the bites of indigenous snakes and spiders and the stings of scorpions. There are facilities in many parts of the United States that stock antivenin for exotic snakes and spiders that may enter the country inadvertently (such as among produce), as pets, or for scientific research or display (as in zoos). Local and regional poison control centers know what antivenin products are available and how to obtain them.

Most antivenins are cultivated from the blood of horses so it is important to know a person's allergy history. Allergic reaction to antivenin is not uncommon. Even in people who have a known ALLERGY to horses, however, the antivenin may be lifesaving. Generally in such a situation the administration of ANTIHISTAMINE MEDICATIONS and EPINEPHRINE will mitigate the allergic response to allow the antivenin to be effective. Serum sickness, an immune reaction to the antigens and blood proteins present in products derived from nonhuman blood, may also occur. Serum sickness generally begins one to two weeks after administration of the antivenin and runs its course over about three weeks. The risk for allergic reaction and serum sickness increases with higher doses of antivenin.

See also ANTIBODY; ANTIGEN; HYPERSENSITIVITY REACTION.

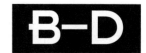

bioavailability The amount of a DRUG's active ingredient the body absorbs and the length of time it takes for that ingredient to cause an effect in the body. A common means of determining bioavailability is to measure the concentrations of the drug in the BLOOD circulation or in the URINE at certain time intervals. Doctors know the spectrum of bioavailability and calculate DOSAGE to obtain the desired therapeutic concentration of the drug.

For most drugs the spectrum of activity provides adequate therapeutic levels and tests to measure the drug's concentrations are not necessary. NARROW THERAPEUTIC INDEX (NTI) drugs such as the anticoagulant warfarin, the antiarrhythmic digoxin, and HORMONE supplements such as levothyroxine (thyroid hormone) require diligent assessment and monitoring because the margin between therapeutic and toxic is very close. The doctor may also assess the drug's bioavailability through observation of clinical changes, such as an INFECTION that improves with antibiotic therapy or BLOOD PRESSURE that drops with antihypertensive medications.

For the most part pharmaceutically equivalent drugs (generic drugs) have consistent bioavailability across manufacturers and are interchangeable from this perspective. The exceptions are NTI drugs, for which doctors and pharmacists recommend staying with the same brand name of drug for the duration of treatment. Which brand does not matter so much as that the brand remains consistent. This is because even minute variations in the manufacturing process, as is inherent in different formulations of the same drug product, affect the way the body absorbs and metabolizes the drug. Other factors that influence bioavailability are interactions with foods, other drugs, and MEDICINAL HERBS AND BOTANICALS. Health conditions such as gastrointestinal MALABSORPTION, renal failure, or LIVER FAILURE, as well as the person's age and weight, and metabolic disorders, also affect bioavailability.

See also EFFICACY; GENERIC DRUG; HALF-LIFE; THERAPEUTIC EQUIVALENCE.

bioequivalence A DRUG that has the same biological effect in the body as a substance the body makes naturally (such as a HORMONE supplement) or two or more drugs that have the same BIOAVAILABILITY and EFFICACY. Bioequivalence is a significant concern with NARROW THERAPEUTIC INDEX (NTI) drugs, which require precise and consistent dosing, as well as with generic drugs.

A GENERIC DRUG, which is a different chemical formulation of equivalent active ingredients compared to the innovator (original) drug, is not necessarily bioequivalent to the INNOVATOR DRUG. That is, the same drug product from different manufacturers may contain the same amounts of active ingredient though not the same inactive ingredients or different proportions of inactive ingredients. The extent to which these differences influence bioavailability (the amount of the active ingredient that enters the body) varies among classifications of drugs and is especially crucial with NTI drugs.

The US Food and Drug Administration (FDA) establishes and regulates the parameters of bioequivalence. Drugs that are bioequivalent must fall within a specific range for the amount of time it takes for each drug to enter and remain in the BLOOD circulation.

See also DRUG INTERACTION; *ORANGE BOOK, THE*; THERAPEUTIC EQUIVALENCE.

cytochrome P450 (CYP450) enzymes A group of about 60 endogenous enzymes (enzymes the body produces) that participate in the METABOLISM of drugs. The CYP450 enzymes also participate in lipid (notably cholesterol) and steroid HORMONE synthesis. Most of the CYP450 enzymes that are active in DRUG metabolism are in the LIVER and the SMALL INTESTINE. The CYP450 enzymes function as catalysts to facilitate the processes by which the drug transforms from its initial chemical structure to the biochemical forms that have action in the body. Each of the CYP450 subtypes, also called isoforms or isoenzymes, metabolizes certain drugs or groups of drugs.

Hormones, antibodies, and foods affect the activity of CYP450 enzymes. Interactions among them may block or enhance a drug's activities; these effects may be beneficial or harmful. Some drug treatment regimens for complex conditions such as HIV/AIDS work by manipulating CYP450 enzyme activity to take advantage of beneficial interactions. Harmful interactions may manifest as adverse drug reactions such as toxicity or unpleasant side effects.

Individuals may express CYP450 activity differently—that is, known variation exists among individuals in the ways CYP450 enzymes function. These variations in CYP450 expression factor into individual responses to medications, at least partially accounting for why one drug may be more or less effective than another drug in the same drug family for a particular individual.

See also ALCOHOL INTERACTIONS WITH MEDICATIONS; ANTIBODY; PHARMACODYNAMICS; PHARMACOKINETICS.

dosage The therapeutic course of a DRUG, encompassing the drug's DOSE (amount of the drug taken), the frequency of the doses, the health condition and status of the person (including age and gender), and the total length of time the drug the person needs to take the drug. For many drugs there are standard dosages that are applicable to most people. The doctor or pharmacist calculates dosages for people who fall outside the standard range, and for NARROW THERAPEUTIC INDEX (NTI) drugs (drugs for which the margin between therapeutic and toxic is very close). People who may fall outside the standard range of dosage for many drugs are the very young, the very old, those who are extremely underweight, those who are extremely overweight, those who have multiple health conditions, and those who take numerous medications.

See also AGING, EFFECTS ON DRUG METABOLISM AND DRUG RESPONSE; PEAK LEVEL; THERAPEUTIC LEVEL; TROUGH LEVEL.

dose The amount of a DRUG a person takes or receives at a single time. A dose falls within a recommended therapeutic range for the drug, the person's condition, and the person's personal health circumstances (including age and gender). An excess of this amount is an OVERDOSE, which can have serious and even fatal consequences.

See also AGING, EFFECTS ON DRUG METABOLISM AND DRUG RESPONSE; DOSAGE; PEAK LEVEL; THERAPEUTIC LEVEL; THERAPEUTIC WINDOW; TROUGH LEVEL.

drug Any product that, when it enters the body, changes the function of the body in some way. Drugs such as ANTIBIOTIC MEDICATIONS work by killing BACTERIA within the body, for example, and antiarrhythmia drugs work by altering the electrical activity of the HEART. As the mainstay of modern medicine, drugs exert therapeutic actions to treat numerous health conditions.

See also ADVERSE DRUG REACTION; ALCOHOL; DRUG INTERACTION; INVESTIGATIONAL NEW DRUG (IND); OFF-LABEL USE.

drug interaction An effect or action that occurs in the body as a consequence of taking two or more drugs that does not occur when taking any one of the drugs alone. Drugs may interact with each other, OVER-THE-COUNTER (OTC) DRUGS and products, vitamin and mineral supplements, MEDICINAL HERBS AND BOTANICALS, and foods. Most DRUG interactions are inadvertent, occurring when a person takes an OTC medication with prescription medications, for example, or when a doctor prescribes a new medication without knowing all of the other medications a person is taking. The latter circumstance becomes a particular challenge when a person must receive urgent care in a clinic, hospital emergency department, or other setting in which the provider is someone other than the person's regular health-care provider.

Some drug interactions are neutral or even beneficial, such as when one medication potentiates (increases or enhances) or mitigates the action of another in a known and predictable way for a therapeutic effect. Such effect occurs, for example, with the combination of codeine (a narcotic PAIN reliever) and promethazine (Phenergan), an antiemetic medication (reduces NAUSEA). Though an effective pain reliever, codeine tends to cause nausea, but promethazine offsets this effect. And though promethazine alone has no analgesic (pain-relieving) effects it does potentiate, or intensify, the actions of codeine on the CENTRAL NERVOUS SYSTEM as well as mitigate its tendency to cause nausea. Other drug interactions can lessen or intensify the effects of one or more of the involved drugs in ways that are detrimental, either by causing adverse actions in the body or preventing the therapeutic effects of one or any of the drugs. Certain ANTIBIOTIC MEDICATIONS, for example, diminish the effectiveness of oral contraceptives (birth control pills).

It is important for every doctor, dentist, or other health-care provider who prescribes a DRUG for an individual to know all of the drugs, prescription and over-the-counter products (including herbal remedies and natural products) that the person is taking.

Most drug interactions occur as the result of a family of enzymes responsible for drug METABOLISM. These enzymes, called CYTOCHROME P450 (CYP450) ENZYMES, are abundant in the SMALL INTESTINE and the LIVER. CYP450 enzymes in the small intestine initiate the process of metabolism to allow molecules of the drug's active ingredient to pass into the BLOOD circulation. The blood carries the molecules to the liver, where the CYP450 enzymes there complete metabolism. There are numerous subtypes of CYP450 enzymes, each responsible for specific metabolic activity for certain drugs. Some drugs work by inducing and others by inhibiting particular CYP450 enzyme subtypes, which in turn affects the metabolism of other drugs. Other drug interactions may occur when the chemicals the drugs contain interact in some fashion. Iron and calcium in foods, vitamin supplements, and ANTACIDS bind with some antibiotics in the STOMACH, for example, preventing the antibiotic from becoming absorbed and entering the blood circulation.

The potential for drug interaction is extensive. The more medications a person takes, the higher the risk for drug interaction. A useful safeguard is to ask the pharmacist when picking up a prescription what other drugs and foods might interact with it. Even when foods do not directly interact with drugs, they may affect the drug's absorption into the body.

See also ADVERSE DRUG REACTION; ALCOHOL INTERACTIONS WITH MEDICATIONS; ANTIEMETIC MEDICATIONS; CONTRACEPTION; ILLICIT DRUG ABUSE; OVERDOSE; PRESCRIPTION DRUG ABUSE.

COMMON DRUG/DRUG AND DRUG/FOOD INTERACTIONS		
This Drug	**In Combination with This Drug or Food**	**Consequence of Interaction**
anticoagulant medications (heparin, warfarin) antiplatelet medications (cilostazol, clopidogrel, dipyridamole, ticlopidine)	aspirin GINGKO BILOBA	further decreases clotting response of the BLOOD, raising risk for bleeding
	large quantities of spinach vitamin supplement containing VITAMIN K	increases ability of blood to clot, diminishing effectiveness of ANTICOAGULANT THERAPY
ANTIFUNGAL MEDICATIONS (fluconazole, griseofulvin, itraconazole, ketoconazole)	ALCOHOL of any kind (including in medications such as cold and flu products)	increases the risk for liver failure

This Drug	In Combination with This Drug or Food	Consequence of Interaction
beta blockers (acebutolol, atenolol, betaxolol, bisoprolol, carteolol, carvedilol, esmolol, labetalol, metoprolol, nadolol, penbutolol, pindolol, propranolol, sotalol, timolol)	oral antidiabetes medications	decreases effectiveness of oral antidiabetes medications masks presence of HYPOGLYCEMIA
	H2 blockers	reduces liver's ability to metabolize beta blocker, allowing potentially toxic levels to accumulate in the blood circulation
	MAOI antidepressants	increases MAOI level; high risk for toxicity
	cigarette smoking	reduces effectiveness of beta blocker
H2 ANTAGONIST (BLOCKER) MEDICATIONS (cimetidine, famotidine, ranitidine, nizatidine)	antifungal medications	reduces absorption and effectiveness of antifungal medications
	oral antidiabetes medications INSULIN	increases effectiveness of antidiabetes medications, raising risk for hypoglycemia
	beta blockers	increases effectiveness of beta blockers, raising risk for bradycardia and HYPOTENSION
	tricyclic antidepressants (amitriptyline, desipramine, imipramine, nortriptyline)	increases antidepressant level in blood circulation, raising risk for serotonin syndrome
metronidazole (Flagyl)	alcohol of any kind (including in medications such as cold and flu products)	action similar to that of disulfiram (antabuse)
	lithium	lithium toxicity
	anticoagulant and antiplatelet medications	further decreases clotting response, raising the risk for bleeding
monoamine oxidase inhibitor (MAOI) ANTIDEPRESSANT MEDICATIONS (isocarboxazid, phenelzine, selegiline, tranylcypromine)	beta blockers foods high in tyramine (beer, red wine, processed cheeses, smoked meats, avocados, bananas, raisins, cured foods) GINSENG CAFFEINE in beverages or medications	sudden, rapid, and very high surge in BLOOD PRESSURE (potentially fatal)

This Drug	In Combination with This Drug or Food	Consequence of Interaction
oral antidiabetes medications	alcohol	decreases effectiveness of oral antidiabetes medication
	CORTICOSTEROID MEDICATIONS thiazide diuretics aspirin and other salicylates MAOI antidepressants NONSTEROIDAL ANTI-INFLAMMATORY DRUGS (NSAIDS) sulfonamide antibiotics warfarin	increases effectiveness of oral antidiabetes medication
quinolone antibiotics (ciprofloxacin, levofloxacin, ofloxacin, trovafloxacin) tetracycline antibiotics (doxycycline, minocycline, tetracycline)	ANTACIDS dairy products calcium supplements iron supplements	chemical binding in stomach prevents absorption of antibiotic
beta-hydroxy-beta methylglutaryl–coenzyme A (HMG-CoA) reductase inhibitor (statin) lipid-lowering medications (atorvastatin, fluvastatin, lovastatin, pravastatin, simvastatin)	grapefruit juice	decreases liver's ability to metabolize statins
	antibiotic and antifungal medications	various adverse reactions
	oral contraceptives (birth control pills)	reduced effectiveness of the oral contraceptive

efficacy The ability of a DRUG to produce a predictable effect in the body. Many factors influence a drug's efficacy, from foods and other drugs to health conditions and a person's metabolic characteristics. An individual's age, weight, gender, and level of activity also may affect the rate at which a drug enters, and how long it stays in, the BLOOD circulation. Efficacy is a key factor in determining a drug's potential effectiveness to treat a particular condition in a specific individual. Some drugs have greater efficacy in younger people, for example. Other factors that are also relevant include BIOAVAILABILITY and BIOEQUIVALENCE.

See also CYTOCHROME P450 (CYP450) ENZYMES; THERAPEUTIC WINDOW.

formulary A list of the prescription drugs a health plan or insurance company, including state and federal health insurance programs, will cover. Typically a committee of physicians and pharmacists makes the determinations about what drugs appear in the formulary and why. Factors for consideration include

- the DRUG'S EFFICACY
- whether generic products are available
- similarity to other drugs that are less expensive or have fewer side effects
- NARROW THERAPEUTIC INDEX (NTI) status
- the need for the drug within the insurer's patient population
- whether over-the-counter forms of the drug are available
- the drug's approved uses

Most insurers update their formularies at least annually. An insurer may pay a smaller percent-age of the cost for a nonformulary drug or may choose not to cover (pay for) nonformulary drugs at all except within the parameters of specifically defined criteria. A doctor may prescribe a drug that is not on the formulary even though the insurer may refuse to pay for it. The person may still receive the drug by paying for the prescription. Drug formularies help establish consistent prescribing practices as well as control costs for the insurer.

See also GENERIC DRUG; *ORANGE BOOK, THE*; OVER-THE-COUNTER (OTC) DRUGS; PHARMACOPEIA; SIDE EFFECT.

generic drug A DRUG that has BIOEQUIVALENCE and THERAPEUTIC EQUIVALENCE to its INNOVATOR DRUG (the first drug to receive approval for use). Generic drugs became significant in the health-care industry in the 1970s when manufacturing requirements and procedures became standardized and patents began to expire on innovator drugs, converging factors that opened the market for competition within the pharmaceutical industry. Most generic drugs are significantly less expensive than their innovator counterparts, and most states have laws allowing pharmacies to substitute generic drugs when filling prescriptions unless the prescribing provider specifies otherwise. The intent behind such laws is to provide consumers with cost-effective alternatives for prescription drugs. Generic products are also available for many OVER-THE-COUNTER (OTC) DRUGS, allowing consumers to choose either generic or trade name products.

The US Food and Drug Administration (FDA), the federal regulatory agency that approves drugs for use in the United States, establishes the criteria for potency, purity, consistency, and efficacy all drugs must meet. These criteria are the same for innovator and generic drugs. Generic drugs may also have trade names, which manufacturers often use to establish brand recognition and brand loyalty for marketing purposes. For example, Elavil and Endep are trade names for amitriptyline, a commonly prescribed tricyclic antidepressant. The manufacturer of an innovator drug may also produce and market generic versions of the drug when the innovator drug's patent expires.

In nearly all circumstances a person may take any manufacturer's product, generic or innovator drug, and experience the same therapeutic effects. The only exception is with NARROW THERAPEUTIC INDEX (NTI) DRUGS, in which the margin between the therapeutic dose and the toxic dose is exceedingly small. People who take NTI drugs should always take the same product, whether the innovator drug or a generic drug. Variations in the drug's inactive ingredients can affect how the body absorbs the drug, which can have therapeutic significance with NTI drugs.

In its electronic document *THE ORANGE BOOK*, the FDA maintains a list of newly approved generic drugs, updated each month, and a list of all generic drugs available in the United States. *The Orange Book* is available at the FDA's Web site (www.fda.gov/cder/ob).

See also INVESTIGATIONAL NEW DRUG (IND); LEGEND DRUGS; OFF-LABEL USE; SCHEDULED DRUG.

half-life The length of time it takes for the body to metabolize or eliminate from the body 50 percent of the amount of a DRUG a person takes or receives. Drug half-life is an important factor in determining appropriate DOSAGE and for treating OVERDOSE. Drug half-life also helps the doctor know when to expect to begin to see the effects of the drug. The calculation of drug half-life is logarithmic. Drug informational literature, packaged with prescription drugs, provides general information about the drug's half-life that is generally adequate for most clinical circumstances. A doctor may conduct BLOOD tests to measure the levels of a drug in an individual's blood circulation over a period of time as a means of indirectly assessing half-life, though this is seldom therapeutically necessary.

See also BIOAVAILABILITY; CYTOCHROME P450 (CYP450) ENZYMES; EFFICACY; METABOLISM; PEAK LEVEL;

THERAPEUTIC LEVEL; THERAPEUTIC WINDOW; TROUGH LEVEL.

imported drug A DRUG or pharmaceutical product not manufactured in the country of purchase. Countries may have differing requirements for testing and product safety for the manufacture and distribution of drugs within their borders. In the United States the Food and Drug Administration (FDA) has regulatory authority over drug production and distribution and establishes the standards for bringing drugs into the country.

The Internet has dramatically broadened access to foreign markets for drugs. Many Americans are drawn to Internet purchasing because of the ease and convenience and because imported drugs are often less expensive than the same drugs purchased in the United States. However, health experts caution that drugs purchased through locations in other countries, either by mail order or via the Internet, may not meet US quality standards for purity, potency, and safety and may not be legal to bring into the country.

The FDA supports the National Association of Boards of Pharmacy's Verified Internet Pharmacies Web site, www.nabp.net. This system provides another way for consumers to verify the legitimacy of online pharmacies.

See also GENERIC DRUG; INVESTIGATIONAL NEW DRUG (IND).

innovator drug The first DRUG containing its specific active ingredients to receive approval for use from the US Food and Drug Administration (FDA). An innovator drug's patent protects the drug from market competition, giving its manufacturer exclusive right to produce and sell the drug. The innovator drug's manufacturer generally has invested significant time and money in the drug's development, testing, and approval process. Only when the patent expires may competing pharmaceutical manufacturers produce and market a generic version of the innovator drug.

See also GENERIC DRUG; INVESTIGATIONAL NEW DRUG (IND).

investigational new drug (IND) A new DRUG in the final phases of development for which the US Food and Drug Administration (FDA) grants restricted approval for use in clinical testing, emergency treatment, or transportation across state lines. Typically the use of an IND must meet one of three requirements:

- The person to receive the IND enrolls in a clinical research study that is evaluating the drug's effectiveness, benefits, and risks among the drug's intended patient population.
- The person to receive the IND has a serious or life-threatening condition the IND is being developed to treat, and there are no ongoing clinical research studies in which the person can enroll.

- The person to receive the IND has a serious or life-threatening condition the IND is being developed to treat, and the FDA is in the process of reviewing the drug's clinical research data.

The most commonly used INDs are antibiotics used to treat multiple-drug-resistant infections and drugs to treat cancer. On its Web site the FDA maintains lists of current INDs by type of drug and information about how to gain access to unapproved drugs (www.fda.gov).

See also ANTIBIOTIC RESISTANCE; OFF-LABEL USE; ORPHAN DRUG.

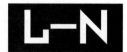

L–N

legend drug   In the United States, any DRUG that requires a physician or other appropriately licensed health-care provider (such as a dentist, optometrist, or podiatrist) to write a prescription and a pharmacist to dispense the medication. The federal approval and regulatory process determines which drugs are legend drugs, the labels of which must carry the admonition, "Caution: Federal law prohibits dispensing without a prescription." Each state further regulates the prescribing and dispensing of legend drugs, though practices are fairly consistent across states. Such regulation includes the kind of information that must appear on the dispensing label and the manner in which the pharmacist must discuss the drug's intended benefits and potential risks with the person receiving the medication. It is common to refer to legend drugs simply as prescription drugs.

See also OFF-LABEL USE; OVER-THE-COUNTER (OTC) DRUGS; SCHEDULED DRUG.

low-cost prescription programs   Need-based programs, usually under the sponsorship of major pharmaceutical manufacturers, that make certain prescription medications available to people who lack insurance coverage for prescription medications or who cannot otherwise afford to obtain them. Most low-cost prescription programs have income limitations for enrollees and many require that a doctor refer the person and that the person receive the medications through delivery to the doctor's office. Doctors, hospitals, and pharmacies maintain information about current programs and their enrollment requirements.

Some organizations, such as the American Association for Retired Persons (AARP), also have membership prescription programs that make drugs available to members at a significant dis-count from regular retail prices. Doctors' offices and clinics hospitals also often have drug samples that pharmaceutical representatives leave. Some programs offer prepaid prescription cards and other kinds of membership promotions for people who do not have insurance to cover prescription drugs but exceed the income levels for low-cost prescription plans. Whether these programs truly save money on prescription drugs depends on the amount and kinds of prescription drugs an individual takes.

See also HEALTHY PEOPLE 2010; ORPHAN DRUG.

narrow therapeutic index (NTI)   A very close margin between the concentration in the BLOOD circulation of a DRUG that is therapeutic and the concentration that is lethal (deadly). Pharmacists generally express the therapeutic index as a ratio between the median effective DOSE (ED50) and the median lethal dose (LD50). A drug has a narrow therapeutic index when there is less than a twofold difference between the ED50 and the LD50. With NTI drugs even very small changes in the dose, variations in product potency, or changes in the person's health status can result in toxic levels of the drug with harmful or fatal consequences.

The current standard of practice is to maintain the course treatment with the same drug product rather than substituting across brand and generic products as commonly and safely occurs with non-NTI drugs. Some doctors prefer to use specific brand name products when prescribing NTI drugs. Some states mandate a nonsubstitution standard via law or regulatory code, requiring pharmacies to dispense the original drug product. Some clinical studies support such caution though others suggest that, at least with some NTI drugs, generic substitution maintains therapeutically acceptable consistency for potency and EFFICACY.

The current standard of practice calls for close monitoring of blood concentrations until the drug reaches the desired therapeutic level, with routine blood tests to monitor blood concentration over time, when the person begins taking a new drug, and when there is a change in the person's health status (including significant change in body weight). Once the blood concentration of the drug reaches a steady state with the drug at a therapeutic level the NTI becomes less of a concern.

**COMMONLY PRESCRIBED
NARROW THERAPEUTIC INDEX (NTI) DRUGS**

aminophylline	carbamazepine	clindamycin
clozapine	cyclosporin	digoxin
disopyramide	isoproterenol	levothyroxine
lithium	metaproterenol	phenytoin
prazosin	primidone	procainamide
quinidine	valproic acid	warfarin

See also BIOAVAILABILITY; BIOEQUIVALENCE; *ORANGE BOOK, THE;* PEAK LEVEL; THERAPEUTIC LEVEL; THERAPEUTIC WINDOW; TROUGH LEVEL.

off-label use Taking a DRUG for a purpose other than that for which it has received regulatory approval. In the United States the Food and Drug Administration (FDA) requires pharmaceutical manufacturers to demonstrate the safety and efficacy of a drug before approving it for use. Once a drug receives FDA approval, however, doctors may legally prescribe it for uses that are consistent with current standards of care. The FDA does not regulate how doctors prescribe or individuals take approved drugs.

Additional beneficial effects of a drug often emerge after the drug has been in use for some time and doctors begin to notice those effects. For some of these drugs the additional effects are so significant that prescribing the drug for them subsequently becomes an approved use. In other situations the drug becomes widely known for its additional effects but the manufacturer does not conduct further studies or seek FDA approval for them.

Off-label use is most common when treating conditions for which conventional therapies are limited or unsuccessful, especially when the condition is progressive or chronic such as MULTIPLE SCLEROSIS, PARKINSON'S DISEASE, CANCER, and CHRONIC PAIN syndromes. Doctors may also turn to off-label use when prescribing medications for children because many drugs receive approval without having been tested for safety and EFFICACY in children. A doctor's decision to prescribe a drug off-label draws from available clinical study results, clinical observations, and best practices standards. It is important for a person considering off-label use of a drug to fully understand the potential benefits and risks of such use as well as the drug's possible side effects and adverse reactions.

See also ADVERSE DRUG REACTION; INVESTIGATIONAL NEW DRUG (IND); SIDE EFFECT.

Orange Book, The A document the US Food and Drug Administration (FDA) maintains that lists all the drugs, prescription and over-the-counter, that have FDA approval for use in the United States. As of 2005 *The Orange Book* is available only as an electronic document (www.fda.gov/cder/ob) on the FDA's Web site (print editions are no longer obtainable). An individual may download the document in a printable format to produce a paper copy, if desired.

The FDA updates *The Orange Book* daily. These updates provide, among other kinds of information, the most current information about newly approved generic products. *The Orange Book* lists drugs by proprietary (trade or brand) name, active ingredient, and patent holder. Listings identify the INNOVATOR DRUG (first drug that received approval) and any GENERIC DRUG also approved for use as well as provide information about the status of the product's patent.

See also FORMULARY; INVESTIGATIONAL NEW DRUG.

orphan drug A DRUG to treat a rare condition. The US Orphan Drug Act of 1983 (ODA) established criteria in the United States to encourage pharmaceutical manufacturers to investigate new drugs and continue to produce approved drugs to treat conditions, such as HUNTINGTON'S DISEASE and some forms of MUSCULAR DYSTROPHY, that affect fewer than 200,000 people. The underlying premise of an orphan drug is that its sales will not generate enough revenue for its manufacturer to recover the costs of its development and testing, a circumstance that makes research and production unappealing to pharmaceutical manufacturers. The ODA establishes mechanisms of financial support for pharmaceutical manufacturers through grants and tax relief, in return for which the manufacturer agrees to produce and market the drug. Additional grants are available to support research about rare diseases. In 2005 there were approximately 1,400 drugs with orphan drug status. The US Food and Drug Administration (FDA) Office of Orphan Products Development (OOPD) oversees orphan drug research.

See also INVESTIGATIONAL NEW DRUG (IND); OFF-LABEL USE.

outdated drug A DRUG that is past the manufacturer's listed expiration date. An outdated drug may be less effective than the unexpired product or may be harmful. Drugs deteriorate over time. Some drugs have short effective periods, particularly those that require refrigeration. Other drugs maintain potency for years. The US Food and Drug Administration (FDA) requires pharmaceutical manufacturers to determine the length of time a drug remains at full potency and to incorporate an expiration date into the drug's labeling information. In general, pharmacists recommend not using a drug after one year from the date it was opened or removed from its original packaging (including preparation or repackaging as a prescription).

No matter what a DRUG's official expiration date, do not use or take products that are discolored or obviously deteriorated (such as tablets that are crumbling) or when there is damage to the container (such as a crack in a tube or a broken lid).

Factors such as exposure to heat, light, moisture, and air may hasten deterioration, causing a drug to become less effective even before its expiration date. It is important to store drugs in their original or prescription containers and in the appropriate environment. Many people keep medications in a bathroom medicine cabinet, which, though convenient for remembering to take medications at the prescribed times, is a less than ideal environment. Most bathrooms are small and enclosed and experience extreme variations in

heat and humidity as a result of people bathing or showering. Pharmacists recommend storing drugs, prescription and over-the-counter, in a cool, dry, dark location unless the label specifies other storage requirements, such as refrigeration.

See also EFFICACY; OVERDOSE.

overdose Consumption of a quantity of a DRUG in excess of its recommended DOSE or of a combination of drugs that results in potentiated effects from any or all of the drugs. Overdose may occur with prescription or OVER-THE-COUNTER (OTC) DRUGS. The consequences of an overdose may range from no apparent symptoms to potentially life-threatening adverse effects. The severity of the consequences depends on numerous factors, including the person's age, health condition, amount and kind of drug, whether the person also consumed ALCOHOL, and to some extent whether the overdose is intentional or unintentional.

Seek immediate medical help for any suspected overdose. Call 911 or the US national poison control hotline at 800-222-1222. Do not induce vomiting unless a health professional so advises. Keep the package or container and any remaining DRUG for positive identification.

Unintentional overdose may occur when a person

- misreads or misunderstands the dosage instructions
- forgets having taken a dose and takes another
- takes one drug thinking it is another drug
- takes multiple drugs that have the same ingredients
- takes a prescription drug and an over-the-counter (OTC) drug that have the same active ingredient
- takes multiple drugs that interact in ways that intensify the effects of one or more of the drugs taken
- drinks alcohol or uses illicit substances when taking the medication

A high risk for overdose exists among young children who spend extended periods of time with older caregivers such as grandparents. Many older people have difficulty with child-resistant drug packaging or set out their medications to remember to take them. Brightly colored tablets and capsules are attractive to young children who think they are candy. The coatings on many pills contain sugar to mask unpleasant flavors during the time the pill is in the person's mouth and to aid in making the pill easy to swallow. A child may experience life-threatening poisoning from taking only a few pills, far fewer than would cause adverse effects in an adult. Medications to treat HEART conditions and iron supplements are among the most hazardous drugs for overdose in children. Overdose of acetaminophen and aspirin may cause permanent LIVER FAILURE or RENAL FAILURE

COMMON DRUG OVERDOSE SYMPTOMS	
Type of Drug	**Common Symptoms**
acetaminophen	initial: NAUSEA, VOMITING, excessive sweating later: ABDOMINAL PAIN, HEPATOMEGALY, JAUNDICE, LIVER FAILURE, RENAL FAILURE
ANTIHISTAMINE MEDICATIONS (brompheniramine, cetirizine, clemastine, diphenhydramine, doxylamine, fexofenadine, loratadine, meclizine, promethazine, tripelennamine, triprolidine)	initial: extremely dry mucous membranes and SKIN, flushing, difficulty urinating, agitation, confusion later: seizures, extreme HYPERTENSION, ARRHYTHMIA, COMA
aspirin, salicylates, and NONSTEROIDAL ANTI-INFLAMATORY DRUGS (NSAIDS)	initial: TINNITUS, vomiting, FEVER, rapid HEART RATE, rapid BREATHING, confusion, HALLUCINATION later: kidney failure, HEART FAILURE, coma, gastrointestinal bleeding
BARBITURATE (pentobarbital, phenobarbital, secobarbital)	initial: drowsiness, lack of coordination, slurred speech, depressed breathing, slow heart rate later: coma, RESPIRATORY FAILURE
BENZODIAZEPINES (alprazolam, chlordiazepoxide, clorazepate, diazepam, flurazepam, lorazepam, oxazepam, prazepam, temazepam, triazolam)	initial: drowsiness, blurred vision, agitation, confusion, hallucinations, depressed breathing, HYPOTENSION later: loss of CONSCIOUSNESS, coma
digoxin	initial: nausea, confusion, blurred vision later: irregular heart beat, CARDIAC ARREST
iron (ferrous gluconate, ferrous fumarate, ferrous sulfate, multiple vitamin and mineral supplement products containing iron)	initial: nausea, vomiting, metallic taste in MOUTH, chills, HEADACHE, dizziness, flushing later: rapid heart rate, hypotension, coma
NARCOTICS (codeine, fentanyl, hydrocodone, hydromorphone, meperidine, methadone, morphine, oxycodone)	initial: drowsiness, hypotension, depressed breathing, pinpoint pupils later: respiratory failure
tricyclic ANTIDEPRESSANT MEDICATIONS (amitriptyline, desipramine, doxepin, imipramine, nortriptyline, protriptyline, trimipramine)	initial: irregular heart rate, nausea, vomiting, DIARRHEA, hypotension later: seizures, psychotic behavior, arrhythmias, extreme HYPERTENSION, cardiac arrest

requiring LIVER TRANSPLANTATION or KIDNEY TRANS-PLANTATION.

Symptoms and Diagnostic Path

The symptoms of drug overdose vary according to the drug or drugs involved and may range from agitation to lethargy to loss of CONSCIOUSNESS. Some symptoms are immediate, such as slowed BREATHING and HEART RATE with narcotic overdose, and others develop over time, such as JAUNDICE, resulting from liver damage. Prompt medical treatment is essential whenever there is cause to suspect overdose. The kinds of symptoms a person has can suggest the general nature of the toxicity (narcotic, cholinergic, hepatotoxic) though it is important to identify as quickly as possible what drug or drugs the person has taken.

Treatment Options and Outlook

Treatment focuses on removing or neutralizing the drug, when health-care providers are reasonably certain what drug or drugs the person has taken. Gastric lavage ("STOMACH pumping") is the common method for attempting to remove ingested (swallowed) drugs. It is effective only within 30 to 60 minutes of ingestion; after this time any swallowed substances have passed from the stomach into the SMALL INTESTINE. Gastric lavage involves inserting a nasogastric tube through the NOSE and down the back of the THROAT into the stomach to withdraw the stomach's contents and flush the stomach with liquid. Sometimes the doctor will infuse a solution of activated charcoal, which is highly absorbent, to help prevent more of the drug from entering the BLOOD circulation. Doctors do not agree about the effectiveness of gastric lavage for improving the person's risk for complications of overdose, and gastric lavage itself carries risks for esophageal perforation (damage to the wall of the ESOPHAGUS) and aspiration of stomach fluids into the LUNGS.

Antagonists, also called antidotes, are available to reverse the effects of some kinds of drugs. They include

- naloxone, which counteracts NARCOTICS
- N-acetylcysteine, which counteracts acetaminophen

- physostigmine, which counteracts some antihistamines
- flumazenil, which counteracts BENZODIAZEPINES

Other treatment targets symptoms and provides supportive care until the body can metabolize enough of the drug for blood concentrations to drop below toxic levels. Such support might include MECHANICAL VENTILATION when breathing is impaired or dialysis for kidney failure. The extent of permanent damage or the likelihood of death depends on the drug and the amount as well as how quickly the person receives treatment.

Risk Factors and Preventive Measures

Child-resistant containers and storing medications in locked cabinets or drawers out of the reach of children are important measures for preventing accidental overdose in children. Adults should store drugs in their original containers and check the container before taking a dose of the drug. Particularly with prescription drugs repackaged in pharmacy containers, it is easy to grab the wrong bottle and take one drug thinking it is another. Contact the pharmacist or doctor if there are unusual symptoms after taking any drug. It is also crucial for the prescribing doctor and the dispensing pharmacist to know all of the drugs a person is taking, prescription and OTC (including MEDICINAL HERBS AND BOTANICALS).

See also ADVERSE DRUG REACTION; AGING, EFFECTS ON DRUG METABOLISM AND DRUG RESPONSE; ALCOHOL INTERACTIONS WITH MEDICATIONS; CYTOCHROME P450 (CYP450) ENZYMES; HEPATOTOXINS; POISON PREVENTION.

over-the-counter (OTC) drug In the United States, a DRUG that is available for purchase without a prescription and that does not require a pharmacist to dispense. However, US laws do require OTC product labels to list the product's active ingredients, main inactive ingredients, strength, recommended DOSAGE, significant side effects (such as drowsiness), and any health conditions a person might have in which the person should not take the drug. Furthermore these drugs must meet drug purity, consistency, and safety standards. OTC drugs are available in a wide variety of retail locations. Most OTC products come in child-resistant packaging. Tablets and cap-sules may come in bulk or single-dose packaging.

The US Food and Drug Administration (FDA) oversees the approval of new OTC drugs, which must meet the general criteria that:

- The drug's benefits outweigh its risks.
- A person can take the drug to treat a self-diag-nosed condition (such as HEADACHE or seasonal allergies).
- The drug has a low risk for abuse.

Many OTC drugs are lower-dose versions of approved prescription drugs and thus have exten-sive clinical history that demonstrates their relative effectiveness and safety. Though OTC drugs are generally safe to take without a doctor's oversight of either the drug's use or the condition the person is taking the drug to treat, people who regularly take prescribed or doctor-recommended medica-tions should ask the doctor or pharmacist about possible problems or interactions.

All drugs have potential side effects, adverse reactions, and interactions. OTC drugs may inter-act with each other or with prescription drugs the person is also taking. Unintentional OVERDOSE may occur when taking a prescription drug and an OTC drug or when taking multiple OTC drugs that con-tain the same ingredients. This is a particular haz-ard when taking cold and flu products with ALLERGY relief products, when taking PAIN relief products with cold and flu products, and when taking prescription drugs to treat OSTEOARTHRITIS with pain relievers or cold and flu products. Many cold and flu products contain an antihistamine and an ingredient to relieve pain and FEVER, such as acetaminophen or ibuprofen. Prescription med-ications for osteoarthritis are often NONSTEROIDAL ANTI-INFLAMMATORY DRUGS (NSAIDS), the same classi-fication of drug as OTC pain relievers such as ibuprofen, ketoprofen, and naproxen. It is impor-tant to read product labels carefully and ask the pharmacist about any possible interactions with other medications.

See also ADVERSE DRUG REACTION; ALCOHOL INTER-ACTIONS WITH MEDICATIONS; GENERIC DRUG; LEGEND DRUG; *ORANGE BOOK, THE*; SCHEDULED DRUG; SIDE EFFECT.

peak level The maximum concentration of a DRUG in the BLOOD circulation. The peak level corresponds in part to the drug's route of administration, chemical composition, and rate of METABOLISM. A drug's peak level may occur within minutes to several hours of taking or receiving it. Injectable drugs enter the blood circulation rapidly; oral medications (taken by MOUTH) take longer to reach the blood as they must first go through digestion. Foods and liquids also consumed affect the rate of digestion and absorption, as do other factors such as the person's activity level, age, body weight, and any health conditions.

A drug's peak level establishes the upper limit of the drug's therapeutic range. For most drugs it is not necessary for the doctor to determine peak level and TROUGH LEVEL (lowest concentration) as the drug's informational literature provides the expected levels. Improvement in the person's symptoms or condition is clinical evidence that the drug DOSAGE is therapeutically appropriate. The doctor may more closely monitor blood concentrations for NARROW THERAPEUTIC INDEX (NTI) drugs, for which the peak and trough levels are critical. Because the goal of most medication therapy is to achieve a fairly constant level of the drug in the blood circulation, peak and trough levels are primarily significant at the onset of treatment.

See also HALF-LIFE; ROUTES OF ADMINISTRATION; THERAPEUTIC LEVEL.

pharmacodynamics The actions of drugs within the body. Drugs enter and act within the body by binding with cell receptors, specialized fragments of proteins that instruct the cell to take or not take specific actions. This binding process, called selectivity, limits and directs the effects of drugs. Pro-teins are the basic components of the body's biochemical messengers, hormones and neurotransmitters. The interactions they initiate are often intricate cascades that influence numerous biochemical processes (such as ion passage for cell communication) as well as DNA encoding and transcription (cell function and replication). Numerous factors influence the unfolding of these cascades, from a person's general health status and existing health conditions to other drugs the person is taking. For example, INSULIN RESISTANCE and DIABETES affect the energy accessible to cells to carry out the functions of cellular METABOLISM, altering the processes and outcomes of receptor binding. Through different mechanisms HYPOTHYROIDISM slows and HYPERTHYROIDISM accelerates cellular metabolism, also affecting receptor binding. Pharmacodynamics gives doctors and pharmacists the ability to assess how individuals may react to specific drugs, depending on their unique health profiles.

See also ALCOHOL INTERACTIONS WITH MEDICATIONS; BIOAVAILABILITY; CYTOCHROME P450 (CYP450) ENZYMES; HORMONE; NEURON; NEUROTRANSMITTER; PHARMACOKINETICS.

pharmacokinetics The timing of a DRUG's absorption, METABOLISM, action, and excretion. Pharmacokinetics is an element of DOSAGE determination and the EFFICACY of a drug. Many variables unique to an individual influence the rate of a drug's entry into, stay within, and passage from the body. Mathematical calculations that integrate the drug's characteristics (such as form and strength) with an individual's health circumstances allow doctors and pharmacists to tailor medication therapy regimens specific to the individual's needs.

See also ALCOHOL INTERACTIONS WITH MEDICATIONS; BIOAVAILABILITY; BIOEQUIVALENCE; CYTOCHROME P450 (CYP450) ENZYMES; PHARMACODYNAMICS.

pharmacopeia A professional and regulatory compendium of information about drugs, including their formulations, dosages, and therapeutic uses, that establishes manufacturing, safety, EFFICACY, and prescribing standards. The US Pharmacopeia (USP) is a formal and official document as well as a process for maintaining quality standards across the spectrum of pharmaceutical manufacturers, pharmacies, and health-care organizations (such as practices, clinics, care facilities, and hospitals) after a drug receives approval from the US Food and Drug Administration (FDA). Drugs and products such as dietary supplements that bear the indication "USP-verified" or include "USP" with the product name meet USP standards. Other countries have similar pharmacopeia (commonly spelled "pharmacopoeia" outside the United States) structures.

See also FORMULARY; *ORANGE BOOK, THE*.

placebo An inert substance that has no biological, chemical, or other action within the body, taken with the intent of producing a therapeutic effect. The placebo effect refers to the sense of improvement of symptoms an individual may experience when taking or using a product that has no active ingredients. Researchers often use placebo products when testing new drugs, particularly medications such as PAIN relievers (ANALGESIC MEDICATIONS), in which the assessment of effectiveness has a subjective component.

See also INVESTIGATIONAL NEW DRUG (IND); MIND-BODY CONNECTION.

route of administration The method by which a person takes or receives a DRUG. The common routes administration are oral (by MOUTH), sublingual (beneath the tongue), injection, topical, transdermal, and rectal. Women may use some drugs intravaginally. Some drugs are available only in certain forms, such as injectable. Many drugs are available in numerous forms. Factors that influence the selected route of administration include the drug's formulation and the person's ability to take or receive a particular form of the drug. For example, a young child or person who has difficulty swallowing or is experiencing NAUSEA and VOMITING may better handle a drug adminis-

ROUTE OF DRUG ADMINISTRATION		
Route	Forms	Entry Mechanism
injection	intravenous (IV), intramuscular (IM), subcutaneous (SC)	IV: into a VEIN, direct entry to the BLOOD circulation IM: into a MUSCLE; rapid absorption into the blood circulation SC: into the fatty tissue beneath the skin; slow absorption into the blood circulation
oral (*per os* or PO)	tablet, capsule, liquid	digestion breaks down the product, with absorption usually in the SMALL INTESTINE
rectal	suppository	Soft carrier wax melts, drug becomes absorbed into the blood circulation through the wall of the RECTUM
sublingual (SL)	tablet, liquid	dissolves under the tongue, becoming absorbed into the blood circulation through the mucosa of the MOUTH
topical	cream, ointment, gel, lotion, spray	intended to remain within the layers of the SKIN
transdermal	patch, cream, ointment	intended to be absorbed through the skin into the blood circulation

tered by transdermal patch, injection, or rectal suppository. Injection allows the most rapid delivery; other forms allow slower entry of the drug into the BLOOD circulation.

See also BIOAVAILABILITY; PHARMACOKINETICS.

scheduled drug   In the United States a DRUG that has strict prescribing and availability criteria because of its potential for ADDICTION or abuse, as the federal Uniform Controlled Substance Act (UCSA) of 1970 specifies and regulates. Some substances are scheduled drugs (also called controlled substances) because they have no medicinal or therapeutic value yet may cause considerable harm or death when used, such as HEROIN and lysergic acid diethylamide (LSD). The UCSA establishes five levels of control for such drugs, indicated by a Roman numeral on the drug package's label.

Each level of control has specific requirements for ordering, storing, prescribing, dispensing, and destroying the scheduled drugs within its definition; in general the distribution system is a closed one in that every individual who handles a scheduled drug must account for that drug's passage through his or her contact. The US Drug Enforcement Agency (DEA) oversees compliance with UCSA regulations. Though state provider licensing regulations designate prescribing authority for scheduled drugs, a provider must have a DEA license to prescribe scheduled drugs.

Schedule I drugs are available only to researchers. Schedule II drugs require a written prescription for each quantity of drug received. Schedule III and schedule IV drugs require a written or oral prescription and are refillable from the original prescription up to five times within six months if the provider authorizes refills. Under federal law schedule V drugs do not require a prescription though states may otherwise regulate their availability.

SCHEDULED DRUGS		
Schedule	**Common Drugs**	**Definition**
schedule I	HEROIN, LSD, mescaline, methylenedioxymethamphetamine (MDMA), methaqualone, racemoramide, tilidine, trimeperidine	no accepted medical use high risk for abuse unsafe for use
schedule II	amobarbital, AMPHETAMINE, COCAINE, codeine, glutethimide, hydrocodone, hydromorphone, levorphanol, meperidine, METHADONE, methylphenidate, morphine, oxycodone, oxymorphone, pentobarbital	limited medical use high risk for abuse high risk for physical or psychological dependence
schedule III	amobarbital, amphetamine, anabolic steroids, BUPRENORPHINE, chlorphentermine, codeine compounds, GLUTETHIMIDE, hydrocodone compounds, phenmetrazine	accepted medical use moderate risk for abuse moderate risk for physical or psychological dependence
schedule IV	BENZODIAZEPINES, CHLORAL HYDRATE, meprobamate, paraldehyde, pemoline, pentazocine, phenobarbital, propoxyphene compounds, zolpidem	accepted medical use low risk for abuse low risk for physical or psychological dependence

schedule V	codeine COUGH preparations, dihydrocodeine, diphenoxylate	accepted medical use
		negligible risk for abuse
		negligible risk for physical
		    dependence, low risk for
		    psychological dependence

See also ILLICIT DRUG USE; LEGEND DRUG; OVER-THE-COUNTER (OTC) DRUGS; PRESCRIPTION DRUG ABUSE.

side effect   An action other than the intended therapeutic effect of a DRUG. Side effects may be neutral, beneficial, or harmful. Many side effects are so common as to be expected, such as DIARRHEA with certain ANTIBIOTIC MEDICATIONS (which occurs because antibiotics kill BACTERIA, including the bacteria that normally reside in the gastrointestinal tract to aid in digestion). Some side effects are temporary, such as drowsiness when first beginning treatment with ANTIDEPRESSANT MEDICATIONS (which affect neurotransmitters and functions of the CENTRAL NERVOUS SYSTEM) and NAUSEA at the onset of therapy with antihypertensive medications (which affect the autonomic NERVOUS SYSTEM). A harmful side effect (one that has serious or long-term health consequences) is an ADVERSE DRUG REACTION. It is important to know what side effects can occur with all medications a person is taking, for each individual drug as well as for the drugs in combination with each other. In the United States federal and state laws require product package inserts or label information to contain brief information about possible side effects.

See also ALCOHOL INTERACTIONS WITH MEDICATIONS; DRUG INTERACTION; NEUROTRANSMITTER; OFF-LABEL USE.

therapeutic equivalence In pharmacology, drugs that have the same active ingredients in the same forms and have the same actions within the body. The US Food and Drug Administration (FDA), which oversees DRUG approval in the United States, refers to such drugs as bioequivalent with matching EFFICACY and safety profiles. Therapeutically equivalent drugs may have superficial differences such as in appearance (shape or color) and the inactive ingredients that serve as the vehicle to contain the active ingredient. However, they must have the same BIOAVAILABILITY and efficacy.

The FDA has adopted a BIOEQUIVALENCE standard based on a statistical methodology in which the time it takes for each drug to reach its maximum concentration in the BLOOD circulation and the amount of time the drug remains at a THERAPEUTIC LEVEL in the blood circulation differ by no more than 20 percent. In its official listing of approved drugs, *The Orange Book,* the FDA identifies all drugs with alternate products as "A" drugs (therapeutically equivalent) or "B" drugs (not therapeutically equivalent).

Health-care providers other than pharmacists sometimes use the term therapeutic equivalence in the context of different drugs within the same classification that have similar effects—for example the drugs fluoxetine and sertraline, both of which are selective serotonin reuptake inhibitors (SSRIs) to treat DEPRESSION. Though these drugs act in similar ways to achieve a similar therapeutic effect, they do not have the same active ingredients.

See also; GENERIC DRUG; INNOVATOR DRUG.

therapeutic level The amount of a DRUG in the BLOOD circulation that is necessary to achieve and sustain the desired effect for treatment, which is usually a steady state with little variation between the drug's PEAK LEVEL and TROUGH LEVEL. Doctors calculate dosages to achieve a therapeutic level, factoring the person's age, body weight, and other medications with which interactions are possible. For most drugs, blood drawn at any time provides the needed information about the drug's concentration in the blood. At the onset of medication therapy or when taking a drug that has a NARROW THERAPEUTIC INDEX (NTI), blood tests taken to measure both peak and trough levels may provide more useful information to assess whether the drug is at therapeutic level. It often is valuable to tell the doctor or the lab the time of the last DOSE of the medication, which may help to determine whether doses are spaced appropriately.

See also CYTOCHROME P450 (CYP450) ENZYMES; DOSAGE; EFFICACY; THERAPEUTIC WINDOW.

therapeutic window The DOSAGE range within which most of a DRUG's likely population will experience the expected EFFICACY and therapeutic value of the drug. The therapeutic window is important to doctors when they calculate dosages, providing a clinically valid starting point for most people. Individual characteristics such as other health conditions, other medications being taken, body weight, and activity level help the doctor determine where within the therapeutic window is the most appropriate point to choose the starting dosage.

See also PEAK LEVEL; THERAPEUTIC LEVEL; TROUGH LEVEL.

trough level The amount of a DRUG in the BLOOD circulation at the drug's lowest therapeutic concentration. Generally the trough level occurs immediately before the person is due to take the next DOSE of the drug. The trough level helps the doctor determine if the dosage is appropriate to achieve the desired therapeutic effect and is useful information primarily at the onset of treatment. The goal of most medication therapy is a steady state of the drug's concentration in the body, at which there is little difference between the drug's PEAK LEVEL (highest concentration in the blood circulation) and trough level.

Trough level is an especially important measure for NARROW THERAPEUTIC INDEX (NTI) drugs (drugs for which the margin between therapeutic and toxic is very close) such as theophylline (to treat ASTHMA), certain ANTIBIOTIC MEDICATIONS, cyclosporine for IMMUNOSUPPRESSIVE THERAPY, some antiseizure medications, and many antiarrhythmia medications.

See also HALF-LIFE; THERAPEUTIC LEVEL.

NUTRITION AND DIET

The science of nutrition concerns itself with the ways in which foods influence health and disease. A health-care practitioner who specializes in nutrition may be a registered dietitian (RD), registered nurse (RN), physician (MD or DO), naturopathic physician (ND), pharmacist (RPh or PharmD), or chiropractor (DC). The general term nutritionist is in common use to identify a health-care professional who specializes in matters of nutrition but does not consistently designate specific education, training, qualifications, or credentials.

This section, "Nutrition and Diet," presents an overview discussion of nutritional concepts as they relate to health, health risk factors, and preventive health measures. The entries in this section focus on the broad picture of how nutrition and diet influence health and disease. The section, "Lifestyle: Obesity and Smoking," provides discussion and content of nutritional topics that relate to WEIGHT LOSS AND WEIGHT MANAGEMENT.

Making the Connection between Diet and Health

Though the mechanisms of nutrition remained unknown until the early 20th century, doctors were quite familiar with the diseases of nutritional deficiencies. Ancient Egyptian physicians identified the disease now called SCURVY, which for centuries was the bane of sailors who spent months to years at sea on ships with no fruits or vegetables to supply needed vitamins and minerals. Biscuits and salt pork sustained life but they did not support nutrition. Not until the middle of the 18th century did ships' surgeons recognize that citrus fruits (namely lemons, limes, and oranges) could cure as well as prevent scurvy among sailors.

Among the most famous names in medical nutrition is John Harvey Kellogg (1852–1943), a late-19th-century American physician and surgeon whose belief that diet was the foundation of good health launched what would become one of the world's largest and most successful cereal companies. Kellogg came up with a recipe for a simple, nutritious breakfast food to serve at the sanitarium where he was at the time the director: cornflakes. The product based on the recipe became itself an American institution. Kellogg implemented many practices based on nutrition during his tenure at the sanitarium, gaining prominence for them in a time when other medical alternatives were fairly nonexistent.

In the flood of transforming discoveries sweeping the practice of medicine, diet was not especially exciting and its connections to health unproven. Researchers discovered aspirin, INSULIN, antibiotics, immunizations, and ANESTHESIA. Surgeons invaded the belly, chest, and cranium. Kellogg, himself a talented surgeon, developed a number of surgical techniques and the instruments to carry them out. Though Kellogg's cornflakes became a national phenomenon, doctors did not pay much attention to the role of diet—the kinds and amounts of foods people eat—in health unless they were treating conditions resulting from or that caused NUTRITIONAL DEFICIENCY or toxicity.

About the time John F. Kennedy became US president, researchers established the first diet–disease correlation, that between cholesterol and

---

HEALTH CONDITIONS RESULTING FROM NUTRITIONAL DEFICIENCIES

BERIBERI	MALNUTRITION
NIGHT BLINDNESS	OSTEOPOROSIS
PELLAGRA	pernicious ANEMIA
RICKETS	SCURVY

CARDIOVASCULAR DISEASE (CVD). Following shortly was the first official recommendation to limit consumption of a particular food, eggs, as an effort to prevent disease. In the decades since, research has confirmed a tight and intricate relationship between DIET AND HEALTH, and diet-related health conditions became the focus of renewed effort to identify nutritious, healthful foods.

HEALTH CONDITIONS LINKED TO DIETARY FACTORS

ATHEROSCLEROSIS	BREAST CANCER
cervical dysplasia	CERVICAL CANCER
COLORECTAL CANCER	CORONARY ARTERY DISEASE (CAD)
DENTAL CARIES	HYPERLIPIDEMIA
HYPERTENSION	OBESITY
PERIPHERAL VASCULAR DISEASE (PVD)	PROSTATE CANCER
STOMACH CANCER	type 2 DIABETES

Current Challenges and Future Directions

A key challenge today is the rapidly changing understanding of the relationships between nutrition and health and between nutrition and disease. Though a general range of nutrient intake is adequate for most healthy adults, it is becoming increasingly clear that individual variations in NUTRITIONAL NEEDS and nutrient intake can make the difference between health and disease. The medical community is in transition in regard to nutritional recommendations, shifting from the system in place since the early 1940s to methods of NUTRITIONAL ASSESSMENT that take individual variations more into consideration. Current research is exploring the ways in which NUTRIENTS may serve to lower health risk factors, such as for CVD and diabetes, over the length of the lifespan.

aging, nutrition and dietary changes that occur with Nutritional needs and dietary choices change across the spectrum of age. Diet and nutrition also influence the processes of aging and the status of health.

Food Choices and Lifelong Health

Health experts recommend BREASTFEEDING for infants, in most circumstances, from birth through at least six months of age if possible. Breast milk fulfills 100 percent of an infant's NUTRITIONAL NEEDS, provided the mother is meeting her own nutritional needs, and provides the infant with extended immune coverage until his or her own IMMUNE SYSTEM develops enough to become protective. Infants for whom breastfeeding is not practical or appropriate should receive fortified formulas that meet their nutritional needs. Cow's milk does not provide adequate nutritional value and contains higher amounts of sugars than infant formulas.

The nutritional needs of the toddler and older child focus on supporting proper growth and development. Children who learn to make nutritious food choices, including portion size, early in life are likely to make such choices the mainstay of diet throughout life. Healthy children do not require vitamin or mineral supplements and should take them only when a doctor recommends them.

A critical health problem among children is OBESITY, which sets the stage for a plethora of health challenges that can have lifelong consequences. Researchers are identifying in children, especially teens, diseases formerly the exclusive territory of middle age such as type 2 DIABETES, OSTEOARTHRITIS, and ATHEROSCLEROSIS. Nutritious EATING HABITS are an important component of weight management. However, children should not go on "diets" or have food intake restricted without precise instructions from a doctor or nutritionist.

Health Changes and Nutrition

Beginning in middle age people start to experience physical changes that alter their ability to digest foods and absorb NUTRIENTS. The STOMACH produces less acid, and foods may stay in the stomach longer before being digested enough to progress to the SMALL INTESTINE. The stomach also produces less intrinsic factor, a biochemical essential for the absorption of vitamin B_{12} (cyanocobalamin). Dental conditions and changes to the gums (such as PERIODONTAL DISEASE) may result in lost TEETH and difficulty chewing. Perceptions of taste and smell may change, altering the desire for certain foods. Other changes include a generalized slowing of the metabolic rate, which affects digestion and nutrient absorption, and a decreased need for nutrients (fewer calories).

Health conditions with metabolic consequences, such as diabetes and GALLBLADDER DISEASE, become more prevalent with advancing age. Health conditions for which nutrition plays a role, such as CARDIOVASCULAR DISEASE (CVD), also become more prevalent. Other chronic health conditions may accelerate the body's use of certain nutrients. Both men and women begin to experience changes in BONE DENSITY and BONE mass in middle age, women in an especially pronounced manner after MENOPAUSE. Without proper vitamin D and calcium intake, OSTEOMALACIA and OSTEOPOROSIS are significant threats to bone health.

The very old (80 and older) may have mobility, independence, and economic issues that prevent them from eating appropriately. Debilitating conditions such as ALZHEIMER'S DISEASE, DEMENTIA, and PARKINSON'S DISEASE are more common among the elderly. NUTRITIONAL DEFICIENCY and MALNUTRITION can develop rather quickly, initiating a cascade of health consequences that can be difficult to reverse. It is important for caregivers and health-care providers to monitor dietary intake and nutrition in the elderly, to make sure food and nutrient consumption is adequate. Basic NUTRITIONAL ASSESSMENT should be a component of most visits to the doctor and of every ROUTINE MEDICAL EXAMINATION.

Maintaining Healthy Nutrition Across the Age Spectrum

Healthy eating habits support the body in maintaining optimal health at any age. In combination with appropriate daily physical exercise, adequate nutrition often is the difference between full recovery and prolonged or incomplete recovery from health conditions that arise. These lifestyle factors also lower the risk for numerous health conditions.

See also CARDIOVASCULAR DISEASE PREVENTION; DIET AND HEALTH; LIFESTYLE AND HEALTH; NUTRIENTS; OBESITY AND HEALTH; PREVENTIVE HEALTH CARE AND IMMUNIZATIONS.

antioxidant A biochemical substance that attracts free radicals, unmatched molecules remaining as the waste byproducts of oxidation functions (energy conversion and release) within the body. Free radicals are associated with numerous health conditions, especially chronic diseases, though researchers do not yet fully understand their roles. Free radicals bind with other molecules, hijacking them from their intended destinations. The resulting rogue molecules do not have legitimate functions within the body and disrupt normal cellular functions. When an antioxidant molecule binds with a free radical, the resulting structure becomes a readily identifiable waste molecule that the body's natural processes then eliminate from the body.

Antioxidants are abundant in fruits and vegetables. The body also synthesizes some antioxidants such as COENZYME Q10. Carotenoids (components of vitamin A), vitamins C and E, the mineral selenium, and phytochemicals such as flavonoids and plant sterols are among the common dietary antioxidants. SOY, GREEN TEA, and GINKGO BILOBA are particularly high in such phytochemicals.

Research suggests antioxidants play a vital role in stopping cancers before they gain any momentum as well as in slowing the progression and damage of chronic conditions such as ATHEROSCLEROSIS and DIABETES.

Though many NUTRITIONAL SUPPLEMENTS contain antioxidants, food-based antioxidants appear to have more potent effects through their numerous though little-understood interactions with one another. One exception is coenzyme Q10, which does not come from dietary sources but rather through processes within the body. Coenzyme Q10 supplements boost coenzyme Q10 levels in the body to have apparently the same effects as endogenous coenzyme Q10. Minerals such as copper and zinc help the body use antioxidants more effectively.

See also NUTRITIONAL THERAPY; PHYTOESTROGENS; SUN'S SOUP; VITAMIN AND MINERAL THERAPY.

appetite The sensation of feeling the desire to eat. Appetite represents complex hormonal, neurologic, and environmental interactions that correlate in varying proportions both to HUNGER, the body's physiologic signal that it needs food, and to learned behaviors for eating. Seeing, smelling, and thinking about food often trigger appetite. Many people also feel the desire to eat at conventional meal times, regardless of whether their bodies actually need food. Emotional circumstances may trigger appetite as well, particularly when there is an emotional or habitual connection between eating and feeling comforted.

The Mechanisms of Appetite

Three regions of the BRAIN work in collaboration and counterbalance to regulate appetite: the appetite center, the SATIETY center, and the hunger center. The appetite center resides within the brainstem, the most rudimentary structure of the brain that regulates functions necessary for survival. It responds to external sensory NERVE signals from the body that travel to the brain via the CRANIAL NERVES as well as to nerve signals that come from the cerebral cortex. Because signals from the cerebral cortex arise from activities of cognitive function (such as thought, memory, and emotion), their influence on the appetite center is within conscious control.

The hunger center resides within the HYPOTHALAMUS, a structure of the midbrain that integrates neurologic and hormonal activity to maintain essential body functions. The hunger center responds primarily to the level of GLUCOSE (the form of sugar that is the primary fuel for the body's cells) in the BLOOD, activating the appetite center when the blood glucose level drops. The hunger center's activation triggers a cascade of response from the hypothalamus that includes sending nerve signals to the appetite center and the cerebral cortex to stimulate the desire to eat, hormonal signals to the gastrointestinal tract to begin releasing DIGESTIVE HORMONES (such as gastrin, secretin, cholecystokinin, and pepsin), and neurohormonal signals that result in an increase of acetylcholine, a NEUROTRANSMITTER that facilitates smooth MUSCLE contraction, in the gastrointestinal tract. These events establish a cycle that continues until blood glucose levels rise. Because the hunger center responds to neurohormonal signals related to basic survival, neither it nor its influence on the appetite center is within conscious control.

The satiety center also resides in the hypothalamus near the hunger center. It responds to nerve signals from the hunger center and from the appetite center. As food enters the SMALL INTESTINE for the main phase of digestion, the small intestine releases peptide YY, a HORMONE that signals the satiety center. The satiety center in turn sends nerve messages to the hunger center and to the appetite center, signaling that the body no longer needs to consume food. Concurrently the balance of digestive hormones begins to shift, further signaling the satiety center as well as slowing the signals going to the appetite center.

Appetite Response

Appetite is a powerful mechanism intended to bring food (energy) into the body. Though aspects of appetite represent areas of conscious control, appetite response is not simply an issue of willpower or of survival. Some people eat a small amount, feel satisfied, and stop eating. Other people eat large amounts of food and do not feel satisfied, even when they begin to feel physically uncomfortable because they have eaten more than enough to fill their gastrointestinal tracts. Appetite appears to be a short-term feature of energy management designed to meet the body's daily energy needs; how appetite correlates with the body's available stores of surplus energy (in the form of body fat) remains a mystery.

There is some evidence that continued exposure to the smells of food without eating may signal both the satiety center and the appetite center that the body is consuming enough food, even when a person is only smelling, not eating, food. However, manipulating the appetite is not so easy. Establishing EATING HABITS that provide adequate CALORIE and nutrition intake helps maintain balance among the appetite, hunger, and satiety centers. This is particularly important for WEIGHT LOSS AND WEIGHT MANAGEMENT as well as for overall health maintenance.

See also DIGESTIVE ENZYMES; METABOLISM; OBESITY AND HEALTH; STARVATION.

beriberi   A health condition resulting from long-term deficiency of thiamine (vitamin B_1). Beriberi affects neurologic, musculoskeletal, cardiovascular, and gastrointestinal structures and functions. Though common in developing parts of the world, beriberi occurs primarily in people who have gastrointestinal disorders that interfere with thiamine absorption and in long-term, chronic ALCOHOLISM. A BREASTFEEDING infant whose mother is thiamine deficient may also develop beriberi. Beriberi is also common among people whose primary food is white rice. Thiamine is necessary for cells in the body to convert GLUCOSE to energy and to convert glucose to energy storage forms (fat).

There are two main forms of beriberi: dry and wet. Dry beriberi is more common and affects primarily the NERVOUS SYSTEM and the musculoskeletal system. Wet beriberi affects primarily the cardiovascular system; its most apparent symptom is edema (swelling due to fluid accumulation), which accounts for the "wet" designation. People who have mild to moderate beriberi typically have distinctly one form or the other; people who have moderate to severe disease generally have both forms as the deficiency is severe enough to affect all body functions.

Symptoms and Diagnostic Path
The early symptoms of beriberi are the same for either the wet or the dry form and include

- fatigue
- difficulty concentrating and cognitive dysfunction
- irritability
- loss of APPETITE
- NAUSEA, VOMITING, and CONSTIPATION
- abdominal tenderness

As the condition progresses symptoms become specific for the body system affected. Neurologic and musculoskeletal (dry beriberi) symptoms include

- peripheral NEURITIS (INFLAMMATION of the nerves) or peripheral NEUROPATHY
- PARESTHESIA (disturbances of sensation such as tingling and numbness)
- cramps in the lower legs
- PAIN and weakness in muscles throughout the body
- difficulty walking and rising from a sitting or squatting position

Cardiovascular (wet beriberi) symptoms are those of congestive HEART FAILURE and include

- tachycardia (rapid HEART RATE)
- diaphoresis ("cold sweats")
- edema
- shortness of breath (DYSPNEA)

The diagnostic path begins with a careful assessment of the PERSONAL HEALTH HISTORY with an emphasis on EATING HABITS. BLOOD tests can measure the amount of thiamine in the blood as well as enzyme levels related to thiamine activity in the body. When symptoms are cardiovascular, the doctor is likely to conduct an ELECTROCARDIOGRAM (ECG) and an ECHOCARDIOGRAM.

Treatment Options and Outlook
Treatment is injections of thiamine until blood levels return to normal and symptoms begin to

subside. Cardiovascular symptoms generally improve within 24 hours, though underlying damage to the HEART may be permanent and require subsequent treatment. Neurologic and musculoskeletal symptoms may take several months to completely resolve. Dry beriberi generally resolves without residual complications except in the most severe cases, in which there may be permanent peripheral neuropathy (damage to the PERIPHERAL NERVES). Untreated beriberi is fatal, usually a result of cardiovascular collapse.

Maintenance therapy with vitamin B supplementation helps prevent RECURRENCE, especially in people who are not likely to receive adequate B vitamins from dietary sources. Most people who have thiamine deficiency are also deficient in other B vitamins and should take a vitamin B complex supplement product. People who have gastrointestinal disorders that interfere with their ability to absorb thiamine, such as PEPTIC ULCER DISEASE, may require ongoing thiamine injections.

Risk Factors and Preventive Measures
The sole risk factor for beriberi is inadequate consumption of dietary thiamine. Accordingly, maintaining adequate dietary consumption of foods that contain B vitamins prevents beriberi in most people. Food sources of thiamine include lean meats (notably pork), legumes, watermelon, acorn squash, and whole grains and whole grain products. Grain products such as breads and cereals produced in the United States are fortified with B vitamins, including thiamine. Highly refined and processed foods, especially white rice and white bread, contain minimal amounts of B vitamins, including thiamine, unless they are fortified. B complex vitamin supplements help ensure adequate intake. B vitamins are water-soluble so there is no risk for OVERDOSE.

See also ANEMIA; MALNUTRITION; NUTRITIONAL DEFICIENCY; NUTRITIONAL NEEDS; PELLAGRA; RICKETS; SCURVY; VITAMINS AND HEALTH.

calorie A unit of measure that denotes heat consumption. In nutrition and exercise, calories represent a measure of energy exchange. The calories in foods represent energy the body takes in, and the calories assigned to physical exertion represent energy the body expends. Recommended daily calorie intake guidelines represent the amount of energy a typical adult requires to carry out the activities of normal living. Taking in more calories than one expends results in weight gain (the body stores extra calories as fat), and expending more calories than one consumes results in weight loss (the body draws from stored energy to meet its needs). The steady state of weight maintenance occurs when there is a relative balance between the calories that enter the body and the calories the body uses.

See also METABOLIC EQUIVALENT (MET); NUTRIENTS; NUTRITIONAL NEEDS.

carbohydrate intolerance An enzyme deficiency that results in the body's inability to metabolize one or more forms of carbohydrate. The most common form of carbohydrate intolerance is LACTOSE INTOLERANCE, which affects up to 50 million Americans and results from a deficiency of the enzyme lactase. Other forms of carbohydrate intolerance are much less common though may result from deficiencies of maltase (necessary to metabolize maltose) and sucrase (also called isomaltase, necessary to metabolize sucrose).

The enzyme deficiencies responsible for carbohydrate intolerance may be congenital (absent from birth), acquired through a natural decline in DIGESTIVE ENZYMES through aging, or as a consequence of gastrointestinal disorders such as CELIAC DISEASE. RADIATION THERAPY and CHEMOTHERAPY treatments for cancer also can affect the cells that produce the various enzymes, resulting in enzyme depletion and intolerance of the corresponding carbohydrate.

The symptoms of carbohydrate intolerance often include abdominal cramping, flatulence (gas), and DIARRHEA. Children may fail to gain weight or grow appropriately. The diagnostic path may include an oral carbohydrate challenge, in which the person drinks a solution containing the suspect carbohydrate. BLOOD samples taken at certain intervals measure the amount of the sugar form present in the blood circulation. Because lactose intolerance results IN excessive hydrogen gas production, breath tests to measure hydrogen concentrations in the lungs are often diagnostic for lactose intolerance.

Many people can tolerate small amounts of substances that contain the sugars for which they are lacking enzymes. Avoiding larger amounts keeps symptoms in check. It is important for people who have carbohydrate intolerance to make sure they receive adequate intake of other NUTRIENTS in foods for which they have intolerance or to take supplements that supply them.

See also AGING, NUTRITION AND DIETARY CHANGES THAT OCCUR WITH.

cholesterol, dietary   A sterol substance found in animal-based foods such as meats and dairy products. Dietary cholesterol under scrutiny in the 1970s when research connected high BLOOD cholesterol levels with increased risk for CARDIOVASCULAR DISEASE (CVD), notably ATHEROSCLEROSIS and CORONARY ARTERY DISEASE (CAD). However, subsequent research has determined the true culprit is endogenous cholesterol—the cholesterol the LIVER synthesizes from the components of dietary saturated fats and trans fats. The liver makes about 80 percent of the cholesterol in the blood circulation, and it continues to make cholesterol as long as it receives the source materials (dietary fats) to do so. Dietary cholesterol has almost no role in this process.

Furthermore, researchers recognized it is not the cholesterol itself that is the problem. Cholesterol, which is important to health because it is essential for cell membrane repair and HORMONE production, has the consistency of a waxy liquid and does not dissolve in water or blood. Carrier proteins called lipoproteins, which the liver also produces, bind with cholesterol molecules so they can travel through the bloodstream. The more cholesterol molecules in the blood circulation, the more lipoproteins required to transport them through the blood. When there are high levels of lipoproteins in the blood some tend to "fall out" against the sides of the arteries, eventually forming plaques (hardened patches) that narrow and stiffen the arteries. These plaques are the early stages of ATHEROSCLEROSIS, the foundation of CAD.

There is very little correlation between the cholesterol in foods and the cholesterol in the blood circulation. Rather, the amounts of saturated fats and trans fats in the diet determine blood levels of cholesterol in most people. Cholesterol and saturated fats co-exist in many animal-based foods, however, so a diet heavy in these foods contributes to higher-than-healthy cholesterol and lipoprotein levels in the blood. Health experts recommend limiting dietary cholesterol to 200 milligrams a day for people who have no increased risk for CVD. Doctors may recommend a lower limit for people who have, or have increased risk for, CVD.

See also CARDIOVASCULAR DISEASE PREVENTION; CHOLESTEROL BLOOD LEVELS; DIET AND HEALTH; HYPERLIPIDEMIA; LIFESTYLE AND HEALTH; NUTRIENTS; TRIGLYCERIDE BLOOD LEVEL; TRIGLYCERIDES, DIETARY.

D–H

diet and health The effects foods and EATING HABITS have on health and HEALTH RISK FACTORS. As diet is the primary means by which the external environment enters the internal environment of the body, much research focuses on how diet affects health in general as well as the risk for numerous health conditions. The obvious correlations are those between specific nutrient deficiencies, conditions such as BERIBERI and SCURVY. Other health conditions that have major dietary connections are the diseases that claim the most lives and cause the most disability among Americans: cancer, CARDIOVASCULAR DISEASE (CVD), DIABETES, OBESITY, and OSTEOPOROSIS. Diet—what foods and how much of them a person eats—has emerged as a significant risk factor for these conditions.

On the whole, the body has a remarkable ability to use the substances it receives through diet to conduct the functions of living. This ability in part stems from the processes of METABOLISM that reduce all NUTRIENTS to their absolute basic components, amino acids and sugars that eventually become GLUCOSE. The body's numerous systems then reassemble those components into the substances they require. In large part the body can subsist in reasonable health on a marginal diet. Eventually, however, the shortcomings become problematic and begin contributing to health conditions. For example, a diet low in fruits, vegetables, and whole grains lacks a consistent supply of the vitamins and minerals the body needs to manage its energy needs, maintain immune functions, and regulate body activities. The consequences of inefficient metabolism range from molecular, which may include the accumulation of free radicals or disruptions in protein sequencing of GENETIC CODE, to overt disease such as CVD.

Correlations between diet and disease are sometimes difficult for researchers to quantify. For example, people who eat a diet high in meats and saturated fats have a higher incidence of COLON cancer than people who eat a diet that is primarily vegetarian and low in fat. The reasons for this are imprecise, however, and likely represent an integration of factors of which diet is only one consideration. Other correlations are more precise, such as those that link high dietary saturated fat, high CHOLESTEROL BLOOD LEVELS, and ATHEROSCLEROSIS. Foods also appear to influence mood and behavior, though again the precise mechanisms of these interactions remain unknown.

Diet can bolster health as well. Supplying the body with the nutrients it needs allows it to function with optimal efficiency. In such a state the body's own systems are fully active to resist damage and respond promptly when injury or illness occurs. Health experts believe lifestyle factors such as diet and exercise have the ability to eliminate as much as 85 percent of HEART disease, obesity, and type 2 DIABETES, and reduce the risk for COLORECTAL CANCER, STOMACH CANCER, and possibly BREAST CANCER and PROSTATE CANCER.

See also ANTIOXIDANT; CANCER PREVENTION; CARDIOVASCULAR DISEASE PREVENTION; DIABETES PREVENTION; FOOD SAFETY; HEALTHY PEOPLE 2010; LIFESTYLE AND HEALTH; OBESITY AND HEALTH.

enteral nutrition Nutritional supplementation or replacement when a person cannot acquire the necessary NUTRIENTS by eating, typically administered via a nasogastric tube or surgically inserted tube, commonly called a feeding tube. Long-term enteral nutrition may become a QUALITY OF LIFE issue or an end-of-life concern, especially for those who become unable to make and express their desires. An advance directive allows a person to establish in writing his or her desires about such matters, mitigating family conflict about making the decision on behalf of the person.

Types of Feeding Tubes for Enteral Nutrition

A nasogastric tube is a thin, flexible catheter the doctor inserts through the NOSE, down the back of the THROAT, through the ESOPHAGUS, and into the STOMACH. The insertion process is somewhat uncomfortable but does not require anesthetic, though the doctor generally sprays a topical anesthetic on the back of the throat to numb the gag REFLEX. A nasogastric tube is for short-term use, usually no longer than a few weeks. The nasogastric tube blocks the nostril through which it enters, and becomes irritating to the nasal mucosa as well as the SKIN around the nostril.

Surgically inserted tubes are for long-term use and are generally somewhat sturdier though still narrow and flexible. They enter the stomach or SMALL INTESTINE through an opening in the abdominal wall. The most common type is the percutaneous endoscopic gastrostomy (PEG) tube, also called a gastrostomy tube or G tube, for long-term use. With the person under general ANESTHESIA, the doctor makes a small incision through the abdominal wall for the insertion of the tube. An endoscope passed into the stomach via the throat and esophagus guides the doctor in placing the tube. A small balloon at the tip of the tube, inflated with saline solution, lodges the tube in the stomach. The surgical wound, called a stoma, heals in 7 to 10 days.

A gastric button is an alternative to a PEG tube. After the stoma is completely healed, the person can remove the tube and replace it with a gastric button, a pluglike device that fits into the stoma to block the opening. At feeding times the person (or caregiver) removes the button, reinserts the tube, and administers the enteral nutrition solution. Some people find a gastric button more discreet and less intrusive. A third surgical alternative is a tube placed into the JEJUNUM, the middle segment of the small intestine. A jejunostomy tube, or J tube, may be necessary for a person who has had a GASTRECTOMY (surgical removal of the stomach) such as to treat STOMACH CANCER, or has severe GASTROESOPHAGEAL REFLUX DISORDER (GERD) that negates

a PEG or other gastric tube. Because the small intestine accepts limited volume, enteral nutrition via J tube is a continuous infusion.

Conscientious PERSONAL HYGIENE is essential with either kind of tube to prevent skin irritation (around the nostrils with a nasogastric tube and at the stoma site with a surgically placed tube) and INFECTION (more of a concern with a surgically placed tubes).

Enteral Nutrition Feeding

Enteral feeding may be continuous or intermittent, depending on the person's health status and NUTRITIONAL NEEDS. Enteral nutrition administered via surgically inserted tubes can provide adequate sustenance for years. Commercially prepared enteral nutrition solutions, most of which require a doctor's prescription, are of appropriate viscosity to avoid clogging the tube. They have high nutritional density and are available in various formulations to meet individual nutritional needs. The formula and the person's requirements determine the frequency and rate of infusions.

In some situations doctors may recommend enteral nutrition formulas that are palatable enough to take by MOUTH, typically in situations in which a person has difficulty chewing or swallowing and does not want a feeding tube, or who generally gets adequate nutrition from eating but would benefit from the nutritional boost of an enteral nutrition formula. Some products are available over the counter (OTC) without a doctor's prescription. Because excesses of some nutrients can cause health problems or interfere with prescribed medications, people who are considering such OTC products should discuss the approach with their doctors first.

See also ENDOSCOPY; NUTRITIONAL ASSESSMENT; PARENTAL NUTRITION.

feeding tube   See ENTERAL NUTRITION.

food–drug interactions   See DRUG INTERACTION.

hunger   The body's physiologic indication that it needs energy (food). Hunger occurs when the STOMACH and SMALL INTESTINE are empty and manifests as physical sensations of discomfort and even PAIN that result from contractions of the stomach.

Hunger sends HORMONE and NERVE signals to the APPETITE and hunger centers in the BRAIN, each of which responds with other neurohormonal messages that intensify the physical and psychological urges to eat. Hunger subsides only when the body receives food (in contrast to appetite, which abates after time even when the person does not eat).

See also DIGESTIVE ENZYMES; DIGESTIVE HORMONES; METABOLISM; STARVATION.

hydration   Maintenance of the body's fluid level. About 60 percent of the body's weight is water. The typical adult requires three quarts (two liters) of water daily to remain adequately hydrated. Health experts recommend drinking six to eight cups of water each day to meet this need, though most people acquire much of the water they need through the foods they eat. Many foods, notably fruits and vegetables, have high water content that helps supply the body with water. Soups, sauces, fruit and vegetable juices, and pastas and rice cooked in water also supply fluid to the diet. Health experts consider water a vital nutrient because the body cannot live without it. Though water contains no calories, it does contain trace minerals that are necessary for metabolic functions. A person can survive only about five to seven days without water.

> **Thirst is not a good indication of proper hydration. By the time a person feels thirsty, the body is experiencing significant fluid depletion. In DEHYDRATION, many people do not feel thirsty.**

DEHYDRATION is a serious condition that results from inadequate water consumption, and can occur much more rapidly than expected during intense physical exercise and in hot temperatures as the body loses significant water through sweat. Distance athletes and WEEKEND WARRIORS are at particular risk for dehydration during competition, the former because their efforts are so intense that it is difficult to drink enough water often enough to keep up with water loss and the latter because they often do not realize the intensity of their efforts and fail to properly hydrate before and during competitive activities including swimming and other water sports. Dehydration leads to electrolyte imbalances as the salts in the body become more concentrated, resulting in numerous physiologic consequences including mental confusion and impaired cognitive function, irregular HEART RATE, fluctuations in BLOOD PRESSURE, and MUSCLE cramps.

WATER CONSUMPTION FOR HYDRATION DURING PHYSICAL ACTIVITY

90 minutes before activity: 12 ounces of cold water
15 minutes before activity: 12 ounces of cold water
During activity: 4 ounces of cold water every 15 minutes
15 minutes after activity: 16 ounces of cold water

Fluids that contain sugar or CAFFEINE actually draw water from the body. Excess sugar pulls water into the gastrointestinal tract as it makes its way through the digestive process. Caffeine is a mild diuretic, acting on the KIDNEYS to cause them to extract more water from the BLOOD. Beverages such as sodas (soft drinks) also contain high quantities of electrolytes, which are minerals in the form of salts. These, too, may act on the kidneys to increase the water the kidneys pull from the blood to pass with the URINE.

In a clinical context hydration may refer to the long-term infusion of fluids via PARENTERAL NUTRITION or ENTERAL NUTRITION (feeding tube) into a person who is in a PERSISTENT VEGETATIVE STATE as a means of preserving life.

See also COGNITIVE FUNCTION AND DYSFUNCTION; CONDITIONING; END OF LIFE CONCERNS; HEAT EXHAUSTION; HEAT STROKE.

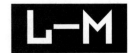

lactose intolerance The inability to digest lactose, a disaccharide sugar in milk and other dairy products. Lactose intolerance occurs because of a deficiency of the enzyme lactase, which is necessary to break down lactose into simpler sugar molecules. It is the most common form of CARBOHYDRATE INTOLERANCE, affecting an estimated 50 million Americans. Lactose intolerance may be congenital (present at birth), occur as a consequence of a disease process that affects the cells that produce lactase (such as CELIAC DISEASE), or develop with aging as the number of lactase-producing cells naturally declines.

Congenital lactose intolerance becomes apparent when a young child begins drinking cow's milk, which is high in lactose. The doctor can usually confirm the diagnosis with a lactose challenge test in which the child drinks a solution that contains lactose. Breath samples taken at certain intervals allow measurement of hydrogen, which increases when lactose remains undigested in the gastrointestinal tract.

Switching to a fortified SOY formula nearly always eliminates symptoms when the child is young. As the child grows older, trial and error will tell whether he or she can eat small amounts of other dairy products such as cheese and ice cream. Many people who have lactose intolerance produce enough lactase to digest small amounts of lactose. Lactase enzymes are available without a doctor's prescription; added to milk, they act on the lactose to split it into its composite sugars. Within 24 hours the milk will be 70 to 90 percent lactose-free. This approach allows the child to benefit from the numerous NUTRIENTS milk and dairy products provide. Lactose intolerance generally does not affect an individual's overall general health, as long as the person acquires necessary nutrients through alternative foods or via supplements.

See also AGING, NUTRITION AND DIETARY CHANGES THAT OCCUR WITH.

malnutrition A state of multiple nutrient depletion that alters body functions. Infants, the elderly, and people who have active cancer, ALCOHOLISM, OBESITY, or chronic health conditions are most susceptible to malnutrition. Malnutrition may develop when a person does not eat enough food, eats a very narrow selection of foods, or eats too much food. Malnutrition is possible with extended adherence to fad diets that limit food types and when the diet primarily contains foods that have low NUTRIENT DENSITY such as "junk" foods. The most severe presentations of malnutrition are the polar extremes of STARVATION and obesity.

In the United States malnutrition resulting from inadequate food or nutrient consumption occurs most often in the chronically ill, the very young, and the very old. Most people who have significant obesity have some degree of nutrient imbalance, not only among the energy NUTRIENTS but also of vitamins, minerals, and other micronutrients. People who have alcoholism, serious chronic health conditions such as HIV/AIDS, or gastrointestinal MALABSORPTION disorders including INFLAMMATORY BOWEL DISEASE (IBD) and CELIAC DISEASE or are also vulnerable to malnutrition.

Symptoms and Diagnostic Path
Early malnutrition can be difficult to detect though initial indications may include dry SKIN, pallor, swollen or bleeding gums, PETECHIAE (pinpoint hemorrhages under the skin), MUSCLE weakness and atrophy, and disturbances of sensory perception (PARESTHESIA) in both inadequate and

excessive nutrient consumption. The diagnostic path includes a comprehensive medical examination, height and weight measurements, careful assessment of EATING HABITS, body composition assessment, and a complete BLOOD count (CBC) as well as other blood tests to measure nutrient levels. A BODY MASS INDEX (BMI) below 17 kilograms per meter squared (kg/m^2) is generally diagnostic of inadequate consumption; a BMI greater than 30 kg/m^2 is generally diagnostic of obesity.

Treatment Options and Outlook

Treatment for malnutrition focuses on correcting the nutritional deficiencies that exist, which usually means generalized nutritional supplementation until symptoms resolve, along with dietary changes to improve overall nutrition. People who have obesity often have significant nutritional deficiencies even though their food consumption may be excessive. The US Department of Agriculture (USDA) publishes a food pyramid with recommendations for food consumption to meet NUTRITIONAL NEEDS. Daily physical activity, such as walking, improves the body's ability to digest, absorb, and metabolize nutrients and also is key to weight management.

The success of treatment depends on the severity of the malnutrition at the time of diagnosis, the status of underlying or contributing causes (such as gastrointestinal or metabolic disorders), the person's age, the availability of nutritious foods, and the ability to feed oneself. Many of the symptoms of malnutrition resolve without residual complications, though severe symptoms may result in permanent damage.

Risk Factors and Preventive Measures

The most significant risks for malnutrition are inadequate food consumption and malabsorption disorders that keep the body from extracting needed nutrients during digestion. Those who cannot easily feed themselves are most susceptible to inadequate consumption. People who diet frequently or follow restrictive eating habits (such as those who follow a vegan diet) are at risk for deficiency in key nutrients normally in the foods they are not eating. APPETITE loss contributes to decreased food consumption in serious chronic conditions such as HIV/AIDS and CHRONIC OBSTRUC-

TIVE PULMONARY DISEASE (COPD). Untreated disorders of specific NUTRIENT DEFICIENCY such as BERIBERI and SCURVY lead to generalized malnutrition.

It is important to eat or provide a variety of foods in the appropriate quantities, as the USDA food pyramid recommends, especially for young children and the very elderly, for whom caregivers sometimes assume intake is nutritionally adequate. Though most healthy children and adults who can feed themselves can acquire the nutrients they need through diet, nutritional supplements can provide a steady and certain source of necessary nutrients for people who have chronic health conditions or who do not eat adequately.

See also AGING, NUTRITION AND DIETARY CHANGES THAT OCCUR WITH; ANEMIA; MINERALS AND HEALTH; OBESITY AND HEALTH; OSTEOPOROSIS; PELLAGRA; VITAMIN AND MINERAL THERAPY; VITAMINS AND HEALTH.

minerals and health Minerals are inorganic micronutrients essential for health and the body's proper development and function. Minerals are abundant in nature and in most foods, and facilitate numerous actions in the body. Six major minerals (also called macrominerals) and nine trace minerals (also called microminerals) are essential for health and the body's proper growth and development; the body cannot survive without them. Numerous other trace minerals are present in the body and presumably important for the body's functions but researchers do not understand their roles. Minerals within the body are also called electrolytes or ions because they are polarized (carry a positive or negative charge).

Major Minerals

The body requires substantial amounts of the major minerals, which are essential for the daily activities that keep the body alive and functional. The body of a person who weighs 160 pounds contains 3 pounds of calcium, 1½ pounds of phosphate, ½ pound of potassium, ¼ pound each of sodium and chloride, and a little over 1 ounce of magnesium.

The major minerals work closely with each other and with the vitamins. For example, calcium, phosphate, and magnesium are essential for BONE mineralization though their passage into the bone requires the presence of vitamin D in the

BLOOD circulation. As well, 85 percent of the body's phosphate is bound to calcium, most of it in the bones. Sodium, chloride, and potassium regulate the contraction of MUSCLE cells (including those in the HEART) and the balance of fluid in the body.

Deficiencies of the major minerals can significantly affect the functioning of the heart, KIDNEYS, neurologic system, bones, and muscles. The most common deficiencies of the major minerals are of calcium, which can result in OSTEOPOROSIS and heart ARRHYTHMIA, and potassium, which occurs most commonly in people who take diuretic medications to treat conditions such as congestive HEART FAILURE and kidney disease.

Mineral toxicities of the major minerals are uncommon though can occur in people who take diuretic medications (when the kidneys keep more of the mineral in the blood circulation, allowing its level to accumulate) and in circumstances of OVERDOSE such as from taking excessive mineral supplements. Overdose of magnesium can disrupt the functions of the neurologic and cardiovascular systems severely enough to be fatal. Some people develop HYPERTENSION (high BLOOD PRESSURE) with long-term dietary excesses of sodium and chloride, though most doctors do not consider this toxicity.

Calcium The hormones PARATHYROID HORMONE and calcitonin, along with the HORMONE form of vitamin D, calcitriol, regulate the amounts of calcium in the blood. Calcium is essential for bone STRENGTH and BONE DENSITY. It is also a key ion (electronically charged particle) with roles in NERVE signals and muscle contraction. Calcium channel blockers are drugs that regulate HEART RATE and function by blocking the passage of calcium ions in the heart muscle (MYOCARDIUM).

Sodium and chloride Sodium and chloride are present in chemical combination with each other. Sodium is a positively charged ion that is abundant in the fluid outside the cells (extracellular fluid) and regulates fluid balance in the body. Chloride is a negatively charged ion that occurs primarily in equilibrium with sodium in the extracellular fluid, assisting with fluid balance. Special molecular sensors in the glomeruli of the kidneys continually monitor the levels of sodium and chloride in the blood circulation, which deter-

mines how much of these minerals the kidneys will reabsorb which in turn determines how much water the kidneys hold for circulation in the blood. Diuretic medications act on the molecular sensors in the glomeruli to limit their ability to reabsorb these minerals.

TABLE SALT

Table salt is sodium chloride, about 40 percent sodium and 60 percent chloride. One teaspoon of table salt contains two grams of sodium and three grams of chloride.

Potassium Potassium is a positively charged ion that is abundant in the fluid within the cells (intracellular fluid). It is a key player in fluid balance within the body, and also in the transmission of nerve impulses across neurons. The kidneys also regulate the amount of potassium in the blood circulation. Long-term diuretic therapy can deplete potassium because potassium passes from the blood along with sodium and chloride though its levels in the circulation are much lower. Chronic VOMITING and DIARRHEA also result in losses of potassium. Chronically low potassium levels cause hypertension, though researchers do not understand the mechanisms of this.

Phosphate This mineral is integral to nucleic acid formation (DNA and RNA) and cell reproduction. It also is a component of numerous enzymes, is necessary for activation of the B vitamins, and participates in energy conversion. Various forms of phosphate bind with lipids to form the primary structure of the cell membrane for every nucleated cell in the body.

Magnesium Magnesium is essential for cellular METABOLISM and energy conversion, influencing the efficiency with which cells use GLUCOSE and serving as a component of numerous enzymes. Magnesium is also essential for initiating the contraction of muscle cells, facilitating nerve signals, integrating certain IMMUNE SYSTEM functions, and regulating blood pressure.

Trace Minerals
Trace minerals are present in the body in barely measurable amounts, though their absence can have far-reaching consequences for overall health. Zinc and copper are essential for HEALING and the

ESSENTIAL MINERALS

Mineral	Dietary Sources
Major Minerals (Macrominerals)	
calcium	dairy products fortified orange juice and soy milk spinach, broccoli, green beans legumes, nuts, tofu canned sardines, salmon, herring (with bones) molasses sweet potatoes (with skin) oranges, raisins, watermelon
chloride	table salt processed foods (as a preservative) pork, ham, beef, chicken, turkey, fish
magnesium	all foods highest in meats, poultry, fish, legumes
phosphate	all foods
potassium	all foods
sodium	table salt processed foods (as a preservative) pork, ham, beef, chicken, turkey, fish
Trace Minerals (Microminerals)	
chromium	pork, ham, beef, chicken, turkey, fish, shrimp raw fruits, vegetables, whole grains
copper	whole grains and whole grain products finfish, shellfish, crab, lobster legumes, tofu nuts, seeds
fluorine	fluoridated drinking water salt water seafood (finfish, shellfish, crab, lobster, kelp)
iodine	iodized table salt salt water seafood (finfish, shellfish, crab, lobster, kelp)
iron	canned clams fortified breads and cereals whole grains spinach, broccoli, peas, green beans, potatoes (with skin), artichokes parsley legumes, tofu

Mineral	Dietary Sources
Trace Minerals (Microminerals)	
iron (continued)	pork, ham, beef, chicken, turkey, fish, shrimp
	raisins
manganese	whole grains and whole grain products
	legumes, nuts, seeds
	finfish, shellfish, crab, lobster
molybdenum	legumes, nuts, seeds
	liver
	whole grains and whole grain products
	fortified breads and cereals
selenium	whole grains and vegetables grown in selenium-rich soil
	salt water finfish, shellfish, crab, lobster
	pork, ham, beef, lamb from animals who graze on selenium-rich land
zinc	oysters, clams, crab, shrimp, lobster
	legumes, nuts, seeds, tofu
	dairy products, especially cheeses
	peas, spinach, broccoli, corn, potatoes (with skin)

formation of new tissues (including growth) and are crucial for oxidative reactions in the cells. The body requires iron to synthesize HEMOGLOBIN, the protein that transports oxygen through the blood circulation. Fluorine strengthens TEETH and bones and increases the resistance of the teeth to bacterial invasion resulting in DENTAL CARIES (cavities). The THYROID GLAND requires iodine to synthesize thyroid hormones, which regulate metabolism. Selenium is a potent ANTIOXIDANT that may be a key player in CANCER PREVENTION. Manganese and molybdenum are essential cofactors for numerous enzymes vital to metabolic functions. Chromium aids metabolism of carbohydrates and fats.

Deficiencies or toxicities of some trace minerals can have significant and potentially fatal consequences for health. Iron deficiency causes ANEMIA, reducing the amount of oxygen that reaches the tissues through the blood circulation. Excessive iron accumulates in organs such as the heart and LIVER, such as occurs with HEMOCHROMATOSIS, eventually causing failure of those organs. Acute iron overdose is often fatal.

WILSON'S DISEASE is a genetic disorder in which the body cannot metabolize copper, allowing copper to accumulate in the heart, liver, PANCREAS, and BRAIN. Unchecked, this accumulation is fatal; treatment is curtailed intake of foods containing copper. High intake of zinc blocks copper metabolism, which is therapeutic in Wilson's disease but hazardous otherwise. Iodine deficiency causes HYPOTHYROIDISM, and iodine excess causes GOITER. Untreated hypothyroidism in a pregnant woman or an infant causes irreversible brain damage. In the United States table salt includes iodine to help ensure adequate iodine intake.

See also CELL STRUCTURE AND FUNCTION; HEALTHY PEOPLE 2010; NUTRITIONAL NEEDS; NUTRITIONAL SUPPLEMENTS; NUTRITIONAL THERAPY; POISON PREVENTION; VITAMINS AND HEALTH.

nutrient density   The nutritional value of a particular food, generally presented as an assessment of the quantity and quality of NUTRIENTS the food delivers per CALORIE. Foods that contain multiple minerals and vitamins per calorie have high nutrient density; those that do not have low nutrient density. Generally the less processed a food is, the higher its nutrient density. Fruits, vegetables, legumes, seeds, whole grains, and nuts have high nutrient density. Prepared dinners, cookies, crackers, chips, candy, and other such food products have comparatively low nutrient density. Some prepared foods, such as cakes and pastries, have relatively little nutritional value beyond the energy forms (carbohydrate and fat) they deliver. Though many prepared foods are not devoid of nutrients, they deliver significantly more calories for comparable nutrient levels. Foods with higher nutrient density also tend to be more filling.

See also EATING HABITS; METABOLISM; NUTRITIONAL NEEDS; WEIGHT LOSS AND WEIGHT MANAGEMENT.

nutrients   Substances that participate in METABOLISM. Macronutrients deliver energy. The three macronutrient groups are carbohydrate, fat, and protein. Micronutrients facilitate the biochemical actions that convert macronutrients into energy. The main groups of micronutrients are vitamins and minerals. Supportive nutrients include phytochemicals (plant-based biochemicals such as flavonoids and plant sterols) and the numerous trace minerals and other chemicals that are present in the body and have roles in metabolism, though researchers do not fully understand those roles. The final nutrient is water. Essential nutrients are those the body must acquire from sources outside itself, such as foods. Other nutrients, though no less important to health, are nonessen-

tial because the body can synthesize them from substances within it.

Macronutrients

The macronutrients—carbohydrates, fats, and proteins—are the body's energy sources. The amounts and ratios of them that an individual needs vary according to age, gender, activity level, and health status. Metabolism reduces all macronutrients ultimately to GLUCOSE. The body stores any excesses (amounts the body does not immediately use for energy) as glycogen and fat, regardless of the source macronutrient. Per gram carbohydrates and proteins yield four calories of energy; fats, which represent stored energy, yield nine calories per gram.

The body must use in some way all of the energy that enters it in the form of food, either through immediate consumption or storage. Glycogen, which the LIVER produces and stores, is an intermediate storage form that can supply about 12 hours of energy. The liver also produces fat, which adipose cells throughout the body store (body fat). The body in healthy balance warehouses enough body fat to supply energy for six to eight weeks.

In 2005 dietary recommendations shifted from a percentage allocation for macronutrient consumption to a stance of moderation in choice with a focus on managing overall CALORIE intake across the spectrum of energy nutrients. Health experts concur that people need a wide variety of nutrients and individual needs vary. Focusing on the quality of foods within each macronutrient group allows people to make choices that meet their personal needs and tastes, yet still meet the nutritional needs of their bodies in healthful ways.

Carbohydrates   Carbohydrates are chemical structures consisting of oxygen, carbon, and

hydrogen. Nutritionists further classify carbohydrates as monosaccharides (single molecule), disaccharides (two molecules), and polysaccharides (multiple molecules). Monosaccharides and disaccharides are simple carbohydrates; polysaccharides are complex carbohydrates. Nearly all foods contain or deliver as a product of metabolism some form of carbohydrate. Monosaccharides and disaccharides convert to energy fairly quickly after consumption; the sugars from fruits and fruit juices and from candies and sodas (soft drinks) can enter the blood circulation within 10 minutes. Polysaccharides such as pastas take longer for the body to digest and metabolize, up to several hours.

Polysaccharides are starches and fibers. Starches are storage forms of glucose the LIVER converts to glycogen. Fibers are structural components of plants that the body cannot digest. Some forms of fiber, such as pectin, are soluble (dissolve in water). These fibers acquire a gel-like consistency in the intestines that bind with lipids (including cholesterol), BILE, and other substances. The primary dietary sources of soluble fibers are fruits, oats, and legumes. Nonsoluble fibers absorb water but do not change consistency. These fibers add bulk to digestive waste in the large intestine, aiding the COLON in moving the waste through and out of the body. Though not itself a nutrient, fiber is essential for the healthy function of the gastrointestinal tract.

CARBOHYDRATES

Monosaccharides		
GLUCOSE	fructose	galactose
Disaccharides		
lactose	maltose	sucrose
Polysaccharides		
cellulose	fiber	glycogen

Enzymes carry out the chemical actions that metabolize carbohydrates to the end form of glucose. Carbohydrate digestion begins in the MOUTH with the aid of amylase, an enzyme in the saliva. Amylase breaks down dietary carbohydrates into smaller polysaccharides and disaccharides. Because the STOMACH does not contain any enzymes that metabolize carbohydrates, the next stage of carbohydrate digestion takes place in the SMALL INTESTINE. The enzymes lactase, maltase, and sucrase break down lactose, maltose, and sucrose, respectively. Lactose and sucrose each produce one molecule of glucose; maltose produces two. From the small intestine the monosaccharides enter the BLOOD circulation. Fructose and galactose travel to the liver where chemical processes convert them to glucose. Depending on the body's needs, the liver may further convert glucose to glycogen for storage.

Fats (lipids) Dietary fats are chemical combinations of carbon and hydrogen atoms that form structures called fatty acids. The number of hydrogen atoms in a fatty acid determines whether the fat is saturated or unsaturated, which is one of the most important features of the fat from a health perspective. A fatty acid's saturation determines how the fat behaves in the body.

Saturated fats, which come primarily from animal-based foods such as meats and dairy, contribute to elevated CHOLESTEROL BLOOD LEVELS, a risk factor for CARDIOVASCULAR DISEASE (CVD). Saturated fats are the primary source material for the liver's production of cholesterol and the carriers that transport them through the blood, lipoproteins. Palm oil and coconut oil are also saturated fats. Saturated fats are solid at room temperature.

TRANSFORMED THINKING ABOUT TRANS FATS

In the 1980s and 1990s researchers and doctors believed trans fats, created through a manufacturing process called hydrogenation that adds hydrogen atoms to unsaturated fatty acid structures to make them more stable in food products, were less harmful for health than the saturated fats they were marketed to replace. However, further research demonstrated that trans fats are instead considerably more harmful to health, causing a rapid and significant rise in blood cholesterol levels and thus dramatically raising the risk for CARDIOVASCULAR DISEASE (CVD). Health experts now recommend avoiding trans fats; and in 2006, US regulations began requiring food labels to list trans fat content.

Unsaturated fats come from plant-based foods. Commonly called oils, unsaturated fats are liquid at room temperature. They are monounsaturated or polyunsaturated, depending on their chemical configurations. Unsaturated fats, in moderation, appear to help lower blood cholesterol levels. Polyunsaturated fats include safflower, corn, and sunflower oils. Monounsaturated fats, which many health experts believe offer the greatest health benefits among the fatty acids, include olive, canola, and peanut oils as well as olives, avocados, almonds, pecans, cashews, and peanuts. Many "vegetable oil" products blend oils from different sources.

Trans fatty acids, or trans fats, are processed fats that contain extra hydrogen atoms to make them more solid at room temperature and more resistant to oxidative degradation than the base fatty acids are in their natural forms. Sometimes called hydrogenated fats, trans fats raise blood cholesterol levels higher and faster than do saturated fats. The most common dietary sources of trans fats are margarines, shortening, and partially hydrogenated cooking oils. Processed baked goods, snack foods, fried foods, and fast foods are common dietary sources of trans fats.

OMEGA-3 FATTY ACIDS AND HEALTH RISK REDUCTION

Research suggests that tipping the balance to favor consumption of omega-3 fatty acids can significantly lower the risk for HEART disease and cancer (especially PROSTATE CANCER and BREAST CANCER) in some people. Eicosapentaenoic acid (EPA) and docosahexaenoic acid (DHA) are two omega-3 fatty acids found in high concentrations in mackerel, salmon, lake trout, herring, sardines, and anchovies. The American Heart Association recommends two servings weekly of any of these fish.

The body requires fatty acids for numerous functions beyond energy, including HORMONE synthesis and cell membrane integrity. Nearly all fatty acids, in foods and in the body, take the form of triglycerides. The essential fatty acids are linoleic acid and linolenic acid, from which the body can synthesize other fatty acids. Linoleic acid is an omega-6 fatty acid; its primary dietary sources are meats, dairy products, and vegetable oils. Linolenic acid is an omega-3 fatty acid; soybeans, flaxseed and soybean oils, nuts, and seeds are its primary dietary sources. The body requires these fatty acids in relative balance. EATING HABITS that disproportionately deliver linoleic acid (saturated fats such as in meats) appear to correlate with increased risk for CVD (notably HYPERTENSION) and some types of cancer (notably hormone induced).

Proteins Dietary proteins, also called peptides, are chains of amino acids; amino acids are chemical structures (molecules) of carbon, hydrogen, oxygen, and nitrogen. Of the hundreds of amino acids in the body, 20 combine in various forms to create the majority of the body's proteins. Nine are essential, meaning they must enter the body from outside sources such as foods. Using these nine amino acids and other substances within the body, the body synthesizes all the other amino acids it needs and combines the amino acids to create proteins. Proteins are key messenger substances in the body. DNA (deoxyribonucleic acid), the GENETIC CODE each nucleated cell contains, is a protein strand. Other proteins carry its instructions to molecules throughout the body, giving the directions for the amino acid sequences that are the foundation of the body's structure and function.

Dietary proteins are also chains of amino acids and are complete or incomplete, according to whether the protein chain contains all nine essential amino acids (complete) or not (incomplete). Animal-based foods (meats, poultry, fish, and dairy) and soybeans provide complete dietary proteins. Plant-based foods provide incomplete proteins, though combining consumption of different plant-based foods can deliver a combination of proteins that are complete. Dietary variety is the most effective way to ensure the body receives adequate amounts of all the essential amino acids.

AMINO ACIDS			
Essential Amino Acids		**Nonessential Amino Acids**	
histidine	isoleucine	alanine	argine
leucine	lysine	asparagine	aspartic acid
methionine	phenylalanine	cysteine	glutamic acid
threonine	tryptophan	glutamine	glycine
valine		proline	serine
		taurine	tyrosine

After consumption dietary proteins undergo digestion and metabolism, processes that break them down to their amino acid structures. The body then reassembles the amino acids into structures it requires for its functions. The body eventually metabolizes excess amino acids to glucose, glycogen, and fat. Though muscles in the body are primarily protein structures, eating large quantities of protein does not build MUSCLE mass; the body uses dietary protein only to supply the components it needs to craft its own proteins. Protein deficiency can be a health concern for vegans, who must take extra care to eat a wide variety of protein-rich plant-based foods to meet their protein needs.

Micronutrients

The key groups of micronutrients are vitamins and minerals, both of which facilitate the processes of energy conversion within the body and are essential for life. Vitamins are organic substances useful to the body only in their whole forms; cooking and processing easily destroy many vitamins. Vitamins are also the source of many antioxidants, biochemicals that remove free radicals (rogue molecules that are the waste byproducts of metabolism) from the body. Researchers believe the cumulative damage free radicals cause contributes to many health conditions, including CVD and cancer. Minerals are inorganic substances abundant in the environment that enter food sources directly (from the soil and water, as with plants) or indirectly (from the plants that animals eat). Minerals remain chemically unchanged from sources to their uses in the body, even when they bind with each other or with other substances.

Supportive Nutrients

Foods contain numerous substances that provide supportive action for nutrients. Key among them is the group called phytochemicals. Among the most prominent of these are the carotenoids, flavonoids, lignans, phenolic acids, phytosterols, PHYTOESTROGENS, and protease inhibitors. Though a number of phytochemicals have achieved recognition for their individual effects on health, the strongest health benefits appear to come from phytochemicals collectively. Health experts recommend going straight to the source for supportive nutrients, acquiring them through fresh fruits and vegetables, legumes, and whole grains.

Other supportive nutrients include minerals such as sulfur; amino acid derivatives such as carnitine and choline; and inositol, a substance the body synthesizes from glucose. Sulfur is present in many animal-based foods and occurs in the body as an ingredient of proteins, some B vitamins, and some hormones. Carnitine, choline, inositol, and numerous similar substances act somewhat like vitamins in the body, though the body synthesizes them.

See also AGING, NUTRITION AND DIETARY CHANGES THAT OCCUR WITH; ANTIOXIDANT; BODY FAT PERCENTAGE; CARBOHYDRATE LOADING; CELL STRUCTURE AND FUNCTION; DIET AND HEALTH; MINERALS AND HEALTH; PHENYLKETONURIA (PKU); STARVATION; TRIGLYCERIDE BLOOD LEVEL; TRIGLYCERIDES, DIETARY; VITAMINS AND HEALTH.

nutritional assessment A clinical evaluation of an individual's nutritional status, typically as part of a ROUTINE MEDICAL EXAMINATION or as a direction of the diagnostic path when evaluating symptoms that suggest NUTRITIONAL DEFICIENCY, MALNUTRITION, gastrointestinal disorders, and systemic (body-wide) disease. Routine nutritional assessment is particularly important for the very young and the very old.

A nutritional assessment begins with measurement of height and body weight; physical examination to detect any signs or indications of nutritional deficiency; and a discussion of the person's EATING HABITS, including the kinds and amounts of food consumed over the course of a day or a week. Basic BLOOD tests can measure the levels of key NUTRIENTS in the blood circulation or nutrients the doctor suspects are deficient (such as iron). The doctor may conduct further tests, depending on the person's health circumstances.

The doctor may also measure UPPER ARM CIRCUMFERENCE, TRICEPS SKINFOLD, WAIST CIRCUMFERENCE, and hip circumference, factors that allow the doctor to quantifiably assess BODY FAT PERCENTAGE as well as loss of MUSCLE tissue in suspected nutritional disorders. From these measurements the doctor or nutritionist can calculate BODY MASS INDEX (BMI), basal metabolic rate (BMR), resting metabolic rate (RMR), and anticipated daily CALORIE requirements based on the person's lifestyle, weight management needs, and unique health circumstances.

See also AGING, NUTRITION AND DIETARY CHANGES THAT OCCUR WITH; DIET AND HEALTH; EXERCISE AND HEALTH; METABOLISM.

nutritional deficiency Inadequate consumption of one or more key NUTRIENTS. Gastrointestinal disorders of MALABSORPTION, such as CELIAC DISEASE and INFLAMMATORY BOWEL DISEASE (IBD), also cause nutritional deficiencies. Long-term, chronic health conditions or their treatments place extended demands on the body's nutrient base. Certain medications may interfere with how the body absorbs or maintains nutrients, such as diuretics ("water pills") which alter the body's mechanisms for retaining magnesium, sodium, potassium, and calcium.

Other treatments such as RENAL DIALYSIS for RENAL FAILURE may remove nutrients from the body. As well, people who have chronic health conditions are not always able to eat properly and thus do not consume adequate nutrients. Vitamin and mineral (micronutrient) deficiencies may develop in people who voluntarily limit their food intake to certain kinds of foods, such as those who follow strict vegan (no animal protein) diets. Fad diets may lead to deficiencies of macronutrients, most commonly protein.

HEALTH CONDITIONS AND CIRCUMSTANCES THAT CAN CAUSE NUTRITIONAL DEFICIENCIES

ALCOHOLISM	anorexia nervosa
BARIATRIC SURGERY	CELIAC DISEASE
COMA	CYCLIC VOMITING SYNDROME
GASTRECTOMY	INFLAMMATORY BOWEL DISEASE (IBD)
MALABSORPTION	PEPTIC ULCER DISEASE
PERSISTENT VEGETATIVE STATE	RENAL DIALYSIS
SHORT BOWEL SYNDROME	STARVATION

Deficiencies are most likely to occur with water-soluble nutrients as the body's stores of these are short-term. Though prompt intervention through dietary changes and nutritional supplementation can easily reverse most nutritional deficiencies, unresolved or untreated nutritional deficiencies can result in serious health conditions such as SCURVY (vitamin C deficiency) and OSTEOPOROSIS (calcium deficiency).

See also DIET AND HEALTH; HEMOCHROMATOSIS; MALNUTRITION; NUTRITIONAL SUPPLEMENTS; WILSON'S DISEASE.

nutritional needs The kinds and amounts of NUTRIENTS the body needs to maintain itself in good health. Research has established minimum levels of many nutrients, and health experts make recommendations for others based on the best available information. The roles of some nutrients remain poorly understood, though the body appears to require the nutrients for proper functioning. A person's nutritional needs change with life stage, lifestyle, PREGNANCY, and health circumstances.

Acknowledging the individualized nature of nutritional needs, the US Department of Agriculture (UDSA), the government agency responsible for establishing guidelines and standards for nutrition and diet, in 2005 revised its gold standard food guide pyramid to present 12 models of recommendations. The different models allow individuals to customize food choices to meet their physical needs and health circumstances, emphasize variety, and incorporate recommendations for

---

NUTRIENT DEFICIENCIES AND THEIR POTENTIAL HEALTH PROBLEMS

Deficient Nutrient	Health Conditions
calcium	OSTEOMALACIA, OSTEOPOROSIS, RICKETS
	MUSCLE cramps
	HEART ARRHYTHMIA
	HYPERTENSION (high BLOOD PRESSURE)
	insomnia
chromium	GLUCOSE intolerance
	peripheral NEUROPATHY
copper	slow HEALING

Deficient Nutrient	Health Conditions
fluorine (fluoride)	DENTAL CARIES (cavities)
iodine	GOITER HYPOTHYROIDISM
iron	iron-deficiency ANEMIA delayed growth and development in children GLOSSITIS (reddened, swollen, painful tongue)
phosphate	BONE DENSITY loss, osteoporosis
selenium	may contribute to hypothyroidism increased susceptibility to certain viral infections
vitamin A	NIGHT BLINDNESS hardening (keratinization) of tissue within the internal organs reduced resistance to INFECTION
vitamin B complex	BERIBERI PELLAGRA pernicious anemia, megaloblastic anemia PARESTHESIA (disturbances of sensory perception) DEPRESSION cognitive dysfunction fatigue, weakness
vitamin C	SCURVY slow healing gum disease, tooth loss
vitamin D	RICKETS, osteomalacia, osteoporosis
vitamin E	hemolytic anemia RETINOPATHY of prematurity ATAXIA, coordination difficulties, muscle weakness, paresthesia
VITAMIN K	easy bruising and bleeding COAGULATION disorders deficits of CLOTTING FACTORS
zinc	ALOPECIA (HAIR loss) HYPOGONADISM night blindness slow healing, lowered resistance to infection loss of APPETITE, altered sense of taste chronic DERMATITIS

physical exercise. Interactive food guide pyramid models are accessible at the USDA's Web site (www.mypyramid.gov). The USDA publication *Dietary Guidelines for Americans 2005* includes discussion of the food guide pyramids and other nutritional information.

Since the 1940s the standard of appropriate nutritional intake for individual nutrients has been the recommended dietary allowance (RDA), which quantifies how much of a nutrient a person should consume to prevent deficiency of that nutrient. Through the decades since, new knowledge and understanding have resulted in the emergence of additional standards that attempt to quantify the normal levels of nutrients necessary for health as well as the lower and upper limits beyond which health problems arise. These now fall collectively under the umbrella term *dietary reference intake (DRI)*. Because most people do not consume the "daily" amount of a nutrient every day the DRI system also takes into consideration variations in eating patterns and nutrient consumption, using formulas that look at nutritional needs over the long term and establishing averages that meet them.

For further discussion of nutritional needs, please see the overview section "Nutrition and Diet."

See also AGING, NUTRITION AND DIETARY CHANGES THAT OCCUR WITH; ANTIOXIDANT; LIFESTYLE AND HEALTH; MINERALS AND HEALTH; VITAMINS AND HEALTH.

nutritional supplements Products that provide additional NUTRIENTS and dietary substances beyond those that enter the body via food consumption. The most commonly taken nutritional supplements, also called dietary supplements, are vitamins and minerals, which are available in combination formulas (multivitamin supplements, multimineral supplements, and multivitamin with mineral supplements) as well as products that contain single nutrients. Some products combine vitamins and minerals with herbal and botanical substances, for example vitamin C with ECHINACEA. The choices among products are nearly endless; the nutritional supplement industry remains a key player in the American economy, with annual sales exceeding $19 billion.

In the United States federal law classifies vitamin and mineral supplements and most MEDICINAL HERBS AND BOTANICALS as dietary supplements. This removes these products from the jurisdiction of the US agency charged with oversight of DRUG safety and EFFICACY, the US Food and Drug Administration (FDA). Though various federal laws regulate matters of safety and efficacy as well as advertising claims of health benefits, testing of supplement products shows wide variation of quality standards across manufacturers and products. This can result in inconsistent doses and effectiveness.

The intent of nutritional supplements should be to augment, not replace, dietary nutrients. Vitamins, minerals, and botanicals do not deliver energy nutrients, though other kinds of nutritional supplements (such as protein supplements) do. Health experts disagree on whether the effect of supplements, especially vitamins and minerals, in the body is the same as that when the same nutrients enter the body from food sources. Some research studies investigating antioxidants, for example, show much higher levels of activity from consumed foods compared to supplements. Other studies show no measurable difference. A common philosophy among nutritionists is "stay close to the earth" because the highest concentrations of nutrients come from fresh fruits, vegetables, and whole grains.

People who have chronic health conditions or take regular prescription medications should check with the doctor or pharmacist before taking nutritional supplements of any kind, as the risk for DRUG INTERACTION is high. As well, some chronic health conditions or the medications taken to treat them have specific effects on how the body absorbs and metabolizes nutrients, increasing or decreasing the need for those nutrients. For such people, doctors may recommend therapeutic nutritional supplementation. For others, most health experts recommend obtaining nutrients from the diet to the extent possible and using nutritional supplements, including vitamins and minerals, only when there are clear and specific reasons to supplement dietary intake. However, research continues to generate new knowledge and understanding of how nutrients affect health and disease, and recommendations continue to evolve. Many people integrate specific nutritional supplements with healthy EATING HABITS.

See also ANTIOXIDANT; MINERALS AND HEALTH; NUTRITIONAL DEFICIENCY; NUTRITIONAL THERAPY; VITAMIN AND MINERAL THERAPY; VITAMINS AND HEALTH.

parenteral nutrition The intravenous administration of NUTRIENTS as a method of supplying appropriate sustenance to a person who cannot meet his or her NUTRITIONAL NEEDS by eating, such as someone who is in a COMA or has a severe swallowing disorder. Parenteral nutrition, called total parenteral nutrition (TPN) when it is a person's sole source of nutrition, is helpful for short-term, intense feeding when ENTERAL NUTRITION is not a viable option. Parenteral nutrition is most successful as temporary supportive treatment such as after extensive surgery or during recovery from major trauma, though sometimes is necessary for longer therapy such as in severe gastrointestinal disease or cancer. In the long term, however, parenteral nutrition cannot deliver all of the nutrients the body needs and, in particular, is lacking in its ability to supply lipids (fats), which the body requires for cell maintenance and energy.

Parenteral nutrition solutions are very irritating to the veins so must be infused into the larger veins deep in the chest. This requires the doctor to insert a percutaneous intravenous catheter (PIC line) into a VEIN in the arm and thread it through the smaller vein to a large vein. An alternative is a Hickman line, in which the intravenous catheter enters the jugular vein at the base of the neck and extends into the superior VENA CAVA, the largest vein in the upper body. Fluids run continuously into either line with the aid of an infusion pump to maintain delivery of the solution at constant rate and pressure.

Some of the complications of extended parenteral nutrition include LIVER FAILURE, RENAL FAILURE, NUTRITIONAL DEFICIENCY (notably of trace minerals and lipids), and MALNUTRITION. INFECTION is also a significant risk, partly because the indwelling catheter provides a pathway for BACTE-RIA to enter the body and partly because the content of parenteral nutrition solutions is very high in GLUCOSE, which attracts and feeds bacteria.

See also END OF LIFE CONCERNS; QUALITY OF LIFE; SWALLOWING DISORDERS.

pellagra A health condition resulting from long-term deficiency of niacin (vitamin B₃). Pellagra is uncommon in the United States, occurring primarily in people who have chronic ALCOHOLISM or gastrointestinal disorders that prevent absorption of dietary niacin (also called niacinamide, nicotinamide, nicotinic acid, or niacinic acid) or of the essential amino acid tryptophan. The body requires niacin for cellular METABOLISM. Tryptophan is a niacin precursor from which the body can synthesize niacin. Niacin is necessary for the energy conversions that take place during cellular metabolism.

Symptoms and Diagnostic Path

Early symptoms of pellagra are those of nonspecific gastrointestinal upset: NAUSEA, VOMITING, and DIARRHEA. Burning in the MOUTH and especially of the tongue is common, with a characteristic gray membranous tissue coating on the gums that continually sloughs or peels. As pellagra worsens, additional symptoms that appear include GLOSSITIS (inflamed tongue) and SKIN RASH that intensifies with sun exposure after which the skin becomes rough, thick, and discolored. A characteristic pattern of this damage often develops around the neck.

At the same time, the lack of niacin causes the mucosa (mucous membrane lining) of the gastrointestinal tract to deteriorate, progressively reducing the ability of the intestines to absorb nutrients; MALNUTRITION results. Niacin deficiency also affects neurons (NERVE cells) and the functioning of the CENTRAL NERVOUS SYSTEM, resulting in behavioral disturbances, delusions, confusion, and DEMENTIA. Disturbances of neuromuscular function include rigidity and involuntary activation of reflexes. The diagnostic path includes BLOOD tests to measure the levels of niacin and tryptophan in the blood circulation. The diagnosis is primarily clinical, however, based on the presenting symptoms and their response to treatment with niacin supplementation.

Treatment Options and Outlook
Treatment is immediate supplementation with niacin, usually in the form of niacinamide, and correction of EATING HABITS to restore foods to the diet that provide niacin. At therapeutic doses niacin often causes uncomfortable symptoms such as SKIN flushing and tingling; the niacinamide form, a slightly different chemical structure, does not. Both chemical forms provide the body with the niacin the cells need for energy conversion. Though many of pellagra's symptoms are reversible, those affecting the skin often result in permanent changes that are sometimes disfiguring. Untreated pellagra results in multisystem organ failure that is usually fatal.

Risk Factors and Preventive Measures
Pellagra develops as a consequence of niacin deficiency; thus adequate niacin intake prevents pellagra. Most people can obtain sufficient niacin supplies through the foods they eat. Meats, poultry, and other animal-based proteins contain high amounts of tryptophan, which the body converts to niacinamide. Asparagus, mushrooms, potatoes, spinach, peanuts and peanut butter, and legumes contain high amounts of niacin.

People who eat large quantities of corn and foods made with corn flour and who do not eat other kinds of foods, are at high risk for pellagra. The niacin in corn is not available through digestion. Other people at high risk for pellagra are those taking long-term treatment with isoniazid for TUBERCULOSIS or who have chronic CIRRHOSIS (the LIVER is fundamental in converting tryptophan to niacinamide).

See also ANEMIA; BERIBERI; DELUSION; NEURON; NUTRITIONAL DEFICIENCY; NUTRITIONAL NEEDS; RICKETS; SCURVY; VITAMINS AND HEALTH.

rickets A health condition that results from long-term deficiency of vitamin D, also called calciferol or ergocalciferol, in which the bones cannot absorb calcium or build new BONE tissue. The body makes most of the vitamin D it requires from cholesterol and sunlight. Dietary sources of vitamin D are primarily those that contain added supplements such as dairy products, orange juice, and some SOY-based food products. Cod liver oil naturally contains ergosterol, a form of vitamin D called D_2, as do oily fish such as salmon and sardines (though not in as high a concentration as cod liver oil). Supplemental vitamin D also interacts with cholesterol to form calcitriol.

The LIVER manufactures cholesterol, the base for vitamin D, and sends a certain amount for storage in the cells of the SKIN. Exposure to the sun's ultraviolet B (UVB) rays activates a series of chemical changes that convert the stored cholesterol molecules to a HORMONE form of vitamin D called calcitriol. The liver and the KIDNEYS also par-

PELLAGRA SYMPTOMS		
Gastrointestinal	**Dermatologic**	**Neurologic**
DIARRHEA	bullae (blisters)	anxiety
GASTROINTESTINAL BLEEDING	erythema	DEMENTIA
GLOSSITIS	hyperpigmentation	DEPRESSION
loss of APPETITE	PHOTOSENSITIVITY	disorientation
MALABSORPTION	thickened SKIN	ENCEPHALOPATHY
NAUSEA		HALLUCINATION
stomatitis		irritability
VOMITING		PARANOIA

ticipate in these chemical changes. In combination with PARATHYROID HORMONE, calcitriol maintains a steady level of calcium in the BLOOD circulation. This balance allows the gastrointestinal tract to absorb calcium from dietary sources and the bones to accept calcium from the supply circulating in the blood.

Rickets develops when a long-term deficiency of vitamin D results in decreased dietary absorption of calcium. To meet its extensive needs for calcium, an important ion for numerous cellular functions, including proper contraction of the MUSCLE cells of the HEART, the body draws calcium from the bones. The bones demineralize and weaken. The long bones, notably those in the legs, bow. Doctors generally use the term *rickets* to refer to this disease process in children and the term OSTEOMALACIA to refer to this disease process in adults.

Symptoms and Diagnostic Path

The primary symptoms of rickets are bowed legs and a protruding belly (the result of weakened abdominal muscles). Deformities may develop at the epiphyses, or growth plates, of the bones, forming characteristic knobs and bumps. The diagnostic path includes X-rays to assess the density and mineralization of the bones and blood tests to measure the levels of calcium, phosphorus, and parathyroid hormone in the blood circulation. The doctor will also take a thorough PERSONAL HEALTH HISTORY including EATING HABITS.

Treatment Options and Outlook

Prompt vitamin D supplementation generally reverses most circumstances of mild to moderate rickets with little residual damage. Moderate to severe rickets, which is fairly uncommon in the United States, may result in consequential deformities of the pelvis, rib joints, and knee and ankle joints. Proper nutrition usually maintains adequate vitamin D intake.

Risk Factors and Preventive Measures

Most people will synthesize (make) all the vitamin D their bodies require with regular modest sun exposure, about 20 minutes to the face and arms four or five days a week. The farther from the equator a person lives, the longer sun exposure is necessary because the intensity of the sun's ultraviolet radiation diminishes. The ideal exposure is that which is just less than what results in mild SUNBURN. Doctors recommend multiple short exposures (5 to 15 minutes several times a day) to reduce the risk for sunburn. Applying sunscreen before going in the sun, though a prudent and recommended measure to prevent sun-related skin damage when engaging outdoor activities, prevents ultraviolet rays from penetrating the skin. People who have dark skin require longer periods of sun exposure.

Some health experts recommend that people who live in regions where the hours of sunlight drop below 12 hours a day (such as above 40 degrees latitude in the Northern Hemisphere, which includes locations north of the US cities San Francisco, Denver, St. Louis, Indianapolis, Philadelphia, and New York City) take vitamin D supplement. It is important to remain within the recommended dosage guidelines, however, because vitamin D is a fat-soluble vitamin that can accumulate in the body to reach toxic levels.

The antiseizure medication phenytoin increases the body's METABOLISM of calcidiol, one of the intermediary vitamin D forms. People who take this medication may need therapeutic vitamin D supplementation, particularly if they do not spend much time outdoors. Young children who live in inner city areas where smog is a problem have increased risk for rickets even when they spend time outdoors because the smog acts to filter the sun's ultraviolet rays.

See also ANEMIA; BERIBERI; FANCONI'S SYNDROME; MALNUTRITION; NUTRITIONAL DEFICIENCY; NUTRITIONAL NEEDS; PELLAGRA; SCURVY; VITAMINS AND HEALTH.

satiety The sensation of fullness and satisfaction after eating a meal. Satiety represents a convergence of physical, physiologic, and emotional factors. The physical sensation of fullness occurs when enough food fills the STOMACH to stretch its walls. The stretching activates NERVE and HORMONE sensors that then send physiologic signals to the APPETITE and satiety centers in the BRAIN and to receptors in the SMALL INTESTINE and the HUNGER center in the HYPOTHALAMUS. These signals slow or stop the release of hormones and neurotransmitters necessary for digestion and initiate the release of other hormones and biochemicals that have roles in absorbing NUTRIENTS into the BLOOD circulation and further METABOLISM of those nutrients.

Research indicates that foods high in protein result in reaching physical satiety the most rapidly. Foods high in fat take much longer to trigger physical satiety. These findings imply that eating the proteins in a meal first, such as meats or legumes, may curb the appetite, whereas eating the fats or carbohydrates in a meal first may extend appetite. Each circumstance has advantages, depending on an individual's health and weight management situation.

The emotional component of satiety comes when the meal has satisfied desires for certain characteristics of food such as textures, flavors, and quantity. Emotional satiety results in nerve signals to pleasure receptors in the cerebral cortex as well as to the brain's appetite and satiety centers. This is the most variable factor of satiety, influencing whether a person eats not enough or too much. Emotional eating is a significant dimension of WEIGHT LOSS AND WEIGHT MANAGEMENT.

See also EATING HABITS; FOOD CRAVINGS; NEURO-TRANSMITTER.

scurvy A health condition that results from long-term deficiency of vitamin C (also called ascorbic acid). Vitamin C is essential for the formation of collagen, a fibrous protein that is the foundation for connective tissue throughout the body and the framework for BONE tissue. Collagen is integral to the walls of BLOOD vessels. Collagen also is an essential component of SCAR tissue, necessary for wound HEALING. Without vitamin C, a water-soluble vitamin the diet must provide on a relatively daily basis, the body cannot produce collagen.

Symptoms and Diagnostic Path

The most common symptoms of scurvy are bleeding gums and loose TEETH. Other symptoms include low grade FEVER, extended or lack of wound healing, PETECHIAE (pinpoint hemorrhages beneath the SKIN), and internal hemorrhage. ANEMIA is often the indication that there is bleeding somewhere in the body. The diagnostic path includes blood tests to measure the amount of ascorbic acid in the blood circulation as well as in the white blood cells (leukocytes) along with a careful PERSONAL HEALTH HISTORY that includes information about EATING HABITS.

Treatment Options and Outlook

Treatment for scurvy is vitamin C supplementation, which generally restores vitamin C levels and eliminates symptoms after about a week of treatment. In all but the most severe cases, scurvy is completely curable. Doctors generally recommend continued vitamin C supplementation to prevent RECURRENCE. Because vitamin C is water-soluble, there is no risk of toxicity with such prophylaxis. Increasing dietary consumption of foods that contain vitamin C, notably raw fruits and vegetables, helps maintain adequate intake.

FOODS HIGH IN VITAMIN C	
bell peppers (especially red)	broccoli
brussels sprouts	cabbage
cantaloupe	grapefruit
kiwi	lemons
limes	mango
oranges	spinach
strawberries	sweet potatoes
watermelon	

Risk Factors and Preventive Measures

Scurvy occurs only as a deficiency of vitamin C, thus adequate vitamin C consumption prevents scurvy. People who have increased risk for scurvy are those who have chronic ALCOHOLISM, chronic health conditions that interfere with the digestion or absorption of NUTRIENTS, and the very elderly who may not receive adequate nutrition through diet because they cannot or do not eat properly. Fruit and vegetable juices are easy substitutions for whole fruits and vegetables. Many juices are fortified with additional vitamin C and other nutrients.

See also BERIBERI; FANCONI'S SYNDROME; LEUKO-CYTE; MALNUTRITION; NUTRITIONAL DEFICIENCY; NUTRI-TIONAL NEEDS; PELLAGRA; RICKETS; VITAMINS AND HEALTH.

starvation The most severe state of MALNUTRITION resulting from extended lack of food and nutrition. An otherwise healthy adult may lose up to 50 percent of body weight before organ systems fail and death occurs. Total starvation that persists beyond about 10 to 12 weeks is usually fatal. In the United States starvation most commonly occurs as a consequence of severe illness, severe gastrointestinal disease, prolonged COMA, and anorexia nervosa. In parts of the world where food supplies are limited, starvation results from famine and causes millions of deaths every year.

The body attempts to survive starvation by dramatically slowing METABOLISM. HEART RATE and BREATHING rate slow, BLOOD PRESSURE and body temperature drop, and BLOOD flow to nonvital structures diminishes. The body turns to tissues such as MUSCLE and most organs outside the CENTRAL NERV-OUS SYSTEM, breaking them down into chemical products that it can use as NUTRIENTS. Consequently emaciation, in which the body looks gaunt and wasted, is a key characteristic of starvation.

Treatment for starvation is aggressive nutritional supplementation to restore the body to a state such that organ systems begin to function. It can take several weeks for the gastrointestinal system to be able to manage solid foods, during which time PARENTERAL NUTRITION can provide sustenance. ENTERAL NUTRITION can deliver concentrated nutrients to address emerging NUTRITIONAL DEFICIENCY disorders. Full recovery may take six months or longer, depending on what underlying health conditions exist.

See also EATING DISORDERS; NUTRITIONAL SUPPLE-MENTS.

triglycerides, dietary Chemical structures that contain three fatty acids in combination with glycerol. Triglycerides are the most common forms of fat in foods and in the body. The body uses triglycerides primarily for energy. Dietary triglycerides circulate in the BLOOD along with triglycerides the LIVER synthesizes from carbohydrates and fats the body does not use for immediate energy. Some triglycerides then go to cells for use as energy and others go to adipose (fat) cells for storage.

The liver also uses dietary triglycerides to synthesize (make) lipoproteins, the carrier proteins that transport cholesterol and fats through the bloodstream to cells throughout the body. Low-density lipoproteins (LDLs) and very low-density lipoproteins (VLDLs) have higher levels of triglycerides than high-density lipoproteins (HDLs). Elevated levels of LDLs and VLDLs in the blood circulation correlate to increased risk for CARDIO-VASCULAR DISEASE (CVD), HEART ATTACK, and STROKE.

Triglycerides are present in a wide range of foods, notably animal-based foods and oils and fats. Reducing overall food consumption so the calories in balance with the calories out and reducing the amount of refined carbohydrates (sugars) in the diet are the most effective way to reduce blood triglyceride levels. Daily physical exercise helps the body more efficiently metabolize nutrients and increases the consumption of triglycerides as an energy source. A small percentage of people have a genetic disorder of lipid METABOLISM that causes them to have high amounts of triglycerides in their blood circulation. Lipid-lowering medications may then be necessary to bring triglycerides levels down.

See also CARDIOVASCULAR DISEASE PREVENTION; CHOLESTEROL, DIETARY; CHOLESTEROL BLOOD LEVELS; GENETIC DISORDERS; HYPERLIPIDEMIA; TRIGLYCERIDE BLOOD LEVEL.

vitamins and health Vitamins are organic micronutrients essential for health and the body's proper growth, development, and function. They interact with each other or with other biochemicals in the body, functioning as cofactors or coenzymes to carry out activities of energy conversion (METABOLISM) though do not themselves provide energy to the body. With the exception of vitamin D, dietary sources provide the vitamins the body requires.

There are 12 vitamins that are essential for health. The 8 B vitamins and vitamin C are water soluble; the body cannot stockpile stores of them (except in limited accumulations within the BLOOD circulation and the LIVER) and thus requires regular consumption to maintain levels adequate to support health. Most healthy people can obtain the vitamins their bodies need for normal functioning through dietary sources. Vitamins A, E, D, and K are fat soluble; the body stores excess amounts of these vitamins in adipose (fatty) tissue and draws from these supplies when dietary intake does not meet needs.

Vitamin deficiency may develop when dietary consumption is inadequate, as a result of gastrointestinal disorders that interfere with nutrient absorption or owing to interactions with medications. Chronic health conditions may drain the body of important NUTRIENTS, including vitamins. Untreated vitamin deficiency can cause potentially serious health conditions such as SCURVY, RICKETS, and NIGHT BLINDNESS.

Vitamin toxicity occurs most commonly as a consequence of excessive vitamin supplementation and can have serious or permanent consequences. Metabolic disorders and medications that interfere with vitamin metabolism are also common culprits. Vitamin toxicity is more common with the fat-soluble vitamins because they accumulate in the body. Vitamin toxicity also is possible with extreme overconsumption of water-soluble vitamins, usually the result of higher levels in the blood circulation than the body can excrete.

Vitamin toxicity is more likely to occur when taking a multiple vitamin supplement and individual supplements that supply significantly greater than the needed amounts of certain vitamins. Vitamins A; E; and the B vitamins niacin (B₃), pantothenic acid (B₅), pyridoxine (B₆), and folic acid (B₉) present the greatest risk for toxicity.

Vitamin A (Retinol)

Vitamin A is essential for proper functioning of the photoreceptor cells (rods and cones) of the RETINA, maintains the health of the SKIN, and appears to have some antiviral capabilities. It is also crucial for growth and development in children. The liver stores vitamin A, a fat-soluble vitamin, and releases it into the blood circulation as the body needs it. The primary dietary sources for vitamin A are foods that supply beta-carotene, which the body converts to retinol. Such foods include yellow vegetables and fruits, green leafy vegetables, egg yolks, and fish liver oil.

Vitamin A deficiency results in disturbances of vision, including impaired dark adaptation (slowing of the ability of the eyes to adjust to changes in lighting) and night blindness. In children, vitamin A deficiency can stunt growth and impair cognitive development. These developmental disruptions can have permanent consequences, although vitamin A deficiency severe enough to cause such disruptions is rare. Other consequences of vitamin A deficiency generally improve when levels of vitamin A return to normal.

Vitamin A toxicity nearly always results from taking high doses of vitamin A supplement and can occur as acute OVERDOSE (taking an extremely large dose at one time) or chronic overdose (excess that accumulates over time), usually the result of over-supplementation. Treatment with retinol medications, such as for severe ACNE, also can result in vitamin A toxicity. In adults the effects and symptoms of vitamin A toxicity are reversible and generally resolve within a few weeks of stopping supplementation or therapeutic retinol.

Vitamin B Complex

The eight B vitamins, called the vitamin B complex, work in close synchronization with one another and have key roles in many functions in the body. Each B vitamin further has specific functions, dietary sources, deficiency level, and toxicity level. In general the B vitamins are essential for energy conversion (metabolism of carbohydrates and fats) and other functions of cellular metabolism, erythropoiesis (making new red blood cells), and maintaining the epithelium (skin and mucous membranes). The liver stores some of the B vitamins for a short time. Food sources of the B vitamins include meats, poultry, fish, eggs, leafy green vegetables, fruits, whole grains, brown rice, and fortified grain products such as cereals and breads (regulations in the United States require such fortification).

Deficiencies of B vitamins affect many functions of the body. Most often deficiencies of the B vitamins occur collectively, though specific deficiency disorders are BERIBERI (thiamine deficiency), PELLAGRA (niacin deficiency), and pernicious ANEMIA (cyanocobalamin deficiency). In the United States vitamin B deficiencies generally result from chronic health disorders, ALCOHOLISM, and MALABSORPTION disorders. In such circumstances it often is necessary for the person to take therapeutic vitamin B supplements, either B complex or specific B vitamins, to compensate.

Toxicity of B vitamins is uncommon though can occur when taking excessive vitamin supplements and in some metabolic disorders; it is most likely to develop with niacin (B_3), pantothenic acid (B_5), pyridoxine (B_6), and folic acid (B_9). Though most symptoms resolve when vitamin B intake returns to normal, vitamin B toxicities can result in permanent neurologic and skin damage.

Vitamin B_1 (thiamine) Thiamine converts carbohydrates into GLUCOSE and is a coenzyme in the synthesis of acetylcholine, a NEUROTRANSMITTER important for cognitive functions in the cerebral cortex and MUSCLE coordination throughout the body. Prolonged thiamine deficiency causes beriberi.

Vitamin B_2 (riboflavin) Riboflavin is a key player in macronutrient metabolism (fats, carbohydrate, and proteins) as well as in energy conversion at the cellular level (cellular oxidation). It is essential for growth and development in children, facilitates erythropoiesis (formation of new red blood cells), and helps support the health of the retina.

Vitamin B_3 (niacin) Niacin exists in two forms: nicotinic acid and niacinamide (also called nicotinamide). In either form it facilitates the metabolism of carbohydrates (glycolysis) and functions of cellular energy conversion. Niacin also helps maintain the structure of the epithelium (skin and mucous membranes). The body synthesizes some niacin from the essential amino acid tryptophan. Prolonged niacin deficiency causes pellagra. Niacin has emerged as an effective therapy for mild to moderate HYPERLIPIDEMIA, reducing CHOLESTEROL BLOOD LEVELS as effectively as some lipid-lowering medications.

Vitamin B_5 (pantothenic acid) Pantothenic acid is essential for metabolizing amino acids and fats to carbohydrates, and works in collaboration with folic acid and biotin for various functions related to cellular energy conversion. The liver uses pantothenic acid in the synthesis of hormones and cholesterol. Canning and freezing destroy pantothenic acid.

Vitamin B_6 (pyridoxine) Pyridoxine facilitates HEMOGLOBIN production, conversion of tryptophan to niacin, and carbohydrate metabolism. Other forms of vitamin B_6 are pyridoxal and pyridoxamine; all forms of vitamin B_6 convert to the coenzyme pyridoxal-5'-phosphate (PLP) in the body. Health conditions that increase the body's specific use of and need for pyridoxine include alcoholism, END-STAGE RENAL DISEASE (ESRD) with RENAL DIALYSIS, serious BURNS, major surgery, GASTRECTOMY or BARIATRIC SURGERY, and chronic CIRRHOSIS. People who smoke and women who take oral contraceptives (birth control pills) are at high risk for pyridoxine deficiency.

Vitamin B₇ (biotin) Biotin works in close alliance with folic acid and pantothenic acid, and is important in metabolizing macronutrients, especially carbohydrates and fats, from food during digestion. Sulfa-based ANTIBIOTIC MEDICATIONS can prevent the body from absorbing biotin from foods during digestion.

Vitamin B₉ (folic acid) Folic acid, also called folate, is essential for the formation of new blood cells (HEMATOPOIESIS) and works in conjunction with cyanocobalamin to repair DNA. Folic acid is crucial for normal development of the neurologic system in the early EMBRYO; prophylactic folic acid decreases NEURAL TUBE DEFECTS by up to 80 percent. Folic acid also participates in cellular energy conversion cycles.

FOLIC ACID PREVENTS NEURAL TUBE DEFECTS

Folic acid is so effective at preventing NEURAL TUBE DEFECTS that doctors urge all women who could become pregnant, regardless of whether they are planning PREGNANCY and especially if they are taking oral contraceptives (which deplete folic acid), to take a folic acid supplement that delivers 400 micrograms daily. Folic acid is crucial for the closure of the neural tube, the rudimentary CENTRAL NERVOUS SYSTEM that develops in the EMBRYO about 14 days after CONCEPTION.

Vitamin B₁₂ (cyanocobalamin) Cyanocobalamin, also called cobalamin, is essential for the formation of myelin, the protein coating that protects NERVE fibers. It also participates in DNA repair (nucleic acid synthesis), erythropoiesis (formation of new red blood cells), and folic acid metabolism. Intrinsic factor, which the stomach produces, is essential for absorption of cyanocobalamin. Health conditions that diminish intrinsic factor production, such as PEPTIC ULCER DISEASE, and circumstances such as bariatric surgery or gastrectomy, significantly reduce the body's ability to absorb cyanocobalamin and often require supplementation via vitamin B₁₂ injections. The ability to produce intrinsic factor diminishes with age, increasing the risk of deficiency.

Vitamin C (Ascorbic Acid)

The body requires vitamin C to create collagen, a protein critical for the formation of connective tissue and in healing (the formation of scar tissue). Collagen forms the foundation of the SKELETON over which the bones develop. Vitamin C is also necessary for production of serotonin, a vital neurotransmitter, and aids in the dismantling of cholesterol for excretion in the BILE. The body absorbs significantly more iron in combination with vitamin C; health experts recommend eating combinations of foods that contain these substances and taking iron supplements with a glass of orange juice. Citrus fruits are the primary dietary source of vitamin C.

LIMEYS

British sailors of the 19th century acquired the nickname "limey" when the British Navy began including limes in sailors' rations while at sea. Citrus fruits are high in vitamin C, which prevents SCURVY. Limes hold up better in storage than other citrus fruits. Before this practice, half or more of a ship's crew often died before returning home from a long sea voyage.

Long-term vitamin C deficiency results in scurvy, a condition of collagen depletion with symptoms that affect the musculoskeletal, neurologic, and immune systems. Vitamin C deficiency is rare in modern times. Increasing dietary consumption of foods high in vitamin C is usually adequate to restore vitamin C levels and reverse symptoms. Though vitamin C is a water-soluble vitamin, it can accumulate to toxic levels with excessive supplementation. The symptoms of vitamin C toxicity (NAUSEA, DIARRHEA, and sometimes anemia) improve immediately when vitamin C consumption returns to normal.

Vitamin C is also a powerful ANTIOXIDANT with roles in healing and preventing diseases. Much research has explored these roles in recent decades, and numerous studies support vitamin C's ability to expedite recovery from viral infections such as COLDS (though vitamin C cannot prevent such infections). Doctors may recommend vitamin C supplementation for people recovering from major surgery, serious burns, and significant dental procedures.

Vitamin D (Calciferol)

Without vitamin D, the body cannot use calcium. Vitamin D is unique among vitamins in that the body can manufacture it as a process of photosynthesis (exposure to sunlight) that converts a form of cholesterol stored in the cells of the skin into vitamin D. Only a small portion of vitamin D enters the body from dietary sources (namely, fortified dairy products) in the form of vitamin D_2 (ergocalciferol) or vitamin D_3 (cholecalciferol). The circulating, active form of vitamin D is calcitriol, which functions as a HORMONE. Calcitriol, in tandem with PARATHYROID HORMONE, regulates the amount of calcium in the blood. This regulation determines the availability of calcium to the bones. Vitamin D also influences IMMUNE SYSTEM functions important for fighting tumors.

Vitamin D deficiency affects bone structure, preventing bone tissue from accepting new calcium and allowing calcium to leave the bones to enter the blood circulation. Vitamin D deficiency can cause rickets in children and OSTEOMALACIA in adults. Both are conditions of demineralization that are reversible with vitamin D supplementation, though severe rickets may result in residual deformity particularly of the pelvis. Sustained vitamin D deficiency in adults leads to OSTEOPOROSIS, an irreversible loss of bone tissue.

Vitamin D toxicity may develop with excessive consumption from vitamin supplements, which can be supplementation within normal limits in healthy people who get adequate vitamin D from dietary sources and is a particular risk among people who take megavitamins. The toxic level is fairly low. Vitamin D toxicity is also a risk in people who are receiving treatment for HYPOPARATHYROIDISM. Excessive levels of vitamin D affect calcium reabsorption in the kidney (HYPERCALCEMIA) and often cause kidney stones (NEPHROLITHIASIS) that can result in permanent damage to the KIDNEYS.

Vitamin E (Tocopherol)

A fat-soluble vitamin, vitamin E's most important function is as an antioxidant. It blocks the reaction of free radicals to produce more free radicals and some metabolism of fatty acids. Vitamin E also maintains the integrity of erythrocytes (red blood cells), which are vulnerable to damage, in the blood circulation. Though vitamin E has a reputation for a wide range of actions in the body to prevent diseases such as cancer and CARDIOVASCULAR DISEASE (CVD); to treat conditions such as FIBROCYSTIC BREAST DISEASE; and to enhance physical ENDURANCE, LIBIDO, and reproduction, research has thus far failed to support these claims. Some research suggests that excessive amounts of vitamin E may in fact contribute to the development of certain cancers. Much research remains under way to better understand the roles of vitamin E in health and in disease.

Vitamin E deficiency may occur in disorders of fat absorption or metabolism though is quite rare. When present vitamin E deficiency may result in hemolytic anemia. Vitamin E toxicity is also uncommon and nearly always occurs in people who take excessive amounts of vitamin E supplements. Vitamin E toxicity can have deleterious effects on the mechanisms of COAGULATION, leading to hemorrhage.

Vitamin K (Quinone)

BACTERIA in the SMALL INTESTINE synthesize 80 percent or more of the VITAMIN K the body needs and uses. The other 20 percent comes from plant-based foods, notably spinach, broccoli, and other dark green vegetables. The bacterial form of vitamin K is menaquinone; the plant form of vitamin K is phylloquinone. Vitamin K is essential for the activation of several CLOTTING FACTORS (VII, IC, X) and prothrombin, which regulate the blood's ability to clot.

Vitamin K deficiency may occur in disorders that interfere with the absorption of fats into the body, such as GALLBLADDER DISEASE and gastrointestinal malabsorption disorders. Long-term antibiotic therapy can significantly reduce the bacteria count in the small intestine, restricting the body's ability to synthesize vitamin K. Anticoagulant medications such as warfarin work by blocking the action of vitamin K. Untreated vitamin K deficiency can result in life-threatening hemorrhage. Vitamin K toxicity is rare and occurs nearly always when taking vitamin K supplements. It can cause JAUNDICE and, when severe, permanent BRAIN damage. Some multivitamin supplements

ESSENTIAL VITAMINS AND THEIR DIETARY SOURCES

Vitamin	Dietary Sources
A (retinol)	carrots
	butternut squash, acorn squash, pumpkin
	spinach, turnip greens, chard
	broccoli
	mangos
	beef liver
B_1 (thiamine)	fortified breads and cereals
	pork, beef, ham, chicken, turkey, fish, eggs
	brewer's yeast
	dairy products
	legumes
	peas, corn, green beans, potatoes (with skins)
B_2 (riboflavin)	fortified breads and cereals
	dairy products
	pork, beef, ham, chicken, turkey, liver, fish, eggs
	oysters, clams, shrimp
	mushrooms
B_3 (niacin)	fortified breads and cereals
	dairy products
	pork, beef, ham, chicken, turkey, liver, eggs
	tuna, cod, halibut, bluefish, shrimp
	peas, corn, sweet potatoes, potatoes (with skins), spinach, broccoli
	peanuts
B_5 (pantothenic acid)	fortified breads and cereals
	mushrooms
	broccoli
	avocados
B_6 (pyridoxine)	fortified breads and cereals
	potatoes (with skin)
	bananas, apples, oranges, watermelon, grapefruit and grapefruit juice, avocados, prunes and prune juice
	legumes
	pork, beef, ham, chicken, turkey, liver, fish (especially tuna), eggs
	seeds, nuts, peanut butter
B_7 (biotin)	fortified breads and cereals
	brown rice, barley, oatmeal, whole wheat
	soy products
	cauliflower
	egg yolks, liver
	tuna, finfish

contain vitamin K; unless a doctor specifically recommends vitamin K supplementation, however, most people should not take supplements that contain vitamin K.

See also CONTRACEPTION; MINERALS AND HEALTH; NUTRITIONAL SUPPLEMENTS; NUTRITIONAL THERAPY; VITAMIN AND MINERAL THERAPY.

Vitamin	Dietary Sources
B_9 (folic acid)	fortified breads and cereals
	spinach, okra, greens
	asparagus, broccoli, corn, green beans, sweet potatoes, potatoes (with skins)
	tomatoes and tomato juice
	legumes
	tofu
	seeds, nuts, peanut butter
	eggs
B_{12} (cyanocobalamin)	fortified breads and cereals
	pork, beef, ham, chicken, turkey, liver, fish, eggs
	shrimp, oysters, clams
	dairy products
C (ascorbic acid)	citrus fruits and juices: oranges and orange juice, lemons, limes, grapefruit and grapefruit juice
	watermelon, strawberries, cantaloupe
	papaya, mangos, tangerines, guava
	broccoli, kohlrabi, cabbage, cauliflower
	spinach, greens
	bell peppers
D (calciferol)	sunlight
	fortified dairy products, orange juice, and soy milk
E (tocopherol)	polyunsaturated oils
	egg yolks
	spinach, greens
	almonds, walnuts, pecans, cashews
	peanuts and peanut butter
	seeds (sunflower, flax)
	whole grains and whole grain products
	wheat germ
K (quinone)	spinach, lettuce other than iceberg
	broccoli, cabbage, kale, kohlrabi
	alfalfa (especially sprouts), oats, rye, whole wheat and whole wheat products

FITNESS: EXERCISE AND HEALTH

Exercise has emerged as a significant factor in nearly all facets of health, both in terms of maintaining overall health and in reducing risk for health conditions and injuries. A health-care practitioner who specializes in fitness-related care may be a doctor (MD or DO), certified physician assistant (PA-C), registered physical therapist (RPT), chiropractor (DC), or exercise physiologist. Doctors who specialize in treating injuries and conditions related to physical activity may be board-certified in sports medicine, family practice, orthopedics, or physiatry (rehabilitation medicine). Education, certification, and credentialing are less consistent for other fitness practitioners such as fitness trainers and athletic trainers who primarily work outside the health-care delivery system to help individuals develop exercise regimens for preventive or therapeutic purposes.

This section, "Fitness: Exercise and Health," presents an overview discussion of physical activity as it relates to health maintenance, health risk factors, health conditions, and preventive health measures. The entries in this section focus on the broad picture of how physical activity and inactivity influence health and disease. The section "Lifestyle: Obesity and Smoking" features discussion and entries about fitness and exercise topics that relate to WEIGHT LOSS AND WEIGHT MANAGEMENT. The section "The Musculoskeletal System" contains discussion and comprehensive entries about the structure, function, health, and health conditions of the bones, muscles, and joints.

Making the Connection between Physical Activity and Health

Researchers provided the first substantive correlation between physical inactivity and health in the 1970s when clinical and epidemiologic studies linked sedentary lifestyle with premature death due to health conditions such as CORONARY ARTERY DISEASE (CAD) and HYPERTENSION (high BLOOD PRESSURE). Health experts subsequently issued the first formal recommendations for incorporating regular physical exercise into daily lifestyle as a means of preventing the development of CARDIOVASCULAR DISEASE (CVD). These recommendations were much the same as current recommendations for minimal physical activity for adults, which are

- physical activity for a total of 30 minutes a day at moderate intensity at least 5 days a week and preferably every day
- physical activity for 20 minutes at a time at vigorous intensity on 3 or more days of the week

Research has continued to strengthen the evidence for these recommendations. However, most Americans fall short of meeting them. The 1996 US Surgeon General's report *Physical Activity and Health* found that 25 percent of Americans do not participate in any physical activity beyond the requirements of daily living, and 60 percent exercise less than the minimum recommendations for health. Among youth between the ages of 12 and 21, about 25 percent engage in physical activity at a level that meets minimum recommendations for health, 50 percent participate in regular physical activity at vigorous intensity, and 25 percent are physically inactive.

Many adults start exercise programs and then do not continue them, most commonly because they begin with activities that support the FITNESS LEVEL they want to achieve rather than those geared to their current fitness level. Such an approach often results in discomforts; minor injuries such as blisters, sore muscles, and aching joints; and discouragement because the body is not ready for such activity. It is important to start at the current fitness level and steadily work up to the desired fitness level. The health benefits of exercise become apparent within two weeks of starting an exercise regimen and progress as physical activity continues. Conversely, the health benefits of physical activity diminish significantly two weeks after stopping an exercise regimen and are gone after two months of physical inactivity.

Though the overall health benefits of exercise far outweigh the risks, a few health risk factors do increase with physical activity, notably those for exercise-related injuries and REPETITIVE MOTION INJURIES. However, most such injuries are preventable through proper WARMUP, preparation, protective items, and technique during activity. Furthermore, maintaining a high fitness level reduces the risk for many other kinds of injuries because regular exercise increases BONE DENSITY, MUSCLE STRENGTH, FLEXIBILITY, and balance.

HEALTH RISKS ASSOCIATED WITH EXERCISE

ACHILLES TENDON INJURY	ANKLE INJURIES
BLISTER	CHAFING
CHARLEYHORSE	EPICONDYLITIS
FRACTURE	KNEE INJURIES
MUSCLE and JOINT soreness	ROTATOR CUFF
SHIN SPLINTS	IMPINGEMENT SYNDROME
SPRAINS AND STRAINS	SYNOVITIS
TENDONITIS	

Prescription: Exercise

Until the 1970s bedrest was the standard prescription for convalescence after significant health conditions ranging from herniated disk (HERNIATED NUCLEUS PULPOSUS) and KNEE INJURIES to HEART ATTACK and major surgical operations. Rest, according to prevailing medical wisdom, allowed the body to heal itself. With the collection of evidence of physical inactivity's harmful effects on health in general growing in the late 1960s, doctors began to question the value of the "rest to recover" approach and to implement gradual physical activity as part of a person's recuperation plan. Doctors observed that people who engaged in limited physical active early in the course of their recovery, such as sitting in a chair or walking to the bathroom, in the days immediately after an OPERATION or a heart attack improved faster and felt better than those who remained on bedrest. Doctors also noted that early mobility, now a

mainstay of recuperation, reduced PULMONARY EMBOLISM (PE) and DEEP VEIN THROMBOSIS (DVT)—BLOOD clots in the LUNGS and the inner veins of the legs, respectively—which are risks with surgery and major injury.

By the mid-1980s supervised and graduated physical activity was the core of structured cardiac rehabilitation programs, and today exercise is a component of treatment regimens for numerous health conditions. Structured physical rehabilitation programs are now also the standard of care for people who have musculoskeletal injuries, operations, and conditions. The typical multidisciplinary health-care team includes professionals who specialize in returning the body to optimal function.

HEALTH CONDITIONS INFLUENCED BY PHYSICAL ACTIVITY AND INACTIVITY

ASTHMA	ATHEROSCLEROSIS
ATHLETIC INJURIES	BREAST CANCER (certain forms)
CARDIOVASCULAR DISEASE (CVD)	CHRONIC FATIGUE SYNDROME
CHRONIC PULMONARY OBSTRUCTIVE DISEASE (COPD)	COLORECTAL CANCER
CORONARY ARTERY DISEASE (CAD)	CONSTIPATION
DIABETES	DEPRESSION
HYPERLIPIDEMIA	FIBROMYALGIA
INSULIN RESISTANCE	HYPERTENSION
OBESITY	INTERMITTENT CLAUDICATION
OSTEOPOROSIS	OSTEOARTHRITIS
PROSTATE CANCER	PERIPHERAL VASCULAR DISEASE (PVD)

Fitness for Health: Public Health Goals

The US federal government adopted formal interest in and support for physical fitness in the 1950s, when President Dwight D. Eisenhower (1890–1969) formed the President's Council on Youth Fitness in response to published scientific data that America's youth were significantly less physically fit compared to European youth. Each US president after Eisenhower strengthened and broadened the role of government agencies to study exercise and educate the public about the relationship between EXERCISE AND HEALTH.

Through the 1970s and 1980s these initiatives expanded to encourage extended physical fitness and sports activities in the schools and support businesses and corporations in promoting exercise and fitness programs and opportunities among employees. Health agencies such as the National Institutes of Health (NIH) and health organizations such as the American Heart Association (AHA) and the American Diabetes Association (ADA) espoused exercise and fitness as preventive measures as well as adjuncts for clinical treatment regimens. In 1990 and in 2000 the US Centers for Disease Control and Prevention (CDC) the US government's health promotion and prevention agendas for Americans, the Healthy People 2000 and HEALTHY PEOPLE 2010 initiatives, incorporated daily physical activity for youth and adults among their priority areas with the overriding objective of preventing health conditions and reducing overall premature deaths that result from physical inactivity.

KEY HEALTHY PEOPLE 2010 PHYSICAL ACTIVITY GOALS

- Reduce the proportion of adults who engage in no leisure-time physical activity.
- Increase the proportion of adolescents and adults who engage regularly, preferably daily, in moderate physical activity for at least 30 minutes per day.
- Increase the proportion of adolescents and adults who engage in vigorous physical activity that promotes the development and maintenance of cardiorespiratory fitness three or more days per week for 20 or more minutes per occasion.
- Increase the proportion of adults who perform physical activities that enhance and maintain muscular STRENGTH and ENDURANCE.
- Increase the proportion of adults who perform physical activities that enhance and maintain FLEXIBILITY.
- Increase the proportion of US public and private schools that require daily physical education for all students.
- Increase the proportion of work sites offering employer-sponsored physical activity and fitness programs.
- Increase among children, adolescents, and adults the proportion of trips made by walking.
- Increase among children, adolescents, and adults the proportion of trips made by bicycling.

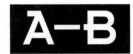

aerobic capacity   The maximum amount of oxygen the body can extract from ambient air (the air of the normal environment) and use during physical activity, expressed as $\dot{V}O_{2max}$ in terms of milliliters of oxygen per kilogram of body weight per minute (mL/kg/min). Because men have larger LUNGS and thus greater surface area for oxygen exchange, all other factors being equal men have greater aerobic capacity than women. Higher $\dot{V}O_{2max}$ correlates with increased ability to sustain high-intensity exercise for an extended time, such as during ENDURANCE activities. People who participate in athletic events at a competitive level, amateur or professional, typically have higher aerobic capacity in general and a significantly higher $\dot{V}O_{2max}$ in the activity of specialty such as bicycling, cross-country skiing, distance running, and swimming. Aerobic capacity is a key indicator of cardiovascular fitness.

REPRESENTATIVE AEROBIC CAPACITY MEASUREMENTS ($\dot{V}O_{2MAX}$)	
sedentary woman	38 milliliters per kilogram per minute (mL/kg/min)
aerobically fit woman	60 mL/kg/min
sedentary man	42 mL/kg/min
aerobically fit man	80 mL/kg/min

Researchers believe the foundation of aerobic capacity is genetic; some people are born with greater aerobic capacity potential, and with sustained AEROBIC EXERCISE at a competitive level they are able to maximize that potential for high $\dot{V}O_{2max}$. A sedentary (physically inactive) person who undertakes a planned, progressive program of aerobic exercise can often improve his or her aerobic capacity by 20 to 30 percent. Such improvement is significant from a health perspective because there is a strong correlation between low aerobic capacity and increased risk for CARDIO-VASCULAR DISEASE (CVD). Increasing aerobic capacity consequently lowers CVD risk factors.

Direct measurement of $\dot{V}O_{2max}$ is fairly complex; because of this doctors tend to conduct direct aerobic capacity testing only in people who have pulmonary disease. A pulmonary function testing center conducts direct $\dot{V}O_{2max}$ measurement, for which the person runs on a treadmill or rides a stationary bicycle wearing specialized equipment that measures the exchange of oxygen and carbon dioxide. Calculations using the measurements determine the $\dot{V}O_{2max}$, usually along with other measures that provide a detailed perspective of lung function and lung capacity.

There are several methods for indirectly measuring aerobic capacity, all of which involve performing sustained aerobic exercise such as running or walking for a determined period of time or a known distance. Calculations use the information to project the anticipated $\dot{V}O_{2max}$ for the data. Indirect $\dot{V}O_{2max}$ measurement is less precise than direct $\dot{V}O_{2max}$ measurement but is accurate enough for most people who are engaged in aerobic exercise and want to know, or monitor improvements in, their aerobic capacity.

See also FITNESS LEVEL.

aerobic exercise   Physical activity that raises the HEART RATE to 60 percent of maximum heart rate, called the target heart rate, for a minimum continuous time of 20 minutes.

A general guideline for approximating one's target heart rate is the "talk test." At target heart rate, a person should be able to speak. A person who cannot talk during exercise is likely exceeding his or her target heart rate and is working too hard. A person who can carry on an extended conversation or sing during exercise is likely below his or her target heart rate and is not working hard enough for aerobic conditioning.

CALCULATING TARGET HEART RATE

The standard formula for calculating target HEART RATE is 220 minus one's age (an estimated maximum heart rate), then multiplying the result by 60 percent. For example, the target heart rate for a person 35 years old is 111 beats per minute: $220 - 35 = 185 \times 0.6 = 111$.

Aerobic exercise uses the large MUSCLE groups in rhythmic, repetitive activity that increases the body's consumption of oxygen, and is the core of cardiovascular CONDITIONING. Regular aerobic exercise improves the all-around efficiency of the cardiovascular system including

- more powerful contractions of the HEART to pump BLOOD out to the body
- the ability of the LUNGS to exchange carbon dioxide for oxygen
- the ability of the muscles in the body to contract with power and force
- the ability of the blood vessels to dilate (open) to carry more blood with each beat of the heart
- lower BLOOD PRESSURE as a result of reduced resistance to the flow of blood

Health experts recommend a minimum of 30 minutes of aerobic exercise three days every week and encourage more. At the onset of an aerobic exercise program a person is likely to achieve target heart rate quickly because the heart is not accustomed to working in such a way. It is important to stay at the target heart rate for as long as possible, which may not be a full 20 minutes at first. As the FITNESS LEVEL and AEROBIC CAPACITY improve, it takes longer to reach and becomes easier to maintain one's target heart rate.

People who want to increase their fitness levels should increase both the length and frequency of their exercise sessions, for example 45 minutes of aerobic activities five days a week. The higher a person's aerobic capacity, the more effort the person must exert to achieve and maintain his or her

target heart rate. Competitive athletes and people at high aerobic capacity may derive greater benefit from exercising at a target heart rate that is 70 to 80 percent of maximum heart rate.

Among the most familiar and popular aerobic activities are running, swimming, cross-country skiing, and bicycling. Brisk walking (five miles per hour) is aerobic as well. Sports such as basketball, volleyball, soccer, and singles tennis also provide an aerobic workout. Participating in aerobic exercise at less than an aerobic level (below target heart rate) provides numerous health and fitness benefits, too, as part of maintaining a physically active lifestyle.

AEROBIC ACTIVITIES

basketball	bicycling
climbing stairs	cross-country running
cross-country skiing	dancing
handball	ice skating
inline skating	jogging
jumping rope	racquetball
roller skating	rowing
running	snow shoeing
soccer	spinning
stair-stepping	stationary cycling
swimming	tennis (singles)
volleyball	walking

See also CARDIAC CAPACITY; EXERCISE AND HEALTH; FLEXIBILITY; LIFESTYLE AND HEALTH; OBESITY AND HEALTH; RESISTANCE EXERCISE; STRENGTH; WEIGHT LOSS AND WEIGHT MANAGEMENT.

aging, changes in physical ability and fitness needs that occur with   As a person grows older, his or her physical capabilities, STRENGTH, FLEXIBILITY, AEROBIC CAPACITY, exercise needs, metabolic rate, body composition, and risk for injury change.

Children and Exercise

Children require physical activity for proper development and growth. BONE and MUSCLE development relies in part on the stimulation from resistance activities such as walking and running. Preschool-age children tend to be on the go constantly. However, many develop fairly sedentary habits by the time they reach school age, with activities such as watching television, using the computer, and playing video games replacing physical activities. Numerous clinical research studies correlate such physical inactivity with the rise in childhood OBESITY AND HEALTH conditions such as type 2 DIABETES, HYPERLIPIDEMIA, and OSTEOARTHRITIS that typically do not appear until middle age or later.

Health experts recommend an hour a day of moderate physical activity for children and adolescents, though estimate 60 percent or more do not meet that recommendation. The health risks associated with physical inactivity not only carry into adulthood but appear to be more severe. Aerobic capacity—the body's ability to use oxygen efficiently—reaches its peak in the early 20s and then begins a gradual decline. Muscle mass and BONE DENSITY are also at their peak in the early 20s. Daily physical activity in late ADOLESCENCE appears capable of extending aerobic capacity and musculoskeletal strength well into adulthood.

Older Adults and Exercise

A physically active adult has an aerobic capacity, measured as $\dot{V}_{O_{2max}}$, up to 25 percent greater than a person of comparable age who does not exercise. Such a difference becomes increasingly significant with advancing age. Between age 20 and age 40 aerobic capacity declines 8 to 12 percent. Between age 40 and age 70 aerobic capacity declines about 10 percent per decade. After age 70 aerobic capacity declines 20 percent per decade. When daily physical activity is an element of lifestyle throughout life, the decline in aerobic capacity significantly slows. A 70-year-old who has a moderate to good FITNESS LEVEL (exercises at or beyond the minimum PHYSICAL ACTIVITY RECOMMENDATIONS) has an aerobic capacity comparable to that of a person 10 to 20 years younger.

Such a difference correlates to lower HEART RATE, lower BLOOD PRESSURE, stronger muscles and bones, increased HORMONE sensitivity and endocrine response, smoother and more regular gastrointestinal function, and even greater elasticity to the SKIN. These factors lower the risk for numerous health conditions including HEART disease, HEART ATTACK, STROKE, OSTEOPOROSIS, hip FRACTURE, type 2 diabetes, OBESITY, SEXUAL DYSFUNCTION, and various forms of cancer. Though no clinical evidence as yet supports exercise as a panacea for aging, researchers have

gone so far as to say that lifestyle factors such as daily exercise, nutritious EATING HABITS, and not smoking have the capability to eliminate 85 percent or more of acquired CARDIOVASCULAR DISEASE (CVD). As well, numerous studies affirm the beneficial effects of exercise toward preventing injury and supporting overall health.

Daily physical activity becomes more significant with advancing age also because the body naturally begins to change in ways that diminish LEAN MUSCLE MASS, muscle strength, JOINT flexibility, gastrointestinal function, and hormone sensitivity. Around age 50 hormonal shifts in both men and women result in loss of muscle tissue, with fat often replacing this loss, and bone density. After age 70 muscle strength, bone density, and aerobic capacity decline in men and women alike. In men these changes are less pronounced; in women particularly they can have catastrophic health consequences if not detected and treated. A woman's risks for heart disease and osteoporosis jump after MENOPAUSE, largely the consequence of the drop in ESTROGENS. The risk of hip fracture due to lost bone density rises in men and women alike after age 70. Though daily exercise cannot prevent such changes from occurring, it can mitigate their severity and help maintain good QUALITY OF LIFE.

Older people who have chronic or serious health conditions may have limited ability to participate in physical activities. Conditions such as HEART FAILURE and CHRONIC OBSTRUCTIVE PULMONARY DISEASE (COPD) may limit aerobic capacity, for example. Osteoarthritis and RHEUMATOID ARTHRITIS may restrict movement. Despite the limitations chronic health conditions may impose on physical activity, they also benefit from regular exercise however modest. A health professional such as a physical therapist, an exercise physiologist, or a physiatrist (physician who specializes in rehabilitation medicine) can help develop an appropriate physical activity regimen for a person who has a chronic or debilitating health condition.

See also ANABOLIC STEROIDS AND STEROID PRECURSORS; DISABILITY AND EXERCISE; WEIGHT LOSS AND WEIGHT MANAGEMENT; YOGA.

blister prevention Methods to reduce irritation to SKIN surfaces from friction. The feet are the most common site of blisters acquired during physical exercise. Athletic activities such as racquet sports, rowing, baseball, golfing, bicycling, and sailing expose the hands to friction and the risk for blisters. A BLISTER is the body's attempt to protect itself from friction-generated injury. Fluid accumulates between the layers of the skin, separating the layers and buffering damage to the underlying delicate tissues. The process stimulates the NERVE endings in the skin to send signals of PAIN to the BRAIN. Blister prevention techniques attempt to anticipate sites of excessive friction to cushion them from irritation.

The right footwear can prevent many blisters from developing on the feet. It is important to wear shoes or boots that fit properly and are appropriate for the activity. Shoes that are too loose allow the foot and toes to slide against the inside of the shoe or the shoe to slip up and down on the heel. Shoes that are too tight pinch the toes and trap moisture against the skin. Even the best-fitting shoes or boots may cause blisters if they are not right for the activity. Socks absorb moisture and establish a physical barrier between the foot and the shoe; double-layer socks are most effective for this purpose. Socks should fit snugly and smoothly against the foot, and like shoes or boots should be appropriate for the intended use. People whose feet sweat excessively (HYPERHIDROSIS) may want to consult a podiatrist or dermatologist for evaluation and treatment to reduce the amount of moisture their feet produce.

Adhesive bandages, blister pads, moleskin, and other products can provide additional protection for areas that are particularly vulnerable to blisters, such as the back of the heels, the toes, and any parts of the foot that rub against the shoe. Some people apply petroleum jelly or antibiotic ointment to "hot spots." Other people find dusting the feet with foot powder or cornstarch, or applying a dry lubricant, helps keep the feet dry and smooths their movement within the shoes.

Athletic gloves, appropriate for the activity and that fit properly, can similarly protect the hands from friction and moisture. It is important for the glove to fit without bunching or pinching, otherwise the glove itself will become the cause of blisters. Rings worn on the fingers, even with gloves, can contribute to blisters by allowing the skin to pinch against them.

A CALLUS (thickened pad of skin) will eventually form at a site that repeatedly blisters, the body's further attempt to protect itself. Once a callus forms the area is much less likely to blister. Working up to a level of activity, such as with running or walking, helps prepare the skin for the exposure it faces. Blisters are more likely to occur when engaging in new activities or at a significantly increased level (such as a competitive event) within a familiar activity.

See also CHAFING; FITNESS LEVEL; PHYSICAL ACTIVITY RECOMMENDATIONS; TINEA INFECTIONS; WALKING FOR FITNESS.

carbohydrate loading The practice of consuming excess quantities of carbohydrates, such as pasta and breads, for a period of time before an athletic or competitive event. The body converts the excess GLUCOSE that results into glycogen, the short-term storage form of glucose held primarily in the LIVER. During exercise when the levels of glucose in the BLOOD circulation drop, the body begins to convert glycogen back to glucose to replenish glucose blood levels. Because carbohydrate loading increases the amount of glycogen the body stores, the athlete can sustain a higher level of energy output for a longer period of time.

The most common approach to carbohydrate loading is to eat primarily carbohydrates for three days before the scheduled event and to reduce the training schedule during that time to allow the body to store, rather than draw from, glycogen. Many top amateur and professional athletes practice some variation of carbohydrate loading, which is most effective for ENDURANCE activities that last two hours or longer. Fitness and nutrition experts also recommend eating a meal that contains both carbohydrates and protein about two hours after intense exercise to help the body replenish the stores of glucose and amino acids it drew from during the physical activity.

See also DIET AND HEALTH; EATING HABITS; NUTRIENTS; NUTRITIONAL NEEDS.

chafing Irritation to the SKIN resulting from clothing and body parts that rub. The areas most vulnerable to chafing are the inner thighs, groin, inner arms and sides of the chest, and front of the chest (especially the nipples). Ill-fitting clothing in combination with moisture is generally the precipitating factor. It is important to wear clothing appropriate for the activity and in most circumstances for the clothing to be snug though not constrictive. High-wicking fabrics in combination with talcum powder and similar products to absorb moisture further reduce the likelihood of chafing. Body lubricants, which form a barrier between clothing and the skin, extend protection for distance activities such as running, hiking, climbing, and bicycling. A CONDITIONING program of steady progress toward fitness goals also helps prepare the body, increasing its resistance to irritation.

See also BLISTER PREVENTION; FITNESS LEVEL; PHYSICAL ACTIVITY RECOMMENDATIONS; WALKING FOR FITNESS.

charleyhorse A sudden, intensely painful MUSCLE contraction, sometimes called a muscle CRAMP. A charleyhorse most often affects the legs and feet and is typically a consequence of electrolyte imbalances, especially deficiencies in magnesium and potassium. A charleyhorse may occur during rest, especially during sleep. A charleyhorse that occurs during exercise often indicated inadequate HYDRATION. Stretching and massaging the affected muscle often relieves the contraction, allowing the muscle to relax. Some people experience relief with ice applied to the area while other people find heat more helpful. Sometimes a degree of discomfort continues for a short time after the cramp subsides. Stretching and WARMUP before beginning exercise help prevent charleyhorses.

See also SHIN SPLINTS; STINGER.

conditioning A planned and consistent effort to establish and maintain, through physical exercise, a FITNESS LEVEL that supports health. Conditioning requires repetitious physical activity that exerts the body for STRENGTH, FLEXIBILITY, and AEROBIC CAPACITY. Physical conditioning may be part of a rehabilitation program for people recovering from serious injury or health condition such as STROKE or HEART ATTACK. Conditioning is also an important component of the lifestyle changes necessary for effective WEIGHT LOSS AND WEIGHT MANAGEMENT.

Building a Conditioning Plan

It is important to build a conditioning plan that starts at the current fitness level and moves in progressive increments toward the target fitness level. There are numerous methods for assessing a person's existing fitness level. Health experts advise a ROUTINE MEDICAL EXAMINATION before beginning a new physical conditioning effort when any of the following circumstances apply

- physically inactive for longer than a year
- over age 50
- BODY MASS INDEX (BMI) over 32
- existing health conditions such as heart disease, DIABETES, OSTEOARTHRITIS, OBESITY, lung disease, or other chronic disorders
- physical limitations or disabilities

The most effective conditioning results occur with an approach that is structured and systematic, with planned activities intended specifically for exercise such as walking, bicycling, light weightlifting, and YOGA. Many people are able to also integrate activities of conditioning into their daily routines, such as walking to work or school and taking the stairs instead of the elevator. People whose jobs are physically active often have the strength and flexibility to accommodate the demands of their job tasks though may lack an overall state of physical fitness. A qualified fitness instructor can conduct a baseline assessment of the person's fitness status and help develop a conditioning plan that integrates work activities with fitness activities. The appropriate clothing, equipment, and technique for specific physical activities help ensure maximum benefit from the activities as well as minimize the risk for injury.

Maintaining a Conditioning Plan

Conditioning is successful when it becomes an element of lifestyle and an aspect of daily routine that incorporates a variety of daily activities that not only improve strength, flexibility, and aerobic

capacity but also are activities a person enjoys. These activities, in combination, maintain the fitness of the entire body. RESISTANCE EXERCISE helps maintain BONE DENSITY and BONE strength, which is particularly important for women who are past MENOPAUSE. Regular physical activity also benefits emotional and psychological well-being. Many people find the commitment to planned exercise allows them time for themselves that provides a calming break from the stresses and pressures of work and family. Many activities also provide opportunities for recreation and social interaction, such as walking clubs, yoga groups, organized bicycling rides, group hikes, volksmarch and other volkssports, and structured classes at a gym or fitness facility.

CALISTHENICS FALLEN FROM FAVOR
Health and fitness experts no longer recommend old-fashioned calisthenics—situps, pullups, and pushups—once the staple of physical fitness programs because the resistance involved is that of body weight, which allows no FLEXIBILITY for either building up to a competence level or increasing the challenge to the body after reaching a level of competence with the exercises. As well, these exercises as taught in the middle decades of the 20th century place undue and potentially harmful strain on the joints and the lower back.

When circumstances interrupt conditioning it is important to get back on track as soon as possible, approaching it as any other integral component of lifestyle. It helps to maintain a modified conditioning effort when possible, such as alternative activities when traveling on business or recreation. Fitness level begins to slip after a week without any exercise at all, though is quickly recoverable with return to the regular physical activities. It is important to reenter the conditioning plan at the current fitness level and work back to the target fitness level.

See also ATHLETIC INJURIES; EXERCISE AND HEALTH; PHYSICAL ACTIVITY RECOMMENDATIONS; TRAINING; WALKING FOR FITNESS; WEEKEND WARRIOR.

cross training The practice of alternating different kinds of exercise to provide a well-rounded workout for the body that establishes and maintains a high overall FITNESS LEVEL. Cross-training exercise typically complements a person's primary athletic activity. Runners may cross train by engaging in swimming to work the upper body, for example, and bicycle one day a week to work different muscles from those that running works in the lower body. Many athletes alternate AEROBIC EXERCISE with RESISTANCE EXERCISE to improve STRENGTH, such as weightlifting, with stretching activities to improve FLEXIBILITY, such as YOGA. The alternation may occur in the form of two or more activities in a single session or alternating activities among different sessions. For example a runner may run one day, lift weights the next day, run the next day, and swim the next day. Cross training also helps reduce the risk for ATHLETIC INJURIES.

See also AEROBIC CAPACITY.

D-E

disability and exercise Regular exercise is important for health and well-being for everyone, and most people are able to participate in physical activities to some degree. Though chronic or debilitating health conditions may limit a person's physical abilities, it is possible to adapt many physical activities to accommodate individual needs. For example, 30 minutes of pushing oneself in a wheelchair is comparable to 30 minutes of walking. In other circumstances health conditions such as moderate to severe CARDIOVASCULAR DISEASE (CVD) may limit AEROBIC CAPACITY; conditions such as CEREBRAL PALSY and OSTEOARTHRITIS may restrict FLEXIBILITY and mobility.

Anyone who has a physical disability should consult with his or her doctor before beginning a new physical activity or exercise plan.

Physical therapists and exercise physiologists, particularly those who specialize in sports medicine, can help people who have disabilities develop effective CONDITIONING or TRAINING plans and modify physical activities to meet their fitness goals and interests. Such modifications may take the form of adaptations in technique or alterations in intensity or duration of activity. Individual circumstances also may require adaptive clothing, shoes, and equipment. Many communities and fitness facilities have special physical fitness programs, including team and competitive events, for people who have disabilities; such programs allow participation at levels that match individual capabilities and interests.

Strengthening and flexibility activities are important for maintaining as much function as possible. Such activities improve BLOOD flow, par-ticularly to the extremities and the SKIN. They also maintain BONE DENSITY and JOINT range of motion, permitting the best mobility possible. Passive exercise (in which a therapist or caregiver guides the person's body gently through structured movements) benefits people who have severely restricted mobility or PARALYSIS such as due to STROKE or SPINAL CORD INJURY.

See also AEROBIC EXERCISE; FITNESS LEVEL; PHYSICAL ACTIVITY RECOMMENDATIONS; RESISTANCE EXERCISE; STRENGTH.

endurance The ability to persist in performing a physical activity. Endurance may refer to AEROBIC CAPACITY (the fitness of the cardiovascular system), the ability to sustain a position over time (such as in YOGA), or the ability to repeatedly and consistently perform a set of movements (such as lifting weights). Endurance is an important element of overall physical fitness that requires an integration of aerobic capacity with STRENGTH and FLEXIBILITY.

Endurance improves with exercise that challenges the body's capabilities at a moderate level, encouraging the muscles to draw energy from glycogen stores and the LUNGS to function at higher efficiency in the amount of air, and consequently oxygen, they take in with each breath. Endurance training emphasizes activities that extend the duration of performance. For aerobic activities this means extending the length of time for TRAINING sessions in incremental fashion, for example increasing distance for running or the duration of holding a yoga pose. RESISTANCE EXERCISE also can improve endurance by increasing the number of repetitions of a resistance activity such as lifting weights or working with resistance bands.

See also CONDITIONING; FITNESS LEVEL.

exercise and health   The correlations between daily physical exercise and health are numerous and solidly affirmed through clinical research studies. In an overarching context physical activity improves the efficiency of metabolic functions at the cellular level throughout the body. Physical exercise further has specific effects on nearly every system of the body, helping the body function with optimum efficiency.

Though researchers do not fully understand the mechanisms within the body through which exercise affects health and disease, they do know that physically inactive people are

- twice as likely to develop CORONARY ARTERY DISEASE (CAD)
- 50 percent more likely to develop HYPERTENSION (high BLOOD PRESSURE)
- up to 6 times more likely to develop type 2 DIABETES between the ages of 18 and 30
- twice as likely to die prematurely for any reason

Many researchers believe that physical inactivity is nearly as significant a risk factor for CARDIOVASCULAR DISEASE (CVD) as cigarette smoking. As well, the correlation between physical inactivity and OBESITY, also a key risk factor for numerous health conditions and premature death, is strong. Though in combination these two risk factors—physical inactivity and obesity—affect every level of bodily function from molecular (metabolic activity) to mechanical (how the body as a whole moves and performs) and are sometimes difficult to separate, exercise alone influences health in distinct ways. People who are overweight yet physically active every day have overall better health and lower risk for serious health conditions such as CVD and type 2 diabetes than people of comparable weight and are physically inactive. Very modest physical activity, such as walking 20 to 30 minutes every day, can result in significant weight loss over time, lowering health risk related to both obesity and physical inactivity.

Evidence conclusively demonstrates that regular exercise, done at least at the minimum level of recommended physical activity

- lowers BLOOD pressure and can reduce hypertension, decreasing the risk for STROKE

- improves INSULIN sensitivity, decreasing the risk for type 2 diabetes and helping stabilize diabetes that already exists
- reduces the risk for COLORECTAL CANCER, BREAST CANCER, and PROSTATE CANCER
- strengthens bones and increases BONE DENSITY, lowering the risk for OSTEOPOROSIS
- increases FLEXIBILITY and STRENGTH, improving mobility and reducing the risks for OSTEOARTHRITIS and injury from falls
- relieves stress and DEPRESSION, improving well-being and the ability to cope with daily difficulties and challenges
- lowers total CHOLESTEROL BLOOD LEVELS and increases high-density lipoprotein (HDL) cholesterol ("good" cholesterol) blood level, reducing the risk for ATHEROSCLEROSIS and CAD
- improves cardiovascular efficiency and lung capacity
- stimulates gastrointestinal activity, shortening the amount of time food takes to complete its journey through the digestive process and decreasing the likelihood of CONSTIPATION and other gastrointestinal disorders

Numerous studies show that modest to moderate physical exercise—30 minutes a day most days of the week—is sufficient to generate measurable health benefits. About 40 percent of Americans meet this objective. Additional exercise increases benefits. It is important to choose a variety of activities that are enjoyable, convenient (logistically feasible and require minimal preparation), within an individual's skill range, and safe within the context of any existing health conditions. Structured activities—even when structure is as basic as setting aside 30 minutes each day to walk—helps give exercise a sense of priority in a person's life, which encourages ongoing participation. Nevertheless, all efforts to increase physical activity in daily living, however small or brief, improve health and QUALITY OF LIFE. Consistency maintains fitness most effectively.

See also CHOLESTEROL, ENDOGENOUS; DIET AND HEALTH; EATING HABITS; HEALTH RISK FACTORS; LIFESTYLE AND HEALTH; METABOLISM; NUTRITIONAL NEEDS; OBESITY; OBESITY AND HEALTH; PHYSICAL ACTIVITY RECOMMENDATIONS; SMOKING CESSATION.

fitness level   The ability of the body to perform physical activity. Fitness encompasses AEROBIC CAPACITY (cardiovascular fitness), STRENGTH, and FLEXIBILITY. These three components combine to help configure a person's LEAN MUSCLE MASS, BODY FAT PERCENTAGE, and BODY MASS INDEX (BMI), which are key risk factors for numerous health conditions, including CARDIOVASCULAR DISEASE (CVD) and DIABETES. A high fitness level, indicating daily physical exercise, reduces numerous HEALTH RISK FACTORS. Conversely a low fitness level, indicating physical inactivity, correlates to increased health risk.

Exercise physiologists use various scales to quantify an individual's fitness level. Some assessment scales emphasize cardiovascular fitness and others measure general fitness. CONDITIONING, which targets overall fitness status, and TRAINING, which prepares a person for a particular event or activity often at a competitive level, are structured methods to improve a person's fitness level.

People whose fitness levels are "very poor" or "poor" do not receive enough physical activity to support their bodies in health and are at increased risk for injury and health disorders. A "moderate" fitness level meets general PHYSICAL ACTIVITY RECOMMENDATIONS to support health, weight management, and reduction of health risk factors. People who have a "good" fitness level enjoy optimum benefit from physical activity. People who have a "very good" fitness level dedicate focused effort to physical fitness and are often athletes who participate in organized or competitive events.

As with EATING HABITS and nutrition, fitness level represents an integration of physical exercise into lifestyle such that activity is an inherent component of daily living. Many people can find ways to increase physical exercise through their daily activities, which can be as effective as structured exercise and makes the most of available time. Activities such as gardening, cleaning house, washing the car, mowing the grass (especially with a nonmotorized mower), and walking whenever possible are among the many ways to increase physical exertion on a daily basis that result in improved fitness level over time. Though physical activity recommendations and fitness level classifications may appear daunting to people who are not presently active and whose lives are busy, fitness is the accumulated result of numerous and daily small physical efforts that pay off in big ways when it comes to health as well as satisfaction with how one feels and looks.

See also BODY SHAPE AND CARDIOVASCULAR DISEASE; EXERCISE AND HEALTH; LIFESTYLE AND HEALTH; OBESITY; OBESITY AND HEALTH; WALKING FOR FITNESS; WEEKEND WARRIOR; WEIGHT LOSS AND WEIGHT MANAGEMENT.

flat feet   A structural circumstance in which the ligaments in the foot do not support the bones to form an appreciable arch. The arch of the foot helps cushion the foot's structure during impact. Young children normally have flat feet until regular walking and running strengthens the muscles and ligaments of the feet, a process that typically occurs between the ages of 3 and 10 years. Unless there is an underlying deformity, there is no medical reason to attempt to treat flat feet in young children because it is the normal state of the feet.

Adults sometimes speak of having "fallen arches," a casual term that refers to stretching and loosening of the foot ligaments that sometimes occurs with increasing age. Flat feet that develop in such a way are more common in people who are physically inactive and overweight. Extra body weight stresses the feet's structure in the absence

GENERAL FITNESS LEVEL CLASSIFICATIONS

Fitness Level	Activities	Duration	Frequency
very poor	very little physical activity beyond that required for daily living (sedentary)	brief	seldom
poor	may walk at work, to and from the mailbox, and for tasks such as grocery shopping	one to two hours combined each day done	one to three days a week
moderate	walks one or two blocks at a time walks up two flights of stairs without shortness of breath some regular physical activity required at work (such as lifting or walking)	two to three hours combined each day done	three to five days a week
	YOGA, TAI CHI, or structured stretching exercises	10 to 20 minutes each day done	one to three days a week
	walk or casual bicycle ride for pleasure	20 to 30 minutes each day done	one to two days a week
good	walks for or more blocks at a time walks up three or more flights of stairs without shortness of breath job requires moderate physical activity	three or more hours combined each day done	four to five days a week
	participates in structured exercise activity	30 to 60 minutes combined each day done	three to five days a week
	yoga, tai chi, or structured stretching exercises	10 to 20 minutes combined each day done	three days a week
	lifts weights or works out with resistance bands	30 to 45 minutes combined each day done	three days a week
	brisk walk, moderate bicycle ride, run, or swim	30 to 90 minutes combined each day done	two to three days a week
very good	walks distances greater than ½ mile with ease walks up multiple flights of stairs without shortness of breath	one to three hours combined each day done	six or seven days a week
	lifts weights or works out with resistance bands	30 to 45 minutes combined each day done	three days a week
	job requires steady, moderate to vigorous physical activity	six to eight hours combined each day done	three to five days a week
	yoga, tai chi, or structured stretching exercises	10 to 30 minutes combined each day done	three to five days a week
	engages in moderate to vigorous aerobic activities or participates in competitive events	two to three hours combined each day done	two to five days a week

of physical exercise that would strengthen the muscles and ligaments.

Many adults who have flat feet have no discomfort or other symptoms and do not need treatment. Flat feet become problematic only when they cause abnormal pronation (side to side movement of the foot with impact), which can alter the alignment of the leg and thus affect the ankles, knees, and hips. For flat feet that cause discomfort, treatment is a combination of properly designed and fitted shoes along with shoe orthotics that support the inner surface of the arch area and the heel, stabilizing the foot during movement. Foot care experts typically further recommend a structured approach of planned, progressive physical activity to strengthen the structures of the foot as a component of an overall WEIGHT LOSS AND WEIGHT MANAGEMENT strategy. Rarely, flat feet may require surgery to tighten ligaments and realign the bones.

See also CONDITIONING; LIGAMENT; MUSCLE; OBESITY AND HEALTH; STRENGTH; SURGERY BENEFIT AND RISK ASSESSMENT; TALIPEDES.

flexibility   The ease with which MUSCLE groups and joints allow movement. Flexibility is an integral though often undervalued component of overall physical fitness.

Fitness experts advocate stretching and WARMUP before and after physical activity, even that which is work related, to prepare the body for activity and reduce the risk for injury. Lack of use, injury, surgery, and health conditions such as OSTEOARTHRITIS may limit range of motion (the ability of a JOINT to move through the full scope of its capability). Exercises that improve range of motion include stretches and movements that prepare the joints for physical activity. YOGA, TAI CHI, and qigong also improve flexibility. Flexibility extends the ability of the body to participate in and benefit from strengthening and AEROBIC EXERCISE. Cycling and swimming combine the benefits of flexibility, strengh, and aerobic workouts.

See also AGING, CHANGES IN PHYSICAL ABILITY AND FITNESS NEEDS THAT OCCUR WITH; AEROBIC CAPACITY; ATHLETIC INJURIES; CONDITIONING; ENDURANCE; FITNESS LEVEL; STRENGTH; TRAINING; WEEKEND WARRIOR.

metabolic equivalent (MET) A unit of measure for the amount of oxygen the body uses during physical activity. One MET is equivalent to the oxygen an adult requires when sitting quietly for one minute. A four-MET activity, such as brisk walking or riding a bicycle on a level surface, requires four times the amount of energy (oxygen consumption) as the one-MET activity of sitting quietly. An eight-MET activity, such as running or riding a bicycle uphill, requires eight times as much energy as sitting quietly. METs are the basis for calculating the number of calories that particular activities burn. Activities that require three to six METs are considered to be of moderate intensity and burn 3.5 to 7 calories per minute. Activities that require greater than six METs are considered to be of vigorous intensity and burn more than 7 calories per minute.

Knowing an activity's MET value helps an individual calculate how long to participate in that activity to meet a desired level of CALORIE consumption. For example, a person who wants to burn 150 calories a day (the minimum recommendation for adults) may choose to walk at three and half miles per hour, a four-MET activity, for 40 minutes or run at five miles per hour, an eight-MET activity, for 20 minutes, depending on the desired level of intensity.

See also AEROBIC CAPACITY; AEROBIC EXERCISE; BODY MASS INDEX (BMI); CONDITIONING; FITNESS LEVEL; PHYSICAL EXERCISE RECOMMENDATIONS; TRAINING; WALKING FOR FITNESS.

metabolism The processes through which cells convert NUTRIENTS to energy. In the most basic sense, metabolism is the point of transition from energy intake (food consumption) to energy expenditure (molecular conversion). Multiple mechanisms within the body regulate the complex chemical interactions that constitute metabolism, with the HYPOTHALAMUS and the endocrine system taking the lead roles. Hormones such as THYROXIN (T4), which the THYROID GLAND produces, and INSULIN, which the ISLETS OF LANGERHANS in the PANCREAS produce, determine the rate at which cells convert GLUCOSE (one of two fuel sources for cells) to energy. The hormones of the body's stress response—CORTISOL, EPINEPHRINE, and NOREPINEPHRINE—also can accelerate metabolism, usually as a short burst; though in times of trauma the STRESS RESPONSE HORMONAL CASCADE can alter the body's metabolism on a long-term basis as a mechanism to facilitate HEALING.

The common perception of metabolism is as a rate that represents a balance between calories consumed and calories expended. Metabolism may also refer to the processes that occur during digestion to convert foods and drugs into chemical molecules the body can use. Metabolism has two primary modes: anabolism and catabolism. Anabolism is energy expended toward construction (building tissue) and catabolism is energy expended toward destruction (breaking down tissue). Energy needs increase when a person is recovering from major surgery, injury, or illness, as the processes of healing engage the body in extra anabolic (constructive) effort.

Measuring Metabolic Rate

The fundamental measure of metabolism is the basal metabolic rate (BMR), which identifies the amount of energy, in terms of calories, that the body requires over 24 hours to function at absolute rest. Nutritionists and exercise physiologists generally use mathematical formulas to calculate BMR because its actual measurement is complex and requires an overnight stay in a special lab to capture measurements at precisely the point of minimal metabolic activity. A common formula for estimating BMR is the Harris-Benedict equation. There are separate equations for women and for men, accommodating gender differences in the ratio of LEAN MUSCLE MASS to body fat.

Easier to measure directly is the resting metabolic rate (RMR), which provides similar information about the body's energy requirements at minimal activity. Many exercise physiology clinics can measure RMR. More sophisticated methods are available that allow determination of precise metabolic measures for elite athletes as well as for people who have severe health conditions. Most people expend 50 to 75 calories per hour at rest, so a rough generalization of metabolic rate is 1,200 to 1,800 calories. The larger a person, the higher his or her metabolic rate, whether body size results from MUSCLE mass or fat accumulation. However, increased muscle mass further raises the metabolic rate because muscle cells use more energy than fat cells in the normal course of their functions. Men generally have higher metabolic rates than women because their bodies have larger muscles and greater lean muscle mass.

Metabolism and Weight Management

From a practical perspective either RMR or BMR presents the body's energy needs in terms of calories, allowing an individual to estimate daily energy use (CALORIE expenditure) to tailor daily calorie intake. Activity factors and injury factors further determine the body's overall energy expenditure and intake needs. A person whose lifestyle is sedentary, for example, uses less energy and consequently requires less intake than a person whose lifestyle includes daily physical exercise. However, the metabolic rate decreases at about 5 percent per decade between the ages of 25 and 75, largely because lean muscle mass decrease; thus at age 75 a person requires about a third fewer calories each day than at age 25. Without a comparable increase in exercise, the difference can amount to a weight gain of four to seven pounds a year. Regular physical activity boosts the metabolic rate by maintaining a higher percentage of lean muscle mass.

Metabolic Response to Trauma

When the body experiences significant physical trauma, such as due to BURNS or major injuries, its natural stress response initiates metabolic changes that allow the body to rapidly convert protein to amino acids (and subsequently to glucose) for the body to use as energy. Major surgery may also initiate this response. The purpose of the metabolic response to trauma is to muster every available resource for healing; the result is rapid destruction (catabolism) of muscle tissue. During healing the metabolic rate rises significantly, reflecting the body's efforts to repair and reconstruct damaged tissue (anabolism). However, the rate of catabolism may be up to 10 times that of anabolism, establishing an imbalance that makes it difficult for the body to replace its protein stores.

Intensified nutritional support in combination with physical exercise (particularly RESISTANCE EXERCISE) can expedite muscle tissue restoration and help metabolism return back to normal. The most effective nutritional support incorporates a high-protein diet (up to two times the recommended dietary allowance) and NUTRITIONAL SUPPLEMENTS to supply increased amounts of certain B vitamins that are essential for cellular energy production and the efficiency with which cells can use glucose. Physical activity stimulates muscle cells to improve the efficiency with which they contract and relax, and encourages development of new muscle tissue. Sometimes doctors may prescribe hormones to further stimulate muscle growth.

Metabolic Disorders

Metabolic disorders are health conditions that alter the function of the body's metabolic, or energy-producing, pathways. Among the most common metabolic disorders are DIABETES, HYPERTHYROIDISM, HYPOTHYROIDISM, and PHENYLKETONURIA (PKU). Though doctors understand the mechanisms of most metabolic disorders, the causes remain largely unknown. Genetic factors play a significant role and may be the sole cause of certain metabolic conditions such as glycogen-storage disorders (which affect the body's ability to metabolize carbohydrates) and lipid-storage disorders (which affect the body's ability to metabolize fats).

Doctors commonly refer to genetic-based conditions as inborn errors of metabolism. Many of these disorders affect the function of specific enzymes that facilitate the conversion or storage of nutrients to energy within the metabolic pathway. The consequence may affect the body as a whole or the activity of specific kinds of cells such as muscle cells or nerve cells (neurons). Researchers do not know the extent to which genetic factors influence acquired metabolic conditions such as hyperthyroidism, hypothyroidism, and type 2 diabetes.

Symptoms of metabolic disorders vary depending on how the disorder affects metabolism and may include

- neurologic deficit and development delays
- CARDIOMYOPATHY
- hearing loss
- vision disturbances
- myoclonus
- seizures
- weakness or movement difficulties
- failure to thrive

Inborn disorders of metabolism may not become apparent until a child is several months to several years old, by which time the condition often causes significant damage to organ systems. Newborn screening for some such disorders, such as PKU, is common in the United States and many other countries. Early detection of PKU and many other metabolic disorders allows treatment or management, such as enzyme replacement therapy or dietary restrictions, to prevent the condition from causing damage. However, most genetic disorders of metabolism are not curable at present.

Hormone replacement therapy is the treatment for hypothyroidism and insulin-dependent diabetes.

Confirming the diagnosis of metabolic disorders may be as simple as common blood tests, such as for diabetes or hypothyroidism, or may require sophisticated laboratory procedures and genetic (DNA) testing. There are no known methods of prevention for most metabolic conditions. Lifestyle factors such as diet and daily exercise can influence, and often prevent or reduce the severity of, type 2 diabetes.

DISORDERS OF METABOLISM	
acid lipase disease	coenzyme A deficiencies
DIABETES	Fabry disease
G6PD DEFICIENCY	galactosemia
gangliosidoses	Gaucher disease
HEMOCHROMATOSIS	hyperoxaluria
HYPERTHYROIDISM	HYPOTHYROIDISM
lipidoses	metachromatic leukodystrophy
mitochondrial myopathies	muscular dystrophies
Niemann-Pick disease	OBESITY
oxalosis	PHENYLKETONURIA (PKU)
Tay-Sachs disease	WILSON'S DISEASE

Continuing advances in genetic and molecular research are allowing scientists to identify gene mutations that underlie a number previously poorly understood syndromes with symptoms of impaired physical and intellectual development. Researchers are hopeful that new findings will result in GENE THERAPY approaches to remedy or prevent the defective metabolic functions.

See also ANABOLIC STEROIDS AND STEROID PRECURSORS; CELL STRUCTURE AND FUNCTION; EXERCISE AND HEALTH; HORMONE; METABOLIC EQUIVALENT (MET); NUTRITIONAL NEEDS; VITAMINS AND HEALTH; WEIGHT LOSS AND WEIGHT MANAGEMENT.

P–R

physical activity recommendations The guidelines health and fitness experts suggest as minimum standards to maintain a FITNESS LEVEL that supports good health and reduces HEALTH RISK FACTORS for conditions such as CARDIOVASCULAR DISEASE (CVD), type 2 DIABETES, OSTEOPOROSIS, OSTEOARTHRITIS, and OBESITY. General physical activity recommendations emphasize AEROBIC EXERCISE to improve AEROBIC CAPACITY because this is the foundation for physical fitness.

The amount of physical activity necessary to have a positive effect on health is less than people commonly perceive. Recent research findings demonstrate that when it comes to exercise, a little goes a long way. Though more is nearly always better, the baseline recommendations for physical activity to support health are modest. To achieve and maintain a moderate fitness level health experts recommend healthy adults engage in

- 30 minutes of moderately intense physical activity on five days of each week

  and

- 20 minutes of vigorous physical activity on three days of each week

WARMUP and stretching should open and close every activity session, improving FLEXIBILITY and lowering the risk for injury. Walking is an ideal activity for exercise of moderate intensity and has the added advantage of being easy for most people to incorporate into their daily lifestyle routines. Walking is also a good RESISTANCE EXERCISE, improving BONE DENSITY. Short sessions, such as 5 to 10 minutes at a time, that add up to 30 minutes over the course of a day are as effective as a single, continuous 30-minute sessions.

Vigorous physical activities are those which raise HEART RATE to 60 percent of maximum for 20 minutes or longer and consume 7 calories or more (eight metabolic equivalents [METs]) per minute. Running, bicycling, swimming, cross-country skiing, jumping rope, step aerobics, aerobic dance, rowing, and stair stepping are among the numerous activities capable of accomplishing this objective. Vigorous physical exercise is most effective when it continues for 20 minutes or longer. Most vigorous exercise also incorporates resistance, increasing MUSCLE STRENGTH and mass as well as supporting BONE density.

Meeting these recommendations increases energy expenditure by 1,200 to 1,400 calories each week, helping with WEIGHT LOSS AND WEIGHT MANAGEMENT. For a person striving to lose weight, exercising at the recommended level can allow weight loss of 18 to 21 pounds over the course of a year without a change in the number of calories consumed. Exercise in combination with nutritious EATING HABITS that maintain dietary intake at the recommended level further expedites weight loss. Adding physical activity beyond these recommendations, which health experts encourage, further improves physical fitness and aerobic capacity and lowers health risk factors for HYPERTENSION (high BLOOD PRESSURE), HYPERLIPIDEMIA, ATHEROSCLEROSIS, CORONARY ARTERY DISEASE (CAD), and INSULIN RESISTANCE.

Health experts recommend a minimum of 60 minutes of moderate physical activity daily (seven days a week) for children and adolescents. Research findings support the belief that such a level of physical activity provides health benefits that extend well into adulthood. Among these benefits are strong bones, cardiovascular efficiency, flexible joints, and healthy BODY MASS INDEX (BMI). Regular physical activity during childhood appears to further reduce risk factors for numerous health conditions in adulthood, even when activity eases. Children for whom daily exercise is a part of lifestyle are far more inclined to maintain physical activity as a priority in adulthood.

See also EXERCISE AND HEALTH; HEALTHY PEOPLE 2010; METABOLIC EQUIVALENT (MET); NUTRITIONAL NEEDS; WALKING FOR FITNESS.

protein loading The practice of consuming increased quantities of protein, such as in meats, for a period of time before an athletic event. Some athletes who participate in activities that require MUSCLE STRENGTH eat high amounts of protein to help build muscle mass. Though the body requires amino acids, which it acquires from dietary proteins, to repair and maintain tissues of all kinds throughout the body, including muscle tissue, a typical diet that contains about 15 percent protein generally meets the body's protein needs.

Excessive quantities of protein consumed in the diet, like excesses of dietary fats and carbohydrates, eventually becomes first GLUCOSE and then glycogen (short-term energy storage) and fat (long-term energy storage). Some studies suggest that long-term excessive protein consumption (usually of protein supplements) can strain the filtering mechanism of the KIDNEYS and can cause kidney damage. However, these findings are inconclusive, particularly in people who have normal kidney function and have no significant health conditions.

Nutrition and fitness experts recommend eating a meal that contains primarily carbohydrates and protein about two hours after intense exercise or a competitive event to help the body more quickly replenish the stores of glucose and amino acids it drew on during the physical activity. Most health experts do not recommend protein loading before an event or a competition, and recommend protein supplements only for people who cannot obtain adequate dietary protein because of health conditions.

See also CARBOHYDRATE LOADING; DIET AND HEALTH; NUTRIENTS; NUTRITIONAL NEEDS; NUTRITIONAL SUPPLEMENTS.

resistance exercise Physical activity, also called resistance TRAINING, in which the muscles exert effort against pressure, such as lifting weights. Resistance exercise, often called weight training when it involves the use of weights, enlarges and strengthens muscles and decreases body fat. It also improves the ability of the bones to retain calcium, maintaining BONE DENSITY and STRENGTH. Resistance exercise is particularly important for women over the age of 50, as BONE loss that can lead to OSTEOPOROSIS becomes a significant concern after MENOPAUSE. Health and fitness experts recommend resistance exercise two or three days a week, alternating with AEROBIC EXERCISE for a comprehensive fitness program.

BIG MUSCLES

Some people desire and other people dread the prospect of bulky muscles. Conventional resistance exercise is more likely to disappoint the former and please the latter. Though resistance exercise decreases the number of fat cells in MUSCLE tissue to give the muscles firmness and definition, it does not generate monster muscles.

A methodical approach exercise physiologists call progressive overload is the key to effective resistance training. Progressive overload is the practice of periodically increasing the difficulty of resistance as MUSCLE groups develop strength and become accustomed to the established resistance level. Most people should increase resistance every six to eight resistance exercise sessions, or about every two weeks. When working with weights, progressive overload can take place by increasing the amount of weight (intensity), the number of repetitions (duration), or the number of sessions (frequency). Many people combine these approaches. Resistance bands, another popular method of resistance exercise, come in different resistance levels, though generally the same concepts of progressive overload apply.

Each resistance exercise session should include multiple sets with rest periods of one to two minutes between each set. Rest, which allows the muscles to recover and "learn" the exercise (muscle memory), is a crucial component of a resistance exercise program. For most people, 20 to 40 minutes of resistance exercise is sufficient. Athletes in training for events or a competitive season may engage in longer sessions. Some people move from one muscle group to the next within each session; other people focus on one muscle group in each session, working a different muscle group the next session.

Resistance exercise also encompasses activities that exert pressure against the musculoskeletal system, such as walking and running, which some people refer to as impact exercise. Nonimpact activities such as moderate to intense bicycling and cross-country skiing challenge the musculoskeletal system in the same fashion as working out with weights. These activities further build strength and increase FLEXIBILITY.

RESISTANCE ACTIVITIES	
body bar	free weights
pullups	pushups
resistance bands	running
walking	weight machine

See also AEROBIC CAPACITY; ENDURANCE; FITNESS LEVEL; HEALTHY PEOPLE 2010; PHYSICAL ACTIVITY RECOMMENDATIONS.

shin splints PAIN along the tibia, the area in the lower leg commonly called the shin. Shin splints are common among people who participate in physical activities such as walking, running, marching, and hiking. Pain is the primary symptom, often occurring at the start of the activity, subsiding as the activity continues, and returning up to several hours after the activity ends. The affected area of the leg is tender to the touch.

Simple shin splints seldom require a doctor's attention; treatment is rest. Many people find ice, applied two or three times a day for 20 minutes eases the pain. NONSTEROIDAL ANTI-INFLAMMATORY DRUGS (NSAIDS) can relieve INFLAMMATION. Full HEALING takes three to four weeks; it is important to avoid the responsible activity during this time. Substituting nonimpact activities, such as bicycling and swimming, can help maintain FITNESS LEVEL or continue a training regimen during the healing period.

Because the pain of shin splints can be intense, people often worry about stress FRACTURE. Stress fracture is much less common than shin splints and occurs with extensive, repeated trauma over time or when TRAINING for an event bumps up the level of intensity, whereas shin splints is a soft tissue injury that typically occurs when starting a new activity after a period of inactivity.

Properly fitted footwear appropriate for the activity in combination with proper technique can reduce the risk for shin splints and other repetitive trauma injuries. Some people benefit from shoe orthotics, devices that correct pronation (the angle of the foot on impact). However, hard surfaces such as pavement and concrete challenge even the best footwear and technique. Rest from the activity at the first signs of shin splints can avert extended down time.

See also ATHLETIC INJURIES; CONDITIONING; FLAT FEET; SPRAINS AND STRAINS.

sports drinks and foods Specialty products marketed as beneficial for replenishing NUTRIENTS during and after exercise. Though many people use these products, most do not need or derive much benefit from them. Health and fitness experts recommend following nutritious EATING HABITS to maintain the body's level of nutrients at optimal level and maintaining adequate HYDRATION by drinking sufficient water before, during, and after exercise. Sports products are most helpful for people who exercise at high intensity for extended periods of time, such as those who participate in competitive ENDURANCE events such as randonneuring, climbing, triathlon, or marathon. In such circumstances, using these products to supplement nutritional needs can provide a steady source of energy to fuel the body's intensified activity.

Products and nutritional supplements that contain ephedra (which is banned in the United States) or the Chinese herb ma huang, which are STIMULANTS, may cause dangerous ARRHYTHMIA (irregularity of the HEART RATE).

Many energy and sports drink products contain high amounts of sugars, which can deliver an energy boost in the form of simple carbohydrates. They also deliver significant calories. Some products also contain CAFFEINE or herbal STIMULANTS such as GINSENG. Sports and nutrition bars may be primarily carbohydrates as well, though some products contain a mix of carbohydrates, proteins, and fats that can provide quick nutrition when eating other foods is impractical. It is important to read product labels carefully.

See also DIET AND HEALTH.

stinger   An injury to the brachial plexus, the large NERVE cluster that branches from the SPINAL CORD to innervate the shoulder, arm, and hand.

An injury that causes numbness on both sides of the body suggests SPINAL CORD damage and requires immediate medical attention. Only medical personnel should attempt to move a person who has a possible SPINAL CORD INJURY.

A stinger, also called a burner, is a common injury in contact sports and occurs when a blow or intense pressure displaces the neck and the compresses the cervical nerve roots between the cervical vertebrae (spinal bones in the neck). The compression causes symptoms that include sharp burning or stinging and numbness. Though the discomfort can be severe, it generally goes away within minutes. Occasionally symptoms may continue for up to several weeks. An isolated stinger leaves no residual damage, though repeated stingers can cause permanent damage to the nerves. The injury at the neck affects the shoulder and arm on the opposite (contralateral) side.

See also ATHLETIC INJURIES; NEURITIS; NEUROPATHY.

strength   The ability of a MUSCLE to engage in physical activity, particularly resistance activity. Common measures of strength are the abilities to move weight (such as in weightlifting) or to exert force against pressure (such as in bicycling or rowing). Strength improves through repetitious actions that generate force against muscle fibers as they contract and relax, which causes them to enlarge as well as become more efficient in their use of oxygen. Muscles exposed to consistent exercise develop denser networks of capillaries, facilitating rapid oxygen exchange, and larger mitochondria capable of expanded functions. Mitochondria are the "engines" of the cell, performing multiple metabolic tasks that allow cells to generate and use energy. As muscles become stronger and larger, they require more challenge

in the form of increased weight or resistance to maintain their strength.

PAIN is a signal that the body has reached its limit or is injured. Stop a strengthening activity at the first indication of pain. Rest five minutes and try the activity again. If the pain persists, stop the session and implement relief measures such as rest and ice to the area.

When exercising with weights it is important to start at an appropriate level for both the amount of weight and number of repetitions and work up to the desired level. Excessive weight can cause injury and inadequate weight does not challenge the muscles. In general, a person should be able to perform 8 repetitions with a particular weight, feeling some resistance though no PAIN with each repetition. When it becomes easy to do 12 to 15 repetitions, the muscle group is ready for an increase in weight. At the new weight, start again with 8 repetitions and increase as the repetitions become easier to perform. Fewer repetitions with heavier weight builds muscle mass and increases strength faster than more repetitions with lighter weight, though the latter builds ENDURANCE. Specific weight TRAINING regimens may have different guidelines.

The body itself can become the source of weight and resistance. Exercises such as curls, pushups, pullups, and squats use the body's weight to generate resistance against movement. The drawback to these exercises is that body weight is inflexible as the source of resistance; one cannot built up to or increase the effect.

Physical activities that use large muscle groups in repetitious activity also use the body's weight as resistance against gravity (such as with walking and running) or against equipment and gravity (such as with cycling and rowing). Aerobic activities such as swimming further tone muscles and improve AEROBIC CAPACITY though are not as effective for strengthening. A person can expect to see a 20 percent increase in strength after two months and a 40 percent increase in strength after four to six months of consistent strength training.

Many factors influence how strong muscles can become, key among them being regular participa-

tion in strengthening activities (such as RESISTANCE EXERCISE), FITNESS LEVEL, FLEXIBILITY, and the range of motion of the joints. Additional factors that may become important for competitive athletes include individual genetic characteristics and physical structure, which influence the manner and rate at which muscle fibers contract, relax, and recover. Rest is an important element of resistance exercise or strength training. Most regimens alter body regions, such as upper body one day and lower body the next day or rotate strengthening activities with endurance activities.

Strength exercises are particularly important for adults over age 65, helping sustain a high percentage of LEAN MUSCLE MASS as well as to maintain BONE DENSITY and BONE strength. Lean muscle mass naturally declines with advancing age, with fat cells replacing muscle cells. Activity that challenges the muscles encourages conversion of fat to muscle, improving lean muscle mass. Changes in HORMONE levels in the body, particularly in women after MENOPAUSE, cause changes in the amounts of calcium in the BLOOD circulation that regulate how much calcium enters and leaves the bones. Regular muscle activity improves calcium distribution mechanisms, keeping more calcium in the bones.

See also AEROBIC EXERCISE; CONDITIONING; DISABILITY AND EXERCISE; PHYSICAL ACTIVITY RECOMMENDATIONS; WEIGHT LOSS AND WEIGHT MANAGEMENT.

training The process of improving the body's FITNESS LEVEL through targeted, repetitive physical activity that has specific goals. Training also may refer to the preparation necessary for an event such as a race or a circumstance such as a sports season. The premise of training is to gradually escalate the challenge to the muscles for improved STRENGTH and FLEXIBILITY and to increase AEROBIC CAPACITY for improved ENDURANCE.

Building a Training Regimen
A typical training regimen emphasizes preparation for the dominant activity, for example running or playing tennis. Flexibility, strength, and AEROBIC EXERCISE target measurable improvement in the activity's performance. A runner may strive for a faster pace, a tennis player may aim for a stronger serve or backhand. Short, focused sessions are most effective at the onset of a training regimen,

with incremental increases in intensity and duration as ability and fitness improve. It is important to have specific, stepped goals and methods for measuring progress toward them. Goals should accommodate competitive as well as personal factors. A new runner might establish first level goals of achieving a 12-minute mile and completing a 5-K race or organized running event, for example. Proper nutrition and HYDRATION are essential as well.

Most people benefit from the advice of experts in their chosen activities, such as by taking classes, joining clubs, or researching training methods in books and on the Internet. Such advice can jumpstart a training regimen, getting to the core of methods with proven effectiveness as well as reducing the likelihood of injury. The most common injuries that occur early in a training regimen are those related to doing too much too fast or to inadequate WARMUP. Such injuries are generally preventable through proper technique and include MUSCLE soreness, blisters, CHAFING, and SPRAINS AND STRAINS.

TIPS FOR SUCCESSFUL PHYSICAL TRAINING

- When starting a training regimen, begin slowly and aim for steady improvement.
- Establish specific goals and methods for measuring progress toward them.
- Start and end every training session with WARMUP exercises and stretches.
- Vary activities to let the body recover, keep interest, and improve overall fitness.
- Increase intensity and duration in increments as ability and fitness improve.
- Eat nutritiously and drink water often.
- Enjoy the chosen activities.

Maintaining a Training Regimen
Once a person reaches his or her desired training level, it is important to continue varying activities and intensity levels to provide a mix of challenges for the body. Some people alternate types of activities each day, for example doing an aerobic activity one day and weight training or resistance training the next. Other people prefer to mix it up within each exercise session.

It is also important to let the body rest. Competitive athletes often incorporate "time off" from their primary sports into their training regimens, using other activities to exercise their bodies in different ways. A runner or bicyclist may swim and jump rope for aerobic exercise, for example. Rest allows the body to heal any minor injuries as well as to recover its capacity to perform, particularly after participation in a competition or organized event.

Philosophies differ on the optimal approach to final preparation for a competitive or organized event. Many sports trainers recommend backing off on training for 5 days before the event, engaging in light activity to keep the body flexible but not at such a level as to exert the muscles or aerobic capacity. A bicyclist training for a century ride (100 miles), for example, may do an 85- to 100-mile ride 10 days before the event, ride 30 to 45 miles every other day until 5 days before the event, and not ride again until the event. A tennis player may engage in two-a-day sessions until the week before a match, drop to a couple days of light volley practice, and then rest until the match. The premise behind this approach is to let the body fully recover and prime itself at its optimal performance level; thus may also minimize the risk for injury. A competitive athlete may choose to consult or work with a personal trainer who can tailor specific training activities, including nutrition and hydration, for his or her individual needs.

Clothing, Equipment, and Technique

The proper clothing, equipment, and techniques are important for safety as well as performance in any training regimen. Every activity has specialized items that are either necessary or make the activity easier and safer to perform. Safety equipment, such as helmets and EYE protection, is crucial in many activities. The right clothing, such as padded bicycle shorts or walking shoes, cushions and protects the body. Proper technique is essential for improvement toward performance goals as well as to reduce the risk for injury. It is important to choose equipment and clothing that is appropriate for the activity and that fits the individual.

See also ATHLETIC INJURIES; PHYSICAL ACTIVITY RECOMMENDATIONS; RESISTANCE EXERCISE; WEEKEND WARRIOR.

walking for fitness A planned approach for improving and maintaining overall physical fitness and health through walking. Health and fitness experts believe walking is the ideal exercise for people of nearly any age, FITNESS LEVEL, and health status. Walking is also an excellent component of any WEIGHT LOSS AND WEIGHT MANAGEMENT strategy. Everyday walking is a good means for becoming consistently more active. Walking for fitness takes walking to the next level, integrating it into one's individual lifestyle as an activity in its own right. Though walking alone will allow most people to reach the minimum recommended level of physical activity, walking in combination with other physical activity such as lifting weights (RESISTANCE EXERCISE and STRENGTH exercise) and swimming or bicycling (moderate to vigorous AEROBIC EXERCISE) provides a more vigorous workout.

As with any physical activity, it is important to dress appropriately and plan a gradual progression of pace and time. Clothing should fit comfortably enough to allow free movement but not be baggy. Fabrics that wick moisture minimize CHAFING. Though 100 percent cotton is comfortable for casual wear, it is not a good fabric for exercise because it tends to absorb rather than wick away moisture. Wet clothing contributes to BLISTER formation, chafing, and chilling. There are technical fabrics on the market, available in casual as well as athletic styles, that pull perspiration away from the body to keep the SKIN surface dry. Shoes should be designed for walking and fit snugly without pinching or gapping. Double-layer walking socks absorb friction to help prevent blisters.

A person whose lifestyle is physically inactive may want to start with a relaxed pace of two miles per hour, walking for 5 to 15 minutes at a time. Health experts recommend minimum physical activity sufficient to use 150 calories each day (1,000 calories a week). Sustained periods of exercise that raise the HEART RATE and BREATHING rate for 20 minutes at a time or longer help develop AEROBIC CAPACITY. BODY MASS INDEX (BMI) influences the pace and time necessary to reach this goal. As well, varying the walking pace and time achieves this goal in different ways depending on a person's interests and circumstances (such as time constraints). A general guideline is to increase the intensity of exercise no greater than 10 percent per week. Pushing to reach a higher level of intensity increases the risk for injury.

The accompanying table shows the approximate energy output (number of calories burned) for different paces and times at representative BMIs for individuals at healthy weight (BMI range 18.5 to 24.9), at overweight (BMI range 25 to 29.9), and at OBESITY (BMI 30 and above). The higher one's BMI, the more calories required to perform the activity. The slower the pace, the more time walking necessary to meet the minimum recommended daily activity level for calories consumed in physical exercise. A pedometer, a computerized device that clips to a belt or the edge of a pocket, functions as a timer and counts strides to measure pace and distance. Many pedometer models also calculate calories consumed and average pace.

See also AGING, CHANGES IN PHYSICAL ABILITY AND FITNESS NEEDS THAT OCCUR WITH; BLISTER PREVENTION; CONDITIONING; DISABILITY AND EXERCISE; OSTEOPOROSIS; PHYSICAL ACTIVITY RECOMMENDATIONS; SHIN SPLINTS; WEEKEND WARRIOR.

warmup Stretches and light-intensity movements that prepare the muscles and joints for physical activity. Warmups increase BLOOD flow to

WALKING FOR FITNESS: APPROXIMATE ENERGY OUTPUT

Walking Pace	Walking Time	Walking Distance	Energy Used (Calories)		
			BMI 22 (healthy)	BMI 27 (overweight)	BMI 32 (obesity)
2 mph (relaxed)	15 minutes	½ mile	43.75	53.75	63.75
2 mph (relaxed)	30 minutes	1 mile	87.5	107.5	127.5
2 mph (relaxed)	45 minutes	1½ miles	131.25	161.25*	191.25*
2 mph (relaxed)	1 hour	2 miles	175*	215	255
3 mph (moderate)	15 minutes	¾ mile	57.5	70	83.75
3 mph (moderate)	30 minutes	1½ miles	115	140	167.5*
3 mph (moderate)	45 minutes	2¼ miles	172.5*	210*	251.5
3 mph (moderate)	1 hour	3 miles	230	280	335
4 mph (brisk)	15 minutes	1 mile	87.5	106.25	126.25
4 mph (brisk)	30 minutes	2 miles	175*	212.5*	252.5*
4 mph (brisk)	45 minutes	3 miles	262.5	318.75	378.75
4 mph (brisk)	1 hour	4 miles	350	425	505
5 mph (fast)	15 minutes	1¼ miles	137.5	170*	202.5*
5 mph (fast)	30 minutes	2½ miles	275*	340	405
5 mph (fast)	45 minutes	3¾ miles	412.5	510	607.5
5 mph (fast)	1 hour	5 miles	550	680	810

Passes minimum daily physical activity recommendation

the muscles, bringing more oxygen and enhancing the ability of the BLOOD to carry away metabolic wastes, such as lactic acid, that result when MUSCLE cells contract. Fitness experts recommend 10 to 15 minutes of warmup before activity and 5 to 10 minutes of the same warmup routine after activity. Warmup stretches and movements after activity, sometimes called cool-down, ease the transition of the muscles back to a less intense level.

A general approach to a warmup is to begin with either the feet or the head and gently move and stretch each group of muscles, taking 5 to 7 minutes to cover the entire body. Then spend another 5 to 10 minutes slowly engaging in the planned activity, easing the muscles into the patterns of its movements and efforts. Some people run in place for a few minutes to loosen the muscles and joints. YOGA postures are effective for stretching and FLEXIBILITY. After the activity, repeat the process in reverse. Spend about 5 minutes going slowly through the movements of the activity, then take 5 to 7 minutes to stretch and sequentially move the muscles in groups for the entire body.

See also CONDITIONING; FITNESS LEVEL; HYDRATION; TRAINING.

weak ankles A circumstance in which the ligaments and muscles of the ankles are lax, failing to provide the ankle with the stability it requires to support the body during physical exercise. Weak ankles often result from physical inactivity though may also occur after injury or surgery to the ankle. Excessive body weight exacerbates the situation. A weak ankle has a tendency to allow the foot to roll inward or outward, presenting risk for sprain (stretched LIGAMENT) or ACHILLES TENDON INJURY. A planned program of structured exercise to strengthen the ankle's ligaments and muscles, coupled with weight loss if indicated, improves weak ankles for most people. Properly fitted shoes that provide good support for the foot further improve the ankle's stability. Some people benefit from wrapping or taping the ankles before activity.

See also CONDITIONING; FLAT FEET; MUSCLE; PHYSICAL THERAPY; SPRAINS AND STRAINS; TENDON; WEIGHT LOSS AND WEIGHT MANAGEMENT.

weekend warrior An individual who participates in intense physical activities on the weekends but gets very little physical activity during the week. There is a tendency to make the most of available free time by doing as much activity as possible. The risk of injury, especially soft tissue injuries such as SPRAINS AND STRAINS, is much higher with this pattern of exercise. WARMUP is especially important to help relax and the muscles and prepare them for activity. Proper nutrition and HYDRATION before, during, and after exercise is essential.

Many people slip into weekend warrior patterns because they do not have time during the work week to participate in exercise activities at the same intensity level. However, even short periods of moderate exercise improve STRENGTH, FLEXIBILITY, and stamina to make weekend activities more enjoyable as well as reduce the risk for injury. People who participate in competitive events or strenuous physical activities on the weekends can bump up their level of daily activity by running stairs, lifting hand weights, and doing stretching and strengthening exercises. The greatest health benefits come from a pattern of regular activity. Health experts recommend daily walking at a minimum (30 to 45 minutes, five to seven days a week).

Some soreness and aches are reasonable to expect after a weekend of intense activity or a competitive event. Ice or heat often provide relief. However, most such discomforts should be gone within a day or two. Those that linger to the next weekend or that limit function may indicate an injury that a doctor should evaluate.

See also ATHLETIC INJURIES; CONDITIONING; EXERCISE AND HEALTH; PHYSICAL ACTIVITY RECOMMENDATIONS.

HUMAN RELATIONS

The area of human relations covers the interactions between people as those interactions affect overall health, specific health conditions, and QUALITY OF LIFE. *Practitioners who provide services within human relations may be psychologists, social workers, mental health nurse practitioners (MHNPs), professional counselors, school counselors, and organizational development specialists.*

This section, "Human Relations," presents an overview discussion of the general relationship between human interaction and health and entries about specific issues within human relations. The section "Psychiatric Disorders and Psychologic Conditions" presents entries about the health and health conditions of thought and emotion. The section "The Nervous System" contains content about the health and health conditions of the structures of the BRAIN and nerves.

Human Interactions and Health
The diagnostic models of many Eastern health systems evaluate an individual's temperament and overall circumstances in conjunction with, as well as on equal standing with, physical signs such as PULSE and body temperature. Interest in how people and their interactions with one another as well as with their environments entered the realm of Western medicine's empirical evidence model in the 1950s when research began to confirm correlations between factors such as stress and health conditions such as CARDIOVASCULAR DISEASE (CVD). Other associations rapidly emerged, quantifying and substantiating the complex relationships among health, disease, attitudes, and satisfaction with life circumstances.

Social relationships are crucial in the human experience, ranging from the limited though sometimes intense interactions of in the workplace to lifelong friendships to the emotionally and physically intimate partnerships of romantic partners to the bonds of family. Relationships are the framework of culture and society, around the world and across generations. They are essential to health and often play roles, directly and indirectly, in the development of disease.

Interventions to Treat or Prevent Disease
Awareness of the interactions between social relationships and health provides opportunity to prevent adverse effects. Stress is perhaps the classic example, as much research in recent decades has illuminated the numerous and varied effects of emotional and psychologic stress on physical health. Stress may arise from any aspect of human relations or social settings, from family to work, and may manifest through diverse expressions ranging from outwardly explosive anger or acts of VIOLENCE to inwardly ravaging disease processes such as CVD. Sustained emotional stress can maintain BLOOD PRESSURE and HEART RATE at higher than normal levels for extended periods of time, potentially altering the function of the cardiovascular system in negative and permanent ways. Recognizing and learning to manage the underlying factors responsible for such stress may mitigate the physiologic and health consequences.

At the other end of the spectrum is growing awareness of the extent to which a person's spiritual beliefs and cultural traditions affect the perceptions of health and disease as well as receptiveness to treatments. Health-care providers are quick to point out that despite the astonishing technologic advances of recent decades, much of modern medicine remains more art than science.

How people feel about themselves, their health situations, the partnerships and relationships in their lives, and their reasons for living may ultimately have greater significance in preventing and treating health conditions than medications, surgeries, and high-tech therapies.

adolescence The stage of emotional and mental development that marks the transition from childhood to adulthood, accompanying the physical transition that occurs with PUBERTY. By adolescence an individual has the physical appearance and characteristics of an adult, including sexual maturity and reproductive capability though does not yet have complete neurologic development and psychologic and emotional maturity.

Though most of the health issues of concern in adolescence may occur at any age, some may be difficult to distinguish from the normal turbulence of this developmental period. The risk for some health conditions is highest during adolescence, such as ACCIDENTAL INJURIES and SEXUALLY TRANSMITTED DISEASES (STDS), because adolescence represents a unique convergence of an intense desire to explore adult behaviors with an immature sense of consequences. During adolescence most Americans learn to drive, start dating, and begin working, all of which are important steps in the transition to independence and adult responsibilities yet expose young people to new risks.

Though the general age of consent (legal adulthood) is 18 in the United States (though 21 for ALCOHOL purchase and consumption), the age of consent for health-care services and medical treatment varies among states. Some states grant the right to receive health-care services and medical treatment for certain circumstances (such as mental health, CONTRACEPTION, PREGNANCY, and SEXUAL HEALTH) as early as age 14 though require the authorization of a parent or legal guardian for surgery, invasive diagnostic or therapeutic procedures, and most nonemergency health-care services until the child reaches age 18. Hospitals, health-care providers, and public health agencies know the limits and constraints of applicable laws and regulations, which are subject to change as a consequence of legislation (new laws) or legal rulings (court cases).

HEALTH CONCERNS COMMON IN ADOLESCENCE	
ACCIDENTAL INJURIES	ACNE
ALCOHOL abuse	BODY DYSMORPHIC DISORDER
cigarette smoking	CONDUCT DISORDER
DEPRESSION	EATING DISORDERS
GENERAL ANXIETY DISORDER (GAD)	OBESITY
OBSESSIVE–COMPULSIVE DISORDER	OPPOSITIONAL DEFIANT
(OCD)	DISORDER
PEER PRESSURE	SEXUAL ASSAULT
SEXUAL HEALTH	SEXUALITY
SEXUALLY TRANSMITTED DISEASES	substance abuse
(STDS)	SUICIDAL IDEATION AND
trauma	SUICIDE
unintended PREGNANCY	VIOLENCE

See also PARENTING; PEER PRESSURE; SECONDARY SEXUAL CHARACTERISTICS; SEXUAL ORIENTATION; YOUTH HIGH-RISK BEHAVIOR.

anger and anger management Anger is a natural, intense emotion of displeasure that represents an interaction between the limbic system, which directs the body's emotional responses, and the frontal lobes of the cerebral cortex, which both interpret information and initiate conscious behavior in response. The frontal lobes are also the source of conscious inhibition, the innate mechanisms that control extremes in emotional expression and behavior. Anger's expression is normal and essential and may span the spectrum from irritation to rage.

Anger results in physiologic changes within the body. The STRESS RESPONSE HORMONAL CASCADE releases surges of CORTISOL, EPINEPHRINE, and NOREPI-

NEPHRINE—the stress hormones. This cascade causes BLOOD vessels throughout the body to constrict, raising BLOOD PRESSURE. It also causes HEART RATE to go up and BREATHING rate to increase. These changes can take place within seconds, though the body takes much longer to return to normal.

Anger can become a personal health issue or a social problem when its expression is inappropriate or when it is a persistent state of being. On the health front, prolonged elevations of the stress hormones can cause permanent changes in the cardiovascular system. Numerous research studies linking prolonged anger in particular with CORONARY ARTERY DISEASE (CAD). The suppression of anger can also result in physical manifestations such as chronic HEADACHE, chronic gastrointestinal symptoms such as NAUSEA or DIARRHEA, or clinical DEPRESSION.

The inappropriate expression of anger that involves aggressive or violent words or actions may also risk the well-being of others. Such expressions may include prolonged yelling, throwing things, physically fighting with others, acts of road rage, acts of VIOLENCE, and in other ways lashing out. ALCOHOL abuse and substance abuse often contribute to inappropriate anger or anger expression.

INAPPROPRIATE EXPRESSIONS OF ANGER

getting into fights	hitting
passive–aggressive behavior	persistent yelling or tirades
placing blame	pretending nothing is wrong
reckless or erratic driving	swearing and abusive
tantrums (at any age)	language
throwing or breaking things	

Anger management is the structured effort to express anger in appropriate, constructive ways through learned responses and behaviors. Therapists and psychologists can teach methods to iden-tify circumstances that trigger anger and appropriate ways of expression through approaches that may include

- COGNITIVE THERAPY to change the way a person thinks about anger
- BEHAVIOR MODIFICATION THERAPY to change a person's actions and behaviors
- discussion of underlying worries, fears, and issues that may contribute to feeling angry
- problem-solving and communication skills

People who are unable to control anger and their behavior responses through therapy may have a psychiatric disorder called intermittent explosive disorder, which often improves with selective serotonin reuptake inhibitor (SSRI) medication treatment. The SSRIs are ANTIDEPRESSANT MEDICATIONS that extend the presence of serotonin, a NEUROTRANSMITTER, in the BRAIN. Serotonin is key in the movement of electrical impulses among brain neurons responsible for mood and emotion.

Some people also benefit from alternative and complementary approaches such as HYPNOSIS and BIOFEEDBACK and from relaxation methods including MEDITATION and YOGA. Regular physical exercise reduces stress, provides an outlet for physical tension, and induces the release of endorphins and enkephalins, biochemicals in the brain that cause feelings of pleasure. Health conditions that can cause changes, sometimes sudden, in a person's anger response and anger management ability include serious illness or injury, STROKE, BRAIN TUMOR, degenerative neurologic conditions such as ALZHEIMER'S DISEASE, and TRAUMATIC BRAIN INJURY (TBI).

See also CHILD ABUSE; DOMESTIC VIOLENCE; ELDER ABUSE; EXERCISE AND HEALTH; PROBLEM-SOLVING AND CONFLICT RESOLUTION; STRESS AND STRESS MANAGEMENT.

C

child abuse Actions by parents and other caregivers that endanger a child's physical and emotional well-being. Child abuse affects about 1 million children in the United States each year, 1,200 of whom die as a result of the abuse they experience. In many countries child abuse is both a health concern and a legal matter. In the United States federal law establishes basic legal criteria that define child abuse; each state further describes the actions that meet such criteria and may extend the criteria to include additional circumstances of abuse. There are four basic types of child abuse:

- Neglect occurs when the parent or caregiver fails to provide for the child's basic needs such as appropriate nutrition, clothing, shelter, medical care, and physical and emotional attention. Examples of neglect include grossly unsanitary living conditions, persistently depriving a child of meals, locking a child in a room or out of the house, and leaving a child alone and unattended for extended periods of time.

- Physical abuse occurs when a child receives injuries, regardless of whether the parent or caregiver intended to cause harm. Examples of physical abuse include harsh physical discipline, hitting, shaking, kicking, and choking.

- Sexual abuse occurs when there is inappropriate physical contact of a sexual nature between a parent or caregiver and the child. Examples of child sexual abuse include fondling, indecent exposure, incest, and rape.

- Emotional abuse occurs when the words or actions of the parent or caregiver impair the child's sense of self and value. Examples of emotional abuse include persistent threatening, yelling, criticizing, and ostracizing.

Typically an abused child experiences more than one type of abuse; emotional abuse is nearly always a component of any other type of abuse. Child abuse may also occur when parents or caregivers fail to take action to prevent harm or injury to the child, including intervening to stop the abusive actions of another parent or caregiver.

Signs of Child Abuse
Indications of child abuse may be physical or behavioral. Signs that suggest neglect and child abuse include

- unexplained bruises, BURNS, fractures, or other physical injuries

- weight and size significantly less than appropriate for age

- steals food or has an extremely unhygienic appearance

- flinching, ducking, and other fearful behavior in response to sudden movements from adults

- nightmares and unusual fears

- inappropriate sexual knowledge or behavior

- symptoms of SEXUALLY TRANSMITTED DISEASES (STDS)

A sudden, unexplainable change in a child's behavior is a warning sign that bears investigation because it can indicate any number of serious issues, from abuse to physical illness to ILLICIT DRUG USE. A child often will not acknowledge that a parent or caregiver is abusive. Children depend on their caregivers and may fear retribution from the abuser or may not recognize that the behavior or situation constitutes abuse. As well, secrecy is often a key component of abuse, with the abuser threatening the child with harm should he or she say anything to others about the abuse.

It is crucial that anyone who suspects a child is being abused, regardless of the person's relationship to the child, notify a health-care provider or other authority. Many communities have anonymous telephone hotlines for reporting suspicions of child abuse.

Detection and Intervention

All communities have child protection agencies and legal mechanisms to safeguard the well-being of children. Most states require health-care providers, educators, and other adults who have frequent interactions with children to report any suspicions or signs of child abuse. Child protection authorities then investigate the situation and may remove, temporarily or permanently, an endangered child from an abusive environment or situation. The longer the child remains in the abusive situation, the more serious and long-lasting the physical and especially emotional consequences.

The safety and health of the child is the priority in circumstances of neglect and abuse. However, because not all neglect and abuse is purposeful, parent education programs that teach PARENTING skills as well as nonabusive methods to manage child discipline and the stress of parenting may help a parent or caregiver change his or her behavior such that it becomes appropriately nurturing and supportive.

See also CULTURAL AND ETHNIC HEALTH-CARE PERSPECTIVES; DOMESTIC VIOLENCE; ELDER ABUSE; FACTITIOUS DISORDERS.

cultural and ethnic health-care perspectives
Awareness of, respect for, and accommodation of the traditions, beliefs, and customs of diverse cultures and ethnicities within the conventional practice of medicine. Factors may include language (non-English speaking), immigration status, views about doctors and personal privacy, and the influence of religious or spiritual beliefs as they relate to the reasons for illness and the role of treatment.

The American model of medicine encourages shared participation between health-care providers and patients. This model expects patients to question what they do not understand. People from some cultures may expect the provider will choose the appropriate therapy and are reluctant to ask any questions. In other cultures families make decisions about health care, sometimes without participation from the person who is receiving the care. These factors influence patient compliance—whether the person carries out the treatment the doctor or other health-care provider recommends. The American model of medicine also has a relative openness about personal privacy and the sanctity of the body, facets of health care that are often distressing or offensive to people of other cultures who may refuse diagnostic or therapeutic procedures unless providers are able to accommodate their customs and beliefs.

Cultural competency is now part of education and training for many health-care professionals in the United States, including physicians, physician assistants, nurses, dentists, and allied health staff. Nearly all hospitals have translators available to overcome language barriers. About 18 percent of the population in the United States speaks a primary language other than English, and cultural and ethnic minorities collectively make up about a third of the US population.

See also AYURVEDA; GENERATIONAL HEALTH-CARE PERSPECTIVES; NATIVE AMERICAN HEALING; SPIRITUAL BELIEFS AND HEALTH CARE; TRADITIONAL CHINESE MEDICINE (TCM).

D–E

domestic violence Actions and behaviors that use aggression, threats, and fear to control another person in a household or partner relationship such as a marriage or dating. Domestic VIO-LENCE has health as well as legal ramifications. In the United States, state laws define the parameters of behaviors that constitute domestic violence.

The National Domestic Violence Hotline—1-800-799-SAFE (7233)—is available tollfree, 24 hours a day, seven days a week, from anywhere in the United States.

Each year more than four million American women seek medical care for injuries resulting from domestic violence. However, either partner may be the abuser. Domestic violence can exist in any domestic partnership, including marriage, nonmarried partners, same-sex partners, and dating. Surveys among American high school and college students suggest violence among dating couples, such as hitting and forced sex, is a serious issue.

Signs and indications of domestic violence in a partnership may be emotional, psychologic, physical, or a combination. Such signs may include

- behaves in a jealous and possessive manner
- attempts to isolate partner from family and friends or monitor visits and activities
- controls finances and other resources such as car keys
- constantly criticizes, uses name calling, and humiliates
- threatens or carries out physical harm to partner, children, friends, or pets

- acts abusively or forcefully in sexual situations; demeans partner
- persistently yells or argues; breaks items in the house

The priority in domestic violence is for the abused person to get away from the situation, which is often difficult. There are the emotional ties of the relationship, however dysfunctional, as well as the practical matters of resources and where to go. Some people are able to go temporarily to the homes of other family members or friends, though sometimes others who know of the violence are reluctant to become involved. More often the circumstance is that the abused person has told no one of the situation and is not willing to do so until a crisis precipitates action. Most communities have public and private agencies and services to support people who are leaving circumstances of domestic violence. Permanent solutions in circumstances of persistent or severe domestic violence are difficult and often require filing appropriate criminal charges against the abuser as well as relocating and re-establishing work and life.

See also ANGER AND ANGER MANAGEMENT; CHILD ABUSE; ELDER ABUSE.

elder abuse Actions by caregivers and family members that endanger the health, well-being, and life of an older person. Many though not all older people who are in situations of abuse are weak or debilitated and depend on those who abuse them, making escape from the abuse difficult or impossible. Elder abuse affects more than two million older adults in the United States each year. There are four basic types of elder abuse:

- Neglect occurs when family members or caregivers fail to provide for the elder's daily needs such as meals, appropriate clothing, assistance with bathing and toileting, administration of medications, and receiving medical care.

- Physical abuse occurs when the elder receives injuries or is in physical peril as a result of the actions of family members or caregivers. Examples of physical abuse include hitting, pushing, exposure to water that is too hot or too cold, physical restraints, and overmedication or undermedication.

- Sexual abuse occurs when there is inappropriate physical contact of a sexual nature between a family member or caregiver and the elder. Examples of elder sexual abuse include indecent exposure, touching of the genitals or forcing the elder to touch the caregiver's genitals, rape, and sodomy.

- Emotional and psychologic abuse occurs when family members or caregivers intimidate, threaten, belittle, or ignore the elder. Stealing from the elder, mismanaging finances, and taking over control of possessions such as a home or car are also forms of emotional and psychologic abuse.

Often the elder experiences more than one type of abuse; emotional and psychologic abuse are almost always present with any other type of abuse. Elder abuse may also result from the failure of family members or caregivers to take actions to prevent harm or injury. Though the dynamic of elder abuse is complex, it is nearly always intentional.

Signs of Elder Abuse

Indications of elder abuse may be obvious or discreet and may be physical or manifest as emotional or psychologic symptoms. Signs of elder abuse may be difficult to distinguish from the symptoms and consequences of health conditions such as STROKE or ALZHEIMER'S DISEASE. Signs that may suggest elder abuse include

- unexplained bruises (especially on the wrists, lower arms, and lower legs), BURNS, scalds, fractures, or other physical injuries

- progressive weight loss

- sunken eyes and dry, loose SKIN

- DECUBITUS ULCER (bed sore)

- health conditions that do not respond as expected with the medications prescribed

- vaginal or anal discharge or bleeding

- SYMPTOMS OF SEXUALLY TRANSMITTED DISEASES (STDS)

- evasiveness or reluctance to participate in social activities

- fearfulness or suspicion

Some conditions of old age, such as Alzheimer's disease, ORGANIC BRAIN SYNDROME, and stroke, may result in aggressive, combative, or otherwise challenging behavior in the older person. Such a circumstance complicates the picture by making it difficult to determine who is the abused and who is the abuser. Patterns of abuse present earlier in life, such as DOMESTIC VIOLENCE between spouses or CHILD ABUSE the elder inflicted on a now-adult child, often continue or may reverse when the person becomes older and unable to live independently. The once-abused child may turn against the now-dependent parent, for example.

It is crucial that anyone who suspects elder abuse report it to health-care or law enforcement authorities for investigation. Many communities have anonymous telephone hotlines for reporting suspicions of elder abuse.

Detection and Intervention

Elder abuse is difficult to detect because it is possible for the elder to remain relatively secluded without raising much suspicion. Older people may be reluctant to report abuse for fear of retribution from the abusive family member or caregiver. Elderly people commonly fear any change that might require a move to a residential care center. As well, many older people have well-established beliefs that what happens in the family stays in the family; there would be irrecoverable loss of pride in revealing abuse at the hands of family members. There are relatively few mechanisms in American culture to safeguard the health and well-being of the elderly, though most states have mandatory reporting requirements for health-care providers and others involved in caring for the elderly when they suspect abuse. When doctors or authorities do detect elder abuse, they often have little choice but to remove the elder from the situation—which is often what the elder fears most. One of the most effective deterrents of elder abuse is social participation—having people visit the older person and getting the older person out to participate in social activities. This approach also provides a break for family members and caregivers, relieving some of the stress that is inherent in providing care for an elder.

See also GENERATIONAL HEALTH-CARE PERSPECTIVES.

end of life concerns The fears and worries that may arise when a person faces the prospect of dying. End of life concerns in regard to health and health care may relate to physical symptoms such as PAIN and loss of function, health-care issues such as feeding tubes and mechanical life support, emotional concerns such as fear of the unknown and leaving loved ones, and legal matters such as medical power of attorney and other advance directives. Cultural and generational factors greatly influence end of life desires and practices, though each person's needs are unique.

The focus of end of life concerns sharpens when a person approaches the end stages of terminal illness. Open communication with health-care providers, family members, and other caregivers establishes clear expectations and intentions around supportive care and medical interventions including pain relief and resuscitative efforts. It also allows a person to make choices and decisions about hospice and other supportive care and to reach closure with loved ones. Sometimes family members have different ideas about what care a loved one might want at the end of life; it is often helpful as well as prudent to put one's wishes in writing.

See also CULTURAL AND ETHIC HEALTH-CARE PERSPECTIVES; GENERATIONAL HEALTH-CARE PERSPECTIVES; GRIEF; QUALITY OF LIFE; SPIRITUAL BELIEFS AND HEALTH CARE.

generational health-care perspectives Awareness of, respect for, and accommodation of the different viewpoints toward health care across generations. Each generation has inherently different expectations around what medical care can accomplish as well as how doctors and hospitals should provide such care. These differences in expectations shape the nature and outcome of many medical interventions, from preventive to therapeutic efforts. Health-care providers must consider these differences when evaluating treatment options and approaches.

People who are today in their 80s lived much of their lives in a time when medical care was limited and doctors came to them to provide care. Most of the drugs, surgical operations, and technologies that are the mainstay of medical treatment today were developed after 1950 and many only since the 1980s. The elderly may view illness as inevitable to certain degree, expect the doctor to take a leadership role in health care, and be unknowledgeable about the ways in which lifestyle influences health and illness.

By contrast, people who are today in their 30s have lived all of their lives in a time in which medicine prevents many of the illnesses that were common causes of death in earlier generations and treats or cures nearly every sort of illness and injury. They have grown up knowing of the health significance of lifestyle factors such as diet, exercise, and cigarette smoking. They may view illness as either avoidable or curable and expect to participate in considering options and making decisions about their health care.

The structure of the practice of medicine to some extent supports generational separations through its model of specialization. The very young—the newest generation—see health-care providers who specialize in meeting the unique needs of infants and children (pediatricians). These doctors and other health-care providers are often around the same age as the parents—the middle generations—and can personally identify with some of the life circumstances and issues they face. The very old—the oldest see health-care providers who similarly specialize in treating health conditions common in or unique to aging (geriatricians). These health-care providers are often significantly younger than the patients they treat and have little personal identification with their perspectives and life circumstances.

Generational perspectives and perceptions influence the point at which an individual will seek medical care for a health concern, which may have significant effect on the outcome of treatment. Many health conditions, from DIABETES to CARDIOVASCULAR DISEASE (CVD) to cancer, are treatable or curable with early diagnosis and treatment. Generational views on what information is private and personal also affect health outcomes.

See also ANTIBIOTIC MEDICATIONS; CULTURAL AND ETHNIC HEALTH-CARE PERSPECTIVES; SPIRITUAL BELIEFS AND HEALTH CARE; VACCINE.

grief Emotions and feelings, often intense, of irretrievable loss. Grief may be a response to the loss of a loved one through death or the end of a relationship or to the diagnosis of a health condition that signifies the end of a certain way of living. It is natural and normal for people to mourn losses of function, potential, and other aspects of their own health as well as to grieve the prospect of their own impending deaths. Some people also experience grief during significant life transitions, such as when a child leaves home.

Though the grieving process, also called bereavement, consists of predictable kinds of responses and feelings, each person handles grief uniquely. The range of emotions associated with grief includes sadness, anger, disbelief, denial, despair, numbness, and guilt. A person may experience some or all of these emotions at varying intensities and periods of time. Grief can be overwhelming and incapacitating, particularly at its onset and in circumstances of unexpected loss. Grief is also important for HEALING from the sense of loss.

A person who is grieving may appreciate support and comfort from others or may prefer to grieve in private. It is important for the grieving person to know others are there, however. Rituals such as funeral ceremonies are among the ways societies deal with grieving in communal ways. Age, culture, and spiritual beliefs are among the many factors that influence the expression and process of grieving.

See also DEPRESSION; END OF LIFE CONCERNS; INTERPERSONAL RELATIONSHIPS; SPIRITUAL BELIEFS AND HEALTH CARE.

interpersonal relationships The partnerships and associations people form with other people. These may include family, friendship, intimate, sexual, workplace, and social relationships. Though the need to socialize is universal, individuals and cultures approach social bonds in different ways. Some people prefer a few close individual partnerships that have a fairly substantial degree of intimacy. Other people prefer to socialize with groups in which there is no distinct pairing or partnering. Such group relationships often form around common interests, ranging from sports and recreational activities to religious beliefs and intellectual or educational pursuits. Gender and generation also influence the ways of socialization and the nature of relationships.

Whatever their configuration, interpersonal relationships are essential for emotional and psychologic health and often also for physical wellbeing. Numerous studies show that people who live in isolation are more likely to develop psychologic conditions such as depression as well as physical health problems. The romanticized notion that one could die of a broken HEART becomes substantiated in reality in situations when people lose their longtime partners, particularly men whose wives die before them. Studies show that even interaction with pets improves emotional stability and satisfaction with life.

Intentional deprivation of interpersonal relationships, such as may occur with CHILD ABUSE, can cause lifelong and sometimes irreparable psychologic damage that inhibits the ability to form friendships and intimate partnerships. Relationships with parents and siblings are the first to form. Family life provides early guidance and teaches the skills a person needs to develop relationships outside the circle of family.

See also AUTISM; DOMESTIC VIOLENCE; ELDER ABUSE; PEER PRESSURE; PROBLEM SOLVING AND CONFLICT RESOLUTION; QUALITY OF LIFE.

parenting The functions and processes of raising a child. Most people grow and change in their roles as parents as their children also grow and change. Parents learn from their experiences and their mistakes. Though one's own parents are often the most dominant role models for parenting, new understandings about childhood development may emphasize a different approach or set of skills for parenting today.

Numerous classes and programs are available—many of which community agencies offer at little cost or no cost—that teach effective parenting skills, appropriate discipline methods, and ways for coping with the unique stresses of each developmental stage from infancy through ADOLESCENCE. Friends and peers who are also raising children often provide alternative ways of looking at and handling specific though universal situations such as tantrums, defiant behavior, dating, and driving.

KEY PARENTING RESPONSIBILITIES

- provide a loving, nurturing, safe environment
- provide adequate nutrition and physical activity
- provide appropriate medical care and dental care
- establish expectations and enforce limits
- listen and respond to the perspectives and concerns the child expresses
- seek help when things get out of hand
- encourage appropriate achievement and express pride in accomplishments

---

Just as there are stages of development for children, there are periods of learning and changing for parents. The needs of children shift as they grow and mature, and it is important for parents to adapt to support and accommodate those shifts and the child's increasing independence. Parents need to relearn supervision and discipline approaches to provide appropriate guidelines with each developmental shift. It is important for parents to be aware of activities in which children may engage that put them at risk. The increasing mobility and technology of the current culture, coupled with the reality that more children than not today grow up in what earlier generations would have perceived as nontraditional households, allows greater independence and access at an earlier age.

Parents also need to balance their careers and social interests with the demands of parenting. It is important for parents to maintain time for their partners and friends, though this is often a challenging and sometimes daunting goal, because it helps them maintain balance overall. It is also important for parents to be able to have time away from their children. As well, staying with other adults helps children develop comfort in knowing their parents can leave and will return.

Many parents worry that they do not give enough of themselves to the functions of parenting, particularly when behavior problems arise. However, behavior is fluid and dynamic and nearly all children engage in some behaviors that distress their parents, teachers, and sometimes even their own friends and peers. Most child development experts agree that whatever the parenting style, flexibility and the ability to "go with the flow" for at least a short time are approaches that help children to find their bearings and move on to more appropriate behaviors. Exceptions, of course, are behaviors that threaten the safety and well-being of the child or others, circumstances that require immediate and appropriate intervention.

See also CHILD ABUSE; INTERPERSONAL RELATIONSHIPS; STRESS AND STRESS MANAGEMENT; WORKPLACE STRESS.

peer pressure The influences of friends, acquaintances, colleagues, and co-workers. Peer pressure may be positive or negative. Though the common perception of peer pressure is of a childhood and ADOLESCENCE phenomenon, the attitudes and actions of others remain influential to varying degree throughout life. One's peers—those with whom a person feels relatively equal—are instrumental in shaping compliance with societal norms and behavioral standards. In the workplace peer pressure becomes the corporate culture, for example. Peer pressure is also a pivotal component of the "one for all" dynamic of military training and performance.

Even in adolescence, a time when individuals are particularly concerned about fitting in and behaving the same as everyone else, peer pressure is more often positive than negative. Friendships, because they develop from shared interests, often reinforce values and behaviors that are desirable within the context of community or family ideals and expectations.

Peer pressure becomes problematic when it induces individuals to think and behave in ways that have negative or adverse consequences. Negative peer pressure may manifest as experimentation with ALCOHOL or ILLICIT DRUG USE, criminal activity, or socially unacceptable attire and appearance. Such manifestations are most common in adolescence because it is a time of vulnerability and searching for self-identity, but it may occur at any point in life. Corrupt and illegal actions within corporations, which periodically become prominent, represent negative peer pressure as well.

Peer pressure is unavoidable. It is a dynamic that shapes conformity with group, societal, and cultural expectations. The key is for individuals to have a strong enough internal framework of integrity to know when those expectations are inappropriate and to be able to stand apart from them when they are.

See also PROBLEM SOLVING AND CONFLICT RESOLUTION; YOUTH HIGH-RISK BEHAVIOR.

problem solving and conflict resolution Skills and methods to resolve differences between individuals and among groups. The essence of problem solving and conflict resolution is to find common ground—shared values, beliefs, goals, intentions, and expectations. From such a platform it is often possible to resolve differences.

There are numerous methodologies for problem solving and conflict resolution, the appropriateness of which depends on the setting and circumstances. Conflicts in the workplace require a different focus from problems in the classroom or challenges in the family, even though the underlying challenges are similar. Regardless of methodology, there are some basic steps common to nearly all settings:

- Isolate the problem: What—not who—accounts for the differences that are creating disagreement and conflict?

- Establish a common base of expectation for resolution: What will improve the situation?

- Agree on steps that will move all parties toward resolution: How will the situation improve?

- Implement the steps, along with a process for assessing the success of each step.

- Reevaluate: Does the solution solve the problem or resolve the conflict?

Personalities and personal agendas often get in the way of objective conflict resolution. It is important to recognize, however, that it is attitudes, behaviors, and actions that are responsible for conflict. These factors are within the ability of an individual to change. People are more willing to make changes when they are able to see the outcome as gaining rather than giving up.

See also ANGER AND ANGER MANAGEMENT; STRESS AND STRESS MANAGEMENT; WORKPLACE STRESS.

S

sexual assault Unwilling, unconsenting, or forced sexual interaction. Sexual assault involves implied or actual use of VIOLENCE to force compliance and is an act of violence, not an act of sexual gratification. Sexual assault is also criminal act and has potentially serious health consequences. Rape is sexual assault in which there is attempted or completed penetration of the VAGINA, ANUS, or MOUTH by the PENIS, finger, or an object. In some states the legal term for penetration other than vaginal is *sodomy*. Incest is sexual assault in which the perpetrator is a family member and may occur as a form of CHILD ABUSE.

Women, men, and children may be the victims of sexual assault. Those at highest risk are women between the ages of 16 and 20. About 100,000 sexual assaults are reported to police in the United States each year, which health experts believe represents perhaps only 1 in 4 of sexual assaults that actually occur. Sexual assault in which the victim is male is even less frequently reported.

Legal Issues of Sexual Assault

Though it is a natural desire to immediately bathe or shower after a sexual assault, it is crucial to first seek medical attention. SEMEN and other bodily fluid samples are essential for identifying the perpetrator of the assault, even when the victim knows the assailant. Hospital emergency departments often have staff (sexual assault nurse examiners) who have special training in obtaining such samples and conducting sexual assault examinations that are in compliance with the standards of legal evidence. Most hospitals have sexual assault advocates and support services they contact who can provide assistance for the victims of sexual assault.

Health Issues of Sexual Assault

Traumatic injury resulting from forceful penetration, SEXUALLY TRANSMITTED DISEASES (STDS), unwanted PREGNANCY, and emotional trauma are the key health issues of sexual assault. Doctors may recommend or administer (with consent) emergency CONTRACEPTION when pregnancy is a possibility. Doctors also typically offer ANTIBIOTIC PROPHYLAXIS as a defense against STDs, with recommended follow-up testing for STDs that have longer incubation periods or are viral, such as HEPATITIS, HIV/AIDS, SYPHILIS, and GONORRHEA.

The emotional consequences of sexual assault can be long lasting and significant. Doctors recommend counseling even when the person does not feel it is necessary. ACUTE STRESS DISORDER and POST-TRAUMATIC STRESS DISORDER (PTSD) are common. Sexual assault may result in prolonged inability to form intimate relationships or enjoy sexual partnerships, either in existing circumstances such as marriage or in subsequent circumstances.

Risk Reduction Measures

Because sexual assault is a criminal act of violence that is often random, it is not possible to completely prevent attack. However, law enforcement officials recommend these measures to reduce the risk for sexual assault

- maintain high awareness of one's surroundings, particularly during times of darkness (including early morning hours especially in the winter)
- when walking alone, walk at a purposeful stride and in the center or closer to the curb side of sidewalks
- do not enter a car, home, or other setting if anything about it seems suspicious

- do not consume so much ALCOHOL when out with a group or on a date that it impairs one's ability to take action to stop unwanted sexual advances

- do not accept or consume "party drugs"

See also DOMESTIC VIOLENCE; ELDER ABUSE; GAMMA HYDROXYBUTYRATE (GHB).

sexual orientation   A continuing or enduring physical and emotional attraction and sexual interest in another person. Most health experts view sexual orientation as a continuum with exclusive heterosexuality (attraction only to people of the opposite sex) at one end and exclusive homosexuality at the other end (attraction only to people of the same sex). Along the continuum are varying degrees of mixed attraction (heterosexual and homosexual), often called bisexuality. Sexual orientation is distinct from an individual's sexual identity and perceptions of SEXUALITY.

Most researchers believe sexual orientation develops in early childhood as a complex interaction of numerous psychologic, biologic, and behavioral factors. However, some researchers believe sexual orientation is purely biologic or genetic, and others maintain that it is purely behavioral. Within these attempts to understand and explain sexual orientation, nearly all researchers agree that whatever its origins, sexual orientation is not a matter of choice. The basis for this agreement is the recognition that sexual orientation emerges before sexual exploration.

The American Psychological Association, American Psychiatric Association, American Counseling Association, and other organizations of health-care professionals affirm that sexual orientation, no matter where it is along the continuum of possible expressions, is simply a dimension of individual experience and definition and adamantly oppose efforts to change sexual orientation (notably homosexuality) through therapy and refute claims that therapy can accomplish such an objective. Rather, mental health professionals hold that the purpose of therapy related to sexual orientation is to help an individual who is uncomfortable with his or her sexual orientation reach a level of understanding and acceptance about it, which may include choices around how to accom-

modate sexual orientation issues and whether to engage in intimate relationships.

See also INTERPERSONAL RELATIONSHIPS; SEXUAL HEALTH.

sexuality   A person's overall attitudes, perceptions, and expressions of sexual identity, SEXUAL ORIENTATION, and sexual behavior, intimate relationships (whether or not those relationships include sexual activity). The organs of reproduction provide the physical basis for gender and sexuality. Other factors, from genetics to biochemistry, add further layers of complexity so that sexuality becomes a fundamental element of human existence along the entire continuum of life. Sexuality plays a significant role in self-esteem and self-confidence, shaping how people perceive themselves, and how they present themselves to others.

Numerous health circumstances affect sexuality, from physical development and aging to injury and illness. Changes in the body's physical appearance shift awareness of sexuality at key life passages such as PUBERTY, PREGNANCY, and MENOPAUSE. Health conditions that affect physical function may affect an individual's interest in or ability to participate in SEXUAL INTERCOURSE and other sexual activity. Among such health conditions are OBESITY, DIABETES, CARDIOVASCULAR DISEASE (CVD), neurologic disorders, STROKE, HEART ATTACK, and CHROMOSOMAL DISORDERS such as TURNER SYNDROME and KLINEFELTER SYNDROME. Because the base of sexuality is inherently linked to the organs of reproduction, conditions (and their treatments) that affect those organs are often especially challenging to sexuality. Treatments that result in physical alterations of the body, such as AMPUTATION and MASTECTOMY, often affect the person's perceptions about his or her physical attractiveness and sexual desire.

See also AGING, REPRODUCTIVE AND SEXUAL CHANGES THAT OCCUR WITH; ERECTILE DYSFUNCTION; INTERPERSONAL RELATIONSHIPS; LIBIDO; SEXUAL DYSFUNCTION; SEXUAL HEALTH.

spiritual beliefs and health care   The influences of an individual's faith on health-care decisions and outcomes. Spirituality is the sense of how one fits within and relates to the scheme of existence, helping define such concepts as the purpose of life. Interactions between the sense of spirit, the mind, and the body provide powerful connections that shape the experiences and expressions of health and well-being as well as of illness and injury.

Faith is often the factor that provides comfort during health crises and confidence that treatment will succeed. Numerous studies show correlations between positive outcomes in serious illness or injury and directed manifestations of belief such as prayer circles, HEALING ceremonies, and spiritual rituals. In some cultures spiritual practices are inseparable from healing. A person's faith or religion (a particular belief structure) may also be the source of acceptance in chronic or terminal health conditions.

As well, religious or spiritual beliefs may guide the kinds of health-care decisions, including diagnostic procedures and treatments, individuals make. For example, a religion's doctrines may proscribe FERTILITY testing, CONTRACEPTION, or the receipt of donor BLOOD (BLOOD TRANSFUSION) or organs.

See also AYURVEDA; CULTURAL AND ETHIC HEALTH CARE PERSPECTIVES; MEDITATION; MIND–BODY CONNECTION; NATIVE AMERICAN HEALING; PRAYER AND SPIRITUALITY; TRADITIONAL CHINESE MEDICINE (TCM).

stress and stress management Stress is any factor that alters equilibrium. Stress management is the effort to manage stress to maintain equilibrium. Stress is a constant and necessary dimension of life. Stress can be physiologic, psychologic, or emotional and often exists in combination.

Physiologic stress maintains vital bodily functions such as BREATHING, HEART RATE, and BLOOD PRESSURE. The STRESS RESPONSE HORMONAL CASCADE instigates the "fight or flight" response that mobilizes the body's resources. The key HORMONE of this cascade is CORTISOL, which the ADRENAL GLANDS secrete. Cortisol influences or regulates numerous physiologic functions, either directly or through the release or suppression of other hormones such as EPINEPHRINE and NOREPINEPHRINE. It also initiates HEALING, stimulating the IMMUNE RESPONSE, and focuses NEUROTRANSMITTER release and NEURON communication in the BRAIN to intensify cognitive function.

The Health Consequences of Excessive Stress

Stress becomes problematic for health when it exists in excess for an extended time. Sustained elevation of the stress hormones damages cells, tissues, and organs throughout the body, most notably those of the cardiovascular system. Indications of prolonged, excessive stress may include

- irritability, moodiness, or outbursts of anger
- worry, crying, or panic attacks
- difficulty sleeping, sleeping too much, or feeling that sleep is not restful
- PALPITATIONS
- frequent HEADACHES
- gastrointestinal distress such as NAUSEA, VOMITING, or DIARRHEA
- increased APPETITE or loss of interest in eating

Elevated cortisol alters the body's ability to produce and use INSULIN, which affects METABOLISM of lipids. Researchers believe this contributes to HYPERLIPIDEMIA and resulting ATHEROSCLEROSIS and may play a role in the development of type 2 DIABETES. Excessive stress may also exacerbate chronic health conditions such as HYPERTENSION (high blood pressure), INFLAMMATORY BOWEL DISEASE (IBS), MULTIPLE SCLEROSIS, PARKINSON'S DISEASE, and DIVERTICULAR DISEASE.

Inappropriate Stress Relief Efforts

People sometimes turn to ALCOHOL, cigarette smoking, and drugs (legal as well as illicit) to relieve stress. Though these approaches may provide relief in the short term, they can have numerous adverse effects on health over the long term. Alcohol is a mild depressant, acting to slow NERVE impulses and neuron function in the brain. Though occasional and moderate alcohol consumption does not present health issues for most people, long-term use of alcohol for stress reduction is both counterproductive and damaging to health. Chronic alcohol consumption has numerous deleterious effects on the body, from LIVER and nerve damage to increased risk for STOMACH CANCER, LIVER CANCER, cognitive dysfunction, memory impairment, and impaired healing. Tobacco, though regular smokers feel it calms them, contains NICOTINE, a powerful and addictive stimulant.

The calming effect of smoking a cigarette is more that of quieting the addictive need than genuine relaxation.

Methods to Manage Stress

The most effective means of managing excessive stress is to reduce its sources to the extent possible. This may require evaluation of the demands of work, family, and other commitments to prioritize them. Much excessive stress results not so much from an individual source but from the cumulative effects of multiple demands. Sometimes simply the process of evaluation reveals potential for change. Though it may not be possible to eliminate the source of the stress, it often is possible to mediate, through various techniques, its ability to cause stress. A key dimension of stress management is the ability to gain control over the circumstances of stress, including personal responses to it.

EFFECTIVE METHODS FOR STRESS RELIEF	
ACUPUNCTURE	AROMATHERAPY
BIOFEEDBACK	BREATHING EXERCISES
COGNITIVE THERAPY	LABYRINTH
MEDITATION	physical exercise
prayer	TAI CHI
VISUALIZATION	YOGA

See also ACUTE STRESS DISORDER; ALCOHOLISM; COGNITIVE FUNCTION AND DYSFUNCTION; GENERALIZED ANXIETY DISORDER (GAD); MEMORY AND MEMORY IMPAIRMENT; POST-TRAUMATIC STRESS DISORDER (PTSD); WORKPLACE STRESS.

support groups People who have in common specific health-care conditions, either as patients or family members and caregivers, who meet to provide information and a safe environment for dialogue about fears, worries, expectations, and other concerns. Hospitals and health organizations often maintain support groups, providing meeting space, structured meeting times, and sometimes a doctor, nurse, therapist, or other health-care provider to serve as moderator or host when the group meets. Other support groups are casual and may meet in a member's home or social setting on either a regular or an ad hoc (as-needed or spontaneous) basis.

A less traditional though sometimes more accessible type of support group is one that communicates through Internet forums and message boards. Such online venues allow people to share their comments and questions any time. Some also feature scheduled presentations from specialists who provide information and answer questions.

See also PSYCHOTHERAPY; STRESS AND STRESS MANAGEMENT.

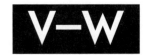

violence Actions of aggression that cause intentional harm to others. Violence may be targeted or random and may occur in the workplace, at school, or in the home (DOMESTIC VIOLENCE). Violence is a leading cause of injury and death in the United States, accounting for nearly two million hospital emergency visits and 20,000 deaths a year. Homicide is also the leading cause of death among pregnant women, claiming about 2,000 lives each year.

Those most vulnerable to injury and death due to violence are young people, primarily men, between the ages of 15 and 24, for whom homicide is the second leading cause of death (and leading cause of death among African Americans). Firearms (mostly handguns) account for nearly two thirds of all homicides in the United States. The most common form of violence against young people is date violence—actions such as hitting, choking, and forced sex. Youth gangs are also often violence oriented.

The long-term consequences of violence include physically disabling health conditions such as TRAUMATIC BRAIN INJURY (TBI) and SPINAL CORD INJURY, which often result in permanent BRAIN damage or PARALYSIS. Psychologic conditions such as ACUTE STRESS DISORDER, DEPRESSION, GENERALIZED ANXIETY DISORDER (GAD), PHOBIA, and POST-TRAUMATIC STRESS DISORDER (PTSD) are also common among people who have experienced violence.

Efforts to reduce violence include recognition of warning signs that a person may be inclined toward violence or is planning an act of violence. Such signs may include

- outbursts of extreme anger or rage
- talk of committing acts of violence
- possession of weapons or destructive devices
- punching, hitting, or choking others in "fun"
- disparaging attitudes and comments toward individuals, ethic groups, or organizations (such as schools, employers, or the government)

Depending on the person's behavior, age, and other circumstances, the appropriate authorities may be able to intervene to thwart potential acts of violence. PSYCHOTHERAPY and BEHAVIORAL MODIFICATION THERAPY may help individuals replace violent reactions and behaviors with behaviors that are more appropriate; therapy can help individuals understand what causes the feelings of frustration or anger that are often behind their violent actions. Psychotherapy and COGNITIVE THERAPY may help people who have experienced violence to develop constructive COPING MECHANISMS.

See also ACCIDENTAL INJURIES; ANGER AND ANGER MANAGEMENT; CHILD ABUSE; ELDER ABUSE; SEXUAL ASSAULT; STRESS AND STRESS MANAGEMENT; SUICIDE IDEATION AND SUICIDE.

workplace stress Tension and pressure among co-workers in the work environment or within individuals as a consequence of work demands. In the work environment people must work together, often in collaborative ways, with people they might otherwise not associate. Though many employers attempt to foster good relationships among employees, co-workers may have little in common beyond specific work qualifications and job skills. More than 25 percent of workers in the United States consider work the most significant source of stress in their lives. About 60 percent of work absenteeism is directly attributable to stress.

Issues in the workplace may include co-workers who do not get along with one another, people who do not pull their share of the workload, heavy workloads, tedious or repetitious work, demanding customers, and short staffing. As well, people may work in jobs that are not a good match for their needs and interests—because such a job may pay more than a better-suited job, offer more lenient time away to deal with children, have health insurance benefits the person or family needs, or be the only work available in a particular location. Physical danger inherent in certain jobs also establishes a high level of emotional stress.

FACTORS THAT CONTRIBUTE TO WORKPLACE STRESS

automation
child care issues
complex, time-sensitive work tasks
co-worker conflict
downsizing and corporate restructuring
family demands
heavy workload
inability to make decisions about work tasks
lack of privacy
noisy work environment
repetitious or tedious work
work unsuited to interests

Work responsibilities are often in direct competition with family responsibilities for a person's time and interest. About 40 percent of American families have only a single parent, resulting in significant stress around child care arrangements and expenses. Even among families in which both parents work, parents find it necessary to juggle work responsibilities and child needs such as illness, health-care appointments, and school activities.

Unmitigated work stress has numerous consequences for both physical and psychologic stress. Stress-related physical conditions may include frequent headaches, IRRITABLE BOWEL SYNDROME (IBS), and ACCIDENTAL INJURIES. Work stress may also contribute to various psychologic conditions in which stress is a significant factor. An extreme of work stress is burnout, in which a person may experience symptoms such as PALPITATIONS, trembling, sleep disturbances, and unprovoked outbursts of anger.

The most effective solutions for work stress combine changes in the work setting with stress management methods. Many people may benefit from career counseling to help them determine what kinds of work or jobs might be more appropriate for their interests and abilities. Sometimes it is necessary to change jobs to relieve work stress. Other approaches may include identifying one specific problem at work that causes stress and coming up with possible solutions.

See also ANGER AND ANGER MANAGEMENT; OCCUPATIONAL HEALTH AND SAFETY; SOMATIZATION DISORDER; STRESS AND STRESS MANAGEMENT; VIOLENCE.

SURGERY

Surgery is the specialty within the practice of medicine in which its practitioners use instruments, devices, and techniques to repair or remove organs and structures affected by congenital defect, injury, or disease processes. Surgical operations are invasive—that is, they enter or open the body in some way.

Two health-care disciplines merge within the arena of surgical operations: ANESTHESIA and surgery. Physicians who administer anesthesia are anesthesiologists (MDs or DOs). Registered nurses who have advanced practice education and certification in anesthesiology are certified registered nurse anesthetists (CRNAs). Anesthesiologists may also choose to further specialize in PAIN management care.

Physicians who perform surgical operations are surgeons, with further designation according to the surgeon's subspecialization. For example, a surgeon who operates exclusively on structures of the chest except the HEART is a thoracic surgeon; a surgeon who operates exclusively on the heart is a cardiac surgeon. A surgeon who operates exclusively on bones and joints is an orthopedic surgeon.

This section, "Surgery," presents an overview discussion of the concepts and practices of surgery and general entries about surgical operations and their role in diagnosis and treatment of diseases, congenital anomalies, and injuries. Entries about specific operations are in the sections that discuss the relevant body system—for example, the entry for HYSTERECTOMY (an OPERATION to remove the UTERUS) is in the section "The Reproductive System" and the entry for CHOLECYSTECTOMY (an operation to remove the GALLBLADDER) is in the section "The Gastrointestinal System."

Surgery Comes of Age

Early documents from diverse cultures provide evidence that surgery—entering the body for therapeutic purposes—has long been among the treatment options of physicians. Ancient Ayurvedic physicians extracted cataracts, amputated limbs, delivered babies by CESAREAN SECTION, drained pus from infected wounds, removed bladder stones, and even performed what plastic surgeons today call pedicle flap tissue grafts to repair damaged noses. Greek physicians operated on soldiers to repair battle wounds. In Babylonia and Egypt surgeons were distinct from physicians, with clearly defined duties and responsibilities.

Toward the end of the 19th century vastly improved understanding of anatomy (the body's structure) and physiology (the body's functions) encouraged physicians to explore the intentional opening of the body to remove tumors and repair damage such as from injury or disease. Nearly all of the misconceptions perpetuated through centuries evaporated in the evidence researchers acquired through scientific study and dissection of human cadavers. Surgeons boldly ventured into new territory: the inner body. Unfortunately, though surgeons had the knowledge their patients were less than eager to allow its display. Few willingly submitted to the scalpel when the only escape from pain was a fortuitously well-placed upper right to the jaw that delivered UNCONSCIOUSNESS. As well, more people died of INFECTION after surgery than recovered from the operation.

But in the 20th century two advances in medicine converged to make surgery feasible: antisepsis and anesthesia. As a result of these two crucial developments, today surgery is the treatment of first choice for numerous health circumstances. Surgical operations can restore and improve function, improve appearance, repair the damage of traumatic injury, replace dysfunctional organs and structures, remove tumors and infected tissue, and correct potentially life-threatening congenital anomalies. Surgeons in the United States perform more than 25 million operations a year.

SURGERY NOMENCLATURE: TYPES OF OPERATIONS	
Term Ends In	**Operation Is to**
-ectomy	remove a body part or segment of tissue
-ostomy	establish a passage between two structures
-otomy	open an area of the body
-plasty	repair or reconstruct a body part

Anesthesia: Making Surgery Painless

Until the middle of the 19th century surgery was a treatment of last resort, chosen only when the only alternative was certain death. The most effective, albeit unpredictable, anesthesia was a surprise uppercut punch to the jaw that could render a person unconscious long enough for a fast surgeon to complete an operation such as extraction of a bullet or AMPUTATION of a limb. ALCOHOL and opium were the drugs of choice for postoperative pain relief.

The first effective anesthetic agent was ether, administered by having the person breathe fumes as they evaporated from a saturated cloth. Though chemists had compounded ether (sulfuric acid distilled in alcohol) since the 13th century and explored it as a solvent and a sedative for centuries, its properties as an anesthetic did not become known until chemistry students in the early 1800s began using it for entertainment at parties. Their instructors observed that the more ether a person inhaled, the more impervious he or she was to pain. But not until the middle of the century did surgeons begin to explore using ether to intentionally intoxicate an individual to create a state of unconsciousness. In 1842 American physician Crawford Long (1815–1878) used ether to anesthetize a friend, then surgically removed several cysts from the friend's neck. The friend felt no pain and had no memory of the surgery.

Discoveries of similar properties for chloroform and nitrous oxide rapidly expanded anesthesia options. These substances were more effective and less noxious than ether and soon displaced it for operations and dental procedures. Over the latter decades of the 19th century surgeons refined the mechanisms for delivery of anesthetic agents to provide relatively predictable and safe anesthesia during surgery. In the 1880s surgeons experimenting with controlled delivery of anesthetic agents had developed valve-controlled inhalers and the precursor of the endotracheal tube, a tube inserted into the trachea with an air-filled cuff on the end to hold it in place and seal the trachea. By 1930 endotracheal intubation had become the standard method for administering inhalation anesthesia, as it remains today.

Modern anesthetic agents are faster acting, more specific in the effects they achieve, and much safer than their predecessors. Though unpleasant side effects remain possible, anesthesia for most people accomplishes precisely and only the intended purpose. Anesthesiologists and certified nurse anesthetists (physicians and registered nurses, respectively) who specialize in the delivery of anesthesia, carefully administer anesthesia tailored to each individual patient's needs and health circumstances.

Antisepsis: Making Surgery Safe

Though surgeons knew all too well the high rate of death after surgery, it was an obstetrician rather than a surgeon who made the connection between antisepsis and death rates among patients. Hungarian physician Ignaz Philipp Semmelweis (1818–1865) noticed that the death rate in the maternity ward was much higher among women cared for by doctors than by midwives. His investigation led him to recognize that doctors often went directly from performing autopsies (procedures in which midwives had no role) to delivering babies. In 1846 Semmelweis implemented procedures for doctors to wash their hands with chlorinated lime before examining obstetrical patients, and maternal death rates from childbirth FEVER (puerperal fever) plummeted.

It was 20 years later that Louis Pasteur (1822–1895) and Joseph Lister (1827–1912) proved the connection between microscopic "germs" and illnesses such as infection, and by the 1870s antisepsis was the standard of practice not only for childbirth but also for surgery and other treatment modalities. Today surgeons and other members of the surgical team follow stringent HAND WASHING (scrubbing) procedures, and wear sterile gowns and gloves in the operating room. The widespread use of ANTIBIOTIC MEDICATIONS has further reduced the risk for postoperative infection.

THE SURGERY TEAM

A typical surgery team today includes the
- primary surgeon
- assisting surgeon or physician assistant; may be several depending on the type of operation
- scrub nurse or surgery technician (also called surgical technologist)
- circulating nurse
- anesthesiologist or certified nurse anesthetist
- perfusionist for certain surgeries

Breakthrough Research and Surgical Advances

The last half of the 20th century saw surgery surge to the forefront of treatment options for numerous health conditions, revolutionizing care as well as survival for heart disease, cancer, CONGENITAL ANOMALY, and major trauma. OPEN HEART SURGERY and ORGAN TRANSPLANTATION are now conventional treatment options. Among the most exciting advances in surgery in recent years has been the evolution of MINIMALLY INVASIVE SURGERY, operations that use tiny video cameras to display the operative site on a monitor similar to a television screen. The surgeon operates using the display for visual guidance, much like a sophisticated video game. Through small incisions, called ports, the surgeon inserts tiny instruments. Minimally invasive surgery reduces the need for large, open incisions, decreasing patient discomfort and recovery time. Operations that were once major ordeals have become fairly minor procedures. Surgeons look forward to a future in which minimally invasive surgery becomes the standard for nearly all kinds of operations.

ambulatory surgery Surgery, sometimes called same-day or outpatient surgery, in which the person comes to the hospital or AMBULATORY SURGERY FACILITY the day of the surgery, has the OPERATION, and goes home without an overnight stay in the hospital. Often the operation uses MINIMALLY INVASIVE SURGERY procedures such as endoscopic methods (laparoscopy, arthroscopy), which greatly reduce the size of the incision and the amount of trauma the body experiences during operation. Minimally invasive surgery techniques allow a rapid course of recovery in the immediate postoperative period as well as over the longer term. Surgeons also can perform numerous OPEN SURGERY procedures on an ambulatory surgery basis. People tend to feel more comfortable recovering in their own homes and often require lower doses of PAIN medications during their recovery. As well, a shorter stay reduces the risk for NOSOCOMIAL INFECTIONS (infections acquired from exposure to BACTERIA in the hospital environment) and more quickly returns a person to regular activities.

Because each person's rate of recovery is unique, some people more quickly return to CONSCIOUSNESS from sedation or general ANESTHESIA and to function from regional anesthesia to engage in basic activities such as drinking fluids and going to the bathroom. Underlying health conditions also influence how quickly a person is ready to leave after ambulatory surgery. Hospitals and ambulatory (outpatient) surgery facilities are equipped and staffed to handle medical emergencies that may arise and are prepared for a person to stay overnight in a hospital should circumstances warrant additional care or observation. The person returns to his or her surgeon for follow-up care such as wound check, suture removal, and dressing changes.

See also ANALGESIC MEDICATIONS; ENDOSCOPY; LASER SURGERY; POSTOPERATIVE PROCEDURES; PREOPERATIVE PROCEDURES; SURGERY BENEFIT AND RISK ASSESSMENT; WOUND CARE.

anesthesia The intentional establishment of loss of PAIN sensation or of consciousness to make a surgical OPERATION possible. Anesthesia may be local, regional, or general, depending on the operation and on the individual's health circumstances and preferences. Doctors sometimes use local and regional forms of anesthesia to treat severe or CHRONIC PAIN not related to surgery.

Anesthesia today is very effective as well as safe. There are several types of anesthesia and numerous anesthetic agents. The anesthesiologist or anesthetist selects the types and agents according to the operation and the person's health conditions and health status, and may combine types and agents to achieve the desired anesthetic effect. The risks of anesthesia vary with the type and agent though are generally minimal.

Individual response to anesthetic agents varies, so the anesthesiologist or anesthetist very closely monitors the person's vital signs and level of anesthesia throughout the operation. After the operation monitoring continues in the postanesthesia care unit (PACU), also called the recovery room, until the person has emerged from anesthesia enough to go to a hospital room or for discharge home (AMBULATORY SURGERY).

Local Anesthesia
Local anesthesia numbs a small area of the body for minor operations such as removal of a LIPOMA (benign tumor of fatty tissue) or NEVUS (SKIN lesion such as a mole). The surgeon generally administers local anesthesia by injection into and surrounding

the site of the operation. Local anesthetic agents block the ability of neurons (NERVE cells) to send nerve signals, preventing the perception of pain. Some local anesthetic agents contain EPINEPHRINE, a vasoconstrictor that reduces bleeding.

The effect of a local anesthetic may last from 20 minutes to 12 hours or longer, depending on the agent and the extent of infiltration of the area. Surgeons sometimes use local anesthetic to infiltrate the area of an operative site at the end of the operation to provide extended pain relief. Surgeons may combine local anesthesia and conscious sedation to reduce anxiety and improve the person's level of comfort during and after the operation. Some amount of a local anesthetic enters the BLOOD circulation and can cause sensations such as lightheadedness or a feeling that the lips are buzzing.

COMMON LOCAL AND REGIONAL ANESTHETIC AGENTS

benzocaine	bupivacaine	chloroprocaine
etidocaine	lidocain	emepivacaine
prilocaine	procaine	ropivacaine
tetracaine		

Regional Anesthesia

Regional anesthesia is an injection that infiltrates nerves to blocks pain signals from a large area of the body. An anesthesiologist or anesthetist administers regional anesthesia. The most common forms of regional anesthesia include

- regional nerve block, in which the anesthesiologist or anesthetist administers a single injection of the anesthetic agent into or around a major nerve to block sensation from the fingers, hand, arm, toes, foot, or leg
- caudal, in which the anesthesiologist or anesthetist administers a single injection of the anesthetic agent into the caudal canal in the sacrococcygeal (tailbone) region of the spine to block sensation in the pelvis and perineum
- epidural, in which the anesthesiologist or anesthetist places a thin catheter into the space surrounding the SPINAL CORD and injects the anesthetic agent, potentially as a steady flow or repeated times, to block sensation from the point of injection downward for operations on the lower abdomen and lower extremities

- spinal, in which the anesthesiologist or anesthetist administers a single injection of the anesthetic agent directly into the CEREBROSPINAL FLUID around the spinal cord to block sensation from the point of injection downward for operations on the abdomen and lower extremities

Many of the anesthetic agents are the same for regional anesthesia as for local anesthesia. As occurs with local anesthetics, a small amount of the anesthetic agent enters the blood circulation and can cause mild effects such as HEADACHE or TINNITUS (ringing in the ears). These effects generally go away within an hour. Because caudal, epidural, and spinal anesthesia affect the pelvic region and the muscles of the BLADDER, the surgeon may instruct placement of a urinary catheter until the anesthetic wears off. The surgeon may sometimes leave the epidural catheter in place for 24 to 48 hours for postoperative administration of light anesthesia or ANALGESIC MEDICATIONS for pain relief.

Regional nerve blocks, caudal anesthesia, and epidural anesthesia may take up to 20 minutes to become effective. Spinal anesthesia takes effect immediately. Though regional anesthesia blocks only the sensory nerves, movement of the anesthetized region is difficult because the lack of sensation makes the affected body parts feel heavy and uncontrollable. A person has adequately recovered from regional anesthesia when he or she can safely walk or regains preanesthesia sensation or movement of the affected area.

Complications are rare with regional anesthesia though may include prolonged labor during CHILDBIRTH, irritation or bleeding at the injection site, drop in BLOOD PRESSURE, and post-anesthesia headache (with epidural or spinal anesthesia). Infection and injury to the nerves are possible though extremely rare. Recovery from regional anesthesia is generally uneventful and fairly rapid.

Conscious Sedation

Conscious sedation alters a person's awareness of pain and activities taking place to and around him or her. With conscious sedation a person generally can answer questions, respond to instructions, and tell the doctor whether he or she is experiencing pain or discomfort though has little or no memory of the operation and events surrounding it when full consciousness returns. Surgeons often use conscious sedation to improve a person's comfort and reduce anxiety during minor operations, usually in combination with local or regional anesthesia. Usually an anesthesiologist or anesthetist administers the sedative medication intravenously with ongoing monitoring of the person's response to the medication, level of awareness, and vital signs such as BREATHING rate, HEART RATE, and blood pressure.

Rarely, a person may experience NAUSEA or headache after conscious sedation. More rarely, a person may have distressing memories of the operation. Though a person appears to return to normal consciousness quickly, the medication may remain at a level in the blood circulation that affects perception and function for 24 hours after its administration. Doctors caution people to avoid driving or performing activities that require alertness and coordination for at least 24 hours after conscious sedation.

POTENTIAL DRUG INTERACTIONS WITH ANESTHESIA

Many prescription medications, OVER-THE-COUNTER (OTC) DRUGS, NUTRITIONAL SUPPLEMENTS, and MEDICINAL HERBS AND BOTANICALS can interfere with anesthesia or BLOOD clotting. It is important to tell the surgeon of all such medications and products. The surgeon or the anesthesiologist may request the person to stop taking certain drugs or herbs for a period of time before and sometimes also after surgery.

General Anesthesia

General anesthesia establishes a state of deep UNCONSCIOUSNESS in which the anesthetic agents circulate in the body to block pain signals, prevent movement, and block memory of the operation. The anesthetic agents may be gases the person inhales or medications (such as sedatives, hypnotics, and MUSCLE relaxants) the anesthetist or anesthesiologist injects intravenously. An endotracheal tube inserted through the MOUTH, into the THROAT, and to the top of the trachea allows the anesthesiologist to seal the airway to prevent foreign matter from entering the LUNGS, as the anesthetic suppresses the COUGH REFLEX that would normally keep mucus and debris from entering the trachea. The endotracheal tube also ensures

that oxygen and anesthetic gases directly enter the lungs. General anesthesia is the standard for operations on the upper abdomen and chest as well as for many major orthopedic operations. In some circumstances the anesthesiologist may combine epidural or spinal anesthesia with general anesthesia. Many general anesthesia agents are fast acting and short lived, allowing rapid anesthetic induction as well as quick recovery.

COMMON GENERAL ANESTHETIC AGENTS		
Inhaled		
enflurane	halothane	isoflurane
methoxyflurane	nitrous oxide	
Injected		
etomidate	KETAMINE	methohexital
propofol	thiopental	

Sophisticated equipment allows precise and safe administration of inhaled anesthetics, including ongoing adjustments of carbon dioxide and oxygen concentrations. The anesthesiologist or anesthetist continuously monitors the person's vital signs, including breathing rate, oxygen saturation, heart rate, blood pressure, and body temperature. The most common side effects of general anesthesia are nausea, VOMITING, a slow return to normal bowel activity, and a prolonged sense of grogginess. The anesthesiologist or anesthetist can administer medications to ease or relieve these symptoms. Sore throat is a common complaint after general anesthesia, a consequence of the endotracheal tube.

Though most general anesthetic agents do not persist in the body at functional levels beyond 24 to 36 hours, many people feel they are not quite themselves for several days after general anesthesia. Postoperative analgesic medications can exacerbate this perception. Walking, to the extent possible, and stool softeners help BOWEL MOVEMENT return to normal. Allergic reaction to anesthetic agents is uncommon but occurs, so it is important to tell both the surgeon and the anesthesiologist or anesthetist of any allergies, including to foods. Smoking, certain prescription medications, ILLICIT DRUG USE, and ALCOHOL consumption affect the ways in which various anesthetic agents function in the body.

It is important to avoid driving or engaging in activities that require focused attention (including making important decisions and signing legal documents) until it is clear that the effects of general anesthesia have completely worn off.

A rare but potentially life-threatening complication of general anesthesia is malignant hyperthermia, in which the person's body temperature rises rapidly and high, muscles become rigid or SPASM, and heart rate and blood pressure vacillate wildly and widely. Doctors believe malignant hyperthermia has a genetic foundation because it occurs in families, though the precise genetic involvement remains unknown. Death as a complication of general anesthesia, though possible, is very rare. Continued advances in anesthetic agents and administration techniques are improving the experience and safety of general anesthesia.

See also NEURON; POSTOPERATIVE PROCEDURES; PREOPERATIVE PROCEDURES; SURGERY BENEFIT AND RISK ASSESSMENT; WOUND CARE.

blood autodonation A practice in which a person donates his or her own BLOOD for potential self-use during a major OPERATION or health emergency such as major trauma. The hospital or blood bank stores the blood for specific and sole use by the person. The person may authorize the hospital or blood bank to release the blood for general use as components (such as ALBUMIN and PLASMA) if he or she does not require it, though guidelines vary according to the procedures in place for collecting autodonated blood. Testing procedures for autodonated may be less stringent than for general BLOOD DONATION because only the donor will receive the blood.

Most people who choose autodonation do so out of concern about the potential for INFECTION such as HEPATITIS acquired from general donation blood. Though screening procedures and tests make the blood supply as safe as possible, the risk of such infection remains a possibility. Autodonation also eliminates the risk for transfusion reaction, which may occur when donor blood carries antibodies that activate an IMMUNE RESPONSE in the recipient. Pretransfusion testing can detect most but not all of these scenarios. Autodonation also ensures the availability of blood for people who have uncommon blood types.

See also ANTIBODY; BLOOD TRANSFUSION; BLOOD TYPE.

bloodless surgery Specialized techniques that allow surgeons to perform major operations to avoid the need for BLOOD TRANSFUSION. Many people oppose BLOOD transfusion on the basis of religious beliefs and others because they have concerns about the safety of donated blood. Though stringent screening and testing procedures for donated blood have minimized the risk of acquired INFECTION from the US blood supply, a slight risk of this remains for whole blood and certain blood products.

Performing surgery when blood transfusion is not an option requires careful planning. When the OPERATION is elective (nonemergency) the person can prepare by taking medications such as ERYTHROPOIETIN (EPO) to boost his or her ERYTHROCYTE (red blood cell) production and donating his or her own blood in advance of the surgery for use if a transfusion becomes necessary. Having more erythrocytes means the blood can carry more oxygen, which encourages HEALING. It also allows the surgeon to administer intravenous fluids during surgery to maintain adequate fluid volume without concern for diluting the blood to the extent that ANEMIA develops.

During the operation, whether elective or emergency, the surgeon can use methods to collect any blood the person loses, filter it, and return it to the person instead of transfusing donor blood. Surgeons also use precision techniques that minimize blood loss when they perform bloodless operations. Sometimes these techniques are time consuming, which makes the surgery more expensive. However, many of the surgical techniques surgeons use for bloodless surgery have become standard for all operations of the same type because they reduce the risk for postoperative infection and encourage more rapid healing and recovery.

Emergency bloodless surgery can be more of a challenge, particularly when there are bleeding injuries that deplete the blood supply even before surgery begins. Fluid expanders sometimes can maintain the body's fluid level without impairing the blood's ability to carry oxygen. Bloodless surgery techniques and blood recycling become essential when the operation is an emergency.

See also BLOOD AUTODONATION; SPIRITUAL BELIEFS AND HEALTH CARE.

endoscopic surgery See MINIMALLY INVASIVE SURGERY.

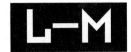

Langer's lines   The natural linear pathways, also called cleavages, of the fasciae fibers (connective tissue layer beneath the SKIN that covers the muscles) throughout the body. Langer's lines resemble a topographic map when overlaid on an outline of the human body. Each person has a unique configuration of Langer's lines, though general patterns are common across individuals. Alignment with relevant Langer's lines is one of several factors a surgeon considers when planning an OPERATION's incision. Surgical incisions that parallel Langer's lines tend to require less suturing and to heal with less obvious scarring than incisions that run counter, and particularly perpendicular, to Langer's lines. Wounds from cuts or punctures are often more severe when they occur in opposition to Langer's lines, tending to gape and tear more than wounds that parallel Langer's lines. The RASH or eruptions of some skin conditions, such as PITYRIASIS rosea, follow Langer's lines.

See also DERMATOME.

laparoscopic surgery   See MINIMALLY INVASIVE SURGERY.

laser surgery   Any OPERATION in which the surgeon uses a device that focuses high-intensity lightwaves that generate heat to cut or ablate (destroy) tissue. *Laser* is an acronym for "light amplification by stimulated emission of radiation." Lasers came into common use in medicine and surgery in the 1960s; the first applications were for the repair of detached RETINA.

The lightwave emission of a laser differs from ordinary light because it is

- all one wavelength (monochromatic)
- organized and unified

- directional and concentrated

There are different types of lasers, classified according to the mechanism by which they produce lightwaves, the length of the lightwaves, and the pattern of emission (continuous or pulsed). The different wavelengths and pulse patterns of emitted light permit targeted use of lasers from making incisions (cutting) to treating discolorations of the SKIN such as a port wine stain BIRTHMARK. The laser's lightwave determines what tissues will absorb the light and what tissues will allow the light to pass through them. For example, the BLOOD in blood vessels absorbs the yellow light of the pulsed laser, though the pigment of light-colored skin does not. Most lasers emit lightwaves in the infrared spectrum; the "cool" lasers emit lightwaves in the ultraviolet spectrum.

Laser lightwaves, like other lightwaves, can travel via fiberoptics, allowing the surgeon to direct the laser emission to a specific location, even one that is deep within the body. Laser surgery requires the surgeon to complete specialized training and requires specialized equipment and facilities for safe use.

Surgical lasers have increased options in all areas of surgery but have revolutionized two areas of treatment in particular: ophthalmologic (EYE) surgery and dermatologic (skin) surgery. The surgeon can so precisely focus and target the laser's beam that any incidental damage to surrounding tissue is nearly nonexistent. Laser surgery incisions tend to heal with minimal scarring. The heat the laser generates kills BACTERIA on the skin at the incision site, reducing the risk for postoperative INFECTION. As well, the intense heat instantly seals blood vessels to reduce bleeding at the site of the incision, making the surgical laser the instrument

265

TYPES OF SURGICAL LASERS

Laser Type	Characteristics	Surgical Application
argon gas	shallow penetration moderately hot only pigmented tissues and fluids absorb the lightwaves	dermatologic procedures refractive surgery (vision correction) coagulate bleeding BLOOD vessels
carbon dioxide (CO_2)	shallow penetration very hot only pigmented fluids absorb the lightwaves	instead of scalpel for incisions vaporize tissue (including tumors) dermatologic procedures such as SKIN resurfacing
neodymium:yttrium-aluminum garnet (Nd:YAG)	deep penetration moderately hot all fluids in the body absorb the lightwaves	fiberoptic transfer to locations within the body vaporize or shrink tumors remove pigmented lesions remove tattoos
pulsed dye	shallow penetration moderately hot tunable wavelength	port wine stain and other vascular birthmarks

of choice for BLOODLESS SURGERY as well as for treating vascular disorders of the skin such as birthmarks.

Because the intense light the laser generates can burn the RETINA and cause permanent blindness, people undergoing laser surgery as well as the surgeon and other members of the surgical team must wear EYE protection when the laser is in use.

Laser surgery has the same risks as conventional surgery for bleeding and infection, and carries additional risk for BURNS and related damage. A laser can permanently discolor the skin, particularly the skin of people of color (notably African Americans, Asian Americans, and Hispanic Americans). Lasers may also cause burns of the skin. Though laser surgery makes many operations easier and more comfortable, it is important to choose a surgeon who is qualified to perform laser surgery and to fully understand the potential benefits and risks of laser surgery compared to conventional surgery.

See also LASER SKIN RESURFACING; MINIMALLY INVASIVE SURGERY; OPEN SURGERY; PHOTOTHERAPEUTIC KERATECTOMY (PTK); REFRACTIVE SURGERY; SURGERY BENEFIT AND RISK ASSESSMENT; TATTOOS.

minimally invasive surgery Any OPERATION in which the surgeon uses an endoscope and specialized instruments to enter the body through small incisions, called ports. An endoscope is a lighted, flexible tube with a tiny camera at the tip that sends visual images of the operative site to a monitor similar to a television screen. The endoscope is specialized for the procedure, such as a laparoscope for operations within the abdominal cavity.

The surgeon watches the images on the screen rather than seeing the operative site directly. Minimally invasive surgery is in contrast to OPEN SURGERY, in which the surgeon makes an incision large enough to allow direct access to the operative site. Surgeons must receive specific training in the minimally invasive procedures they perform, which require special equipment and instruments. Surgeons sometimes combine minimally invasive procedures with LASER SURGERY, assisted open surgery, or other operative techniques.

Recovery time is typically faster and less painful than with open surgery as there is less intrusion into the body. Many minimally invasive surgery operations are ambulatory surgeries that do not require an overnight stay in the hospital. As is the case with any surgery, minimally invasive procedures carry some risk for ANESTHESIA complications, bleeding, and INFECTION.

See also AMBULATORY SURGERY; ENDOSCOPY; SURGERY BENEFIT AND RISK ASSESSMENT.

open surgery Any surgical OPERATION in which the surgeon makes an incision that allows direct access to the operative site. An open surgery incision may be quite large. Until the emergence of MINIMALLY INVASIVE SURGERY procedures in the 1980s open surgery was the standard of surgical treatment for nearly all operations. Surgeons today can perform many operations with minimally invasive techniques, reserving open surgery for circumstances in which the surgeon needs the broad exposure open surgery provides. Such circumstances include OPEN HEART SURGERY for operations such as CORONARY ARTERY BYPASS GRAFT (CABG) and heart valve replacement, open THORACOTOMY for operations on the LUNGS, open laparotomy for major operations on the structures of the abdomen such as the GALLBLADDER and intestines, and ORGAN TRANSPLANTATION. Common risks of any surgery include bleeding and INFECTION, which are somewhat more likely with open surgery than with minimally invasive surgery. As well, recovery and recuperation take longer with open surgery, generally 4 to 12 weeks, depending on the type of operation. Open surgery may also leave a more noticeable SCAR after HEALING.

See also ANESTHESIA; LASER SURGERY; SURGERY BENEFIT AND RISK ASSESSMENT.

operation A surgical procedure to enter the body and conduct a repair, remove a tumor, or in some other way alter a structure or organ. A surgical operation takes place under sterile conditions in a controlled environment, an operating room, used exclusively for surgery. Minor operations may take place in AMBULATORY SURGERY centers and specialized surgical clinics; major operations take place in hospitals that have sophisticated facilities and experienced staff to provide care before, during, and after surgery. Though traditionally the term *surgery* has applied to the medical specialty of

COMMON SURGICAL OPERATIONS	
Surgical Operation	**Purpose**
adenoidectomy	remove chronically infected and enlarged adenoids
APPENDECTOMY	remove an inflamed or infected APPENDIX
ATHERECTOMY	remove ATHEROSCLEROTIC PLAQUE deposits from within arteries
BLEPHAROPLASTY	repair or reconstruction of the eyelids
CHOLECYSTECTOMY	remove the GALLBLADDER
colectomy	remove part or all of the COLON
COLOSTOMY	create a passage from colon through the abdominal wall

Surgical Operation	Purpose
craniotomy	operations on the BRAIN and related structures, PITUITARY GLAND
cystectomy	remove the urinary BLADDER
ENDARTERECTOMY	remove an occlusion from an ARTERY
EPISIOTOMY	incision to widen the vaginal opening during CHILDBIRTH
GASTRECTOMY	remove part or all of the STOMACH
hernioplasty	repair of a HERNIA
HYSTERECTOMY	remove the UTERUS
LAMINECTOMY	remove a vertebral disk
laparotomy	operations on structures of the abdomen such as the intestines, LIVER, appendix, uterus, OVARIES, FALLOPIAN TUBES
LARYNGECTOMY	remove the larynx
lobectomy	remove a lobe of the LUNGS
MASTECTOMY	remove a BREAST
NEPHRECTOMY	remove a kidney
nephrotomy	remove a tumor or remove kidney stones
OOPHORECTOMY	remove ovaries
ORCHIECTOMY	remove a testicle
OTOPLASTY	repair or reconstruction of the outer EAR
pneumonectomy	remove an entire lung
PROSTATECTOMY	remove the PROSTATE GLAND
resection	remove (excise) a portion of a structure
RHINOPLASTY	repair or reconstruction of the NOSE
RHYTIDOPLASTY	repair or reconstruction of the face (facelift)
salpingectomy	remove a fallopian tube
SPLENECTOMY	remove the SPLEEN

Surgical Operation	Purpose
THORACOTOMY	operations on structures within the chest except the HEART
tonsillectomy	remove chronically infected and enlarged tonsils
TRACHEOSTOMY	create a passage from the TRACHEA through the surface of the neck
TYMPANOPLASTY	repair or reconstruction of the TYMPANIC MEMBRANE (eardrum)
VASECTOMY	remove a segment of the VAS DEFERENS

surgery, many people now use the terms *operation* and *surgery* interchangeably.

See also ARTHROSCOPY; BARIATRIC SURGERY; CARDIAC CATHETERIZATION; CATARACT EXTRACTION AND LENS REPLACEMENT; CESAREAN SECTION; ENDOSCOPY; JOINT REPLACEMENT; LASER SURGERY; MINIMALLY INVASIVE SURGERY; MOHS' SURGERY; PLASTIC SURGERY; REFRACTIVE SURGERY; SURGERY BENEFIT AND RISK ASSESSMENT; TUBAL LIGATION.

organ transplantation The surgical replacement of a nonfunctioning vital organ with a functional organ acquired from a donor. Most donor organs are allogeneic, also called deceased donation or cadaver donation, in which a specialized surgical team removes the donated organs after a person's death when the person has previously authorized, or when the person's family authorizes at the time of the person's death, organ donation. In some circumstances a person may make a living organ donation to another person, such as for kidney, lung lobe, and partial LIVER. US surgeons perform almost 27,000 organ transplantations each year, nearly 7,000 of which are organs from living donors. The most commonly transplanted organs are KIDNEYS and livers. However, approximately 89,000 people remain on waiting lists for donor organs.

TRANSPLANTED ORGANS AND TISSUES		
BONE MARROW	CORNEA	HEART
ISLETS OF LANGERHANS cells	kidney	LIVER
lung	PANCREAS	SKIN
SMALL INTESTINE	stem cells	

Organ Allocation and Acquisition
Organ transplantation transitioned from experimental to mainstream in the 1980s, riding a wave of technologic advances and the success of cyclosporine, the first effective immunosuppressive DRUG. In 1984 the US Congress passed the National Organ Transplant Act (NOTA), which established the Organ Procurement and Transplantation Network (OPTN) to ensure consistency and equity in the allocation of deceased donor organs. OPTN is a not-for-profit organization that is a collaborative union of public and private organizations. The United Network for Organ Sharing (UNOS) administers OPTN under contract to the US Department of Health and Human Services. Hospital transplant programs across the United States determine a person's eligibility for transplantation, then submit the person's name and health data (such as organ needed and blood type) to the UNOS database.

A regional organ procurement organization (OPO) receives notification from hospitals and other health-care providers when deceased donor organs become available within its geographic boundaries. The OPO coordinates the effort to match the organs with appropriate donors, initiating a "match run" from the UNOS database. The match run identifies prospective transplant recipients waiting for the particular kind of organ, the medical urgency of the transplant need, the general health circumstances, and the geographic proximity of the donor organ to the prospective recipient. The matched names go on a list for the organ, ranked in order of need. UNOS generates a new match run each time an organ becomes available, specific for each kind of organ, so a waiting recipient may appear on several lists and in different rankings relative to others on the same list.

The available organ goes to the waiting recipient who is the best match on as many criteria as possible. For organs such as the HEART and LUNGS, geographic proximity is a critical factor because the window of opportunity for transplantation is so short. Body size may be important for organs such as the liver, heart, and lungs. Typically gender and ethnicity or race are not factors for vascularized organ transplants unless they influence body size. Financial status is not a consideration under any circumstances. Living donor transplants are not subject to OPTN/UNOS procedures but rather are coordinated privately between the donor and the recipient.

Organ Transplantation Surgery

Transplantation of vascularized (solid) organs is major surgery that may require the organ recipient to be prepared for surgery within hours of notification that an organ is available. Time is especially critical for heart, lung, and heart–lung transplantation. In most transplant operations the surgeon transplants a single organ. Combination transplantations are becoming more common, however, with surgeons transplanting together heart and lung, SMALL INTESTINE and liver, or kidney and pancreas. The operation to transplant a single organ may take three to five hours; combination transplants may take longer. The transplant recipient may remain hospitalized for several weeks after surgery, depending on the organ, rate of recovery, and overall health status.

With some organs, such as kidneys, the surgeon can leave the native organ in place and transplant the donor organ in an adjacent location. This is a heterotopic transplant. The surgeon may also choose to remove the recipient's native, diseased organ and transplant the donor organ in its place, such as the liver. This is an orthotopic transplant. One approach is not necessarily easier or more effective than the other for either the surgeon or the recipient. Circumstances that shape the decision include the recipient's general health status, anatomic characteristics, and the organ being transplanted.

Life after Transplantation

The course of recovery after transplantation varies with the organ transplanted, age, and overall health circumstances. Most organ transplant recipients are able to return to previous work, recreational, and lifestyle activities they enjoyed before experiencing the health circumstances that made their transplants necessary, usually within two to three months. Transplant recipients do require ongoing medical assessment and care, which may consist of doctor visits every few weeks for the first 6 to 12 months after the transplant and every 6 to 12 months indefinitely, depending on the organ transplanted and general health status.

The key health risks after transplantation are primary organ failure and organ rejection. Primary organ failure occurs when the organ does not function after transplantation. The organ may start to function and then stop or may never begin functioning. Some organs, such as the kidneys, may take several weeks to several months to start functioning or to function normally, which is the usual course of events for them and does not necessarily indicate that the transplant has failed. It is not unheard of for a kidney transplant recipient to require renal hemodialysis after the transplant OPERATION, and hemodialysis remains a therapeutic option when a transplanted kidney does fail. Primary organ failure of the heart, lungs, or liver is a medical emergency that requires retransplantation as soon as possible. Numerous and often collusive factors may account for primary organ failure of a transplant.

Organ rejection occurs when the recipient's IMMUNE SYSTEM produces antibodies that attack the transplanted organ and is a process rather than an event. Every transplant experiences rejection to some degree because rejection represents the body's natural IMMUNE RESPONSE. Organ rejection may be acute or chronic. Acute rejection develops rapidly and may present symptoms similar to a viral INFECTION such as the flu, though often there is tenderness or PAIN at the site of the transplant. Acute rejection requires immediate medical treatment with immunosuppressive agents to attempt to subdue the immune response and minimize damage to the organ. Episodes of acute rejection are common in the first year after transplantation and can occur months to years later. A single episode of acute rejection is seldom enough to cause organ failure, especially when treatment is prompt.

IMMUNOSUPPRESSIVE AGENTS TO MINIMIZE ORGAN REJECTION

Induction and Antirejection (up to 30 days)

Atgam	basiliximab
daclizumab	methylprednisolone
muromonab CD3	rapamycin
Thymoglobulin	

Maintenance (long-term)

azathioprine	cyclosporine
mycophenolate mofetil	prednisone
rapamycin	tacrolimus

Chronic organ rejection represents the steady and slow consequences of the immune system's efforts to eliminate the organ, which the immune system perceives as an "intruder." At present the standard of treatment to minimize organ rejection is lifelong IMMUNOSUPPRESSIVE THERAPY, taking drugs that suppress the immune response. Doctors monitor immune status and transplanted organ function with regular BLOOD tests. The risks of long-term immunosuppression include increased vulnerability to infection (such as COLDS, flu, and OPPORTUNISTIC INFECTIONS), which may require ANTIBIOTIC PROPHYLAXIS or ANTIFUNGAL MEDICATIONS. Long-term immunosuppression also increases the risk for lymphoma and MULTIPLE MYELOMA, two cancers of the immune system; when detected early these cancers are easily treatable. Immunosuppressive agents also have numerous drug interactions and potential side effects.

Organ Donation

Nearly anyone can be an organ donor. Most US states incorporate organ donation permission on driver's licenses. A driver's license is the most common form of identification Americans carry, and MOTOR VEHICLE ACCIDENTS are the most common cause of unexpected death. As well, organ donation authorization forms are available at hospitals, medical centers, doctor's offices, public health departments, and other providers of health-care services. Some states also have donor registries. A person age 18 or older can authorize organ donation for himself or herself; a parent or legal guardian must authorize organ donation for a person under the age of 18. It is also a good idea for a person who desires to donate his or her organs after death to let a close relative or friend know of this intention. Such knowledge eases the decision-making process family members may face.

Doctors must follow accepted standards of practice for determining when BRAIN DEATH (irreversible loss of complete BRAIN function) has occurred or the person is pronounced dead, after which they may seek the family's permission to proceed. The removal of donated organs, called organ retrieval or organ harvesting, takes place in an operating room under sterile conditions. The window of opportunity for transplanting a donated organ ranges from 4 hours after harvesting for a heart, 6 hours for lungs, 12 hours for liver, and to up to 24 hours for a kidney. Special preservative solutions and methods (such as pulsatile perfusion, which moves chilled preservative fluid through the organ) help keep organs viable until transplantation.

NO COST FOR DONOR ORGANS AND TISSUES
Federal law in the United States prohibits buying and selling human organs and tissues. Organs and tissues for transplantation must come from donors. The expenses associated with organ transplantation are those of medical care before and after the transplantation and for the transplant operation and its related costs (such as for hospitalization). There is no cost for being on the organ donor registry or for donor organs and tissues.

Surgeons carefully remove organs to preserve them as intactly as possible. Harvesting of hearts and lungs must be take place before the heart stops, which requires certification of brain death and often life support to maintain oxygenation and BLOOD circulation until the organ retrieval team can remove them. When doctors cannot use the entire organ, they sometimes can make use of key parts. For example, a heart that has significant myocardial damage due to HEART ATTACK may have healthy valves, which doctors can harvest for heart valve replacement. There is no cost to the person's family for harvesting donated organs, nor is there disfiguration of the donor's body. Under US medical confidentiality laws, the donor remains anonymous to the recipient and the recipient remains anonymous to the donor's family.

Availability of donor organs remains the most significant challenge for organ transplantation, which has become the standard of care for END-STAGE RENAL DISEASE (ESRD), end-stage HEART FAILURE, and end-stage LIVER FAILURE. The need for donor organs is about four times greater than the availability. The US government maintains a Web site (www.organdonor.gov) to provide information updates about organ donation and a downloadable organ donor card. Another Web site (www.transplantliving.org) provides comprehensive information from OPTN/UNOS about the entire organ transplantation process, from eligibility for transplantation to life after receiving a transplant.

See also ANESTHESIA; BLOOD TRANSFUSION; CIRRHOSIS; EPSTEIN-BARR VIRUS; GRAFT VERSUS HOST DISEASE; HEART TRANSPLANTATION; ISLET CELL TRANSPLANTATION; KIDNEY TRANSPLANTATION; LIVER TRANSPLANTATION; LUNG TRANSPLANTATION; SKIN REPLACEMENT; SURGERY BENEFIT AND RISK ASSESSMENT.

patient controlled analgesia (PCA) The postoperative self-administration of intravenous (IV) PAIN relief (analgesic) medication. PCA requires an IV (a thin catheter inserted into a VEIN), a PCA pump that contains a special syringe with the pain medication, and a PCA control button. Each time the person depresses the PCA button the PCA pump releases a certain amount of pain medication from the syringe into the IV. Most people feel pain relief within a few minutes of pressing the button.

The PCA pump can release medication only according to the amount and frequency for which it is programmed, no matter how often the person presses the button, so there is no danger of receiving too much. An alarm on the PCA pump notifies nursing staff when the amount of medication in the syringe gets low or when there is any disruption of the pump's proper function. The PCA pump may also be programmed to deliver a steady flow of pain relief medication, with extra medication released with the button as the person needs it to maintain comfort.

Numerous studies show that people tend to have less anxiety about postoperative pain and pain relief and use less pain relief medication with PCA. As well, appropriate pain control facilitates faster HEALING. Within a few days after an OPERATION most people are able to switch to oral (by MOUTH) pain medications.

See also ANALGESIC MEDICATIONS; SURGERY BENEFIT AND RISK ASSESSMENT.

plastic surgery Any surgical OPERATION to alter the appearance of a body area or part. Plastic surgery may be reconstructive (re-creates or repairs a body part that is damaged or missing) or cosmetic (changes physical appearance for reasons of personal preference). Though both disciplines encompass elective operations, the US health-care system considers reconstructive surgery to be medically necessary; therefore, health insurance plans typically pay for reconstructive operations. Cosmetic surgery operations are not medically necessary and health insurance plans seldom pay for them.

In some circumstances the nature of a plastic surgery operation overlaps between cosmetic and reconstructive. For example, a person may desire RHINOPLASTY (NOSE alteration) because of dissatisfaction with the nose's appearance, though the surgeon's examination leads to the discovery that the person also has a deviated septum, which affects BREATHING and the health of the SINUSES. A person may seek plastic surgery to alter the perception of aging that arises from drooping eyelids, and then discover the eyelids obscure the field of vision.

Reconstructive Surgery

Reconstructive surgery rebuilds missing or lost structures with the goal to restore function. The loss may be due to numerous factors that include CONGENITAL ANOMALY, traumatic injury, BURNS, disease processes, and surgical treatment for conditions such as cancer. Reconstructive surgery is often complex and requires multiple operations to achieve the desired result. Reconstructive operations performed in childhood may need revision as the child grows. Reconstructive surgeons may coordinate care and treatment with surgeons and physicians in other specialties such as orthopedics (bones and connective tissues) and neurology (nerves). Doctors often request a plastic surgeon to suture or otherwise repair LACERATIONS and wounds to the face or hands. Plastic surgeons perform about five million operations a year in the United States.

MOST COMMON RECONSTRUCTIVE OPERATIONS

BREAST reconstruction	CONGENITAL ANOMALY reconstruction
laceration repair	operations on the hands and fingers
SCAR revision	tumor removal

Cosmetic Surgery

Cosmetic surgery alters appearance for aesthetic reasons and can have profound psychological and emotional benefits. US plastic surgeons perform more than nine million cosmetic surgery procedures a year, with Americans spending more than $8 billion to have them performed. Surveys suggest people who undergo cosmetic surgery are generally satisfied with the results, perceiving improvements in self-image and social interactions. Realistic expectations are especially important when making cosmetic surgery decisions. Some cosmetic operations, such as RHYTIDOPLASTY (facelift), have long-lasting though not permanent effects because the SKIN and connective tissues continue to undergo natural changes with aging.

MOST COMMON COSMETIC OPERATIONS

abdominoplasty	augmentation mammoplasty
BLEPHAROPLASTY	body contouring after significant
liposuction	weight loss
RHYTIDOPLASTY	

Plastic Surgery Benefits and Risks

The benefits of plastic surgery often encompass improved function, appearance, and self-image or self-esteem. Specific benefits vary with the operation and often are not entirely apparent for weeks to months after the operation when HEALING is complete. As with all operations, plastic surgery operations entail risk. General risks include excessive bleeding during or after surgery, postoperative wound INFECTION, PNEUMONIA (a complication of general ANESTHESIA), unpredictable SCAR formation, and unsatisfactory or unexpected results. Death during or as a complication of plastic surgery is very rare though can occur. Cigarette smoking, DIABETES, and PERIPHERAL VASCULAR DISEASE (PVD) can limit peripheral BLOOD circulation, slowing healing and increasing the risk for complications.

It is not possible for the surgeon to guarantee the outcome of a plastic surgery operation. People sometimes have unrealistic expectations for what the operation can achieve, leading to dissatisfac-

tion with the results. It is crucial to thoroughly understand what the operation can and cannot accomplish and the full spectrum of potential complications and risks; it is equally important to select a qualified (board-certified) plastic surgeon who is experienced in performing the desired operation and who performs surgeries in an appropriately credentialed and licensed facility.

PLASTIC SURGERY OPERATIONS

abdominoplasty	augmentation mammoplasty
BIRTHMARK removal or reduction	BLEPHAROPLASTY
	body contouring
brachioplasty	BREAST reconstruction
brow lift	cervicoplasty
facial implants	HAIR transplantation
laceration repair	LASER SKIN RESURFACING
lip augmentation	lipoplasty
liposuction	mastopexy
mentoplasty	OTOPLASTY
panniculectomy	platysmaplasty
POLYDACTYLY correction and reconstruction	reduction mammoplasty
	RHINOPLASTY
RHYTIDOPLASTY	SCAR revision
sclerotherapy	SKIN graft
SYNDACTYLY release	tissue flap surgery

See also BARIATRIC SURGERY; BOTULINUM THERAPY; CHEMICAL PEEL; DERMABRASION; HAIR TRANSPLANTATION; LASER SURGERY; SMOKING CESSATION; SURGERY BENEFIT AND RISK ASSESSMENT; WOUND CARE.

postoperative procedures The events that take place to guide a person's safe and comfortable recovery from ANESTHESIA and to initiate effective PAIN relief after a surgical OPERATION. When the operation is over the person goes to a postanesthesia care unit (PACU) where staff monitor vital signs (HEART RATE, BREATHING rate, BLOOD PRESSURE, and body temperature) and emergence from anesthesia. A person who has had regional or general anesthesia may remain in the PACU for two to four hours, until he or she regains the ability to use the anesthetized region of the body or regains CONSCIOUSNESS.

It is common and normal to feel disoriented when first coming out of anesthesia. Many people who have had general anesthesia do not realize the operation is over. It is also normal to feel chilled and to experience discomfort, numbness, or pain. The surgeon may infiltrate the operative site with a local anesthetic to provide localized pain relief for 12 to 24 hours after the operation or place tiny catheters in the surgical wound to instill a continuous irrigation of a local anesthetic for extended pain relief. Most often the person is already receiving analgesic medications to relieve pain and generally receives PATIENT CONTROLLED ANALGESIA (PCA) during the recovery period. When fully stable the person may go to a room in the hospital, if an overnight stay in the hospital is necessary, or home to recover and recuperate. Before discharge the PACU staff provide instructions for WOUND CARE, pain management, possible complications such as unusual bleeding, and follow-up appointments with the surgeon.

See also PREOPERATIVE PROCEDURES; SURGERY BENEFIT AND RISK ASSESSMENT.

preoperative procedures The events that take place to prepare a person for a surgical OPERATION. Preoperative procedures for elective (nonemergency) operations may begin several days to a week before the scheduled surgery with activities such as

- preoperative consultation with the surgeon or a member of the surgeon's staff to discuss the preparations for surgery, including any revisions to routine medications, dietary restrictions, LAXATIVES or ENEMA, or SKIN-cleansing procedures as well as expectations for the operation's outcome and the anticipated recovery period
- signing of informed consent documents that specify, in detail, the planned operation and the reasons for it, the scope of surgery the surgeon may perform, and the operation's possible complications and risks
- routine BLOOD tests to assess blood cell counts, HEMOGLOBIN level, COAGULATION (clotting) times, LIVER function, and kidney function
- possible chest X-RAY, ELECTROCARDIOGRAM (ECG), and other diagnostic testing, depending on the operation and the person's health status and age

- consultation with the anesthesiologist or anesthetist to determine the optimal anesthesia choices for the person's health status and the planned operation
- health insurance preauthorization or financial arrangements

The doctor will provide instructions about not eating for a specified period of time before the scheduled operation, and about taking any daily medications on the day of the operation.

Before signing informed consent documents, it is crucial to fully understand the scope of the planned OPERATION, the expected benefits of the operation, the anticipated course of recovery, and possible complications and risks of the operation and of the ANESTHESIA.

Most people arrive at the AMBULATORY SURGERY FACILITY or hospital surgery unit several hours before the scheduled time of the operation. In preparation for the operation, a person undresses and puts on a surgical gown. The preoperative nurse starts an intravenous (IV) infusion to maintain HYDRATION and to administer medications. Surgical staff may apply electrodes to the chest to monitor HEART RATE, place a BLOOD PRESSURE cuff around the arm to monitor blood pressure, and place a PULSE oximeter over the tip a finger to monitor blood oxygenation. Some surgical facilities allow a family member or close friend to be present during these early preparations. The surgeon or assistant surgeon often visits the person before sedation or anesthesia begins to confirm the person's identity, the planned operation, and the location of the operative site (such as left leg or right BREAST). Other staff may also make these same confirmations to prevent errors. Many surgeons use a marking pen on the skin to identify the operative site. As the time for the operation to begin draws near, most people receive a sedative for relaxation and comfort.

See also POSTOPERATIVE PROCEDURES; SURGERY BENEFIT AND RISK ASSESSMENT.

S

surgery benefit and risk assessment Objective evaluation of the reasons and expectations for a surgical OPERATION. Surgery is a common therapeutic approach today, with surgeons in the United States performing more than 25 million operations a year. Risks and complications related to surgery and ANESTHESIA have declined dramatically over the past three decades, making surgery one of the safest and most effective treatments for many health conditions. However, surgery is often not the only therapeutic option for a particular condition or health circumstance. It is important to fully understand

- the specific operation the surgeon recommends and why
- the expected benefits of the operation
- other surgical operations that might also treat the problem
- the possible nonsurgical treatments for the condition
- the potential risks of the operation itself
- how the operation's risks compare to the risks of other treatment options (including nontreatment) for the condition

Some people need time to think through their options, the reasons the surgeon recommends the operation, and the possible complications of the operation. There is usually no hurry to schedule an elective operation, though symptoms such as PAIN may make the scheduling timely. It is often helpful to write down questions and concerns, then schedule an appointment with the surgeon to discuss them before making the decision to proceed with surgery.

The surgeon who will perform the operation should be qualified and experienced. Many hospitals are teaching centers where surgical residents (trained physicians who are learning advanced skills in surgery) participate in operations. They do so under the direction and close supervision of the primary surgeon. Teaching hospitals are required to obtain signed permission for staff who are in training (physicians, nurses, and ancillary staff) to participate in care delivery, including surgery. As well, for most operations the surgeon has at least one other surgeon assisting him or her. A person should know who will actually be performing the operation and the other doctors who will be assisting because these are factors that may influence the outcome of the surgery.

Surgery Benefits

The benefits of surgery are numerous and mostly specific to the planned operation. In general, surgery corrects or repairs defects, injuries, functions, or appearance. Surgery may be lifesaving, as in major trauma or CORONARY ARTERY BYPASS GRAFT (CABG), and is the first line of treatment for many forms of cancer. Surgery may also be palliative, such as to reduce pain, pressure, or other discomforts that may occur in chronic health conditions such as NEUROPATHY or terminal cancer. It is important to discuss with the surgeon the anticipated or hoped for benefits of the recommended operation.

POTENTIAL BENEFITS OF SURGERY	
correct congenital defects	improved appearance
relieve intractable PAIN	improved function
treat injuries or conditions	removal of tumors

277

Surgery Risks

All operations have general as well as specific risks. General risks include excessive bleeding, wound INFECTION, PNEUMONIA, and death resulting from unanticipated crisis during the operation (such as HEART ATTACK or STROKE). Surgeon error is also a risk for any operation.

Personal health factors that increase surgical and anesthetic risks include cigarette smoking, ALCOHOL use, OBESITY, DIABETES, CHRONIC OBSTRUCTIVE PULMONARY DISEASE (COPD), HYPERTENSION (high BLOOD PRESSURE), CYSTIC FIBROSIS, and CORONARY ARTERY DISEASE (CAD). Numerous medications (including herbal products, over-the-counter products, and illicit drugs) can interfere with anesthesia, BLOOD clotting, or HEALING.

Age alone does not increase risk for surgical complications. However with advancing age the likelihood of numerous health conditions increases, many of which can remain undetected until a stress such as anesthesia or surgery brings them to the forefront of the person's health picture. Such health conditions may include type 2 diabetes, ATHEROSCLEROSIS, CAD, renal (kidney) disease, LIVER disease, and sometimes hypertension.

POSSIBLE RISKS OF SURGERY	
ANESTHESIA reaction	death
excessive bleeding during or after surgery	failure of the OPERATION to resolve the condition
intestinal adhesions	need for BLOOD TRANSFUSION
nerve injury	outcome other than expected
PNEUMONIA	unacceptable SCAR appearance
worsening of health condition	wound INFECTION

Second Opinion Consultation

A second opinion is an assessment from another specialist who provides treatment for the same condition for which the surgeon recommends an operation. The specialist is often another surgeon though may practice in a different subspecialty of surgery. For example, a person considering back surgery as treatment for HERNIATED NUCLEUS PULPOSUS ("ruptured disk") may have a surgery recommendation from an orthopedic surgeon and seek a second opinion from neurologist, as both specialties treat back problems. A person may also seek a second opinion from a specialist who is not a sur-

geon, who may recommend nonsurgical treatment options.

Because there are often numerous options for treating a particular health problem and surgery is inherently invasive (a treatment that enters the body), health experts recommend a second opinion consultation for most elective (nonemergency) operations. People sometimes worry that seeking a second opinion will offend the first surgeon in some way. However, current standards of practice support second opinions, and surgeons are themselves often the first to recommend them. Some health insurance plans require second opinion consultation for certain, and sometimes all elective, operations.

The second opinion surgeon or physician should

- be board-certified in an appropriate and relevant specialty

- practice in a different group or facility from that of the first surgeon

- know the consultation is for a second opinion

ELECTIVE OPERATIONS FOR WHICH HEALTH EXPERTS URGE A SECOND OPINION CONSULTATION	
adenoidectomy	cancer operations
carpal tunnel surgery	CATARACT EXTRACTION AND LENS REPLACEMENT
CHOLECYSTECTOMY	
CORONARY ARTERY BYPASS GRAFT (CABG)	DILATION AND CURETTAGE (D&C)
	HERNIA repair
hemorrhoidectomy	HYSTERECTOMY
JOINT REPLACEMENT	knee surgery
MASTECTOMY	PROSTATECTOMY
tonsillectomy	vein ligation and stripping

The surgeon or physician providing the second opinion consultation will require medical records, diagnostic procedure reports, laboratory test results, and other information relevant to the condition. The doctor will conduct a thorough examination of the person, then discuss the findings and his or her professional opinions about the possible treatments. The second opinion may or may not support the initial recommendation for the operation. The person may choose which physician or surgeon will provide the recommended care. A complex health circumstance may require multiple consultations from different specialists, in which case it may be helpful to have one's primary-care doctor assist in sorting through the options, benefits, and risks.

Informed Consent

Informed consent documents describe in detail the proposed operation, reason for the operation, recommended anesthesia options, expected benefits, and possible complications and risks. Informed consent is required before the operation may begin for all surgeries except in certain life-threatening circumstances. The informed consent documents should contain no surprises or new information; if they do, it is important to discuss the situation with the surgeon before signing them. In some circumstances the surgeon may request advance permission to perform a more extensive operation than planned, depending on the findings during the surgical operation. This permits the surgeon to do what needs to be done in a single operation rather than having the person go through a second procedure.

See also CANCER TREATMENT OPTIONS AND DECISIONS; QUALITY OF LIFE.

wound care The care necessary, including cleansing and dressing changes, to keep surgical incisions, or wounds, healthy as they heal. Most surgical wounds heal quickly and without complication and require very little care beyond keeping them clean and dry for one to five days after surgery. Redness at the incision line is normal, though the surgeon should evaluate any redness that extends farther than one half inch from the incision because this may indicate INFECTION. Sometimes there is bruising (ECCHYMOSIS) around the incision site, which typically heals in about a week.

By the fifth postoperative day the edges of the wound should be adhered to each other, with or without an obvious scab. Most scabs fall off 10 to 14 days after surgery, which indicates the incision is fully closed and about 85 percent healed. Factors that influence HEALING include DIABETES, cigarette smoking, and OBESITY.

Full healing is complete in three months. The SCAR may at first appear reddened and raised, though after about six months most scars are flush with the SKIN's surface and are pink or white. A scar generally continues to fade over time and remains lighter in color than the surrounding skin. Incisional scars are more sensitive than the surrounding skin to sun exposure and should be protected with SPF (sun protective factor) 30 sunscreen or clothing to prevent SUNBURN.

Skin Closures

A surgeon closes a surgical wound from the inside out, typically using fine sutures (threads that sew the tissue edges together) to bring together the layers of MUSCLE, FASCIA, and subcutaneous fat. These sutures, commonly called stitches, dissolve over 5 to 7 days as the tissues heal. The surgeon may use sutures, staples (small wires that pull together the edges of the skin), glue, or adhesive strips to close the final layer of the skin. The method of closure depends on the incision's location and length, the tension on the skin edges, and the surgeon's preference. The surgeon may use a combination of closure methods for large or abdominal incisions. The surgeon must remove staples and nondissolving sutures, typically 3 to 10 days after the OPERATION, though often recommends leaving the adhesive strips in place until they fall off on their own, usually in about 5 days. Staple or suture removal is quick and usually does not hurt, though some people find the minor pulling and tugging sensations uncomfortable or disconcerting.

Dressings and Dressing Changes

At the end of the operation the surgeon will place a surgical dressing over the incision site. The dressing is typically absorbent, as it is normal for the wound to bleed a little, and may be a pressure dressing to limit the amount of bleeding. The surgical dressing stays on for 24 hours, after which the surgeon, if the person stays overnight in the hospital, or the person may remove it. A larger incision may require replacement dressings for the next 72 hours, after which most incisions remain uncovered though some surgeons may instruct that the incision site remain covered for a longer period. When applying a fresh dressing, it is important to wash the hands with warm water and soap before touching bandages or the surgical wound. The surgeon may instruct the application of an antibiotic ointment. The surgeon will remove nondissolving skin sutures or staples 3 to 10 days after the operation, after which the incision is fairly well healed.

Postoperative Complications

Infection is the most common postoperative wound complication. Rarely a surgical wound may bleed. Though some degree of bleeding at the incision for the first 24 hours after surgery is normal for most operations, bleeding that saturates the bandage requires immediate assessment by the surgeon or hospital nursing staff. Extended irritation at the incision site (redness farther than one half inch from the incision), pus, and FEVER are early indications of infection that the surgeon needs to evaluate. Obesity, diabetes, and PERIPHERAL VASCULAR DISEASE (PVD) can affect the circulation of BLOOD in the body, particularly to the limbs. People who have these conditions should be alert to changes in the surgical wound that could suggest infection.

Discomfort or PAIN is a common and expected complication for a period of time after the operation, the severity and duration of which depends on the kind of operation. Restricting use of the operated area minimizes discomfort. The surgeon will prescribe appropriate ANALGESIC MEDICATIONS to relieve pain.

Return to Bathing or Showering and Normal Activities

Most surgical wounds are closed enough to permit showering 24 to 48 hours after surgery. Getting the incision wet does not affect the skin closures (sutures, staples, or adhesive strips). Bathing (sitting in a tub of water) should wait until the incision is completely healed (2 to 3 weeks), unless it is possible to sit in the water without getting the incision wet. Soaking in bath water softens the skin at the incision's edges and may allow BACTERIA to gain entrance, causing infection. The full return to normal activities depends on the operation and the person's individual rate of healing and can take place anytime from a few days to 3 months.

See also SURGERY BENEFIT AND RISK ASSESSMENT.

NOSOCOMIAL WOUND INFECTION

About 500,000 of the 27 million Americans who undergo surgery every year develop postoperative wound infections. About 25 percent of postoperative infections are nosocomial (also called iatrogenic)—that is, they occur as a consequence of exposure to pathogens in the hospital environment. Proper wound care minimizes the risk for INFECTION of any kind and supports optimal HEALING.

LIFESTYLE VARIABLES: SMOKING AND OBESITY

The two lifestyle variables that have emerged in recent years as the key causes of preventable disease are smoking and OBESITY. Each represents a complex mingling of contributory factors, many within the reach of individual control. These variables span health-care specialties; practitioners in nearly all fields of medicine address health issues that derive from either or both. Between them, smoking and obesity account for nearly all preventable HEART disease and many types of cancer.

This section, "Lifestyle Variables: Smoking and Obesity," presents an overview discussion of smoking and obesity as they contribute to health conditions. The entries in this section focus on the health consequences of smoking and obesity, including weight management topics. The section "Nutrition and Diet" features an overview discussion and entries that focus on the broad context of nutrition and diet in health and the development of health conditions. Similarly the section "Fitness: Exercise and Health" features an overview discussion and entries that focus on the broad context of physical activity in health and the development of health conditions.

Lifestyle and Smoking

Cigarette smoking attained social status in the 1920s when soldiers returning from World War I brought their habit home with them. Cigarette smoking became fashionable across social strata, a mark of sophistication and success. But as early as the 1940s doctors recognized that many of their patients who had heart disease or lung disease, including LUNG CANCER, were smokers. Numerous research studies soon confirmed and detailed the specific health risks of smoking, which are extensive. In 1964 the US Surgeon General released the landmark report, *Smoking and Health: Report of the Advisory Committee to the Surgeon General of the Public Health Service,* which presented in fairly stark detail the known and suspected health conse-quences of cigarette smoking. The report's publi-cation was a wake-up call for doctors as well as the general public, nearly 45 percent of whom were smokers.

Over the next 40 years concerted education efforts resulted in cutting the number of smokers nearly in half. However, the health consequences of smoking skyrocketed. CARDIOVASCULAR DISEASE (CVD) became the leading cause of death, and ciga-rette smoking was identified as the leading cause of CVD. Lung cancer became the leading cause of death from cancer, and cigarette smoking was identified as the leading cause of lung cancer.

Over the decades, research unequivocally linked cigarette smoking with oral cancer, laryn-geal cancer, ESOPHAGEAL CANCER, PANCREATIC CANCER, BLADDER CANCER, PROSTATE CANCER, RENAL CANCER, STOMACH CANCER, and LIVER CANCER. Cigarette smoking proved responsible for most nonallergic ASTHMA, CHRONIC OBSTRUCTIVE PULMONARY DISEASE (COPD), and chronic BRONCHITIS. Researchers also affirmed that ENVIRONMENTAL CIGARETTE SMOKE (sec-ondhand smoke) caused these same health condi-tions in nonsmokers and was also responsible for most chronic upper respiratory conditions in chil-dren.

By the early 2000s many cities in the United States outlawed cigarette smoking in public build-ings and restaurants went smoke-free or estab-lished separate dining areas for smokers and nonsmokers. Hospitals also banned smoking. By

2004—40 years after the first surgeon general's report on smoking and health—48 million American adults remained smokers, fewer than a quarter of the US adult population, and the number of new smokers reached an all-time low. Nonetheless, cigarette smoking remains the leading cause of CVD, cancer, chronic lung disease, and premature death in the United States.

Lifestyle and Obesity

Cultural and social perceptions strongly influence the extent to which people understand the health risks and consequences of obesity, representing a complex intertwining of personal accountability and societal pressures. Until the 20th century being overweight was a sign of personal prosperity and even a hallmark of health. The corpulent individual was one who could afford unlimited access to food and indulged in its luxury. No correlation as yet existed to link obesity with common and debilitating ailments such as "dropsy" (the generalized edema of congestive HEART FAILURE) and "quinsy" (ANGINA PECTORIS, a symptom of CORONARY ARTERY DISEASE [CAD]). As doctors began to recognize the health implications of obesity a key challenge that emerged was that of convincing people of the connections between health, longevity, and body weight.

Despite what now amounts to decades of scientific evidence, misperceptions persist about the roles of EATING HABITS, food choices, and daily physical activity in WEIGHT LOSS AND WEIGHT MANAGEMENT efforts. Furthermore, food is essential for life—unlike cigarettes and ALCOHOL, which also influence health. One cannot simply stop eating as one can stop smoking or drinking alcohol (which are not easy accomplishments themselves). As is the case with cigarette smoking, the health consequences of obesity accumulate slowly over decades, lulling a person into believing that nothing adverse is happening in his or her body. The first recognition that obesity is a health problem often comes when the doctor diagnoses a health condition such as OBSTRUCTIVE SLEEP APNEA or HYPERTENSION and prescribes weight loss among the treatment recommendations.

For many people with class 2 or 3 obesity, the prospect of losing enough weight to have an effect on health is daunting if not overwhelming and often requires medical assistance. Yet even the loss of 10 or 20 pounds over six months, a goal most people can reach simply by adding 30 minutes of walking to every day's activities, makes a measurable difference in health. Health improvements are apparent almost immediately and extend as weight loss continues. Some people are able to stop taking medications to treat conditions such as hypertension and type 2 DIABETES when their weight reaches healthier levels.

Between 1990 and 1999 the percentage of American adults who have obesity doubled. In 2001 the US Office of the Surgeon General issued *The Surgeon General's Call to Action to Prevent and Decrease Overweight and Obesity*, another landmark report identifying obesity as a significant as well as preventable cause of hypertension, type 2 diabetes, ATHEROSCLEROSIS, OSTEOARTHRITIS, and numerous types of cancer. Weight loss became an explicit health objective in HEALTHY PEOPLE 2010, the US national agenda for public health improvement. Many health experts believe obesity, which affects more than 55 million American adults, now rivals cigarette smoking for its deleterious effects on health.

A–B

abdominal adiposity The accumulation of body fat around the middle of the trunk, forming the "apple" body shape or the "spare tire" appearance. Abdominal adiposity has emerged as a pattern of fat storage that correlates to an increased risk for CARDIOVASCULAR DISEASE (CVD) and particularly HEART ATTACK. Doctors assess abdominal adiposity using WAIST CIRCUMFERENCE and WAIST TO HIP RATIO measurements. Reducing abdominal adiposity through weight loss correspondingly lowers related health risks. Abdominal adiposity may become a particular concern for women after MENOPAUSE when hormonal influences can shift fat storage patterns within a woman's body.

A person can be of healthy weight and still have abdominal adiposity because abdominal adiposity is a mechanism of fat distribution in the inner tissues of the abdomen such as around the vital organs. A person who is of healthy weight but who has abdominal adiposity often appears to have a somewhat thickened trunk and thin arms and legs, carrying the traditional "apple" body shape even though he or she does not look overweight. In this circumstance health experts recommend more physical activity to lower the BODY FAT PERCENTAGE. With overall reduction in body fat the trunk stores less fat, lowering the health risks associated with abdominal adiposity.

HEALTH CONDITIONS ASSOCIATED WITH ABDOMINAL ADIPOSITY

ATHEROSCLEROSIS	CORONARY ARTERY DISEASE (CAD)
HEART ATTACK	HYPERLIPIDEMIA
HYPERTENSION	ISCHEMIC HEART DISEASE (IHD)
PERIPHERAL VASCULAR DISEASE (PVD)	type 2 DIABETES

See also ASCITES; BODY MASS INDEX (BMI); BODY SHAPE AND CARDIOVASCULAR DISEASE; DIET AND HEALTH; EXERCISE AND HEALTH; HEALTH RISK FACTORS; LEAN MUSCLE MASS; OBESITY; WEIGHT LOSS AND WEIGHT MANAGEMENT.

bariatric surgery Any of several types of surgical operations to achieve rapid and significant weight loss in people who have morbid OBESITY (obesity severe enough to pose an imminent risk to life). People who weigh 100 pounds or more above healthy weight or who have a BODY MASS INDEX (BMI) of 40 or greater are at severe risk for premature death as well as for health conditions due to obesity. At this level, body fat accounts for one third or more of total body weight. People whose BMIs are between 35 and 40 and who also have CARDIOVASCULAR DISEASE (CVD) or OBSTRUCTIVE SLEEP APNEA are also candidates for bariatric surgery because their obesity is a key contributory factor in these conditions. US surgeons perform about 140,000 bariatric operations a year.

Types of bariatric surgery are either malabsorptive or restrictive, according to the mechanism by which they impede the digestive process. The long-term success rate for maintaining weight loss varies with the kind of OPERATION and the person's commitment to lifestyle changes in EATING HABITS and physical exercise after the surgery. In general the amount of weight loss and the extent of complications are both more significant with malabsorptive operations. Bariatric operations include jejunoileal bypass, biliopancreatic diversion, gastric bypass, and gastric banding.

Surgical Procedure

Open bariatric surgery operations are complex, extensive, and may take several hours for the surgeon to perform. Laparoscopic, or minimally invasive, techniques allow the surgeon to operate

BARIATRIC OPERATIONS

Operation	Benefits	Risks and Complications
jejunoileal bypass (seldom performed)	rapid, significant, and sustainable weight loss reduced health risk for CARDIOVASCULAR DISEASE (CVD), DIABETES, and OSTEOARTHRITIS improvement in existing HYPERTENSION and diabetes	OPEN SURGERY high risk for postoperative complications malabsorption disorders and nutritional deficiencies secondary ANEMIA and OSTEOPOROSIS chronic gastrointestinal discomfort and DIARRHEA LIVER FAILURE kidney stones
biliopancreatic diversion biliopancreatic diversion with duodenal switch	rapid, significant, and sustainable weight loss reduced health risk for CVD, diabetes, and osteoarthritis improvement in existing hypertension and diabetes	open surgery moderate to high risk for operative and postoperative complications intolerance for high protein foods resulting in protein deficiency nutritional deficiencies with risk for anemia and osteoporosis gastric ulcers gastric dumping syndrome belching, abdominal cramping, and FLATULENCE chronic, intermittent diarrhea
Roux-en-Y gastric bypass	rapid, significant, and sustainable weight loss reduced health risk for CVD, diabetes, and osteoarthritis improvement in existing hypertension and diabetes	open surgery moderate risk for operative and postoperative complications nutritional deficiencies VOMITING gastric dumping syndrome PEPTIC ULCER DISEASE
vertical banded gastroplasty	laparoscopic surgery reversible rapid and significant weight loss for people who also make appropriate lifestyle changes	slight risk for operative and postoperative complications staple failure occasional gastric dumping syndrome gastric pouch can expand with continued excessive food consumption
adjustable gastric banding	laparoscopic surgery adjustable and reversible rapid recovery and return to normal activities gastrointestinal structure remains unchanged	balloon failure infection at the banding site slower and less consistent weight loss than with other bariatric operations gastric pouch easily expands with excessive food consumption up to 20 percent of people may experience no weight loss

through several small incisions called ports and generally require less time in the operating room. The stay in the hospital after bariatric surgery varies from a day for laparoscopic banding operations to five days or longer for open gastric bypass or biliopancreatic diversion operations. Full recovery and return to normal activities can take several months, though many people are able to return to most routine activities and to work in four to six weeks.

Jejunoileal bypass Jejunoileal bypass is a malabsorption operation. The first weight-reduction operation surgeons performed, the jejunoileal bypass joins the first part of the SMALL INTESTINE's second segment, the JEJUNUM, to the last part of the small intestine's third segment, the ILEUM. This bypasses the stretch of small intestine where most nutrient absorption takes place, rerouting food relatively undigested on a direct path from the STOMACH to the end of the small intestine and into the COLON. Though successful in generating significant weight loss jejunoileal bypass has numerous unpleasant side effects, including chronic and sometimes persistent or severe DIARRHEA, MALNUTRITION, electrolyte imbalance, and small bowel obstruction (ILEUS). Because of the high rate of complications with jejunoileal bypass and the current availability of other weight loss operations, surgeons in the United States seldom perform jejunoileal bypass today.

Biliopancreatic diversion Biliopancreatic diversion combines restriction and malabsorption. Developed as an improvement over jejunoileal bypass, the operation involves removing a portion of the stomach to reduce the volume of food it can hold as well as bypasses the central segment of the small intestine to curtail absorption during digestion. The surgery may be open or laparoscopic (minimally invasive). The first segment of the small intestine, the DUODENUM, connects the stomach to the small intestine and also serves as the conduit through which the PANCREAS channels DIGESTIVE ENZYMES and the GALLBLADDER empties BILE.

In straight biliopancreatic diversion, the surgeon removes the lower two thirds of the stomach and connects the remaining third directly to the ileum, the end portion of the small intestine near

its junction with the colon. The stomach becomes a very small pouch, restricting the amount of food that can enter the gastrointestinal tract. The digestive process bypasses most of the small intestine, limiting absorption.

A variation of this operation is biliopancreatic diversion with duodenal switch. In this operation the surgeon divides the stomach about in half lengthwise, creating a pouch between the ESOPHAGUS and the duodenum. The surgeon then divides the duodenum in half lengthwise and reconstructs it into two narrow, tubelike structures. One of these structures drains digestive enzymes from the pancreas and bile from the gallbladder into the gastrointestinal tract. The surgeon joins the other to the end portion of the ileum near the colon. Biliopancreatic diversion with duodenal switch allows better absorption in the remaining segment of small intestine of NUTRIENTS such as protein, vitamins, calcium, iron, and fat.

Gastric bypass Gastric bypass operations severely restrict food consumption by reducing the size of the stomach to a small pouch that can hold about 0.5 ounce (15 milliliters); the stomach normally holds about 50 ounces (1.5 liters). The most common and successful gastric bypass operation is the Roux-en-Y gastric bypass, a complex operation in which the surgeon divides the stomach to form two segments and reroutes the small intestine. Both segments of the stomach remain functional. The upper segment is a small gastric pouch with a capacity of 0.5 to 1 ounce. The surgeon joins the jejunum to the bottom of the pouch, bypassing the primary absorptive segment of the small intestine. The lower segment of the stomach retains the duodenum, which the surgeon restructures to join the jejunum near the ileum. The duodenum feeds digestive enzymes and DIGESTIVE HORMONES into the jejunum to aid in the absorption of nutrients.

Gastric banding Like gastric bypass operations, gastric banding operations reduce the stomach to a small pouch that can hold about 0.5 ounce and narrow the outlet at the base of the stomach to slow the passage of food from the stomach to the small intestine. Gastric banding significantly limits the volume of food the person can consume; exceeding the limit causes VOMITING. Surgeons

most commonly perform two types of gastric banding operations.

- Vertical gastric banding (VGB), also called vertical banded gastroplasty, partitions the stomach into two vertical segments. Surgical staples separate the segments, leaving a narrow channel between them. The small gastric pouch limits the amount of food the person can consume. A silicone band constricts the channel between the two gastric chambers to significantly slow the flow of food from the upper gastric pouch to the lower segment of the stomach. Food travels through the gastrointestinal tract in the normal way though moves through the stomach much more slowly than normal.

- Adjustable gastric banding (AGB), also called lap banding, partitions the stomach solely through the use of an inflatable silicon band applied so that it creates a gastric pouch that can hold about 1 ounce. A narrow catheter extends from the band to a port implanted beneath the SKIN. The surgeon gradually inflates the balloon with sterile saline during follow-up office visits to increase constriction of the stomach.

Gastric banding operations are laparoscopic, greatly reducing operative and postoperative risks and complications, and have the added benefit of being reversible. Most people return to normal activities within four weeks after the surgery. However, gastric banding has the lowest success rate among the bariatric operations. Weight loss is more gradual than with other operations. Over time the stomach can stretch to hold considerably more volume, depending on how much food the person attempts to consume on a consistent basis. Because food continues to the small intestine and digestion of it remains unaffected, a person who consumes high-CALORIE foods after a gastric banding operation may end up losing little if any weight.

About 80 percent of people who undergo gastric banding operations lose weight after surgery and about 50 percent reach the goal of losing 50 percent of their excessive weight within the first year after surgery. About 20 percent, however, do not lose weight because their lifestyle habits remain unchanged and their stomachs quickly regain capacity.

Risks and Complications

Any bariatric operation is major surgery with inherent risks, including excessive bleeding during or after the operation and INFECTION. Infection in the early postoperative period is a particular risk with any surgery on the gastrointestinal tract. Leakage of gastrointestinal contents into the abdominal cavity can cause PERITONITIS, a potentially life-threatening infection of the membrane that lines the abdominal cavity. Emergency surgery may be necessary to treat peritonitis. BLOOD clots may break free from blood vessels at the operative site, traveling through the body until they lodge in blood vessels too narrow to carry them any farther. Blood clots can occlude (block) arteries or veins anywhere in the body, including the LUNGS (PULMONARY EMBOLISM), BRAIN (STROKE), and HEART (MYOCARDIAL INFARCTION).

Though the risk dying as a consequence of bariatric surgery is less than 1 percent, many people who have OBESITY also have other health conditions that increase their risk profile. It is important to fully understand the risks of surgery compared to the risks of the obesity.

About 50 percent of people who undergo bariatric surgery experience complications after the operation, most of which are manageable postoperatively though may become chronic. Malabsorptive operations that bypass the small intestine have high risk for vitamin, mineral, and protein deficiencies. One in three people who undergo a weight loss operation develops chronic nutritional deficiencies with long-term health consequences such as OSTEOPOROSIS and ANEMIA. One in five requires additional surgery to repair problems such as fistula (abnormal opening) or HERNIA. The rapid weight loss of bariatric surgery triggers GALLBLADDER DISEASE, especially the formation of gallstones, in half of people who undergo bariatric surgery.

Milder common complications include GASTROESOPHAGEAL REFLUX DISORDER (GERD); belching;

chronic gastrointestinal discomfort; and gastric dumping syndrome, a reaction of the gastrointestinal tract to eating high concentrations of sugar (sweets) and protein (meats). Excessive body weight stretches the skin, which may sag and fold after extensive weight loss. About 30 percent of people who undergo bariatric surgery subsequently have PLASTIC SURGERY operations such as panniculectomy and abdominoplasty to remove excess skin after weight loss.

Outlook and Lifestyle Modifications

Most people require four to eight weeks for full recovery from bariatric surgery and return to regular activities. Some people may require longer, particularly those who experience postoperative complications. The changes to the gastrointestinal system that bariatric surgery makes are permanent and alter the way the digestive process functions, sometimes in ways that require ongoing medical care and medications. Many people will also need to continue taking medications to treat conditions they had before surgery, such as HYPERTENSION and DIABETES.

For several weeks to several months, people who have gastric bypass procedures to restrict the size of the stomach must eat liquid or pureed foods to give their gastrointestinal tracts time to adjust. The gastric pouch can hold such a limited volume that it often is necessary to separate eating and drinking by 30 to 60 minutes. As well, the person must thoroughly chew food before swallowing, as the gastric pouch lacks the MUSCLE capacity and size to participate in further breaking down the size of food particles.

Despite the changes to the gastrointestinal system's structure and function, lifestyle factors such as food choices and physical exercise remain important for long-term weight management. The success of bariatric surgery for maintaining weight loss depends on the extent to which an individual makes the necessary changes in these factors. Doctors consider bariatric surgery successful when the person maintains weight loss of 50 percent of excess body weight for five years after surgery. Though many people may lose 100 pounds or more with bariatric surgery, they may remain overweight though at a healthier weight than before surgery.

In general, people who undergo bariatric operations lose 50 percent of excess body weight in the first year after surgery. The rate of weight loss depends on the type of operation and tends to be most dramatic with gastric bypass operations. Weight loss tends to peak around three years after surgery, at 70 to 85 percent of excess body weight. Five years after surgery, however, about 70 percent of people have regained weight to about 50 percent of the excess (which still falls within the parameters for successful surgery) and about 5 percent of people have regained all of their lost weight. Doctors attribute these results largely to continuation of poor eating habits and physical inactivity. Food choices and daily exercise are essential to sustain weight loss over the long term.

Outcome studies of bariatric operations show evidence that people who maintain their weight loss lower their risk for CVD and type 2 diabetes to the same extent as people who lose the weight through nonsurgical methods. Because weight loss is so dramatic, some people are able to manage mild to moderate hypertension and type 2 diabetes through lifestyle alone, ending the need for medications. Researchers believe such findings further support the role of obesity as an independent risk factor for these conditions as well as demonstrate the health value of WEIGHT LOSS AND WEIGHT MANAGEMENT.

See also DIET AIDS; DIET AND HEALTH; DIETING; EATING DISORDERS; LIFESTYLE AND HEALTH; MALABSORPTION; MINERALS AND HEALTH; MINIMALLY INVASIVE SURGERY; NUTRITIONAL NEEDS; OBESITY AND HEALTH; SURGERY BENEFIT AND RISK ASSESSMENT; VITAMINS AND HEALTH.

body fat percentage   The proportion of the body's composition that is fat. Body fat percentage is an indirect indicator of LEAN MUSCLE MASS and correlates to health circumstances such as FERTILITY as well as health conditions such as type 2 DIABETES and CARDIOVASCULAR DISEASE (CVD). The body requires a minimum amount of fat for its functions and activities, generally about 4 percent for men and 12 percent for women. Body fat percentage above 25 percent for men and 32 percent for women correlates with OBESITY. A high body fat percentage in combination with ABDOMINAL ADIPOSITY (the "apple" body shape) portends a particularly high risk for CVD, HEART ATTACK, and STROKE.

BODY FAT PERCENTAGE AND HEALTH RISK

Health Status	Men	Women
at risk for NUTRITIONAL DEFICIENCY	< 4 percent	< 12 percent
lean (athlete or high fitness level), no increased health risk	4 to 15 percent	12 to 22 percent
healthy, no increased health risk	< 20 percent	< 27 percent
overweight, moderate increase in health risk	20 to 25 percent	27 to 32 percent
OBESITY, significant increase in health risk	> 25 percent	> 32 percent

Methods for measuring or approximating body fat percentage include

- BODY MASS INDEX (BMI), a mathematical formula based on weight and height

- skinfold calipers, which measure the thickness of a fold of SKIN (typically at the triceps on the back of the upper arm) to determine the amount of subcutaneous fat

- bioelectrical impedance, which measures the resistance a mild electrical current encounters when passed through the body

- hydrostatic weighing, which uses water displacement to determine body mass

Additional measures that improve the precision of body fat percentage estimates include WAIST CIRCUMFERENCE and WAIST TO HIP RATIO, as these measures increase with excessive body fat. Dual-energy X-RAY absorptiometry (DEXA), an X-ray procedure to determine BONE DENSITY as an assessment of

OSTEOPOROSIS, also provides calculations of body fat percentage and lean tissue mass. No single method provides an absolute measure of body fat percentage.

See also DIET AND HEALTH; EXERCISE AND HEALTH; FITNESS LEVEL; UPPER ARM CIRCUMFERENCE; WEIGHT LOSS AND WEIGHT MANAGEMENT.

body mass index (BMI)   A mathematical measure of total body size and its correlation to health risk. BMI values derive from height (without shoes) and weight (without clothes) measures, with mathematical calculations that convert those measures to a value that reflects overall body size. BMI represents the mass of the body in kilograms per meter squared (kg/m^2) though the common presentation of BMI is simply the numeric value. A low or a high BMI corresponds with increased risk for numerous health conditions. A BMI of 25 or greater is overweight; a BMI of 30 or greater is OBESITY. BMI values apply to men or women who have the same measurements. For example, a

BMI AND HEALTH RISK

BMI	Classification	Health Risk Due to Weight
> 18.5	underweight	may indicate EATING DISORDERS or undernutrition
19 to 24.9	healthy weight	no increased health risk
25 to 29.9	overweight	moderate health risk
30 to 34.9	OBESITY, class 1	significant health risk
35 to 39.9	obesity, class 2	high health risk; INSULIN RESISTANCE or CARDIOVASCULAR DISEASE (CVD) likely
40+	obesity, class 3	severe health risk; DIABETES, CVD, or HYPERTENSION likely

man who is 5 feet 8 inches tall and weighs 175 pounds has the same BMI as a woman who is 5 feet 8 inches tall and weighs 175 pounds.

For most people a high BMI indicates increased body fat. The higher the BMI is above the "healthy" range, the greater the health risk for HYPERTENSION (high BLOOD PRESSURE), type 2 DIABETES, and forms of CARDIOVASCULAR DISEASE (CVD) such as HYPERLIPIDEMIA, ATHEROSCLEROSIS and CORONARY ARTERY DISEASE (CAD). Risk for these conditions further increases when WAIST CIRCUMFERENCE also is greater than 40 inches for men and 35 inches for women, though waist circumference is itself an independent risk factor for the same health conditions. Losing weight drops BMI and reduces health risk.

BMI values may not be accurate in children, the elderly, and performance athletes because body mass may not correctly reflect body composition. The elderly may have more body fat than BMI indicates, with a correspondingly higher health risk. Performance athletes (amateur or professional) typically have higher LEAN MUSCLE MASS (large skeletal muscles) and lower body fat percentages than less physically active people of the same weight; the increased MUSCLE mass raises the BMI even though body fat is lower.

See also ABDOMINAL ADIPOSITY; CHILDHOOD OBESITY; DIET AND HEALTH; EXERCISE AND HEALTH; LIFESTYLE AND HEALTH; NUTRITIONAL ASSESSMENT; NUTRITIONAL NEEDS; OBESITY AND HEALTH; WEIGHT LOSS AND WEIGHT MANAGEMENT.

BODY MASS INDEX (BMI)

BMI Height (inches)	19	20	21	22	23	24	25	26	27	28	29	30	31	32	33	34	35	36	37	38	39	40	41	42	43	44	45
											Body Weight (pounds)																
58	91	96	100	105	110	115	119	124	129	134	138	143	148	153	158	162	167	172	177	181	186	191	196	201	205	210	215
59	94	99	104	109	114	119	124	128	133	138	143	148	153	158	163	168	173	178	183	188	193	198	203	208	212	217	222
60	97	102	107	112	118	123	128	133	138	143	148	153	158	163	168	174	179	184	189	194	199	204	209	215	220	225	230
61	100	106	111	116	122	127	132	137	143	148	153	158	164	169	174	180	185	190	195	201	206	211	217	222	227	232	238
62	104	109	115	120	126	131	136	142	147	153	158	164	169	175	180	186	191	196	202	207	213	218	224	229	235	240	246
63	107	113	118	124	130	135	141	146	152	158	163	169	175	180	186	191	197	203	208	214	220	225	231	237	242	248	254
64	110	116	122	128	134	140	145	151	157	163	169	174	180	186	192	197	204	209	215	221	227	232	238	244	250	256	262
65	114	120	126	132	138	144	150	156	162	168	174	180	186	192	198	204	210	216	222	228	234	240	246	252	258	264	270
66	118	124	130	136	142	148	155	161	167	173	179	186	192	198	204	210	216	223	229	235	241	247	253	260	266	272	278
67	121	127	134	140	146	153	159	166	172	178	185	191	198	204	211	217	223	230	236	242	249	255	261	268	274	280	287
68	125	131	138	144	151	158	164	171	177	184	190	197	203	210	216	223	230	236	243	249	256	262	269	276	282	289	295
69	128	135	142	149	155	162	169	176	182	189	196	203	209	216	223	230	236	243	250	257	263	270	277	284	291	297	304
70	132	139	146	153	160	167	174	181	188	195	202	209	216	222	229	236	243	250	257	264	271	278	285	292	299	306	313
71	136	143	150	157	165	172	179	186	193	200	208	215	222	229	236	243	250	257	265	272	279	286	293	301	308	315	322
72	140	147	154	162	169	177	184	191	199	206	213	221	228	235	242	250	258	265	272	279	287	294	302	309	316	324	331
73	144	151	159	166	174	182	189	197	204	212	219	227	235	242	250	257	265	272	280	288	295	302	310	318	325	333	340
74	148	155	163	171	179	186	194	202	210	218	225	233	241	249	256	264	272	280	287	295	303	311	319	326	334	342	350
75	152	160	168	176	184	192	200	208	216	224	232	240	248	256	264	272	279	287	295	303	311	319	327	335	343	351	359
76	156	164	172	180	189	197	205	213	221	230	238	246	254	263	271	279	287	295	304	312	320	328	336	344	353	361	369

Adapted from U.S. National Heart, Lung, and Blood Institute (NHLBI) Obesity Education Initiative (2005)

childhood obesity The development of unhealthy body weight due to excessive body fat before adulthood (age 18). Childhood OBESITY has numerous health consequences that affect METAB-OLISM, physical growth and development, and PUBERTY. Childhood obesity jumped significantly between 1970 and 2000. Currently 15 percent of US children have obesity. Another 20 percent are overweight, which places them at risk for obesity.

Health experts attribute the rise in childhood obesity primarily to EATING HABITS and physical inactivity. Ongoing health assessment monitoring, such as the periodic National Health and Nutrition Examination Survey (NHANES) and the Behavioral Risk Factor Surveillance System (BRFSS), reveals a steady decline in the level of physical activity among young people, including through physical education programs in the schools. Increasing the physical activity of children as a mechanism for improving long-term health is among the objectives of HEALTHY PEOPLE 2010, the US government's agenda for community health. Researchers also continue to explore other factors that may contribute to obesity. Much attention focuses on the role of genetics and regulation of metabolic processes within the body such as the release and activity of hormones.

Diagnosing Childhood Obesity

Conventional methods of assessing BODY FAT PER-CENTAGE and BODY MASS INDEX (BMI), the standard measures of obesity, are somewhat different for children from those used for adults. A child's body fat varies with developmental stages and growth cycles. Correspondingly, a child's BMI varies according to age and developmental stage. As well, boys and girls have different body fat composition through the end of ADOLESCENCE.

In 2001 the US Centers for Disease Control and Prevention (CDC) developed gender-specific BMI-for-age charts to provide guidelines for assessing underweight, healthy weight, and overweight in children between the ages of 2 and 20. The charts correlate BMI to percentile, a measure of relative comparison that allows monitoring of BMI through the entire course of childhood. The boundary for overweight is the 85th percentile (85 percent of children who are the same age and gender have a lower BMI) and for obesity the 95th percentile (95 percent of children who are the same age and gender have a lower BMI).

Health Implications of Obesity in Childhood

Doctors are seeing INSULIN RESISTANCE, type 2 DIA-BETES, HYPERTENSION (high BLOOD PRESSURE), HYPER-

BMI FOR AGE FOR CHILDREN AND TEENS: KEY PERCENTILE MARKERS					
BMI for Age: Boys/Girls				BMI for Age Percentile	Health Status for Body Weight
2 years	7 years	15 years	20 years		
14.8/14.4	13.7/13.4	16.6/16.3	19.1/17.8	5th	underweight
18.2/18.0	17.4/19.2	23.4/24.0	27.1/26.5	85th	overweight or at risk for overweight
19.3/19.1	19.1/19.6	26.8/28.1	30.6/31.8	95th	obesity

LIPIDEMIA, OSTEOARTHRITIS, and the beginnings of ATHEROSCLEROSIS in an increasing number of children, especially adolescents, who have obesity. These conditions may require treatment with medications and other interventions, the long-term health consequences of which remain unknown. Emotional, social, and self-esteem issues also are common among children who have obesity. The stigma of being "fat" is a difficult challenge for children who are forming their sense of self and are especially sensitive to peer acceptance and rejection. Obesity may result in a young person feeling ostracized in school and having difficulty forming friendships.

Health Implications of Childhood Obesity in Adulthood

Increasing evidence points to long-term health consequences for people who enter adulthood with obesity. Childhood obesity correlates with increased risk for earlier onset in adulthood of insulin resistance and type 2 diabetes, osteoarthritis, hypertension, hyperlipidemia, atherosclerosis, CORONARY ARTERY DISEASE (CAD), STROKE, and certain cancers. An increased risk for these conditions may exist even among people who had childhood obesity yet achieve relatively healthy weight as adults. These health conditions account for significant physical disability and further complications resulting from co-morbidities (the cascading consequences of co-existing, multiple health conditions).

Treatment Approaches and Outlook

Prevention of obesity is the first line of treatment. Routine childhood health examinations monitor a child's growth and development. Intervention for children who have BMI-for-age values near or at the 85th percentile can head off obesity. Lifestyle modifications—nutritious eating habits and increased physical exercise—presented in a positive context represent the most effective approach for long-term weight management. However, obesity is a complex condition that requires individualized assessment and a treatment approach that accommodates the various factors relevant for a child. Counseling and SUPPORT GROUPS may help address DEPRESSION, emotional issues, and family dynamics.

Positive reinforcement must frame treatment approaches for OBESITY in children. Punitive approaches such as withholding food, criticizing the child, and forcing exercise are inappropriate and can have serious emotional and psychologic consequences for the child.

Established obesity is a more difficult challenge for treatment, though lifestyle modifications remain the mainstay of therapeutic approaches. Nutrition education and BEHAVIOR MODIFICATION THERAPY are helpful for older children, especially adolescents. Many health experts recommend involving the entire family in the effort to shift to healthful lifestyle habits. Older adolescents who struggle with obesity may benefit from medications intended to suppress APPETITE. Many eating disorder treatment programs offer comprehensive treatment that targets the child's individual circumstances and needs. BARIATRIC SURGERY, a treatment option for adults who are otherwise unable to treat their obesity, is not usually an option for young people.

There is every reason to believe the health outlook for children who achieve healthy weight and enter adulthood at healthy weight is excellent. Health experts are hopeful that lifestyle modifications implemented early in life will carry through adulthood, helping reduce adult obesity as well.

See also DIET AND HEALTH; EXERCISE AND HEALTH; OBESITY AND HEALTH; QUALITY OF LIFE; WEIGHT LOSS AND WEIGHT MANAGEMENT.

diet aids Products that claim to expedite weight loss. Diet aids may be products proclaimed as APPETITE suppressants (decrease the urge to eat) or products or electronic devices advertised to "burn away" fat. Though most such diet aids have limited or no value, the diet aid industry in the United States generates about $30 billion in annual sales.

Over-the-counter appetite suppressants typically contain diuretics (drugs that increase URINATION), STIMULANTS such as pseudoephedrine (a decongestant) and CAFFEINE, or bulking agents that draw water after consumption and purport to instill a sense of fullness. These kinds of products may have a limited effect to decrease appetite though may have undesired side effects such as agitation and mucous membrane dryness.

Devices that claim to burn energy by stimulating MUSCLE fibers to contract may indeed stimulate muscle contraction but do not generate enough energy to affect the body's metabolic balance. Wraps, creams, and other substances applied to the SKIN that proclaim to "melt away" fat lack scientific basis for their claims. Many diet aids come with diet plans that advise increased exercise and reduced food intake—the only proven method for weight loss.

See also DIET AND HEALTH; DIETING; "FAT BURNERS"; NUTRITIONAL NEEDS; WEIGHT LOSS AND WEIGHT MANAGEMENT.

dieting The practice of temporarily altering one's food intake to achieve weight loss. Dieting approaches typically restrict calories and often food types. Though such approaches are effective for short-term weight loss, they are not sustainable in the long term and many people regain the lost weight in less time than it took to lose it. Weight loss as a component of long-term weight management requires lifestyle modifications that dieting does not accommodate, such as increased physical exercise and EATING HABITS that foster healthful food choices.

Dieting tends to focus on restricting foods that are high in calories, such as carbohydrates and fat. Depriving the body of CALORIE intake forces it to draw from stored energy sources such as glycogen and body fat, though severe calorie restriction (less than 800 calories a day) results in protein METABOLISM and loss of LEAN MUSCLE MASS because protein is easier for the body to convert to GLUCOSE to meet its energy needs. Restrictive dieting is likely to deprive the body of other needed NUTRIENTS such as vitamins and minerals, and commonly results in food cravings for items the diet does not allow.

Some dieting approaches are detrimental to health over time. High-fat, low-carbohydrate diets may achieve short-term weight loss but are likely to result in increased levels of cholesterol and triglycerides in the BLOOD circulation, raising the risk for HYPERLIPIDEMIA and ATHEROSCLEROSIS regardless of weight loss. As well, low-carbohydrate diets cause the body to excrete more water than usual, resulting in weight loss but not loss of body fat. "Yo-yo" dieting, in which weight continually fluctuates, is particularly harmful not only for long-term weight management but also for the glucose–INSULIN balance, generating increased risk for INSULIN RESISTANCE. There is also the tendency to regain the lost weight as well as additional weight as somewhat of a rebound response in the form of excessive eating when the restrictive diet ends.

People who have class 2 or 3 OBESITY, in which adverse health conditions are either imminent or already exist because of excessive body weight, may benefit from a doctor-supervised, short-term restrictive diet as part of an overall weight management approach. However, the most effective form of dieting for sustained weight loss and improved health status is that which combines moderately reduced caloric intake and increased daily exercise. Though weight loss is gradual with such an approach (health experts recommend one half to one pound a week), it is more likely to be permanent because it arises from lifestyle modifications that are themselves sustainable.

See also APPETITE; DIET AND HEALTH; EATING DISORDERS; EXERCISE AND HEALTH; HUNGER; NUTRITIONAL NEEDS; OBESITY AND HEALTH; WEIGHT LOSS AND WEIGHT MANAGEMENT.

eating habits The ways in which an individual approaches food consumption. Eating habits encompass factors such as food choices, the timing and frequency of meals and snacks, portion size, and social practices around eating (such as sitting down as a family to eat meals at the table or eating while watching television). Eating habits affect nutrition, body weight, and body composition.

Why People Eat

Much eating occurs for reasons other than to bring energy and NUTRIENTS into the body. People may eat

- for emotional comfort
- for something to do or social interaction, such as going out to eat
- out of habit, such as because it is meal time
- because other people are eating
- because a particular item of food smells or looks good
- to satisfy a food craving

These eating habits are not always easy to break. Recognizing them is the first step; changing them often requires understanding the reasons behind them. Increasing physical activity helps accommodate extra calories consumed and also provides diversion to direct interest elsewhere.

How—and How Much—People Eat

Portion size is a key factor in healthy eating. Many people overestimate the amount of food that con-

stitutes a serving and underestimate how much food they eat. Product labels specify the number size of servings the package contains. However, much packaging gives the appearance of a single serving when the label specifies several servings. It is important to carefully read labels and to purchase packaged products that truly contain a single serving, that several people can share, or that are easy to store.

Portion sizes are especially difficult to assess for home-cooked meals. For example, a single serving of meat is 3 ounces, about the size of a deck of cards. Yet most people eat a portion that is 8 to 12 ounces or more, which is equivalent to 2½ to 4 servings. A single serving portion of cooked rice or mashed potatoes is 1/2 cup, though the typical serving spoon dishes up more than that. A person who pours a bowlful of cereal with milk for breakfast is likely eating 2 to 4 servings of each. Even a few handfuls of chips eaten from the bag likely constitute 3 or 4 servings. As well, many people feel compelled to eat all the food on their plates.

What People Eat

Nutritional guidelines recommend the highest proportion of foods come from fruits, vegetables, whole grains and whole grain products, and low-fat proteins. However, fats and carbohydrates make up the majority of dietary intake for many people. In the United States the frequency with which people eat in restaurants, sit down as well as fast food, is very high. Though a number of restaurants offer fresh vegetables and fruit and feature "heart healthy" menu choices, restaurant meals tend to be high in both fat and carbohydrate. The same is true of snack foods and prepared foods such as frozen dinners and boxed and canned products.

When People Eat

Eating when hungry is the ideal timing for the body but is often fraught with challenge in real life. Because APPETITE is as much a factor of desire to eat as a signal of the body's need to acquire nutrients, most people have difficulty distinguishing genuine hunger. The urge to eat, particularly when delayed, tends to manifest as overconsumption. Some people try to eat only one meal as a means of controlling how much they eat, though this is a counterproductive effort because when they eat they are so hungry that they eat too much and often less than nutritious foods. Other people may eat full meals at breakfast, lunch, and supper because it is the pattern of eating they have always followed. Snacking between meals and eating on the go are habits that often result in overeating as well as high-fat, high-carbohydrate consumption.

Establishing and Maintaining Health-Oriented Eating Habits

Planning for meals often instills a sense of calm around the process of eating because the planning helps take away the pressure of figuring out what to eat and how to make the meal happen. Household members can take turns being responsible for meals, sharing both the responsibility and the pleasure of the meal. Most people do better nutritionally when they eat five smaller meals spread throughout the day, though personal schedules may make such an approach impractical, or three meals a day with nutritious snacks between.

See also DIET AND HEALTH; FOOD CRAVINGS; NUTRITIONAL NEEDS; WEIGHT LOSS AND WEIGHT MANAGEMENT.

"fat burners"   Products—foods, drinks, supplements, devices, and other items—that proclaim to reduce body fat without exercise or changes in diet. Such products are not effective in this manner; the only method for "burning" fat is for a person to expend more energy through activity than he or she consumes through eating. Some "fat-burner" products contain diuretics (substances that draw fluid from the body to increase URINE output). Some "fat burners" claim to spot-reduce, or eliminate fat in a targeted fashion. For the most part such claims are at best inaccurate and more often deceptive. The body does not draw fat from one location any more than another during weight loss efforts. Rather the body draws fat from fat stores throughout the body. Fat accumulates in larger amounts in certain parts of the body because these areas have more fat cells to accept lipid storage. These areas tend to be the abdomen, hips, buttocks, thighs, and upper arms. When weight loss occurs, correspondingly more fat

leaves these areas. As well, fat loss in these areas is more apparent because the fat collects in layers just underneath the SKIN. Fat loss from the cheeks and neck also appears noticeable early in the weight loss process.

See also DIET AIDS; DIETING; WEIGHT LOSS AND WEIGHT MANAGEMENT.

food cravings   The desire to eat particular foods, typically without correlation to HUNGER or APPETITE. Some people speculate that food cravings suggest certain substances are missing from the diet or from consumption, such as salt when a person craves salty foods. Others believe food cravings originate as signals the BRAIN sends to satisfy its pleasure centers. Changes in HORMONE levels in the body, such as occur during PREGNANCY, appear to initiate cravings for foods in sometimes unusual combinations. Food aversions are also common in pregnancy. Pica is the condition of craving nonfood substances such as dirt or paper and may indicate an iron deficiency.

Other food cravings appear emotionally driven, such as those for comfort foods during times of emotional distress. For the most part, however, there are no clear scientific explanations for food cravings, and everyone experiences them at some time. As long as a person continues to eat an overall nutritious diet, succumbing occasional food cravings has no detrimental effect on health. However, uncontrolled response to food cravings may result in nutritional imbalances and often is a key factor in overeating, overweight, and OBESITY. It may also signal underlying emotional or psychological disturbances.

Controlling food cravings is challenging and highly personalized. Methods that are effective for some people include

- diversionary activities that make succumbing to the craving difficult (such as taking a walk or bicycle ride)

- eating healthful alternatives to the desired food (such as fresh fruit instead of candy or lemon instead of salt for seasoning)

- HYPNOSIS to fortify the resolve to resist the craving

- eating regular meals throughout the day that contain a balance of nutritious foods

- eating a small serving or portion of the desired food, such as a mini-size instead of a full-size candy bar

- BEHAVIOR MODIFICATION THERAPY to gain insight and understanding about the reasons for craving foods

See also ANEMIA; EATING DISORDERS; EATING HABITS; MORNING SICKNESS; SATIETY.

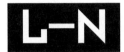

lean muscle mass The amount of body tissue that is lean MUSCLE in contrast to the percentage that is body fat. There is an inverse relationship between lean muscle mass and BODY FAT PERCENTAGE, such that when one increases the other decreases. Lean muscle mass increases with regular physical exercise that challenges muscle fibers to expand. Serious illness or injury, such as significant BURNS or major trauma, may draw protein from lean muscle mass to aid in HEALING, resulting in diminished lean muscle mass. A common method for estimating lean muscle mass is UPPER ARM CIRCUMFERENCE, a measurement of the distance around the middle of the upper arm. It is also possible, though less accurate, to approximate lean muscle mass based on body fat percentage determinations. The X-RAY procedure dual-energy X-ray absorptiometry (DEXA), a diagnostic test that measures BONE DENSITY, also provides data for calculating lean muscle mass.

See also BODY MASS INDEX (BMI); RESISTANCE EXERCISE; WAIST CIRCUMFERENCE; WAIST TO HIP RATIO.

nicotine replacement Products intended to wean a person from NICOTINE otherwise acquired through cigarette smoking. Nicotine is a highly addictive DRUG that occurs naturally in tobacco. Though behavior is an important component of smoking, the addictive quality of nicotine accounts for the difficulty people have in quitting. Nicotine replacement can be fairly effective as an aid for SMOKING CESSATION. The premise is that the nicotine in the product, though less than that in a cigarette, fulfills the body's desire for nicotine when the person stops smoking.

Most nicotine replacement products come in diminishing strength doses so over the course of a typical smoking cessation program (usually 12 weeks) the person takes decreasing doses to ease the body's dependence on the nicotine. Nicotine replacement products include

- transdermal (SKIN) patches, which a person wears for 16 to 24 hours to deliver a steady trickle of nicotine absorbed through the skin
- chewing gums, which deliver doses of nicotine with timed chewing and holding the gum between the gum and cheek for absorption of the released nicotine through the tissues of the MOUTH and into the BLOOD circulation
- lozenges, which release nicotine as they dissolve in the mouth for absorption through the tissues of the mouth and into the blood circulation
- nasal sprays, which deliver nicotine to the membranes inside the NOSE for rapid absorption into the blood circulation
- inhalers, small plastic mouthpieces that hold cartridges containing nicotine a person draws in through the mouth similar to smoking a cigarette; nicotine enters the blood circulation by absorption through the tissues of the mouth (not the LUNGS)

Taking NICOTINE replacement products in combination with one another or while still smoking cigarettes presents a major risk for nicotine toxicity. Symptoms of nicotine overdose include
- **PALPITATIONS**
- **rapid or irregular HEART RATE**
- **NAUSEA**
- **DIARRHEA**

Nasal sprays and inhalers require a doctor's prescription. Transdermal patches and chewing gums are available over the counter as well as by prescription, depending on the strength (nicotine DOSE). With all nicotine replacement products nicotine OVERDOSE can occur if the person combines nicotine products or continues to smoke or use other tobacco products (such as chewing tobacco or cigars) while using a nicotine replacement product. It is important to keep nicotine replacement products, especially gums and lozenges, out of the reach of children.

Other possible side effects include local irritation of the tissues, HICCUPS with the gum or lozenges, and COUGH with any nicotine replacement product except transdermal patches. Some people may develop dependence on the nicotine replacement product, which is more of a risk with nasal sprays and inhalers because these methods deliver nicotine rapidly to the blood circulation in similar fashion as cigarette smoking. The typical course of smoking cessation therapy with nicotine replacement is 12 to 16 weeks and should not extend longer than 6 months.

See also ADDICTION; ANTISMOKING EFFORTS; SMOKING AND HEALTH.

obesity The circumstance of weighing 20 percent or greater in excess of ideal or healthy weight as a consequence of excessive body fat. Doctors consider a BODY MASS INDEX (BMI) of 30 to be the boundary of obesity. In the 1990s health experts classified obesity as a clinical diagnosis as well as an independent risk factor for numerous health conditions, including DIABETES, GALLBLADDER DISEASE, HYPERTENSION (high BLOOD PRESSURE), ATHEROSCLEROSIS, HEART FAILURE, HORMONE-DRIVEN CANCERS of the BREAST and PROSTATE GLAND, and CORONARY ARTERY DISEASE (CAD). Obesity also interferes with INSULIN sensitivity and with HEALING. Many researchers believe obesity is as significant a risk factor as cigarette smoking for CARDIOVASCULAR DISEASE (CVD).

Causes of Obesity

The simple cause of obesity is more intake than outgo—energy from food consumed exceeds energy expended through physical activity. However, the circumstances that establish this imbalance are complex. Lifestyle factors—EATING HABITS and physical inactivity—are key causes of obesity. The extent to which genetic factors influence obesity remains unknown, though researchers have identified gene-directed processes that regulate many of the variables within the body responsible for how the body uses and stores energy. Social, cultural, emotional, and psychologic issues further influence the development of obesity.

Genetic factors Researchers have discovered a number of genes that regulate body functions related to APPETITE and METABOLISM. One is the *ob* GENE, which regulates the production of the HORMONE leptin. Leptin suppresses the HUNGER, appetite, and SATIETY centers in the HYPOTHALAMUS and brainstem. Certain mutations of the *ob* gene result in diminished sensitivity of the leptin receptors to leptin, reducing leptin's effectiveness. Other mutations influence the production of leptin. Leptin also influences the actions of another protein, neuropeptide Y (NPY), that stimulates appetite. Researchers believe mutations of the *ob* gene predispose individuals to obesity because appetite control mechanisms within the body do not function properly. However, these mutations do not unequivocally cause obesity.

Social and cultural influences Many people who meet the diagnostic criteria for obesity do not recognize that their weight has become a health condition with serious consequences if untreated. About two thirds of people who have obesity identify themselves as such; one third perceive themselves as overweight but not to an extent that interferes with health or exceeds their ability to manage by losing weight at will. There is a social tendency to joke about excessive weight, diminishing its significance as a health factor with a corresponding cultural shift toward accommodating larger body size.

Emotional and psychologic factors The reasons people eat often have little to do with hunger or nutritional need. Eating can provide a sense of comfort during times of emotional stress. Overeating is an eating disorder that often has complex psychologic foundations related to issues of self-esteem, control, or psychologic injury such as may occur as a consequence of sexual, domestic, or childhood abuse.

Symptoms and Diagnostic Path

The primary symptom of obesity is significantly increased body size due to excessive body fat. The diagnostic markers for obesity include

- BMI of 30 or greater

- body fat percentage greater than 25 percent for men or 32 percent for women
- WAIST CIRCUMFERENCE greater than 40 inches for men or 35 inches for women

Most people who have obesity meet all three of these diagnostic markers. People who have significantly increased MUSCLE mass, such as performance athletes and bodybuilders, may have a higher BMI without having obesity.

Treatment Options and Outlook

The treatment for obesity is weight loss. Treatment options include lifestyle modifications, BEHAVIOR MODIFICATION THERAPY, medications to suppress appetite, and BARIATRIC SURGERY. Many people experience better results with a combination of treatments; lifestyle modifications are essential for sustained weight management, regardless of other treatments. However, most people who have obesity have tried many weight loss approaches without success.

Noninvasive methods are more likely to succeed for people who have class 1 obesity. The US National Institutes of Health (NIH) recommends aggressive noninvasive treatment for people who have class 2 obesity but who have not yet developed significant co-morbidities (health conditions resulting from and intertwined with obesity). For people who have class 2 obesity and two or more comorbid conditions (such as hypertension and diabetes) and for people who have class 3 obesity, the NIH recommends bariatric surgery. Though bariatric surgery entails significant risks, health experts believe the benefits of extensive weight loss that is possible outweigh the risks of the surgery when body fat percentage exceeds 30 percent (class 3 obesity).

The long-term success of treatment for obesity requires ongoing and continuous management of obesity's numerous and often intertwined causes. For some people weight management remains a lifelong challenge and sometimes a struggle though others are able to achieve and maintain healthy weight.

Risk Factors and Preventive Measures

The key risk factors for obesity are physical inactivity and excessive food consumption. People who are sedentary (get no physical exercise) are at highest risk for obesity. Nutritious eating habits and daily physical exercise are preventive as well as therapeutic. To prevent obesity health experts recommend

- food (CALORIE) intake appropriate for age and physical activity level
- eating foods with high nutrient density, notably fruits, vegetables, whole grains and whole grain products, and low-fat proteins
- minimizing consumption of high-fat foods (such as fast foods and snack items) and empty carbohydrates (such as sodas and sweets)
- a minimum 30 minutes a day of moderate physical exercise such as walking

Preventive efforts are most likely to succeed when all members of the household participate in them.

See also CHILDHOOD OBESITY; CULTURAL AND ETHNIC HEALTH-CARE PERSPECTIVES; EATING DISORDERS; GENERATIONAL HEALTH-CARE PERSPECTIVES; HEALTHY PEOPLE 2010; INSULIN RESISTANCE; LIFESTYLE AND HEALTH; OBESITY AND HEALTH; PEER PRESSURE; SMOKING AND HEALTH; WEIGHT LOSS AND WEIGHT MANAGEMENT.

CLINICAL CLASSIFICATIONS OF OBESITY		
Body Mass Index (BMI)	**Clinical Classification**	**Health Risk**
30 to 34.9	class 1	moderate
35 to 39.9	class 2	serious
40 and above	class 3	severe or morbid

obesity and health   Obesity reached the status of health crisis in the United States in the 1990s. In 2005, one third of Americans—nearly 60 million people—weighed 20 percent or more above healthy body weight, the key clinical marker for diagnosing obesity. An equal number were overweight, weighing 5 to 20 percent above healthy body weight. Many health experts believe obesity is as significant a health risk factor as cigarette smoking, complicit in a broad spectrum of health conditions.

HEALTH CONDITIONS IN WHICH OBESITY CAN BE A FACTOR

ATHEROSCLEROSIS	BREAST CANCER
COLORECTAL CANCER	CORONARY ARTERY DISEASE (CAD)
ENDOMETRIAL CANCER	ERECTILE DYSFUNCTION
GALLBLADDER DISEASE	GASTROESOPHAGEAL REFLUX
HEART FAILURE	DISORDER (GERD)
HYPERTENSION	INSULIN RESISTANCE
MENSTRUAL DYSFUNCTION	OBSTRUCTIVE SLEEP APNEA
OSTEOARTHRITIS	OVARIAN CANCER
POLYCYSTIC OVARY SYNDROME	PROSTATE CANCER
(PCOS)	SEXUAL DYSFUNCTION
STEATOHEPATITIS	type 2 DIABETES

How Obesity Affects the Body and Health

Obesity has numerous negative influences on health. It is the leading cause of HYPERTENSION (high BLOOD PRESSURE) and type 2 DIABETES and is an independent risk factor for the development of ATHEROSCLEROSIS, CORONARY ARTERY DISEASE (CAD), PERIPHERAL VASCULAR DISEASE (PVD), OSTEOARTHRITIS, GALLBLADDER DISEASE, COLORECTAL CANCER, hormone-driven BREAST CANCER, and PROSTATE CANCER. Health risk for these conditions and their complications or consequences increases moderately for overweight and significantly for obesity. In addition to its role as a key risk factor for numerous health conditions, obesity is itself a health condition with significant and potentially fatal consequences when it remains untreated.

Obesity and type 2 diabetes   More than 95 percent of people who have type 2 diabetes are overweight and many have obesity. Increased body fat decreases cell sensitivity to INSULIN, which sets in motion a cascade of adaptations that ultimately overwhelm the body's normal metabolic balance. Cells become resistant to insulin (the prediabetes condition INSULIN RESISTANCE), which requires increasingly higher levels of GLUCOSE in the BLOOD circulation to initiate an appropriate insulin response. The high blood glucose levels essentially "burn out" the cells that form delicate nerves and blood vessels, causing them to die. The resulting irreversible damage manifests as PVD and NEUROPATHY.

In an effort to bring blood glucose levels down, the ISLETS OF LANGERHANS in the pancreas, which contain the cells that produce insulin, pump out increasing amounts of insulin. The environment within the body reaches the state of type 2 diabetes when the islet cells can no longer keep pace with the body's demands. The amount of glucose in the blood circulation ultimately reaches levels that cause symptoms such as excessive thirst and URINATION that represent the body's efforts to rid itself of the excessive glucose. Symptoms that reflect damage resulting from elevated blood glucose also occur, such as vision changes, development of cataracts, tingling or loss of sensation in the feet, and wounds that do not heal.

Obesity and cardiovascular disease (CVD)   Obesity sets the stage for HYPERLIPIDEMIA, the pathologic circumstance of excessive lipids (fatty acids) in the blood circulation. Hyperlipidemia is the foundation of occlusive forms of CARDIOVASCULAR DISEASE (CVD) such as CAD, atherosclerosis, and CAROTID STENOSIS. Obesity is also the primary cause of hypertension, partly as a consequence of obstructive CVD such as atherosclerosis and partly because the pressure excessive body fat places on the arteries, veins, and organs increases the resistance blood encounters as it flows through the circulation and forces the HEART to work harder to pump blood. The increased workload of the heart may lead to HEART FAILURE.

Obesity and osteoarthritis   Excessive body weight places considerable stress on the structures of the musculoskeletal system, most notably the back, hips, knees, ankles, and feet. The CARTILAGE that pads and cushions the joints distorts under such pressure, and over time sustains permanent damage. Physical inactivity exacerbates the situation. Osteoarthritis symptoms dramatically improve with weight loss, however, and much of the temporary damage to the structures of the joints is able to heal.

Obesity and gallbladder disease   Gallstones are three times more common in people who have obesity. Lipids and fatty acids in the blood circulation provide the LIVER with a supply of the material it needs to manufacture cholesterol, a key ingredient of BILE. Ironically, rapid weight loss in someone who has obesity (greater than three pounds per week) also triggers formation of gallstones.

Obesity and cancer   Rates of certain cancers are significantly higher in people who have obesity. The correlation is strongest for hormonally driven cancers such as prostate cancer in men and breast cancer, OVARIAN CANCER, and ENDOMETRIAL CANCER (cancer of the UTERUS) in women. Many health experts believe obesity is a major risk factor for colorectal cancer, particularly in men, though studies are less conclusive than for obesity's correlation with other cancers.

Obesity as an independent health condition   Aside from its role as a contributing factor to numerous health conditions, which doctors call co-morbidity, obesity itself is a disorder with metabolic, cardiovascular, pulmonary, and musculoskeletal symptoms. The presence of obesity alone, setting aside all correlating health conditions, shortens LIFE EXPECTANCY nearly as much as cigarette smoking. People who weigh more than 30 percent above healthy body weight are up to 10 times more likely to die prematurely of any cause. The excessive weight and body mass stresses all structures of the body, pressuring internal organs, including the LUNGS, and affecting their ability to function.

Obesity and Quality of Life

Obesity, notably class 3 (morbid) obesity in which a person weighs 100 pounds or more above healthy weight, has a measurably detrimental effect on QUALITY OF LIFE. This level of obesity presents challenges for finding clothing, seating on airplanes, sitting on chairs, riding in cars, navigating store aisles, and even simply being able to walk to get around for the activities of daily living. These challenges commonly result in social isolation and can be a problem for developing friendships and relationships.

Health conditions that have developed as a consequence of obesity may hinder some weight management efforts, notably physical exercise. It is important to find activities that are enjoyable and to persist in them to the extent that they do not worsen other health conditions. A person who has painful osteoarthritis, for example, may choose to walk for 5-minute periods of time four to six times a day instead of walking for 20 or 30 minutes at a time. The cumulative benefit of the short periods of exercise are as effective and easier to accommodate.

OVERCOMING OBSTACLES

Health conditions that limit mobility may interfere with activities such as grocery shopping, leading to relapses in EATING HABITS. Alternative methods to obtain healthful foods might include hiring a teenage neighbor who can drive to shop on a regular basis or shopping through the online services many grocery stores now offer. For a small fee, such services select the items requested and deliver them to the home.

See also CHILDHOOD OBESITY; DEPRESSION; DIABETES PREVENTION; DIET AND HEALTH; EATING DISORDERS; EXERCISE AND HEALTH; LIFESTYLE AND HEALTH; WEIGHT LOSS AND WEIGHT MANAGEMENT.

S

smoking and health   There are no health benefits and numerous health risks from cigarette smoking. In the 1940s few people, including doctors, recognized the magnitude of health risks associated with cigarette smoking. But 20 years later cigarette smoking was a known and publicly identified risk factor for numerous health conditions and the primary cause of HEART disease and LUNG CANCER. In the 1965 cigarette smoking in the United States peaked with about 45 percent of American adults being smokers; by the early 2000s, only 23 percent of American adults smoked. However, that 23 percent represents 48 million people who have significantly increased risk for CARDIOVASCULAR DISEASE (CVD), chronic lung disease, and cancer. Cigarette smoking remains the leading cause of preventable disease in the United States.

PACK YEARS AND DISEASE RISK

One method of representing the amount of cigarette smoke exposure an individual has had is the "pack year." This calculation expresses the number of packs of cigarettes a person smokes each day times the number of years the person has smoked. A person who has smoked for 10 pack years may have smoked half a pack a day for 20 years, one pack a day for 10 years, or two packs a day for five years. The higher the number of pack years, the greater exposure and more significant the risk of pulmonary and cardiovascular disease.

How Smoking Affects the Body and Health

Cigarette smoking affects every cell in the body beginning within seconds of the first inhalation from a cigarette. NICOTINE contracts BLOOD vessels, increases HEART RATE, raises BLOOD PRESSURE, and activates neurotransmitters in the BRAIN that result in CENTRAL NERVOUS SYSTEM stimulation to produce a combined sense of exhilaration and alertness. With each inhalation of cigarette smoke, tar makes its way to the delicate alveoli deep within the LUNGS, clogging them and preventing them from exchanging oxygen. Other chemicals in the smoke irritate the bronchi, causing an increase in mucus production and narrowing of the bronchial openings. Carbon monoxide beats out oxygen to bind with HEMOGLOBIN in the red blood cells (erythrocytes), cutting by up to 60 percent the amount of oxygen each breath carries into the blood circulation. The combined effects of these actions and the chemicals that enter the bloodstream affect cellular METABOLISM in countless ways. Dozens of these chemicals are carcinogenic; they cause cells within the body to develop into cancers. Some of the effects linger for hours after the cigarette and compound with further smoking.

Cigarette smoking and CVD   The leading health consequence of cigarette smoking is CVD. Repeated exposure to nicotine causes permanent changes in the cells that form the lining of the arteries, making the arteries vulnerable to ATHEROSCLEROTIC PLAQUE deposits and, over time, ATHEROSCLEROSIS, CORONARY ARTERY DISEASE (CAD), and PERIPHERAL VASCULAR DISEASE (PVD). Persistent nicotine exposure also causes the arteries to stiffen and lose FLEXIBILITY. These changes lead to HYPERTENSION (high blood pressure) and increased risk for HEART ATTACK and STROKE. The strain on the heart can eventually cause HEART FAILURE.

Cigarette smoking and cancer   The primary form of cancer associated with cigarette smoking is lung cancer. However, cigarette smoking increases the risk for various forms of cancer, including oral cancer, laryngeal cancer, ESOPHAGEAL CANCER, PANCREATIC CANCER, BLADDER CANCER, PROSTATE CANCER,

BREAST CANCER, RENAL CANCER, STOMACH CANCER, and LIVER CANCER. The burning of a cigarette releases smoke that contains more than 4,000 chemicals, dozens of which are known carcinogens (substances that cause cancer).

CARCINOGENS IN CIGARETTE SMOKE	
acrolein	acrylonitrile
aminobiphenyl	aromatic amines
aromatic nitrohydrocarbons	arsenic
benzene	benzofluoranthene
benzopyrene	butadiene
cadmium	chromium
chrysene	crotonaldehyde
dimethylhydrazine	dibenzacridine
dibenzanthracene	dibenzocarbazole
dibenzopyrene	ethylcarbamate
formaldehyde	hydrazine
hydrocarbons	lead
methylamine	methylchrysene
naphthylamine	nickel
nitropropane	nitrosamines
nitrosonomicotine	phenols
polonium-210 (radon)	quinoline
tar	toluidine
urethane	vinyl chloride

Cigarette smoking and chronic pulmonary conditions Cigarette smoking is the primary cause of numerous chronic pulmonary conditions, including CHRONIC OBSTRUCTIVE PULMONARY DISEASE (COPD), chronic BRONCHITIS, and nonallergic ASTHMA. The damage that results from COPD is irreversible and progressive, often leading to permanent disability.

Cigarette smoking and healing The changes that take place in the cells with cigarette smoking slow cellular metabolism, limiting the ability of cells to grow and divide. These functions are essential for HEALING after injury or surgery. As well, lungs damaged by cigarette smoking are unable to deliver adequate oxygen to the blood circulation, restricting a fuel source necessary for cell function. The effects of cigarette smoking on healing are so significant that most surgeons will not perform elective (nonemergency) operations on people who smoke. It is necessary to be smoke free for two to four weeks to mitigate enough of smoking's deleterious action on cellular function to allow effective healing.

Cigarette smoking, fertility, and pregnancy Cigarette smoking affects sperm production in men and OVULATION in women. Smoking during PREGNANCY limits the amount of oxygen the developing fetus receives, affecting fetal growth and development. The babies of women who smoke during pregnancy tend to be 10 to 20 percent smaller at birth than the babies of women who do not smoke. Low birth weight is a health risk for the infant.

Smoking and Preventable Disease
Nearly all of the health consequences associated with cigarette smoking are preventable by not smoking. People who never smoke enjoy the strongest preventive benefit. People who smoke and quit can, over time, restore their health risk for many conditions to near normal. Health conditions such as COPD, lung cancer, laryngeal cancer, and bladder cancer are rare in nonsmokers. Other factors such as EATING HABITS and physical inactivity contribute to CVD, though not smoking removes a significant factor from an individual's health risk profile.

See also ANTISMOKING EFFORTS; ENVIRONMENTAL CIGARETTE SMOKE; ERYTHROCYTE; LIFESTYLE AND HEALTH; NEUROTRANSMITTER; NICOTINE REPLACEMENT; SMOKING CESSATION; TOBACCO USE OTHER THAN SMOKING.

smoking cessation Efforts to stop smoking. Tobacco contains NICOTINE, the addictive quality of which is comparable to that of HEROIN. As well, cigarette smoking becomes a compelling behavioral element of daily life. Most smokers who attempt to quit make numerous efforts before succeeding for the long term and the risk for relapse remains high for years. Of the 1.8 million American smokers who quit every year, 30 percent remain smoke free for one year.

Several medical interventions can help to smokers break the grip of nicotine, including NICOTINE REPLACEMENT products (such as chewing gums, transdermal patches, inhalers, and nasal sprays) and the prescription medication bupropion (Zyban), which appears to diminish the desire to smoke. Nonmedical interventions include HYPNOSIS and BEHAVIOR MODIFICATION THERAPY. Many smokers are more successful with a combination of methods than with a single approach; those who smoke more than 25 cigarettes a day generally benefit more from a structured smoking cessation program with ongoing support and encouragement from a therapist or through a support group.

TIPS FOR SUCCESSFUL SMOKING CESSATION

• Prepare to stop smoking by eliminating all items associated with smoking such as lighters, ashtrays, and cigarettes.

• Identify places and circumstances where smoking is likely to be irresistible and plan alternatives.

• Purchase NICOTINE REPLACEMENT products before quitting and place them in former smoking places, such as in the bathroom, kitchen, and car.

• Plan a system of self-reward for success in meeting short-term goals.

• Arrange with someone to be available around the clock to call when the urge to light up becomes intense.

• Use stress management techniques such as meditation, yoga, and physical exercise to unwind and relax.

The effect of nicotine remains active in the body for about 20 minutes after smoking a cigarette. For many smokers the time between the last cigarette and what would have been the next cigarette is the most difficult, as the body exerts its demand for the next DOSE of nicotine. After 72 hours the nicotine urge subsides considerably. Each day, week, and month without smoking lessens the body's sense of nicotine dependence. About 75 percent of people who make it one month smoke free are able to stay smoke free for one year. Each year of remaining smoke free increases the likelihood of long-term smoking cessation. It is important to take setbacks in stride, identify and eliminate the trigger for the setback, and quickly resume smoking cessation efforts.

See also ANTISMOKING EFFORTS; SMOKING AND CARDIOVASCULAR DISEASE; SMOKING AND HEALTH; TOBACCO USE OTHER THAN SMOKING.

![T–U]

tobacco use other than smoking Forms of tobacco such as chewing tobacco and smoking cigars. Tobacco use other than cigarette smoking is the primary cause of oral cancers (cancers that involve structures of the MOUTH). The two primary forms of tobacco use other than cigarettes are cigars and smokeless tobacco.

Cigar and Pipe Smoking

Cigar and pipe smoke contains many of the same chemicals and carcinogens as cigarette smoke. Because cigar and pipe smokers hold the smoke in their mouths rather than inhaling it, the structures of the mouth have intense exposure to these chemicals. Long-term exposure to tobacco smoke is detrimental to the gums and TEETH and increases the risk for CARDIOVASCULAR DISEASE (CVD).

Though the risk of LUNG CANCER from smoking cigars or pipes is less than that from smoking cigarettes, it is notably higher than for people who do not smoke at all and in people who smoke three or more cigars a day. People who regularly smoke cigars also have higher risk for PANCREATIC CANCER, laryngeal cancer, and ESOPHAGEAL CANCER. The most significant cancer risks from cigar smoking are cancers of the lips, tongue, cheeks, soft palate (roof of the mouth), floor of the mouth, and gums.

Smoking two to three cigars or more a day raises the risk for CVD nearly as much as cigarette smoking. The NICOTINE in tobacco becomes rapidly absorbed into the BLOOD circulation through the mucous membranes in the mouth. Nicotine stimulates the smooth MUSCLE that makes up the walls of the arteries, causing the arteries to stiffen. Chronic exposure to nicotine also alters the structure of the muscle fibers in the arterial walls, reducing their FLEXIBILITY. These changes cause HYPERTENSION (high BLOOD PRESSURE). The changes to the arterial wall's structure also facilitate the accumulation of arterial plaque and atherosclerotic deposits, leading to ATHEROSCLEROSIS and increasing the risk for CORONARY ARTERY DISEASE (CAD).

Smokeless Tobacco

It is a common misperception, particularly among young people, that smokeless tobacco is safe because there is no smoke involved with its use. This is not true. Smokeless tobacco contains nicotine, which is highly addictive. It can be as difficult to quit using smokeless tobacco as it is to stop smoking. A pinch or dip of smokeless tobacco contains as much nicotine as three cigarettes. Forms of smokeless tobacco include snuff, which is powdery, and chewing tobacco (plugs, twists, and loose leaf).

Smokeless tobacco is particularly damaging to the teeth and gums. After only a few years of regular use, the gum tissue may become structurally unstable, unable to support the teeth. Tooth loss may be unpreventable in such circumstances. The irritation of the tobacco against the gums and cheeks also causes sores that can be painful or can further erode the tissue around the base of the teeth. Tobacco juice permanently stains the teeth yellow or brown and erodes the enamel outer layer, increasing the risk for DENTAL CARIES (cavities) and weakening the teeth.

About four times the concentration of nicotine enters the blood circulation from smokeless tobacco as from cigarette smoking. Nicotine that enters the blood circulation by being absorbed through the tissues of the mouth has the same negative effects on the blood vessels as nicotine that enters the blood circulation through the

LUNGS, raising the risk for atherosclerosis and CAD with prolonged use. As well, smokeless tobacco contains carcinogens that release into the mouth and is the leading cause of oral cancers. Doctors diagnose 30,000 people with oral cancers due to smokeless tobacco use each year in the United States; about 8,000 Americans die each year from such oral cancers.

CARCINOGENS IN SMOKELESS TOBACCO

acetaldehyde	arsenic
benzopyrene	cadmium
crotonaldehyde	formaldehyde
hydrazine	nitrosamine acids
polonium-210 (radon)	tobacco-specific
volatile aldehydes	nitrosamines (TSNAs)
volatile nitrosamines	

See also CARCINOGEN; HALITOSIS; SMOKING AND CANCER; SMOKING AND HEALTH; SMOKING CESSATION.

triceps skinfold A measure of the thickness of a fold of SKIN at the triceps (MUSCLE at the back of the upper arm), which indicates BODY FAT PERCENTAGE. Triceps skinfold thickness is easy for doctors, nutritionists, and fitness professionals to measure as a means of monitoring loss of body fat. A tensioned caliper, placed over a segment of pinched skin at the triceps, measure the skinfold thickness in millimeters. The thickness value corresponds roughly to the body fat percentage. For example, a triceps skinfold measurement of 10 millimeters (mm) corresponds to approximately 10 percent body fat; of 35 mm to approximately 35 percent body fat. The triceps skinfold measurement may also serve as an indicator for adequate nutrition in infants and young children, with less than 5 mm (5 percent body fat) indicating insufficient nutrition.

See also BODY MASS INDEX (BMI); UPPER ARM CIRCUMFERENCE; WAIST CIRCUMFERENCE; WAIST TO HIP RATIO.

upper arm circumference A measurement of the distance around the center of the upper arm, which serves as an approximate measure of LEAN MUSCLE MASS. Upper arm circumference, also called mid-upper arm circumference (MUCA), is one method to estimate appropriate nutrition. The muscles store protein, thus measuring the size of muscles provides an approximation of the body's protein supply. In undernutrition and MALNUTRITION MUSCLE size shrinks because the body metabolizes protein stores to generate energy. Overnutrition (overweight and OBESITY) results in exaggerated muscle size as a consequence of high amounts of fat in the muscle fibers. RESISTANCE EXERCISE such as weightlifting enlarges the upper arm muscles, which can make upper arm measurement less accurate as an assessment of lean muscle mass.

UPPER ARM CIRCUMFERENCE AND HEALTH

Measurement (centimeters)	Health Risk Correlation
<16	MALNUTRITION
16.1 to 18.5	increased risk for undernutrition
18.6 to 22	no increased health risk
22.1 to 25	overweight, moderate health risk
> 25	OBESITY, significant health risk

See also BODY MASS INDEX (BMI); TRICEPS SKIN FOLD; WAIST CIRCUMFERENCE; WAIST TO HIP RATIO; WEIGHT LOSS AND WEIGHT MANAGEMENT.

waist circumference The distance measured around the waist. Doctors define the waist as the imaginary line that circles the body between the umbilicus (belly button) and the crest of the hip bones. Healthy waist circumference is less than 35 inches for a woman and less than 40 inches for a man, regardless of age. Waist circumference is an important measure of health risk for conditions such as OBESITY, INSULIN RESISTANCE, type 2 DIABETES, and forms of CARDIOVASCULAR DISEASE (CVD) such as HYPERTENSION (high BLOOD PRESSURE), HYPERLIPIDEMIA, ATHEROSCLEROSIS, and CORONARY ARTERY DISEASE (CAD). Excessive waist circumference also dramatically increases risk for HEART ATTACK.

Though waist circumference alone increases the risk for health conditions, the risk compounds when it occurs in combination with elevated BODY MASS INDEX (BMI). Health risk rises moderately when BMI reaches 25 and significantly when BMI reaches 30. In combination with waist circumference that exceeds 35 inches for a woman or 40 inches for a man, health risk jumps to the next level. Other risk factors for CVD, such as cigarette smoking and physical inactivity, further increase the likelihood for heart disease, heart attack, and STROKE. Weight loss sufficient to decrease waist circumference also decreases BMI, improving the health risk.

Waist circumference that exceeds 35 inches for women or 40 inches for men when body weight is within the range of healthy (BMI of 18.5 to 24.9) indicates a body fat distribution pattern of ABDOMINAL ADIPOSITY, which reflects increased risk for heart attack and CVD even when no other risk factors for heart disease are present. Doctors recommend modest weight loss (5 to 10 percent), with emphasis on increased physical activity, to reduce waist circumference.

See also HEALTH RISK FACTORS; WAIST TO HIP RATIO; WEIGHT LOSS AND WEIGHT MANAGEMENT.

waist to hip ratio The proportion between the distance around the waist and the distance around the hips (WAIST CIRCUMFERENCE divided by hip circumference). A waist to hip ratio of 0.9 in men and 0.8 in women indicates an "apple" body shape, which reflects an elevated body fat percentage, heralds an increased risk for CARDIOVASCULAR DISEASE (CVD) and HEART ATTACK in particular. The higher the waist to hip ratio, the greater the risk.

WAIST TO HIP RATIO AND HEALTH RISK		
Health Risk	**Men**	**Women**
healthy, no increased risk	0.89 or less	0.79 or less
moderate to significant	0.9 or greater	0.8 or less

WAIST CIRCUMFERENCE, BODY MASS INDEX (BMI), AND HEALTH RISK DUE TO WEIGHT			
Health Risk	**Moderate**	**Significant**	**Severe**
BMI overweight (25 to 29.9)	X		
waist > 35 inches/40 inches	X		
BMI overweight plus waist > 35/40 inches		X	
BMI OBESITY class 1 (30 to 34.9)		X	
BMI obesity class 1 plus waist > 35/40 inches			X

See also ABDOMINAL ADIPOSITY; BODY MASS INDEX (BMI); BODY SHAPE AND CARDIOVASCULAR DISEASE; UPPER ARM CIRCUMFERENCE.

weight loss and weight management The approaches and methods to lose excessive weight and maintain healthy weight after weight loss. Two thirds of Americans weigh more than is healthy, with a corresponding increase in weight-related health conditions such as HYPERTENSION (high BLOOD PRESSURE), type 2 DIABETES, OSTEOARTHRITIS, ATHEROSCLEROSIS, and CORONARY ARTERY DISEASE (CAD). Americans also spend tens of billions of dollars each year on diet programs, books, diet aids, and other weight-loss products. Yet the premise of weight loss and weight management is fairly simple: eat less and exercise more as a matter of lifestyle.

Losing Weight

A weight loss approach that balances decreased food intake and increased exercise can provide steady, sustainable results. Health experts recommend a rate of nonsurgical weight loss that targets no more than a 10 percent drop in weight over no less than six months for optimal success in keeping the weight off long term. Short-term weight loss goals help monitor progress and establish a sense of success. Methods for weight loss include lifestyle modifications, BEHAVIOR MODIFICATION THERAPY, medication therapy, and BARIATRIC SURGERY.

Lifestyle modifications: eating habits and exercise Lifestyle is the cornerstone of weight management. Many people achieve greater success with their weight loss efforts when they join programs that incorporate nutritional control (such as prepared meals or stringent menus) and structured physical exercise (such as group classes). However, fad diets that promise rapid weight loss generally do not produce sustainable results.

It is important for people who need to lose weight to understand portion sizes, NUTRIENT DENSITY, NUTRITIONAL NEEDS, and nutritional food choices that are also palatable. This understanding is essential for incorporating healthy EATING HABITS into long-term lifestyle modifications. Unless under a doctor's supervision and guidance, daily CALORIE intake should never drop below 1,200 calories for women and 1,600 calories for men.

Calorie intake below these levels activates the body's starvation mechanisms, which result in slower METABOLISM and efforts to conserve energy (calories). Daily exercise is essential to increase the body's energy expenditure. During weight loss efforts, increased activity and decreased food consumption combine for the most efficient results.

---

30 MINUTES A DAY = 15 POUNDS A YEAR
One pound of fat is the equivalent of 3,500 calories. Physical exercise at the minimum recommended level of 30 minutes daily typically consumes 150 calories a day. This adds up to nearly 1½ pounds a month, or 15 pounds a year, lost through exercise alone.

Behavior modification therapy Behavior modification therapy may incorporate techniques such as taking smaller portions with the understanding that one can have more if still hungry, extending consumption of a meal over a certain period of time to encourage a slower pace of eating, eating only at the table without reading or watching television, keeping a food and exercise journal, scheduling exercise "appointments," and shopping after eating and only from a list.

Medication therapy Prescription APPETITE suppressants can help people follow portion size and eating recommendations to reduce the amount of calories they consume. Medications tend to become less effective over time. Researchers are uncertain whether this is an issue of physiologic tolerance (the body becomes resistant to the medication's effect) or a matter of becoming accustomed to the medication and more able to overcome its effect. Medication may be an appropriate treatment for people who have a BODY MASS INDEX (BMI) between 30 and 34.9 (class 1 OBESITY) and who have been unsuccessful with efforts to lose weight. The medications to suppress appetite may have significant side effects or DRUG interactions.

Over-the-counter (OTC) diet medications often contain CAFFEINE or a decongestant such as pseudoephedrine. These drugs may mildly suppress the appetite though their long-term use may result in side effects such as agitation and PALPITATIONS. OTC diet products generally provide no greater benefit than diet and exercise alone.

MEDICATIONS TO SUPPRESS APPETITE

Medication	Actions	Possible Side Effects
orlistat (Xenical)	blocks intestinal absorption of fat	frequent or uncontrollable bowel movements deficiency of fat-soluble vitamins (A, D, E, and K)
phentermine (Fastin)	CENTRAL NERVOUS SYSTEM stimulant increases NOREPINEPHRINE levels in the BRAIN, which suppresses the APPETITE and HUNGER centers	dependency PALPITATIONS insomnia DRUG INTERACTION with monoamine oxidase inhibitor (MAOI) antidepressants
sibutramine (Meridia)	increases norepinephrine and serotonin levels in the brain, an action that suppresses the appetite and hunger centers and elevates mood	serotonin syndrome drug interaction with narcotic analgesics, selective serotonin reuptake inhibitor (SSRI) antidepressants, and MAOI antidepressants

Bariatric surgery Weight loss surgery is a drastic measure that becomes a treatment option when an individual's weight exceeds 100 pounds over healthy weight (class 3 obesity) or otherwise directly and immediately threatens health. Most bariatric surgery operations either restrict the size of the STOMACH to limit the volume of consumed food or alter the flow of ingested food to curtail absorption. Surgery for weight loss has numerous risks and potential complications, though may be the therapeutic approach that succeeds for people who have been otherwise unable to reach a healthier weight.

HEALTH BENEFITS OF WEIGHT LOSS

- decrease OSTEOARTHRITIS symptoms
- improve INSULIN sensitivity
- relieve OBSTRUCTIVE SLEEP APNEA
- improve type 2 DIABETES
- increase energy and mobility
- reduce risk for CARDIOVASCULAR DISEASE (CVD)
- relieve chronic BACK PAIN
- improve HYPERLIPIDEMIA
- improve HYPERTENSION
- improve LIBIDO and sexual function
- improve self-esteem
- improve FERTILITY
- reduce risk for cancer
- reduce risk for type 2 diabetes
- relieve GASTROESOPHAGEAL REFLUX DISORDER (GERD)

Maintaining Healthy Body Weight

Weight loss that is gradual and steady generally results from incorporating lifestyle changes that will support sustained weight management. Even small progress makes a measurable difference in health and well-being.

Social and family support Encouragement and support for weight loss and weight management from family and friends is crucial for long-term success, though is often a complex dynamic. Some people find themselves alone in their weight loss efforts because other family members do not want to make the same changes in their own eating habits and physical activity. Other people are able to make weight loss and weight management a family endeavor or to join with friends to support and encourage one another. Positive reinforcement for achievements, however small, is far more effective than criticism.

Relapse and weight gain Relapses of regained weight are common and disheartening. However, the quicker a person recognizes that his or her weight is slipping back toward obesity the easier it is to stop the slide and return to the treatment methods that were effective. Unfortunately many people tend not only to regain lost weight but also to gain additional weight. Such a rebound or "yo-yo" effect is especially detrimental to health. It is important to get back on track with eating habits and exercise as quickly as possible to halt weight gain before it becomes overwhelming to confront.

See also DIET AND HEALTH; EATING DISORDERS; EXERCISE AND HEALTH; OBESITY AND HEALTH.

SUBSTANCE ABUSE

Substance abuse is the use of any DRUG, including ALCOHOL, or other psychoactive substances in ways that are harmful to a person or others whom the person's actions may affect. Health-care practitioners who provide care for people who have substance abuse problems, alcohol or drug DEPENDENCE, and ADDICTION may be physicians (MDs or DOs), psychiatrists (physicians who specialize in psychiatric disorders), psychologists (PhDs), social workers (LSWs), and clinical registered nurse practitioners (CRNPs). Practitioners may be certified substance abuse professionals (SAPs), designating that they have additional education and experience in treating substance abuse (including ALCOHOLISM).

This section, "Substance Abuse," presents an overview discussion of the health implications of substance abuse and alcoholism and entries about substances of abuse, health risks related to substance abuse, and treatment for substance abuse.

From Tonic to Toxin: Opium's Odyssey

Many substances currently restricted because of their high potential for abuse were once in common use. For centuries cultures around the world used opium, the dried sap from the poppy plant, *Papaver somniferum,* to relieve PAIN, induce sleep, and provide INTOXICATION. In 1805 a young pharmacist's assistant, Freidrich Wilhelm Adam Serturner (1783–1841), isolated morphine, opium's most potent ingredient, from opium; 90 years later chemists at the Bayer Company created HEROIN from morphine. For the next decade the most common use of heroin was to treat morphine addiction—clearly a circumstance, in retrospect, of leaping from the frying pan into the fire.

By 1913 the Bayer Company stopped producing heroin, and in the 1920s opium and heroin became illegal in the United States. Federal law regulated the manufacture, sale, and possession of morphine and other medicinal OPIATES. Nonetheless heroin continued to make its way into the United States, and in 1970 its abuse peaked with more than 750,000 Americans addicted. Perhaps not so coincidentally the US Congress passed the Controlled Substances Act, the first comprehensive classification and enforcement legislation for

drugs, in the same year. Through concerted legal, social, and medical efforts heroin abuse declined significantly over the following 30 years, and in 2004 the US Substance Abuse and Mental Health Administration (SAMHA) estimated 166,000 people actively using heroin.

Opiates, and in particular morphine and its direct derivatives, remain the mainstay of analgesia (pain relief) in medical treatment though under tight regulatory control. Tens of millions of Americans use opiates for effective pain management. However, PRESCRIPTION DRUG ABUSE of opiate NARCOTICS such as hydromorphone, hydrocodone, oxycodone, and codeine becomes problematic for about four million of them.

Health Implications of Substance Abuse

Addiction is a condition that develops over time, regardless of the substance or behavior that is the source of the addiction. Social factors compound the health issues of addiction; many people are afraid or reluctant to acknowledge a possible addiction for fear of repercussions in all areas of their lives. Despite advances in understanding addiction in recent years, the perception remains that addiction is a matter of insufficient willpower. However, addiction arising from substance abuse (whether alcohol, NICOTINE, illicit drugs, or prescription drugs) represents a complex entanglement of physiologic, psychologic, and social factors. Many people abuse multiple substances though have a primary substance of abuse.

DRUG SLANG

Drug Name	Slang Names
ALKYL NITRITES	rush, locker room, rave, poppers, snappers
AMPHETAMINES	speed, go-pill, upper
BARBITURATES	yellow jackets, reds, blues, rainbows, downers, barbs, goofballs
COCAINE	coke, snow, flake, blow, big C, lady, nose candy, white, party favors
DEXTROMETHORPHAN	DXM, skittles, candy, c-c-c, dex, DM, Drex, red devils, tussin, velvet
FLUNITRAZEPAM (Rohypnol)	roofies, rophies, roach, rope, forget-me pill
GAMMA HYDROXYBUTYRATE (GHB)	liquid ecstasy, soap, easy lay, vita-G, Georgia home boy
HEROIN	smack, horse, brown sugar, junk, black tar, big H, bag
KETAMINE	special K, vitamin K, super K, keets
lysergic acid diethylamide (LSD)	acid, blotter, trip, hit, sugar cube, microdot, tab, purple haze
marijuana	pot, weed, reefer, mary jane, aunt mary, boom, kif, skunk, herb, dope, gangster
METHAMPHETAMINE	speed, crank, crystal, ice, glass, meth, crystal meth
METHYLENEDIOXYMETHAMPHETAMINE (MDMA)	XTC, X, hug drug, ecstasy, ecstacy
PHENCYCLIDINE (PCP)	angel dust, ozone, wack, rocket fuel, crystal supergrass, embalming fluid, killer joint

Often the break from the addictive behaviors occurs as a consequence of intervention, either by family members and friends or through legal processes such as court-imposed sentencing to a substance abuse program. Unfortunately, such intervention all too often comes at the cost of injury to self or others. Alcohol is a factor in more than half of MOTOR VEHICLE ACCIDENTS in the United States. Other substances that alter perception, judgment, and reaction time further contribute to traffic accidents, which are the leading cause of accidental injury and death. These substances include CANNABIS products (marijuana, hashish, hash oil), as well as STIMULANTS, BARBITURATES, BENZODIAZEPINES, and HALLUCINOGENS.

Two thirds of new HIV/AIDS INFECTION among women in the United States result directly or indirectly from injected drug use: either the woman herself injects illicit drugs or has sexual partners who inject illicit drugs. Intravenous drug use is also the leading means of transmitting infection with HEPATITIS B, hepatitis C, and hepatitis D. Intravenous drug users face numerous other risks including ENDOCARDITIS (bacterial infection of the HEART valves), damaged and destroyed veins, cellulitis (infection of the skin and underlying tissue), MALNUTRITION, and poisoning from the unknown ingredients illicit drugs contain as fillers.

Special Risks: Substance Abuse During Pregnancy
Substance abuse during PREGNANCY poses unique risks for the developing FETUS, which may experience health crises at birth and lifelong health consequences. Among the most toxic substances of abuse is alcohol, which is teratogenic at nearly every stage of pregnancy. FETAL ALCOHOL SYNDROME

(FAS) is the most severe complication of maternal alcohol use during pregnancy. FAS may involve significant physical BIRTH DEFECTS, BRAIN damage, developmental delays, LEARNING DISORDERS, and psychologic conditions.

Infants of women who are addicted to drugs are born addicted themselves, requiring intensive medical care after birth to wean them from the drugs and restore normal body functions. These infants are also often born prematurely, further compromising their health and well-being. Though the teratogenic risks of drugs such as heroin and COCAINE remain unclear, long-term health problems and learning disabilities later in childhood are common.

Babies born to women who smoke cigarettes are characteristically of small birth weight, which researchers believe results from insufficient oxygen in the mother's BLOOD circulation. They also have high risk for failure to thrive, a potentially lethal health circumstance in which the infant does not grow and develop normally but for no discernible medical reasons. Such infants require diligent care and frequent medical attention, and are more vulnerable to infection and illness.

Advances in Knowledge and Treatment

Discovery of opiate receptors in the early 1970s was a huge leap forward in understanding how narcotics work in the brain. Subsequent advances allowed researchers to identify the roles of other neuroreceptors and neurotransmitters and to discover alterations in brain function that occur with specific drugs. Psychiatric disorders also play roles in susceptibility to addiction.

Some research has shown that more than 80 percent of people diagnosed with SCHIZOPHRENIA are also heavy cigarette smokers—addicted to nicotine—have other substance abuse problems or addictions. Researchers do not know whether the addictions increase susceptibility for psychiatric illness or psychiatric illness increases vulnerability for addictions.

The multiplicity of factors that contribute to addiction make its treatment all the more difficult. Of the 20 million Americans who have substance abuse or addiction problems, fewer than 4 million seek treatment. New medications that target specific neuroreceptors have vastly improved symptom relief during DETOXIFICATION and help maintain SOBRIETY after withdrawal for many people. Integrated efforts to educate students and employees about the dangers of substance abuse, coupled with mandatory drug testing in a growing number of environments, appear to have significantly reduced substance abuse in certain settings. Focused therapy that helps people learn new behaviors (BEHAVIOR MODIFICATION THERAPY) and gain insight into the reasons they abuse drugs and alcohol (COGNITIVE THERAPY) seems to be improving the success rate for maintaining sobriety. As well, pharmacologic research is producing new kinds of narcotics that can target specific neuroreceptors in ways that provide therapeutic action (such as pain relief) with low risk for addiction.

addiction A pattern of lifestyle that revolves around obtaining and using drugs. The behaviors of this pattern are compulsive and difficult to resist or overcome, particularly when there is physical DRUG DEPENDENCE. However, addiction can occur with nearly any substance (such as drugs, ALCOHOL, and tobacco) or behavior (such as gambling) that a person feels he or she cannot live without and is willing to take substantial risks to keep the substance or behavior part of everyday life. For most people addiction is a chronic condition for which successful treatment often requires ongoing diligence, participation in SUPPORT GROUPS, and PSYCHOTHERAPY.

Numerous health complications are associated with addiction. Key among them are HEPATITIS and HIV/AIDS among people who inject drugs using shared needles and paraphernalia. MALNUTRITION is common among people who have addictions to alcohol, HEROIN, COCAINE, AMPHETAMINES, and METHAMPHETAMINE. Prime health risks associated with the leading addiction in the United States, cigarette smoking, include CARDIOVASCULAR DISEASE (CVD) and LUNG CANCER.

SUBSTANCES FOR WHICH ADDICTION IS MOST COMMON

ALCOHOL	AMPHETAMINES
BARBITURATES	BENZODIAZEPINES
CANNABIS compounds	COCAINE
DESIGNER DRUGS	HALLUCINOGENS
inhalants	METHAMPHETAMINE
methylphenidate	NICOTINE
OPIATES	organic solvents

Symptoms and Diagnostic Path
Symptoms of addiction are often apparent to family members and friends long before the person who has the addiction recognizes them. Denial of addiction is itself a key symptom. Specific symptoms of addiction vary with the substance that is the source of the addiction and may cover a broad range of physiologic and psychologic characteristics. General symptoms of addiction may include

- agitation or anxiety
- obsessive interest in maintaining or obtaining access to the substance or behavior
- loss of interest in work, family, and social activities
- isolation from others
- dramatic change in physical appearance, such as continuously runny NOSE, bloodshot eyes, or weight loss

Diagnosis of addiction is a complex process that often includes input from a physician, a psychologist or psychiatrist, and a substance abuse specialist. Though BLOOD and URINE tests may provide evidence that a particular substance is in the body, such test results alone do not establish a diagnosis of addiction. The diagnostic path includes physical and psychologic examinations that look for indications of substance abuse, such as needle tracks (injected drugs) or rotted TEETH (methamphetamine), and behaviors that suggest addiction (most possessions have disappeared, poor PERSONAL HYGIENE, fired from multiple jobs or not able to get a job, frequent arrests or other legal problems).

Treatment Options and Outlook
There are numerous approaches to treatment for addiction, most of which have short-term and long-term components. The treatment approach must meet the specific needs of the individual as

well as address the physiologic and psychologic aspects of the substances to which the person has addictions. In the short term, SUBSTANCE ABUSE TREATMENT may require intensive psychologic support and therapy through an outpatient or inpatient substance abuse treatment program.

Treatment may involve medical care for symptoms of WITHDRAWAL SYNDROME resulting from drug dependence, such as NICOTINE REPLACEMENT patches for tobacco dependence, METHADONE or BUPRENOR-PHINE for opiate dependence, and disulfiram for alcohol dependence. Medication therapy may also focus on treating underlying or accompanying psychologic disorders such as DEPRESSION (ANTIDE-PRESSANT MEDICATIONS) and anxiety (ANTIANXIETY MEDICATIONS). Treatment programs typically also include intensive psychotherapy, BEHAVIOR MODIFI-CATION THERAPY, COGNITIVE THERAPY, group therapy, and peer support. These approaches attempt to help people understand their motivations for seeking the effects of the substance of abuse, the behaviors they indulge in to achieve the substance, and the ways in which they can replace those behaviors with others that support nondrug-seeking behaviors.

Relapses are common among people who have addictions. Once established, an addiction remains a powerful compulsion even with treatment and methods to mitigate its strength. Absolute avoidance of the substance or behavior (abstinence) is crucial; most addiction experts agree that people who have addictions cannot experience "just a little" of the addiction's source without succumbing again to the addiction. Though researchers do not fully understand the complexity of addiction's mechanisms, they do know that even small exposure to the source can reactivate the addiction. Long-term REMISSION requires persistence and determination in combination with a strong support network of family, friends, and health-care providers.

Risk Factors and Preventive Measures
Multiple factors contribute to addiction. Among the key risks are

- underlying psychologic conditions such as depression, ATTENTION DEFICIT HYPERACTIVITY DIS-ORDER (ADHD), and POST-TRAUMATIC STRESS DISOR-DER (PTSD)

- intense feelings of anxiety, loneliness, and loss
- PEER PRESSURE
- family history of ALCOHOLISM or substance abuse

Though genetic factors likely exist that contribute to an individual's vulnerability to addiction, researchers believe such factors are multiple and affect numerous processes within the body. As well, some drugs have higher potential for addiction, notably those that produce an intense response to taking them. Such drugs include methamphetamine, heroin, and cocaine.

It often seems, to those outside looking in at addiction, that the simple solution to preventing addiction is making the choice not to use drugs or alcohol. This is an effective solution in many circumstances; the person who is able to avoid the substance does not develop addiction to substances if not taking them. However, the health condition of addiction is complex; one of its most destructive features is its ability to impair a person's capability to make such choices. The consequences of addiction are often severe yet do not deter the pursuit of the addiction's source. The most effective prevention efforts are those that combine education about substance abuse and its negative health effects with measures to help people choose not to use substances of abuse the first time.

See also GENERALIZED ANXIETY DISORDER (GAD); ILLICIT DRUG ABUSE; NALTREXONE; OBSESSIVE–COMPUL-SIVE DISORDER (OCD); PRESCRIPTION DRUG ABUSE; SMOK-ING CESSATION; SCHEDULED DRUG; SUBSTANCE ABUSE PREVENTION; TOLERANCE.

aerosols and glues See ORGANIC SOLVENTS.

alcohol In the context of health and substance abuse a fermented or distilled beverage containing ethanol (also called ethyl alcohol) that, when ingested, has numerous effects on the body, ranging from mild relaxation to INTOXICATION. Alcohol consumption is legal though regulated in the United States by federal and state laws and prohibited by minors (those under age 21). Each state establishes the laws and regulations that govern its alcohol sales. However, access to alcohol is such that underage alcohol consumption is a significant health and social problem. In the United States, alcohol is a factor in more than one third of MOTOR VEHICLE ACCIDENTS. Long-term alcohol abuse contributes to numerous health conditions including permanent birth defects in children exposed to alcohol during fetal development (FETAL ALCOHOL SYNDROME). Alcohol is the most commonly abused DRUG in the United States.

Alcoholic Beverages

From the perspective of intoxication, a drink is merely the vehicle that carries alcohol into the body. The alcohol in a distilled beverage such as gin is no different from the alcohol in beer or wine. What does differ is the concentration of alcohol within the drink. A distilled drink may contain 40 percent alcohol (represented as "80 proof" on the label); a beer is usually 4 percent and wine is 10 to 14 percent. Thus a 1-ounce shot of distilled spirits, 12-ounce glass of beer, and 5-ounce glass of wine all contain roughly the same amount of alcohol. Each of these is a "standard" drink for purposes of assessing alcohol consumption. Alcohol contains 7 calories per gram, 100 to 150 calories per standard drink. Mixers add additional calories. Other than energy, alcohol has no nutritional value.

Alcohol Absorption and Metabolism

Ethanol is a small molecule that the body rapidly absorbs through the STOMACH and SMALL INTESTINE and that, once in the BLOOD circulation, readily crosses the BLOOD–BRAIN BARRIER to affect the BRAIN directly. A person generally begins to feel the effects of alcohol within 10 minutes of ingesting an alcoholic drink; the amount of alcohol in the blood circulation peaks about 45 minutes after consumption. Factors that influence the rate of absorption include carbonation and the presence of food. The alcohol from carbonated alcoholic beverages, such as beer and champagne, enters the blood circulation more rapidly than from non-carbonated alcoholic beverages such as wine. Foods, particularly those high in fat and protein, significantly slow the absorption of alcohol.

Once in the blood circulation, however, alcohol metabolizes at a consistent, predictable rate regardless of its ingested form. The body metabolizes alcohol far more slowly than it absorbs alcohol. Though alcohol METABOLISM varies among individuals, in general the body takes 60 to 90 minutes to metabolize one standard drink's worth of the alcohol. Men tend to metabolize alcohol more quickly than women because they have higher quantities of the enzyme acetaldehyde dehydrogenase, which breaks down acetaldehyde (a harmful toxin) to acetic acid (a harmless waste product) that the body can excrete in the URINE.

Ingesting large quantities of ethanol (alcoholic beverages) or of alcohols other than ethanol such as methanol (wood alcohol) and isopropyl alcohol (rubbing alcohol) is potentially fatal.

Alcohol Intoxication

Intoxication (drunkenness) occurs with alcohol consumption because alcohol, which is chemically a solvent, literally softens the neural membranes (the outermost structure of a NEURON), disrupting their ability to respond to electrical impulses (action potential). The highest concentration of neurons is in the brain; the brain neurons most significantly affected appear to be those of the prefrontal cortex, a part of the brain responsible for coordinating numerous functions of cognition, judgment, memory, and inhibition. From a physiologic perspective these changes and the behaviors that result define intoxication. The return to normal follows the same path in reverse, with the less complex functions returning first as the neural membranes essentially "dry out."

Alcohol also alters the presence and balance of chemicals in the brain. Among them are

- gamma-aminobutyric acid (GABA), an inhibitory NEUROTRANSMITTER that carries NERVE impulses in the cerebral cortex to facilitate processes related to inhibitions

- DOPAMINE, a neurotransmitter that is key for nerve impulses related to mood, emotion, and the perception of pleasure

- glutamate, an excitatory neurotransmitter that increases activity among neurons

Alcohol blocks the actions of GABA and glutamate, suppressing the mechanisms in the brain that inhibit inappropriate behaviors and create a sense of relaxation and calmness. At the same time alcohol increases the presence of dopamine, resulting in feelings of pleasure or even euphoria. With continued, excessive alcohol consumption the brain becomes accustomed to these altered balances and develops reliance on the alcohol to maintain them. At the same time the brain develops TOLERANCE to the presence of alcohol in the blood circulation; it requires higher doses of alcohol to elicit the same neurotransmitter responses.

The physical and mental impairments typically associated with intoxication begins with the most complex skills and progresses to the least complex skills. Because judgment is among the complex skills, by the time a person loses motor function skills (such as balance and coordination) he or she is unable to perceive their deficiencies. Memory storage and retrieval are also high-level skills impaired early in intoxication, accounting for the inability to remember events that happen during intoxication. Long-term, chronic alcohol abuse (frequent, repeated intoxication) alters GENE expression within cells that may result in permanent changes in cell activity.

The uniform standard for legal intoxication in the United States is a blood alcohol concentration (BAC) of 0.08 percent, which represents a measure 80 milligrams of alcohol per deciliter (100 milliliters) of blood. This is the level of alcohol concentration in the blood circulation at which predictable impairments typically occur. However, individuals may appear more or less intoxicated than their BACs suggest because response to alcohol varies.

Health Benefits of Alcohol Consumption

A number of research studies suggest that for most people regular, moderate alcohol consumption—no more than one alcoholic drink daily for women and two alcoholic drinks daily for men—can reduce the risk for CARDIOVASCULAR DISEASE (CVD) such as HYPERTENSION (high BLOOD PRESSURE) and ATHEROSCLEROSIS (fatty deposits in the walls of the arteries). Alcohol affects lipid metabolism, raising levels of high-density lipoprotein (HDL) cholesterol—the "good" cholesterol. It also influences COAGULATION processes, altering the activation of certain coagulation factors in ways that slightly slow blood clotting. Alcohol appears to help relax the smooth MUSCLE of the walls of the arteries,

reducing blood pressure. However, health experts caution that people who do not currently drink should not start; the potential health benefits do not sufficiently outweigh the risks. People who should not drink alcohol under any circumstances include those who are in recovery from ALCOHOLISM and pregnant women. People who take prescription drugs should be cautious because alcohol interferes with numerous medications.

Health Risks of Alcohol Consumption

Alcohol toxicity is a serious risk with bouts of heavy or binge drinking in which a person consumes large quantities of alcohol in a short time. A blood alcohol concentration twice the legally defined level of intoxication, 0.16 percent, results in the state of euphoria commonly associated with being intoxicated. At this concentration in the blood circulation alcohol significantly impairs judgment, physical coordination, and reaction time. A blood alcohol level three times the typical legal limit—0.24 percent—causes extreme confusion and possibly stupor. With a blood alcohol level of 0.35 percent the average person is unconscious; 0.50 percent is often a point of no return leading to RESPIRATORY FAILURE and death.

HEALTH RISKS OF ALCOHOL ABUSE

Short Term

ACCIDENTAL INJURIES	acts of VIOLENCE
alcohol toxicity	impaired cognitive function
impaired judgment	impaired physical
interaction with medications	coordination
reduced inhibition	short-term memory
sleep disturbances	difficulties
slowed reaction times	slurred speech

Long Term

BERIBERI	CARDIOMYOPATHY
CIRRHOSIS	FETAL ALCOHOL SYNDROME
GASTRITIS	GASTROINTESTINAL BLEEDING
HYPERTENSION	LIVER CANCER
LIVER DISEASE OF ALCOHOLISM	NUTRITIONAL DEFICIENCY
PANCREATIC CANCER	PANCREATITIS
STEATOHEPATITIS	STOMACH CANCER

The primary health consequence of chronic, excessive alcohol consumption is alcoholism. Alcoholism is an addiction to alcohol (physiologic and psychologic dependence on alcohol) and is a leading health problem in the United States. Secondary to alcoholism is a high risk for LIVER disease. Because it metabolizes alcohol, the liver is the organ most vulnerable to alcohol's toxic effects. Long-term excessive alcohol consumption also increases the risk for LIVER CANCER, STOMACH CANCER, COLORECTAL CANCER, BREAST CANCER, CORONARY ARTERY DISEASE (CAD), hypertension, and NUTRITIONAL DEFICIENCY.

See also ALCOHOLIC HALLUCINOSIS; CELL STRUCTURE AND FUNCTION; DELIRIUM TREMENS; HEPATOTOXINS; ILLICIT DRUG ABUSE; PRESCRIPTION DRUG ABUSE; SUBSTANCE ABUSE PREVENTION; SUBSTANCE ABUSE TREATMENT.

alcohol interactions with medications The numerous ways in which ALCOHOL intensifies or inhibits the actions and side effects of prescription and OVER-THE-COUNTER (OTC) DRUGS. Alcohol also interacts with illicit drugs though often unpredictably because of their uncertain composition. As well, some drugs interact with alcohol in ways that alter alcohol's METABOLISM and actions in the body. Alcohol-medication interactions are of increasing concern as more than 70 percent of Americans take regular medications and at least 10 percent of them drink alcohol daily.

Liver Enzymes and Drug Metabolism

The LIVER produces CYTOCHROME P450 (CYP450) ENZYMES that metabolize (break down into their chemical components) most drugs that enter the body. The enzymes act at predictable rates for specific substances, one of the key factors in establishing appropriate DRUG dosages. Alcohol–medication interactions occur in two general ways: through competition for the enzymes that metabolize them (short-term or acute alcohol consumption) and through changes in the way the liver produces these enzymes (long-term or chronic alcohol consumption). Because the primary interaction between alcohol and medications occurs at this enzyme level, alcohol affects in some way the actions of nearly all medications.

In the short term, acute alcohol consumption (drinking alcoholic beverages) engages the CYP450 enzymes available in the liver. Consequently fewer enzymes are then available to metabolize other substances such as medications.

This reduced enzyme access extends the amount and length of time other drugs are active in the BLOOD circulation. The result may be an intensified effect of the drug or an ADVERSE REACTION. For example, drinking while taking antihypertensive medications to treat HYPERTENSION (high BLOOD PRESSURE) may cause blood pressure to drop lower than intended, resulting in dizziness or unsteadiness, especially when standing up after lying down (orthostatic HYPOTENSION).

In the long term, chronic alcohol abuse causes the liver to increase activation of CYP450 enzymes, resulting in more rapid metabolism of drugs. The result may be lower levels of drugs in the blood circulation than are necessary to provide therapeutic effects. With antihypertensive medications, for example, this might mean blood pressure remains elevated beyond the level expected for the DOSE of medication. The alteration of enzyme activity may also metabolize drugs in ways that cause toxicity. Adverse reactions are a particular risk among people who regularly drink alcohol but do not divulge the information to their doctors or often to family members because denial is a hallmark of ALCOHOLISM. Altered enzyme activity may continue for weeks to months after stopping alcohol consumption and may be a permanent state when alcohol abuse has been exceptionally long term (over decades).

Direct Interactions between Alcohol and Other Drugs

Consumed alcohol may also directly compete for or bind with neuroreceptors in the BRAIN in ways that interfere with drugs that act on the CENTRAL NERVOUS SYSTEM such as anesthetic agents, ANALGESIC MEDICATIONS (PAIN relievers), ANTIDEPRESSANT MEDICATIONS, ANTIANXIETY MEDICATIONS, MUSCLE RELAXANT MEDICATIONS, antiseizure medications, ANTIPSYCHOTIC MEDICATIONS, ANTIHISTAMINE MEDICATIONS, and hypnotics. The interaction often intensifies side effects such as sleepiness, confusion, and cognitive dysfunction.

Increased Risk for Liver Damage

As the body's clearinghouse for drugs, the liver is especially vulnerable to damage from toxic byproducts of drug metabolism. Though the liver has great capacity to restore itself, the double onslaught of hepatotoxic drugs and alcohol may overwhelm its renewal mechanisms. Alcohol is a potent hepatotoxin; it is a poison that destroys liver cells. Many medications are also hepatotoxic and in combination with alcohol consumption can result in significant liver damage and LIVER FAILURE. Some of the most dangerous drugs in combination with alcohol are those in such common use that many people fail to recognize their potential risks or the frequency with which they take them: acetaminophen and the NONSTEROIDAL ANTI-INFLAMMATORY DRUGS (NSAIDS). These drugs are common ingredients in numerous products to relieve symptoms of COLDS, sinus congestion, menstrual cramps, arthritis pain, and general pain (such as in prescription analgesic medications). It is important to minimize or avoid drinking alcohol when taking products that contain these drugs. Various prescription medications are also hepatotoxic themselves or in combination with alcohol.

See also COGNITIVE FUNCTION AND DYSFUNCTION; DRUG INTERACTION; HEPATOTOXINS; ILLICIT DRUG ABUSE; LIVER DISEASE OF ALCOHOLISM; MEDICINAL HERBS AND BOTANICALS; MILK THISTLE; OVERDOSE; SUBSTANCE ABUSE PREVENTION; SUBSTANCE ABUSE TREATMENT.

alcoholic hallucinosis A state of temporary PSYCHOSIS that may occur after sudden withdrawal of ALCOHOL in a person who has heavily consumed alcohol for an extended time. Typical symptoms include auditory and sometimes visual HALLUCINATIONS, PARANOIA, and vivid nightmares. However, thought processes remain clear, and the person remains fully alert and aware of his or her surroundings. Symptoms do not usually require treatment beyond reassurance that they will soon end, though some people benefit from short-term treatment with a BENZODIAZEPINES such as chlordiazepoxide. Most people recover in 10 to 14 days though some symptoms may linger up to 3 weeks.

See also ALCOHOLISM; ANTIANXIETY MEDICATIONS; DELIRIUM TREMENS; SCHIZOPHRENIA; WITHDRAWAL SYNDROME.

alcoholism A health condition resulting from ADDICTION to ALCOHOL. As with other addictions, alcoholism is a combination of physiologic, psychologic, behavioral, and social factors. About 20 million Americans abuse alcohol, at least half of whom have alcohol addiction (alcoholism). Alcoholism has extensive health and social consequences.

Symptoms and Diagnostic Path
A significant factor with alcoholism is hiding the amount of drinking the person is doing. Indications of excessive drinking are often behaviors that might appear normal in isolation but that in aggregate are problematic. These indications may include

- establishing rituals around drinking
- changing plans or missing appointments to drink
- denying drinking or that drinking is a problem
- drinking alone or seeking ways to drink in secret
- hiding bottles of alcohol in odd places
- needing double shots or multiple drinks to feel the effects of the alcohol

Indications of problem drinking that others notice may include

- frequent absences from work or school
- forgetting people, conversations, or events
- unexplained changes in personality or interests
- disappearing at times throughout the day
- out-of-control drinking episodes that the person denies
- frequent illness or health complaints, especially gastrointestinal conditions

The diagnostic path includes physical and psychologic examinations with an initial screening questionnaire about alcohol use. Health-care providers who treat alcoholism use a variety of such screening and assessment tools. Further testing may include diagnostic procedures to diagnose physical health problems associated with alcohol abuse such as LIVER disease, CARDIOVASCULAR DISEASE (CVD), and gastrointestinal disorders. The doctor may also want to test for DIABETES, as chronic alcohol consumption interferes with the GLUCOSE–INSULIN balance. However, there are no BLOOD tests or other procedures to conclusively diagnose alcoholism. The doctor makes the final diagnosis on the basis of the aggregate findings, including the best determination of the person's drinking patterns and history.

Treatment Options and Outlook

Alcoholism is a chronic, lifelong condition that requires ongoing management to maintain complete abstinence from alcohol. DETOXIFICATION—the process the body goes through to completely eliminate alcohol—takes 5 to 7 days. Medications to ease the symptoms of WITHDRAWAL SYNDROME may include BENZODIAZEPINES and NALTREXONE, which calm anxiety and reduce cravings for alcohol, respectively. After the body is free of alcohol, maintaining sobriety often requires a combination of approaches that may include

- medications such as disulfiram, which prevents the body from metabolizing alcohol, and naltrexone to mitigate alcohol cravings
- individual PSYCHOTHERAPY to gain insight and understanding of the factors that contribute to the desire to drink
- group therapy or SUPPORT GROUPS such as Alcoholics Anonymous to provide opportunity to talk about alcoholism with others who have the condition and to reinforce behaviors to remain drink free

For nearly everyone who has alcoholism, maintaining sobriety (absolute abstinence) requires continued diligence. It is important to seek appropriate intervention to return to sobriety as quickly as possible when relapses do occur. Most alcohol treatment centers and programs also offer support groups and sometimes counseling for family members.

Risk Factors and Preventive Measures

Persistent, regular drinking is the most significant risk for developing alcoholism, because over time the body acquires both alcohol TOLERANCE and alcohol DEPENDENCE. Additive risks include beginning to drink at a young age, family history of alcoholism, genetic composition (separate from family history), and history of psychologic conditions such as ATTENTION DEFICIT HYPERACTIVITY DISORDER (ADHD), DEPRESSION, and BIPOLAR DISORDER. As well, three in four people who have alcoholism are men.

See also ALCOHOLIC HALLUCINOSIS; DELIRIUM TREMENS; FETAL ALCOHOL SYNDROME; HEPATITIS; SUBSTANCE ABUSE PREVENTION; SUBSTANCE ABUSE TREATMENT.

alkyl nitrites Inhaled drugs that rapidly relax smooth MUSCLE and dilate the BLOOD vessels. The alkyl nitrite with therapeutic application is amyl nitrite, a treatment for ANGINA PECTORIS (CHEST PAIN resulting from constriction of the CORONARY ARTERIES). Amyl nitrite requires a physician's prescription in the United States. Other alkyl nitrites have legitimate uses in products such as room deodorizers, adhesive removers, and various types of cleaners. Medicinal amyl nitrite comes in small glass ampules encased in fabric. To use the vial the person snaps or pops the vial within its protective fabric, releasing and breathing the vapors.

As substances of abuse, alkyl nitrites produce euphoria, reduced inhibition, and a sensation of excitement. Inhaled alkyl nitrites also are reputed to intensify sexual experiences because they relax sphincter muscles such as those in the VAGINA and the ANUS. The primary users of alklyl nitrites are adults between the ages of 30 and 50. Abuse of alkyl nitrites has moderate risk for psychologic DEPENDENCE. OVERDOSE of alkyl nitrites can result in ARRHYTHMIA (irregular heartbeat). Alkyl nitrites may aggravate HYPERTENSION (high BLOOD PRESSURE) or intensify the effects of nitrite-based medications to treat cardiovascular conditions such as hypertension and HEART FAILURE.

COMMON ALKYL NITRITES	
amyl nitrite	butyl nitrite
cyclohexyl nitrite	ethyl nitrite
isobutyl nitrite	isopropyl nitrite
methyl nitrite	pentyl nitrite

Long-term use of alkyl nitrites can cause METHEMOGLOBINEMIA, a condition in which the HEMOGLOBIN cannot properly bind with oxygen. Ingestion or injection of alkyl nitrites carries high risk for death. Because alkyl nitrites use tends to encourage high-risk sexual behavior their use results in increased risk for HEPATITIS and SEXUALLY TRANSMITTED DISEASES (STDS) including HIV/AIDS, though alkyl nitrites do not directly cause such infections. Long-term, chronic alkyl nitrites abuse also causes changes in the function of the IMMUNE SYSTEM that may make users more susceptible to INFECTION.

See also CLUB DRUGS; CORONARY ARTERY DISEASE (CAD); DRUG INTERACTION; SUBSTANCE ABUSE PREVENTION.

amphetamines Drugs that stimulate the CENTRAL NERVOUS SYSTEM. Amphetamines belong to the phenylethylamine class of drugs, a large DRUG family that also includes amphetamine-like drugs with similar actions and effects. Amphetamines and amphetamine-like drugs are SCHEDULED DRUGS in the United States, requiring a physician's prescription for legal use and possession. Those that are schedule 2 drugs further must meet narrowly defined treatment criteria. Methcathinone and cathinone, though ingredients of schedule 2 and schedule 3 drugs, are schedule 1 drugs in their pure forms and do not have therapeutic uses.

Amphetamines and amphetamine-like drugs have dual activity in the BRAIN: They increase the release of serotonin, DOPAMINE, and NOREPINEPHRINE; and they block the reuptake of dopamine, norepinephrine, and monoamine oxidase (MAO). These neurotransmitters have numerous roles in brain activities in regard to mental focus, concentration, and mood. Consequently amphetamines and amphetamine-like drugs increase alertness, reduce APPETITE, and establish a sense of confidence and well-being. Therapeutic uses include treatment for NARCOLEPSY, ATTENTION DEFICIT HYPERACTIVITY DISORDER (ADHD), weight loss in morbid OBESITY, and alertness in military pilots.

Abuse of amphetamines and amphetamine-like drugs occurs to take advantage of the euphoria, heightened alertness, and diminished need for sleep. As well, the stimulant effects of these drugs may intensify LIBIDO (sex drive), though ERECTILE DYSFUNCTION is a common SIDE EFFECT of chronic abuse. TOLERANCE develops quickly, escalating the amount of drug necessary to produce the desired effects. Because dopamine is also essential for movement, its presence in excess results in involuntary movements (DYSKINESIA). Short-term side effects that usually go away when the drug leaves the body include trembling, HALLUCINATION, increased perspiration, and HEADACHE. Side effects with long-term use that may be long lasting or permanent include SCHIZOPHRENIA-like PSYCHOSIS,

PARANOIA, SLEEP DISORDERS, DEPRESSION, ARRHYTHMIA, and aggressive behavior. Amphetamines and amphetamine-like drugs have high risk for psychologic DEPENDENCE and ADDICTION with chronic abuse.

**COMMON AMPHETAMINES
AND AMPHETAMINE-LIKE DRUGS**

amphetamine	benzphetamine
cathinone	dextroamphetamine
diethylpropion	mazindol
METHAMPHETAMIN	Emethcathinone
methylphenidate	phendimetrazine
phentermine	

See also BARBITURATES; CAFFEINE; HYPNOTICS; NARCOTICS; NICOTINE; OPIATES; PERFORMANCE-ENHANCING SUBSTANCES; SUBSTANCE ABUSE TREATMENT.

anabolic steroids and steroid precursors Hormones or hormonelike substances taken to increase MUSCLE mass and STRENGTH. Anabolic steroids are class 3 SCHEDULED DRUGS in the United States, legally available only with a physician's prescription. As substances of abuse, anabolic steroids and steroid precursors (substances the body metabolizes into anabolic steroids) are popular among athletes, bodybuilders, people who work in jobs that require physical strength, and people who desire a particular physique. Anabolic steroids are available in injectable forms and oral tablets.

Therapeutic Uses
Therapeutic uses for anabolic steroids are very limited; many anabolic steroid products are illicit. Though most anabolic steroids are androgenic (increase the production of ANDROGENS, the male sex hormones), anabolic steroids that are nonandrogenic (increase muscle mass without intensifying masculine traits) became available in the late 1990s for therapeutic uses. Anabolic nonandrogenic steroids appear to have fewer undesirable side effects, though the full extent of any long-term consequences remains unknown.

Most commonly doctors prescribe a TESTOSTERONE product for androgen supplementation or therapy and a nonandrogenic anabolic steroid to treat growth-related disorders in children.

Therapeutic uses for anabolic androgenic steroids include treatment for certain kinds of BREAST CANCER and TESTICULAR CANCER, and endocrine disorders in which the body does not produce normal levels of testosterone and other androgens. Therapeutic uses for anabolic nonandrogenic steroids include disorders of the PITUITARY GLAND and other conditions (such as chronic RENAL FAILURE) in childhood that result in smaller than normal stature, and circumstances of muscle loss associated with long-term chronic health conditions such as AIDS.

Abusive Uses

Most anabolic steroid abusers are men ages 20 to 40, though anabolic steroid use among teens (boys and girls) and women, especially athletes, is growing. However, athletic organizations worldwide prohibit the use of anabolic steroids and steroid precursors at all levels of competition from high school through professional. At elite levels of competition, sanctioning organizations use URINE and BLOOD tests to detect anabolic steroid use among competing athletes.

There is some use of anabolic steroids, both androgenic and nonandrogenic, as antiaging therapies. These are unproven uses.

Adverse Health Risks and Consequences

Short-term, adverse health consequences of anabolic androgenic steroids are usually reversible (go away after stopping the DRUG) and may include

- enlarged breasts (GYNECOMASTIA), testicle shrinkage, reduced body HAIR, and other feminization characteristics in men
- facial hair, increased body hair, lowered voice, and other masculinizing characteristics in women
- mood swings, emotional volatility, and outbursts of rage
- moderate to severe DEPRESSION
- DELUSION
- ACNE

Long-term, adverse health consequences of anabolic androgenic steroids are often permanent (continue when no longer taking the drug) and may include

- INFERTILITY or sterility
- LIVER damage
- LIVER CANCER
- left ventricular hypertrophy (enlarged left ventricle of the HEART)
- ATHEROSCLEROSIS and CORONARY ARTERY DISEASE (CAD)

In young people who are still growing, anabolic androgenic steroids cause the growth plates in the long bones to close, ending their growth. Other risks of anabolic steroid use may include INFECTION with HEPATITIS, HIV/AIDS, and other diseases acquired through sharing needles to inject the steroids.

COMMON ANABOLIC STEROIDS AND STEROID PRECURSORS

Anabolic Androgenic Steroids

boldenone	chlorotestosterone
clostebol	dehydrochlormethyltestosterone
dihydrotestosterone	drostanolone
ethylestrenol	fluoxymesterone
formebolone	mesterolone
methandienone	methandienone
methandriol	methandrostenolone
methenolone	methyltestosterone
mibolerone	nandrolone
norethandrolone	oxandrolone
oxymesterone	oxymetholone
stanolone	stanozolol
testolactone	TESTOSTERONE
trenbolone	

Anabolic Androgenic Steroid Precursors

androstenediol	androstenedione
DEHYDROEPIANDROSTERONE (DHEA)	norandrostenediol
norandrostenedione	

Anabolic Nonandrogenic Steroids

human growth hormone (hGH)	insulinlike growth factor 1 (IGF-1)

See also AGING, ENDOCRINE CHANGES THAT OCCUR WITH; ANTIAGING APPROACHES; GAMMA HYDROXYBUTYRATE (GHB); HORMONE; INJECTING DRUGS, RISKS OF; PERFORMANCE-ENHANCING SUBSTANCES.

barbiturates DRUGS that depress the functions of the CENTRAL NERVOUS SYSTEM. Barbiturates are SCHEDULED DRUGS in the United States, requiring a physician's prescription for legal use and possession. Some barbiturates are schedule 2 drugs, which strictly limits the reasons for which physicians may prescribe them.

Barbiturates readily cross the BLOOD–BRAIN BARRIER once in the BLOOD circulation and act similarly to ALCOHOL in the ways they affect BRAIN neurons. Though researchers do not know the precise mechanisms through which barbiturates alter brain function, they believe these drugs cause changes in the cell membranes of neurons in a way that alters their action potential (ability to transmit electrical impulses). Researchers do know barbiturates also potentiate (enhance) the presence and activity of gamma aminobutyric acid (GABA), a NEUROTRANSMITTER that regulates many of the brain's inhibitory functions.

Excessive amounts of barbiturates in the blood circulation suppress the respiratory centers in the brain. Barbiturates also slow HEART RATE and lower BLOOD PRESSURE. Combining barbiturates with alcohol is particularly hazardous, as these drugs act in the same ways to depress neurologic function.

Barbiturate OVERDOSE is life threatening and requires emergency medical care. Signs of barbiturate overdose include UNCONSCIOUSNESS, dilated pupils, shallow BREATHING, and slow PULSE.

Barbiturates have numerous therapeutic uses, including sedation during diagnostic and minor surgical procedures, suppression of seizures, and relief of severe anxiety. However, because barbiturates have high potential for ADDICTION and abuse, they are seldom the first line of therapy for most conditions except certain seizure disorders. As drugs of abuse barbiturates are popular for the sense of calm and well-being they can provide and their effectiveness to induce sleep.

THE TRUTH ABOUT TRUTH SERUM

Thiopental, better known by its trade name Pentothal, is a fast-acting barbiturate that produces a trancelike state of semiconsciousness. One effect of this state is the blockade of inhibition, allowing a person to do and say what the conscious mind might block. Psychiatrists first used sodium pentothal expressly for this purpose when treating what was then called battle fatigue in soldiers returning from World War II. Psychiatrists were able to learn the details of the traumatic experiences the soldiers endured and provide therapy to help them cope with their memories. However, a person under Pentothal's influence does not necessarily answer questions truthfully and indeed may sometimes tell lies once the effect of medication removes the inhibition that would otherwise prevent him or her from doing so.

COMMON BARBITURATES	
amobarbital	aprobarbital
butabarbital	butalbital
mephobarbital	methohexital
pentobarbital	phenobarbital
secobarbital	thiopental

Suddenly stopping barbiturates after long-term use can result in serious or lethal complications, resulting from neurotransmitter imbalance in the brain that causes erratic and extreme NERVOUS SYSTEM responses affecting brain function as well as vital functions such as regulation of blood pressure, heart rate, and body temperature.

See also ALCOHOL INTERACTIONS WITH MEDICATIONS; AMPHETAMINES; BENZODIAZEPINES; HYPNOTICS; PRESCRIPTION DRUG ABUSE; SUBSTANCE ABUSE PREVENTION; SUBSTANCE ABUSE TREATMENT.

benzodiazepines Drugs that depress CENTRAL NERVOUS SYSTEM functions. In large part benzodiazepines have replaced BARBITURATES in many therapeutic applications and have numerous therapeutic uses including as MUSCLE relaxants, antianxiety medications, and sleep aids. Doctors also prescribe benzodiazepines to relieve the symptoms of WITHDRAWAL SYNDROME. Benzodiazepines are class 4 SCHEDULED DRUGS in the United States, requiring a physician's prescription for legal use and possession. As drugs of abuse, benzodiazepines are popular for easing the symptoms of "coming down" from other drugs. They may also cause sensations similar to moderate ALCOHOL INTOXICATION. Benzodiazepines are among the most frequently abused prescription medications. Risks of long-term, chronic abuse may result in ADDICTION and symptoms such as HALLUCINATION, trembling, and confusion.

COMMON BENZODIAZEPINES	
alprazolam	chlordiazepoxide
clobazam	clonazepam
clorazepate	clorazepate
diazepam	estazolam
flurazepam	halazepam
lorazepam	midazolam
oxazepam	prazepam
quazepam	temazepam
triazolam	

See also GENERALIZED ANXIETY DISORDER (GAD); HYPNOTICS; PRESCRIPTION DRUG ABUSE.

blood doping Actions to boost the ability of the BLOOD to carry oxygen by increasing the volume of red blood cells in the blood circulation. Red blood cells (erythrocytes) contain HEMOGLOBIN, protein molecules that bind with oxygen molecules in the LUNGS. The two commonly used methods of blood doping are BLOOD TRANSFUSION and ERYTHROPOIETIN (EPO) supplementation. Doctors may use either of these methods therapeutically to treat certain types of ANEMIA and to maintain the level of or hasten the return of blood cells after CHEMOTHERAPY. Blood doping is an abuse of these methods done to improve athletic performance by increasing AEROBIC CAPACITY, typically among athletes who compete in ENDURANCE events. However, athletic organizations worldwide prohibit blood doping at all levels of competition, and many routinely test athletes for evidence of it.

Blood Transfusions
Blood transfusion is usually of packed red blood cells and may be homologous (from a donor) or autologous (the person's own blood). For autologous transfusion, the person may undergo HEMOPHORESIS, in which blood withdrawn from the body undergoes cell separation; the components other than the red blood cells are returned to the blood circulation. The concentrated red blood cells collected via hemophoresis are then refrigerated or frozen to store them until a few days before a competition. The athlete receives his or her own red blood cells back via transfusion, boosting the number of red blood cells in the blood. For homologous transfusion, the athlete receives a transfusion of red blood cells collected from donors.

Erythropoietin (EPO)
EPO is a natural HORMONE the body produces to stimulate the BONE MARROW to produce erythrocytes. EPO supplement, which became available in the late 1980s, is a recombinant hormone that intensifies this action. Injections of EPO thus cause the bone marrow to produce extra red blood cells, increasing their presence in the blood. Because it is far easier than blood transfusion to use in secret, EPO is the favored method of blood doping.

Health Risks and Complications
Risks of blood doping include blood clots that can cause HEART ATTACK or STROKE and increased viscosity (thickness) of the blood, which strains the HEART and can cause CARDIOMYOPATHY and HEART FAILURE. Homologous blood transfusions carry the risk of contracting a bloodborne INFECTION such as

HEPATITIS B and hepatitis C, particularly when donation circumvents usual donor screening and collection procedures to minimize detection of the transfusions.

See also ANABOLIC STEROIDS AND STEROID PRECURSORS; ERYTHROCYTE; PERFORMANCE-ENHANCING SUBSTANCES; RECOMBINANT DNA.

buprenorphine A DRUG administered therapeutically to treat opiate ADDICTION. Buprenorphine is available in two formulations: buprenorphine alone for use during DETOXIFICATION; and buprenorphine in combination with NALTREXONE, an opiate antagonist, for long-term use to help prevent recurrence. In the United States buprenorphine is one of the SCHEDULED DRUGS, available only by prescription from a physician who has completed an approved program for its appropriate use in SUBSTANCE ABUSE TREATMENT.

Buprenorphine for opiate addiction treatment is available as sublingual tablets that dissolve under the tongue, releasing buprenorphine for absorption into the BLOOD circulation through the mucosa of the MOUTH. Administered in this way, buprenorphine has an extraordinarily long HALFLIFE in the body. Because of this, dosing is often every other day in the maintenance phase of treatment. However, it is possible to crush the tablets and mix them with water for injection, which results in a "high" similar to that of HEROIN or other OPIATES. To prevent this, doctors prescribe the buprenorphine with naltrexone formulation (brand name Suboxone in the United States) to help maintain SOBRIETY after initial detoxification when drug cravings may intensify. Very little naltrexone enters the blood circulation through sublingual absorption. However, high amounts enter the blood circulation when dissolved and injected.

Buprenorphine is a synthetic drug that partially binds with opiate receptors, which is enough to activate an opiate response in the body without an intoxication effect. Because of this binding, it is possible to develop a physical DEPENDENCE to buprenorphine. Substance abuse treatment programs taper the dosage over a period of time to wean the body from dependence. Buprenorphine is also available as an analgesic medication (PAIN reliever), which doctors prescribe primarily for pain relief after surgery. Undesired side effects associated with buprenorphine include drowsiness, NAUSEA, CONSTIPATION, and HYPOTENSION (low BLOOD PRESSURE). Buprenorphine OVERDOSE can cause potentially fatal respiratory depression.

See also CYTOCHROME P450 (CYP450) ENZYMES; LEVO-ALPHA ACETYLMETHADOL (LAAM); METHADONE; PRESCRIPTION DRUG ABUSE.

C

caffeine A CENTRAL NERVOUS SYSTEM stimulant. Though not commonly perceived as a DRUG of abuse, caffeine is the most widely used psychoactive drug in the world. The primary sources of caffeine are coffee, tea, and colas. Chocolate also contains some caffeine. A typical cup of coffee contains 100 to 150 milligrams (mg) of caffeine; tea and cola drinks contain 60 to75 mg per serving. Many OVER-THE-COUNTER (OTC) DRUGS, notably those for PAIN relief and relief of menstrual cramps, contain caffeine. Chocolate may contain 3 to 5 mg of caffeine per ounce. Though researchers disagree as to whether caffeine is addictive, many people experience mild withdrawal symptoms when stopping caffeine after long-term consumption of caffeinated beverages. Such symptoms may include HEADACHE, irritability, difficulty concentrating, and cravings for the beverage. Excessive caffeine consumption may cause PALPITATIONS, agitation, and feelings of anxiety.

See also ANALGESIC MEDICATIONS; DYSMENORRHEA; NICOTINE; PERFORMANCE-ENHANCING SUBSTANCES; STIMULANTS.

cannabis The plant *Cannabis sativa*, the source for marijuana, hashish, and hash oil. Cannabis is the most widely used illicit DRUG in the Western world; more than 80 million Americans have used marijuana, the most common form of cannabis, at least once and about 15 million use it regularly. The primary psychoactive chemical in cannabis substances is delta-9-tetrahydrocannabinol, commonly called THC. THC has moderate risk for DEPENDENCE and ADDICTION. ALCOHOL potentiates (enhances and alters) the effects of THC when a person consumes the two drugs together.

Cannabis sativa is among several species of *Cannabis* cultivated in many parts of the world for hemp, the tough fibers of the plant's stem, for use in making rope, floor coverings, nets, and sometimes clothing. Stems and hemp fibers do not contain THC. However, in the United States growth, cultivation, and possession of *Cannabis* are illegal (schedule 1 drug) no matter the reason.

Medical Uses

At present the only accepted medical use of THC is the synthetic formulation dronabinol (Marinol), which doctors may prescribe to treat NAUSEA associated with CHEMOTHERAPY and to improve APPETITE in people who have AIDS. Dronabinol is a schedule 3 drug in the United States; possession and use requires a physician's prescription.

Considerable research has explored the ability of THC to decrease INTRAOCULAR PRESSURE (pressure within the EYE) as a treatment for GLAUCOMA. However, research results have been inconclusive. Though THC (in therapeutic use often referred to as medical marijuana) does lower intraocular pressure the effect lasts only as long as THC is active in the body, about five hours. THC's psychoactive effects make the drug impractical for glaucoma treatment.

Actions and Effects in the Body

THC produces euphoria, heightened or altered sensory perceptions, and a sensation of calm and relaxation. It exerts its psychoactive actions by binding with cannabinoid receptors in the BRAIN. Ordinarily the NEUROTRANSMITTER anandamide binds with these receptors, which are abundant in certain parts of the brain, including the hippocampus, cerebellum, and basal ganglia. The hippocampus regulates memory storage and retrieval for short-term memory. The cerebellum and basal ganglia coordinate and control voluntary motor movement.

THC also binds with neuroreceptors in the brain that affect sensations of pleasure, notably those associated with food and eating. Recent research suggests long-term, chronic use of substances containing THC results in permanent changes to the cannabinoid receptors. Those in the hippocampus seem particularly vulnerable, which researchers believe may account for the long-lasting difficulties chronic marijuana abuses have with short-term memory.

Marijuana

Marijuana is a product formed from the dried leaves and buds of the *Cannabis* plant, which are usually then smoked like cigarettes or in pipes. The psychoactive ingredients, primarily THC, enter the BLOOD circulation rapidly through the LUNGS. The effect lasts about two hours, though THC remains detectable in the blood and URINE for at least 24 hours and up to 10 days after smoking marijuana. Some people mix marijuana with food, in which case THC more slowly enters the blood circulation via absorption through the intestinal mucosa (mucous lining of the SMALL INTESTINE). Most marijuana has a THC content of 5 to 7 percent. A cultivation method that removes the seeds from the plants in their early stages of development results in a particularly potent form of marijuana called sinsemilla, which has a THC content of 10 to 15 percent.

Aside from the neurologic risks of THC, a significant health concern with marijuana is its smoke. Burning marijuana releases more than 400 chemicals, many of which are the same carcinogens (cancer-causing agents) found in cigarette smoke. As well, the smoke is an irritant to the bronchial structures and the lungs. Long-term smoking of marijuana can result in some of the same health problems that result from long-term cigarette smoking such as COUGH, chronic BRONCHITIS and CHRONIC OBSTRUCTIVE PULMONARY DISEASE (COPD). Whether long-term marijuana smoking increases the risk for LUNG CANCER remains unknown, though many researchers believe it has

similar carcinogenic characteristics because it contains many of the same chemicals.

Hashish and Hash Oil

Hashish is the dried and compressed resin extracted from the tops of the *Cannabis* plant. As with marijuana, the most common methods of consumption are smoking (though typically in pipes) and cooking in foods. Its THC content is 5 to 7 percent. Hash oil is an extract of the THC and other cannabinoids (cannabis chemicals) pulled from the flowers of *Cannabis* plants using a solvent. The resulting liquid is thick and concentrated, with a THC content of about 15 percent. The user may place a few drops on an ordinary cigarette or in foods. The effects and their duration for both hashish and hash oil are similar to marijuana.

HEALTH RISKS OF CANNABIS ABUSE

Short Term

altered judgment and relaxed inhibition	anxiety
	cognitive dysfunction
delayed reaction time	dizziness
heightened sensory perceptions	impaired balance and
increased APPETITE	coordination
panic attack	

Long Term

apathy and disinterest in life	delusions
DEPRESSION	IMMUNE SYSTEM suppression
loss of short-term memory functions	PSYCHOSIS

See also COGNITIVE FUNCTION AND DYSFUNCTION; ILLICIT DRUG USE; MEMORY AND MEMORY IMPAIRMENT; SCHEDULED DRUGS; SUBSTANCE ABUSE TREATMENT.

chloral hydrate A hypnotic drug used therapeutically as a sleep aid. Chloral hydrate is a schedule 4 drug in the United States, requiring a physician's prescription for legal use and possession. As a drug of abuse chloral hydrate may be taken alone or mixed with ALCOHOL ("Mickey Finn"). The latter produces a potent sedative as well as amnesiac effect. Such a mixture gained notoriety as a "date rape" concoction in the early decades of the 20th century. When taken at therapeutic dosage chloral hydrate is very safe. However, at high doses, chloral hydrate may produce potentially fatal respiratory depression.

HEALTH RISKS OF CHLORAL HYDRATE ABUSE

Short Term

ARRHYTHMIA	disturbed balance and
dizziness	coordination
HALLUCINATION	impaired motor function
irritability	slurred speech

Long Term

HEART damage	kidney damage
LIVER damage	sleep disturbances

See also FLUNITRAZEPAM; GAMMA HYDROXYBUTYRATE (GHB); HEPATOTOXINS; HYPNOTICS; SCHEDULED DRUGS; SEXUAL ASSAULT.

club drugs Drugs popular for illicit use in settings such as "rave" clubs and at parties. Most club drugs are designer drugs though some are conventional drugs used illicitly. The key risks with club drugs are not knowing what they are when taking them and combining them with ALCOHOL.

Among the most popular club drugs are HALLUCINOGENS such as KETAMINE and METHYLENEDIOXYMETHAMPHETAMINE (MDMA), commonly called ecstasy, and HYPNOTICS such as FLUNITRAZEPAM (Rohypnol), commonly called rophies or roofies, and GAMMA HYDROXYBUTYRATE (GHB). Flunitrazepam and GHB, which are odorless and tasteless, have gained notoriety as "date rape" drugs because they produce amnesia of events that occur during the time of the drug's effectiveness in the body. Other drugs sometimes popular as club drugs include LSD and METHAMPHETAMINE.

Mixing any of these drugs with alcohol is particularly hazardous and can result in potentially fatal respiratory depression.

See also DESIGNER DRUG; MEMORY FUNCTION AND IMPAIRMENT; SCHEDULED DRUGS.

cocaine A DRUG that acts as a CENTRAL NERVOUS SYSTEM stimulant. Cocaine is highly addictive and is a schedule 2 drug in the United States, subjecting its legal use to stringent requirements. The primary therapeutic use of cocaine is as a topical anesthetic applied to the mucous membranes for dental and surgical operations. Cocaine is a popular drug of abuse, and an estimated 35 million Americans have used it at least once.

Extracted from the leaves of the *Erythroxylum coca* plant, cocaine as a drug of abuse produces intense euphoria, energy, and a sense of physical and mental infallibility. The most common method of use is to snort (rapidly inhale) the powdered form of the drug into the NOSE, where absorption through the nasal mucosa (mucous membrane lining of the nose) allows the drug to enter the BLOOD circulation within a few minutes for an effect that lasts two to three hours. Crack cocaine—created by mixing cocaine powder with sodium bicarbonate and water, then igniting the dried mixture and inhaling the smoke—gets the drug into the blood circulation even more rapidly through the LUNGS. Some people dissolve the powder in water and inject the solution intravenously for an instant and intense though short (20 to 30 minutes) effect.

The key risk of cocaine abuse is ADDICTION; about 10 percent of people who try cocaine eventually become addicted. Crack cocaine is particularly addictive. The compulsion to use cocaine is so intense for many people who are addicted that they resort to extraordinary actions to acquire the drug. The person trying to quit cocaine often needs short-term medical support to mitigate symptoms of withdrawal and long-term family and social support to stay off cocaine.

HEALTH RISKS OF COCAINE ABUSE

Short Term

anxiety	diminished ability to feel PAIN
elevated body temperature	HEART ATTACK
HYPERTENSION	PARANOIA
rapid HEART RATE	restlessness, irritability, or agitation

Long Term

ADDICTION	ARRHYTHMIA
chronic nasal congestion	DYSPNEA (difficulty BREATHING)
HALLUCINATION	MALNUTRITION
PSYCHOSIS	runny NOSE (RHINORRHEA)
seizures	SUDDEN CARDIAC DEATH

Though the effects on fetal development when a pregnant woman uses cocaine are uncertain the infant can be born with cocaine addiction, especially if the mother is using crack cocaine. Because many women who abuse cocaine also drink ALCO-

HOL and smoke cigarettes, both of which affect fetal development, health consequences for infants born to cocaine-addicted mothers are often multiple and complex. Infants born addicted to cocaine require extensive medical care until their bodies are free from the effects of the drug. They are also more likely to be born prematurely, increasing the need for medical care during early infancy as well as the risk for lifelong health problems, including developmental delays and LEARNING DISORDERS later in life.

Cocaine abuse may also cause changes in cardiovascular function that can result in sudden HEART ATTACK in users of any age and during any use of the drug, including the first time. Researchers do not know what causes such cardiovascular changes or their precise nature, though speculate the cardiovascular effect is a combination of conductive (ARRHYTHMIA) and ischemic (severely decreased blood flow and oxygen supply to the HEART MUSCLE) circumstances that collude to cause the heart to suddenly stop beating.

See also AMPHETAMINES; ANESTHESIA; ILLICIT DRUG USE; SCHEDULED DRUGS; STIMULANTS; SUBSTANCE ABUSE PREVENTION; SUBSTANCE ABUSE TREATMENT.

delirium tremens A serious medical condition that may develop during withdrawal from ALCOHOL ADDICTION (ALCOHOLISM). The symptoms of delirium tremens are both physical and psychologic; the physical symptoms can be life threatening without prompt medical treatment. Most people who experience delirium tremens (also called DTs) are long-term heavy drinkers who suddenly quit drinking. However, delirium tremens may also occur after a single episode of extreme alcohol consumption in a person who does not often drink heavily.

Delirium tremens develops as a consequence of the BRAIN's inability to restore the balance among the neurotransmitters gamma-aminobutyric acid (GABA), DOPAMINE, and glutamate. Instead the imbalance that resulted from alcohol DEPENDENCE spirals out of control, producing a spectrum of autonomic dysfunctions that affect multiple body systems.

Symptoms begin within a few to 48 hours of alcohol cessation and are often severe from the onset. Symptoms may include

- tremors and seizures
- hyperactive reflexes
- confusion, DELUSION, and HALLUCINATION
- anxiety, irritability, restlessness, and agitation
- tachycardia (rapid HEART RATE), TACHYPNEA (rapid BREATHING), diaphoresis (excessive sweating), and PALPITATIONS
- elevated body temperature and BLOOD PRESSURE
- NAUSEA and VOMITING

Diagnostic tests may include BLOOD tests to measure blood alcohol concentration, LIVER enzyme levels, and complete blood count (CBC).

The doctor may desire other tests to evaluate specific symptoms, such as ELECTROCARDIOGRAM (ECG) for palpitations and tachycardia. Treatment is generally intravenous administration of BENZODIAZEPINES, such as chlordiazepoxide and diazepam, to produce sedation and to help stabilize the NEUROTRANSMITTER balance in the brain because benzodiazepines also bind with GABA neuroreceptors. Without treatment delirium tremens may so significantly disrupt brain function as to cause death. With appropriate and timely treatment, symptoms end in about 72 hours and most people recover completely in 7 to 10 days.

See also ALCOHOL HALLUCINOSIS; NALTREXONE; SUBSTANCE ABUSE TREATMENT; WITHDRAWAL SYNDROME.

dependence The physiologic or psychologic need to continue taking a particular DRUG. In physiologic dependence, predictable changes occur within the body that reconfigure or adapt a particular facet of function and result in the body's reliance on the substance to maintain that function. Often the body then reacts in unpleasant ways (WITHDRAWAL SYNDROME) when the person stops taking the substance. Physiologic dependence ends when the body completely clears all chemical traces of the drug. Drugs often subject to abuse that cause physiologic dependence include ALCOHOL, HEROIN, and opiate NARCOTICS such as morphine, hydrocodone, and oxycodone.

In psychologic dependence taking the drug results in pleasurable sensations and the desire (craving, when intense) to take the substance to obtain them. Though the drug causes chemical changes in the body that result in temporary alterations of function, the drug does not establish any physiologic adaptation. Psychologic dependence can be intense and does not correlate to the drug's presence in the body. Because the body develops TOLERANCE to many drugs taken on a long-term basis (requiring a higher DOSE to achieve the same effect), the longer the person uses the substance the more likely he or she may experience some physiologic and psychologic symptoms when stopping the substance, representing the body's adaptation to the drug's absence. The nature of such symptoms depends on the drug. Drugs often subject to abuse that cause psychologic dependence include COCAINE, AMPHETAMINES, BENZODIAZEPINE drugs, and HALLUCINOGENS.

Though drug dependence is often a key factor in substance abuse and ADDICTION, it is not synonymous with either. Substance abuse and addiction encompass the ways in which people use the drugs and the behaviors in which they engage to obtain the drugs. Physiologic dependence occurs in numerous therapeutic applications—for example, with therapies involving systemic CORTICO-STEROID MEDICATIONS, ANTIDEPRESSANT MEDICATIONS, and antihypertensive medications. As well, a person may develop dependence on a substance commonly abused (such as a narcotic PAIN reliever or antianxiety medication) when taking it to legitimately treat a health condition and yet not abuse or have an addiction to that substance.

Symptoms and Diagnostic Path

Indications of drug dependence vary according to the drug. In a therapeutic context such symptoms reflect achievement of the desired effect of the drug—for example, suppression of the IMMUNE RESPONSE with corticosteroid medications or relief of symptoms with antidepressant medications or pain relief medications. In the context of substance abuse or addiction, indications of drug dependence may include attempts to obtain increasing quantities of the drug, taking the drug inappropriately, and obvious differences in behavior between when taking the drug and when not taking the drug.

Treatment Options and Outlook

Treatment for undesired or unintentional drug dependence, such as with corticosteroid or antidepressant medications, consists of controlled weaning from the drug, a process that may take several weeks to complete. In circumstances in which

there is also substance abuse or addiction, extensive support and treatment such as PSYCHOTHERAPY are also essential. Though physiologic dependence ends when the drug is no longer present in the body, psychologic dependence can persist for weeks, months, or even years after stopping the drug.

Risk Factors and Preventive Measures

The primary risk factor for drug dependence is taking repeated doses of the drug. When doing so is to achieve therapeutic outcomes, drug dependence is desired and appropriate. When the purpose of taking a drug is other than therapeutic, not only is dependence possible but there is a high likelihood for substance abuse or addiction. As such use is detrimental to health, prevention efforts include restricting access to the drug along with education and therapy, if appropriate, to understand the health consequences of continued dependence and behavioral approaches to avoid use of the drug.

See also ANALGESIC MEDICATIONS; ILLICIT DRUG USE; PRESCRIPTION DRUG ABUSE; SCHEDULED DRUGS; SUBSTANCE ABUSE PREVENTION; SUBSTANCE ABUSE TREATMENT.

depressants   Chemicals that slow the activity of the CENTRAL NERVOUS SYSTEM. The primary therapeutic purpose of depressants is to cause sedation or sleep. Most work through actions that directly affect the function of BRAIN neurons, neurotransmitters, and neuroreceptors. Many do so by increasing the activity of gamma aminobutyric acid (GABA), a NEUROTRANSMITTER that slows brain function. Depressants have high potential for DEPENDENCE and ADDICTION. Abruptly ending their use may cause WITHDRAWAL SYNDROME that, with certain drugs, has the potential to be life threatening when symptoms are serious and untreated.

Types of prescription drugs that are depressants include ANTIANXIETY MEDICATIONS, HYPNOTICS, BARBITURATES, and BENZODIAZEPINES. Drugs in these classifications are SCHEDULED DRUGS in the United States, which require a physician's prescription for legal possession and use. Doctors may prescribe them to treat GENERALIZED ANXIETY DISORDER (GAD), panic attacks and PANIC DISORDER, SLEEP DISORDERS, and POST-TRAUMATIC STRESS DISORDER (PTSD).

As substances of abuse, depressants produce INTOXICATION with initial euphoria and subsequent diminished cognitive function. Those who abuse depressants often do so to dull the effects of coming down from other drugs such as METHAMPHETAMINE and COCAINE. The most commonly abused depressants are ALCOHOL and benzodiazepines, notably alprazolam and diazepam. Other commonly abused depressants include the illicit drugs FLUNITRAZEPAM and GAMMA HYDROXYBUTYRIC ACID (GHB).

See also ALCOHOLISM; ILLICIT DRUG USE; PRESCRIPTION DRUG ABUSE; STIMULANTS.

designer drugs Illicit drugs created by altering the molecular structure of existing drugs, usually drugs that are legal but restricted. The designer drug is typically similar to the derivative drug in its actions and effects, though both are often enhanced or intensified in some way. Because "street chemists" (commonly called cookers) manufacture designer drugs in casual settings, these drugs are often of inconsistent potency and purity. There are often dozens of variations on a particular formula, each somewhat different molecularly but all touted as the same drug.

Most designer drugs are CLUB DRUGS produced solely for the purpose of creating an intoxicating or hallucinogenic experience, though some designer drugs are substances people take to improve physical or athletic performance. The risk for OVERDOSE, either from a single unexpectedly potent dose or through combining drugs, is very high. Designer drugs have no therapeutic use.

See also AMPHETAMINES; BLOOD DOPING; HALLUCINOGEN; METHAMPHETAMINE; PERFORMANCE-ENHANCING SUBSTANCES; SUBSTANCE ABUSE PREVENTION.

detoxification The process of eliminating from the body a substance to which a person is addicted. Detoxification causes physiologic changes that restore to normal the way the body functions, reversing the changes that occurred as DEPENDENCE and ADDICTION developed. This process of restoration can cause symptoms such as ABDOMINAL PAIN, JOINT and MUSCLE PAIN, NAUSEA, VOMITING, "shakes" (tremors), and sometimes seizures.

Controlled detoxification, also called medically supervised withdrawal, is the first stage of treatment for DRUG addiction (including ALCOHOL addic-

tion). Many people undergoing treatment for addiction receive medications to mitigate withdrawal symptoms. Detoxification may take as long as 14 days, though the most severe symptoms occur within the first 3 to 5 days for most addictions. Successful recovery from addiction requires further, and often ongoing, treatment that may include PSYCHOTHERAPY, BEHAVIOR MODIFICATION THERAPY, COGNITIVE THERAPY, and intensive family and peer support.

See also ALCOHOLIC HALLUCINOSIS; ALCOHOLISM; INTOXICATION; SOBRIETY; WITHDRAWAL SYNDROME.

dextromethorphan A COUGH suppressant, also called an antitussive, that is a common ingredient in numerous OVER-THE-COUNTER (OTC) DRUGS. These products are the most common sources for abuse, though other sources include illicit dextromethorphan powder or capsules that contain dextromethorphan powder. Though not a narcotic, dextromethorphan binds with certain opiate receptors in the BRAIN and SPINAL CORD (CENTRAL NERVOUS SYSTEM) and has an opioid effect in suppressing the cough REFLEX. Dextromethorphan has low risk for DEPENDENCE or ADDICTION.

At the recommended DOSAGE in cough and cold relief products dextromethorphan effectively relieves cough without significant side effects. When taken in amounts that exceed the recommended dosage dextromethorphan causes NAUSEA, disorientation, HALLUCINATION, and dissociation (perceptions of separating from the physical body). In very high doses, dextromethorphan causes confusion, slurred speech, disturbed vision, tachycardia (rapid HEART RATE), and peripheral PARESTHESIA (tingling and numbness of the fingers and toes). Seizures or fatal ARRHYTHMIA (irregular HEART beat) may also occur with very high doses. Chronic dextromethorphan abuse may result in PSYCHOSIS and permanent neurologic damage to the brain.

Other ingredients in multisymptom products that contain dextromethorphan, such as acetaminophen (an analgesic and antipyretic) and guaifenesin (an expectorant), may cause other undesired side effects. Chronic acetaminophen use or acetaminophen OVERDOSE has high risk for permanent LIVER damage, LIVER FAILURE, kidney damage, and RENAL FAILURE.

HEALTH RISKS OF DEXTROMETHORPHAN ABUSE

Short Term

confusion	disorientation
double vision	HALLUCINATION
NAUSEA and VOMITING	seizures
sudden death	tachycardia (rapid HEART beat)

Long Term

ARRHYTHMIA	BRAIN damage
chronic hallucinations	neuromotor dysfunction

See also ANALGESIC MEDICATIONS; HALLUCINOGENS; HEPATOTOXINS; NARCOTICS; OPIATES; PRESCRIPTION DRUG ABUSE.

disulfiram A medication that blocks the action of the enzyme acetaldehyde dehydrogenase in the second stage of ALCOHOL METABOLISM. This inhibition prevents the conversion of acetaldehyde, a potent toxin, to relatively harmless acetic acid. The consequence is rapid accumulation of acetaldehyde in the BLOOD circulation, causing an array of extremely unpleasant symptoms similar to severe hangover. The intensity of symptoms correlates directly to the DOSE of disulfiram and the amount of alcohol consumed.

Disulfiram, better known by its trade name Antabuse, may be among the treatments for ALCOHOLISM. Though disulfiram is very effective for controlling alcohol consumption, it does not cure alcoholism. Symptoms that occur with the combination of disulfiram and alcohol, called the disulfiram–alcohol reaction, include

- throbbing HEADACHE
- intense thirst and profuse VOMITING
- excessive sweating
- PALPITATIONS and CHEST PAIN

- blurred vision
- HYPERVENTILATION and DYSPNEA (shortness of breath)

Symptoms typically begin about 10 minutes after consuming alcohol and last 60 to 90 minutes. Though disulfiram can be very effective in helping maintain SOBRIETY in people who stringently comply with the conditions of treatment, it can cause severe and potentially life threatening symptoms when alcohol consumption is substantial. Such severe symptoms require emergency medical attention. Among them are tachycardia (rapid HEART RATE), ARRHYTHMIA (irregular HEART rate), seizures, and RESPIRATORY FAILURE.

> Because so many products and substances, including medications, can contain ALCOHOL, health-care providers recommend that anyone taking disulfiram carry a wallet card that identifies them as on disulfiram therapy and the contact information for the prescribing physician.

Abstinence from alcohol prevents symptoms. It is essential to avoid all products that contain alcohol. Common sources of alcohol include alcoholic beverages (beer, wine, mixed drinks), salad dressings, food sauces, cough and cold preparations, any medicinal preparations labeled elixirs, mouthwashes, and some COLD SORE treatments. Topical products that contain alcohol, such as aftershave lotion, may also activate the disulfiram–alcohol reaction. Ingesting alcohol in any quantity in the 12 hours before the first disulfiram dose or up to 14 days after the last disulfiram dose will produce symptoms.

See also INTOXICATION; METHADONE; NALTREXONE.

E–G

ecstasy See METHYLENEDIOXYMETHAMPHETAMINE (MDMA).

ethchlorvynol A sedating hypnotic DRUG, similar in physiologic action and effects to BARBITURATES, doctors may prescribe as a sleep aid to treat insomnia. Ethchlorvynol (brand name Placidyl) has high potential for physical DEPENDENCE and ADDICTION, however, and is seldom the medication of first choice in a therapeutic setting. It is a schedule 4 drug in the United States; possession and use are legal only with a doctor's prescription.

TOLERANCE to ethchlorvynol develops after about one week of taking it regularly, which means the body requires a higher DOSE to achieve the same effect. Taking ethchlorvynol for three weeks or longer often establishes physical dependence; abruptly stopping the drug after this time is likely to result in withdrawal symptoms such as NAUSEA, agitation, HALLUCINATION, tremors ("shakes"), and possibly seizures. It is important to taper the amount of drug over days to weeks to stop taking it. As a drug of abuse, ethchlorvynol produces an intoxicating effect. As with other hypnotics, combining the drug with ALCOHOL enhances the sedating effect and can result in OVERDOSE. People who abuse substances such as METHAMPHETAMINE or COCAINE may use ethchlorvynol to ease the transition between the "high" of the stimulant and the "crash" of returning to normal state.

See also CHLORAL HYDRATE; DEPRESSANTS; HYPNOTICS; PRESCRIPTION DRUG ABUSE; SCHEDULED DRUGS; STIMULANTS; WITHDRAWAL SYNDROME.

fentanyl A narcotic PAIN reliever about 80 times more potent than morphine. Fentanyl's primary therapeutic uses are for intravenous anesthetic during surgery and for analgesia (pain relief) after major operations such as OPEN HEART SURGERY or to treat significant CHRONIC PAIN such as may occur with terminal cancer. Fentanyl is a schedule 2 DRUG in the United States, strictly regulating its legitimate use. Numerous analogs (pharmacologic derivations) of fentanyl are available illicitly, though only a few are available for legitimate use.

As a drug of abuse fentanyl produces effects similar to those of HEROIN though is significantly more potent. The most common method of administration, as with heroin, is intravenous injection (using a needle to inject the drug directly into a VEIN). Other forms of fentanyl subject to abuse are transdermal patches (Duragesic) and a "lollipop" that allows the drug to enter the BLOOD circulation by being absorbed through the mucous membrane of the MOUTH (transmucosal absorption). The risk for OVERDOSE is very high with abuse of these forms of fentanyl, as their structure releases a consistent amount of the drug over an extended period of time and consuming them faster than intended releases excessive amounts of the drug. Fentanyl has a high risk for DEPENDENCE and ADDICTION, with significant withdrawal symptoms when stopping the drug.

See also ANALGESIC MEDICATIONS; ANESTHESIA; ILLICIT DRUG USE; KETAMINE; OPIATES; PHENCYCLIDINE (PCP); PRESCRIPTION DRUG ABUSE; SCHEDULED DRUGS; WITHDRAWAL SYNDROME.

fetal alcohol syndrome A constellation of BIRTH DEFECTS that may occur as a result of a woman's ALCOHOL consumption during the early stages of PREGNANCY. About 6,000 infants are born with fetal alcohol syndrome (FAS) each year in the United States. Up to five times as many more infants are born with symptoms of alcohol exposure during prenatal development, although they do not have

full-blown FAS. Doctors may call incomplete forms of FAS alcohol-related neurodevelopmental disorder (ARND) when symptoms are primarily behavioral and alcohol-related birth defects (ARBD) when symptoms are primarily physical. People sometimes refer to the entire range of these conditions as fetal alcohol spectrum disorders (FASDs), though this is a general rather than a clinical term.

Researchers first identified FAS in 1981 and are still unable to determine any safe level of drinking during pregnancy. Alcohol is highly teratogenic, meaning it has strong capability to cause damage to cells of all types during fetal development. The highest risk for severe birth defects occurs with heavy drinking during the first eight weeks of pregnancy, the time when body systems and organs are developing. The BRAIN and NERVOUS SYSTEM are particularly vulnerable to alcohol toxicity; exposure during any stage of pregnancy may affect whatever neurologic development is occurring at the time. The result may be a range of intellectual, emotional, and behavioral dysfunctions that become apparent as the child grows up.

Symptoms and Diagnostic Path
A collaboration of US health-care agencies convened as the National Task Force on Fetal Alcohol Syndrome and Fetal Alcohol Effects issued diagnostic criteria and guidelines in 2004, under mandate from the US Congress to establish consistent diagnosis. These criteria include

- small head (microcephaly) with structural brain abnormalities apparent with diagnostic imaging procedures
- three unique and characteristic craniofacial anomalies, also called facial dysmorphias: smooth philtrum (no ridges in the upper lip); narrowly placed eyes with short slits (palpebral fissures); and narrow, thin upper lip
- impaired growth (height or weight that remains below the tenth percentile for age)
- mental delays and functional deficits (varied and numerous intellectual, cognitive, and behavioral problems)

Some infants who have FAS also have other birth defects. Prenatal exposure to alcohol may be the affirming factor, though the collective characteristics of FAS are relatively unique to the effects of alcohol. Mild symptoms are sometimes difficult to detect and diagnose, especially when health-care providers do not know the mother's alcohol consumption during pregnancy (as is common in many adoption circumstances). From initial establishment of FAS criteria, the diagnostic path includes further neurologic and psychologic testing to more concisely define the extent of the damage.

Treatment Options and Outlook
Treatment attempts to manage symptoms and the effects of the damage that has occurred. The earlier diagnosis takes place and interventions can begin, the more successful treatment usually is in helping the child reach his or her full potential. Children who have FAS are more likely also to have psychologic conditions such as ATTENTION DEFICIT HYPERACTIVITY DISORDER (ADHD) and CONDUCT DISORDER. The first children diagnosed as having FAS are only now entering adulthood, so doctors do not know the long-term consequences of FAS. People who have mild symptoms and receive aggressive, targeted intervention are often able to function in society with relative success. Those who have severe symptoms may need ongoing care even in adulthood.

Risk Factors and Preventive Measures
The only risk for fetal alcohol syndrome is a woman's consumption of alcohol during pregnancy. FAS is entirely preventable if the woman completely abstains from alcohol during pregnancy, from CONCEPTION to birth. Because more than half of pregnancies in the United States are unplanned, the greatest risk exists for women who are not planning pregnancy but become pregnant.

Extensive education efforts have increased awareness of the dangers of alcohol during pregnancy, among them warning labels placed on alcoholic beverage containers and posted in establishments that serve alcoholic beverages such as restaurants, lounges, taverns, and bars. However, many people, including some health-care providers, still erroneously believe it is safe to drink in moderation during pregnancy. The US

Surgeon General in 2005 issued an advisory stating that there is no safe threshold for alcohol consumption during pregnancy and that the risk for FAS and related conditions increases with the amount and frequency of alcohol a woman consumes during pregnancy.

See also ALCOHOLISM; PRENATAL CARE; SUBSTANCE ABUSE TREATMENT.

flunitrazepam A hypnotic DRUG with sedative actions and effects similar to those of other BENZODIAZEPINES. Flunitrazepam, better known by its brand name Rohypnol or its slang names ropies and roofies, is not legal in the United States, though it is manufactured as a legal drug in other countries. As a drug of abuse flunitrazepam is popular at parties and in clubs. Taken alone it produces a euphoric INTOXICATION. When combined with ALCOHOL flunitrazepam causes incapacitation and amnesia of events that take place while the drug combination is active in the body. Because of this interaction flunitrazepam has gained notoriety as a "date rape" drug. The risks for DEPENDENCE and ADDICTION are moderate.

See also CLUB DRUGS; DEPRESSANTS; DETOXIFICATION; SCHEDULED DRUGS; WITHDRAWAL SYNDROME.

gamma hydroxybutyrate (GHB) An illicit DRUG with depressant and anabolic effects in the body, depending on the amount and frequency taken. GHB originally gained popularity among bodybuilders and athletes for whom STRENGTH and MUSCLE mass are important. Though not a HORMONE, GHB has anabolic effects—that is, it causes an increase in both the number and size of voluntary muscle cells. Its sedative qualities also make GHB an effective sleep aid for people also using other anabolic steroids, which tend to cause sleep disturbances.

As a CENTRAL NERVOUS SYSTEM depressant, GHB functions as a hypnotic with moderate sedating action. Combining GHB with ALCOHOL greatly intensifies this action, resulting in rapid and deep sleep with amnesia; the person does not remember events that occur during the INTOXICATION period. As a consequence GHB has acquired notoriety as a "date rape" drug, used to unknowingly intoxicate others for the purpose of SEXUAL ASSAULT.

GHB is a schedule 1 drug in the United States, indicating that it has no known therapeutic use. A legal, uncontrolled GHB precursor to is 1,4-butanediol, a chemical commonly available as an industrial solvent. 1,4-butanediol metabolizes to GHB after ingestion and has the same effects in the body. Efforts are under way in the United States to reclassify 1,4-butanediol to restrict its availability as well.

See also ANABOLIC STEROIDS AND STEROID PRECURSORS; CLUB DRUGS; DEPRESSANTS; HYPNOTICS.

glutethimide A hypnotic DRUG first used as a substitute for BARBITURATES to treat insomnia and other SLEEP DISORDERS. Glutethimide (brand name Doriden) is highly addictive, and, like barbiturates, poses a significant risk for life-threatening symptoms when taken in excessive amounts. TOLERANCE to the drug (increased amount necessary to produce the same effect) occurs after about a week of regular use; DEPENDENCE may develop after three weeks of regular use. Stopping the drug suddenly after three weeks or longer of regular use often results in withdrawal symptoms that may require medical treatment. Because of its high risk for ADDICTION and OVERDOSE, glutethimide is a schedule 2 drug in the United States and requires a physician's prescription for legal possession and use. Few physicians prescribe glutethimide, however, because other sedatives and hypnotics are as effective with fewer side effects and lower risk for addiction.

See also HYPNOTICS; PRESCRIPTION DRUG ABUSE; SUBSTANCE ABUSE TREATMENT; WITHDRAWAL SYNDROME.

hallucinogens Psychoactive substances that alter the BRAIN's perceptions of sensory experiences. Auditory and visual HALLUCINATION, time disorientation, and altered depth perception are common with hallucinogen abuse. However, not all people who take hallucinogens experience hallucinations. Researchers do not know the precise mechanisms of hallucinogens though believe many of them affect the presence of serotonin, a NEUROTRANSMITTER in the brain. Most hallucinogens are illicit substances; many come from natural sources such as mushrooms and cacti and others are synthesized (created in clandestine laboratories using chemicals). In the United States hallucinogens are SCHEDULED DRUGS; most are schedule 1 drugs because there are no therapeutic applications for their use and they have such high abuse potential.

Short-term, adverse health consequences of hallucinogen use include distortions of reality that may lead to irrational decisions and actions. Rapid mood swings and corresponding changes in behavior are common. The effective action of some hallucinogens may be 10 hours or longer. Long-term, adverse health consequences of chronic hallucinogen use include possible neurotoxicity and death of brain neurons. Some people experience flashbacks—hallucinatory experiences that repeat days, weeks, and sometimes months after hallucinogen use. Occasionally PSYCHOSIS develops in a person who uses hallucinogens extensively. Hallucinogen use does not typically result in DEPENDENCE though may result in ADDICTION (desire to take the DRUG).

Lysergic Acid Diethylamide (LSD)

The original purpose of lysergic acid diethylamide (LSD), first synthesized in 1938, was as a treatment to prevent seizures. However, testing did not bear out this potential. Through incidental ingestion, LSD's developer, Swiss chemist Albert Hofmann (b. 1906), discovered the drug's hallucinogenic capabilities. Because the effects of taking LSD could be remarkably similar to the some types of SCHIZOPHRENIA, researchers subsequently used LSD in clinical research as an effort to better understand this psychiatric disorder. However, LSD proved unable to provide the insights researchers hoped it would. In the 1960s LSD became popular as an illicit hallucinogen.

LSD is a very potent hallucinogen that can remain active in the body up to 12 hours. High doses often generate unpleasant or frightening experiences and tend to produce flashbacks for two to three days after its use. Common initial effects include rapid HEART RATE, NAUSEA, low body temperature, and diaphoresis (cold sweat). Hallucinations begin about an hour after ingestion and may result in bizarre behavior as the person reacts to distorted sensory perceptions. Some people experience intense anxiety and DEPRESSION after the effect of the LSD wears off.

Natural Hallucinogens

Natural sources of hallucinogenic substances are abundant and include plants such as cacti, which contain mescaline, and numerous types of mushrooms, which contain tryptamines such as psilocybin. Some natural hallucinogenic substances are potentially lethal even in small doses. Tryptamine-containing mushrooms grow abundantly in hot, moist environments around the world, including in the United States. The peyote cactus (*Lophophora williamsii*) grows abundantly in the southwestern United States and northern Mexico. The peyote's crowns contain high concentrations of mescaline. The most common methods of ingestion are chewing or eating dried plants or mushrooms or drinking liquid brewed from them. The potency and effect of natural hallucinogens are unpredictable.

Other Drugs with Hallucinogenic Effects
Many substances can generate hallucinatory experiences, particularly when taken in high doses. Hallucinations, especially visual, are common with abuse of many types of AMPHETAMINES and NARCOTICS. Among such drugs are

- METHYLENEDIOXYMETHAMPHETAMINE (MDMA), better known by its slang name ecstasy, a popular amphetamine-based club drug that produces a combination of euphoria and excitation
- KETAMINE, an anesthetic agent seldom used for ANESTHESIA in people because it produces hallucinations and sometimes DELIRIUM
- PHENCYCLIDINE (PCP), a veterinary anesthetic agent that produces intense hallucinations, DELUSION, delirium, and other psychoactive responses in people

These drugs also produce primary effects such as CENTRAL NERVOUS SYSTEM stimulation, analgesia (PAIN relief), and anesthesia (unawareness of sensation). When used as drugs of abuse, the overall effects are often unpredictable. Illicit chemists often mix different drugs together to create variations of these drugs, which are particularly harmful because their actions are unknown in such combinations.

COMMON HALLUCINOGENS

alpha ethyltryptamine (AET)	bufotenine
diethyltryptamine (DET)	dimethyltryptamine (DMT)
KETAMINE	lysergic acid diethylamide (LSD)
mescaline	peyote
PHENCYCLIDINE (PCP)	psilocybin

See also CLUB DRUGS; ILLICIT DRUG USE; HYPNOTICS; NEURON; NEUROTRANSMITTER; SCHEDULED DRUGS; SUBSTANCE ABUSE PREVENTION; SUBSTANCE ABUSE TREATMENT.

hangover Unpleasant physical symptoms that occur as a toxic reaction after excessive consumption of ALCOHOL. These symptoms are most prominent immediately on waking in the morning and may include

- significant HEADACHE
- NAUSEA
- VOMITING
- dizziness and VERTIGO
- PHOTOPHOBIA (aversion to bright light)

Though many remedies profess to prevent or cure hangover, the only prevention is avoiding excessive alcohol consumption and the only cure is time. The folk remedy of consuming an alcoholic drink to relieve hangover does not really end the hangover but instead induces mild INTOXICATION. In a person who is addicted to alcohol (ALCOHOLISM) this restores the effect of alcohol on the balance of neurotransmitters in the BRAIN. However, hangover is an indication that the LIVER's METABOLISM of alcohol has not been able to keep pace with the body's consumption, allowing higher concentrations of aldehyde (a toxin that is the first step of alcohol metabolism) to circulate in the BLOOD. There is some evidence that the herb MILK THISTLE (silymarin) improves liver function so the liver can more efficiently metabolize alcohol.

See also DETOXIFICATION; LIVER DISEASE OF ALCOHOLISM; WITHDRAWAL SYNDROME.

hashish See CANNABIS.

hash oil See CANNABIS.

heroin A narcotic DRUG derived from morphine. Widely used to relieve PAIN when it first became available in the early 1900s, heroin even appeared in over-the-counter pain remedies (as did other OPIATES) marketed to relieve various aches and discomforts. Today, however, heroin has no therapeutic uses and is a schedule 1 drug in the United States, making it legally available only for clinical research. Heroin has very high risk for DEPENDENCE and ADDICTION; heroin addiction presents significant health and social problems in the United States and throughout the world.

Heroin absorbs poorly through the gastrointestinal mucosa; thus its classic method of administration is intravenous injection (injected with a needle directly into a VEIN). Other means of using heroin are injecting it—intramuscular (into a MUS-CLE) or under the SKIN (subcutaneous, also called "skin popping")—snorting it into the NOSE, or smoking it mixed with tobacco or marijuana. These other methods are no less addictive, though snorting and smoking do reduce the risk for contracting bloodborne diseases such as HEPATITIS and HIV/AIDS. Such infections are significant risks with injected drugs of abuse, particularly when users share needles, syringes, and other paraphernalia.

The risk for OVERDOSE is high because heroin's potency and other ingredients are uncertain from DOSE to dose. Most powder sold as heroin is 10 to 70 percent heroin. The remainder may be other number of other substances from sugar to acetaminophen to other illicit drugs or even poisons. Exceptionally pure heroin is also hazardous because it is more narcotic than the person is accustomed to using.

HEALTH RISKS OF HEROIN ABUSE

Short Term

CONSTIPATION	delayed reactions
drowsiness	inability to concentrate
NAUSEA and VOMITING	OVERDOSE

Long Term

ADDICTION	ENDOCARDITIS and other
HEPATITIS, HIV/AIDS, and other	bacterial INFECTION
viral infection	scarring and damage to BLOOD vessels

See also INJECTING DRUGS, RISKS OF; NARCOTICS; SCHEDULED DRUGS; SMOKING AND HEALTH; WITHDRAWAL SYNDROME.

hypnotics DRUGS that induce sleep or cause heavy sedation. Hypnotics are CENTRAL NERVOUS SYSTEM DEPRESSANTS that act primarily to elevate levels of gamma aminobutyric acid (GABA), a NEUROTRANSMITTER that conveys NERVE impulses among BRAIN neurons to slow brain activity. BARBITURATES, most BENZODIAZEPINES, and some ANTIHISTAMINE MEDICATIONS have hypnotic actions.

Short-term health risks of hypnotic use include

- excessive drowsiness or difficulty waking up in the morning
- sense of sluggishness the next day

These consequences and side effects usually go away after the drug is no longer present in the body. Health risks of continued or long-term use of hypnotics may include

- DEPENDENCE on the drug to fall asleep
- ADDICTION
- severe withdrawal symptoms when suddenly stopping the drug, including possible PSYCHOSIS
- profound DEPRESSION
- increased potential for OVERDOSE

Because the body develops TOLERANCE for hypnotics, the margin between a safe amount of the drug and the amount necessary to produce the desired effect narrows with long-term use. This is particularly hazardous with barbiturates and can result in unintended fatal overdose.

COMMON HYPNOTICS

BARBITURATES	BENZODIAZEPINES
CHLORAL HYDRATE	diphenhydramine
doxylamine	ethchlorvynol
GAMMA HYDROXYBUTYRIC ACID (GHB)	GLUTETHIMIDE
meprobamate	methaqualone
METHYPRYLON	paraldehyde
zaleplon	zolpidem

See also SCHEDULED DRUGS; SLEEP DISORDERS; SUBSTANCE ABUSE TREATMENT; WITHDRAWAL SYNDROME.

I

illicit drug use Any use of substances not legal to possess. Many illicit drugs are "underground" drugs that individuals manufacture specifically for illicit use. Some of these drugs may be legal in other countries though are not legal in the United States or in the country in which the person is using them. As well, illicit drugs may be drugs that are legal but the person possessing them does not have legal authorization, such as a physician's prescription.

A significant health concern with illicit drugs is their production. Many drugs that come in loose form (such as HEROIN, COCAINE, METHAMPHETAMINE, and marijuana) are "cut" with various and often unknown substances, including other drugs and sometimes chemicals not intended for human consumption. These fillers, which dilute the DRUG's strength, may alter the actions of the drug or themselves cause effects in the body that are unexpected or toxic. The manufacture of illicit drugs in pill form is also questionable, with potency and ingredients varying certainly from batch to batch and often from pill to pill. Many people who manufacture illicit drugs such as methamphetamine have little knowledge of chemistry beyond that required to produce the drugs, and produce the drugs in less than ideal and often unsanitary conditions.

Other illicit drugs are produced in countries where their use is legal; they are smuggled into the United States and other countries. The production circumstances may or may not be of acceptable standards in terms of the drug's purity and consistency and the cleanliness of the manufacturing environment. Manufacturing inconsistencies, sanitation, and impurities may all pose health risks for people who use drugs smuggled into the United States from other countries. The other significant risk with illicit drugs is the legal consequence for their possession, which may result in jail sentences, fines, and serious consequences for a person's career, family, and lifestyle. In the United States the 1970 Controlled Substances Act (CSA) and its subsequent revisions establish the legality of drugs. Other countries have comparable legislative guidelines.

COMMONLY ABUSED ILLICIT DRUGS

ANABOLIC STEROIDS AND STEROID PRECURSORS	COCAINE
	FLUNITRAZEPAM
GAMMA HYDROXYBUTYRIC ACID (GHB)	hashish
	HEROIN
LSD	marijuana
mescaline	METHAMPHETAMINE
METHYLENEDIOXYMETHAMPHETAMINE (MDMA)	peyote

See also ADDICTION; CLUB DRUGS; DESIGNER DRUGS; STIMULANTS; HALLUCINOGENS; NARCOTICS; OPIATES; PRESCRIPTION ABUSE; SCHEDULED DRUGS; SUBSTANCE ABUSE PREVENTION.

injecting drugs, risks of The potential health consequences of sharing needles and DRUG paraphernalia. Sharing needles allows the passing of BACTERIA and viruses that are in the BLOOD among all individuals who use the needles. Rinsing with water or cleaning with bleach is not enough to prevent INFECTION with many bloodborne pathogens.

Intravenous drug users who share needles and drugs have particularly high risk for infection with bloodborne viruses such as HEPATITIS B, hepatitis C, HIV/AIDS, and for acquiring bacterial infections such as TUBERCULOSIS and MENINGITIS. It is also possible to acquire infection with some SEXUALLY TRANSMITTED DISEASES (STDS).

Needle exchange programs have become effective public health tools for reducing communicable disease transmission among intravenous drug users. Local health departments administer such programs, which give the person a sterile needle and syringe in exchange for a used one. Though it is a common perception that such needle exchange programs inherently encourage intravenous drug abuse, there is little clinical evidence that this is the case. Many substance abuse experts believe needle exchange programs, though they do not overtly encourage users to stop using drugs, do provide regular access to information about treatment programs that allow users who want to stop to find the help they need to do so as well as reduce the risk for disease.

See also SEXUAL HEALTH; SEXUALLY TRANSMITTED DISEASE (STD) PREVENTION; SUBSTANCE ABUSE PREVENTION; SUBSTANCE ABUSE TREATMENT; WITHDRAWAL SYNDROME.

intoxication The presence of ALCOHOL or other DRUG in the body in an amount that alters perception, behavior, thought processes, motor skills, judgment, and other physical or psychologic activities in ways that are dysfunctional or disruptive. From a health perspective intoxication is a state of poisoning. Slang terminology for intoxication includes drunkenness (alcohol intoxication), stoned, high, and buzzed. The primary objective of substance abuse is to achieve a state of intoxication, which continues for as long as the substance responsible for it remains active in the body. In the United States and most countries laws define the legal boundaries of intoxication, beyond which intoxication while participating in certain activities such as driving becomes a criminal offense.

See also DETOXIFICATION; ILLICIT DRUG USE; OVERDOSE; POISON PREVENTION; PRESCRIPTION DRUG ABUSE; SOBRIETY; SUBSTANCE ABUSE TREATMENT.

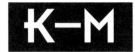

ketamine An intravenous anesthetic agent used primarily in veterinary medicine that has euphoric and hallucinogenic effects when used as a substance of abuse. Ketamine causes a sense of dissociation (separation of one's self from PAIN and other physical sensations associated with surgery), amnesia for events that occur while it is effective in the body, and primarily visual HALLUCINATION that are often quite vivid. Users sprinkle ketamine powder on cigarettes or marijuana and smoke it, snort the powder, or dissolve the powder and inject it intravenously. Excessive doses result in anesthesia-like loss of CONSCIOUSNESS. In the United States ketamine is a schedule 3 drug.

See also ANESTHESIA; CANNABIS; ILLICIT DRUG USE; NARCOTICS; PHENCYCLIDINE (PCP); SCHEDULED DRUGS.

levo-alpha acetylmethadol (LAAM) An oral DRUG to treat narcotic ADDICTION, primarily HEROIN addiction. LAAM is a synthetic product similar in chemical composition as well as action in the body to METHADONE, though a single DOSE is effective for up to 72 hours. In the United States LAAM is a schedule 2 drug. However, a rare but serious SIDE EFFECT of LAAM is damage to the HEART and BLOOD vessels. Because of this, doctors use LAAM primarily when treatment with methadone is not effective.

See also NALTREXONE; SCHEDULED DRUGS; SUBSTANCE ABUSE TREATMENT.

LSD See HALLUCINOGENS.

marijuana See CANNABIS.

methadone A synthetic analgesic (PAIN medication) originally developed as an oral substitute for morphine, a narcotic analgesic, during World War II. Methadone binds with opiate receptors in the BRAIN in the same way as does morphine, though methadone's chemical structure differs from that of morphine and methadone's effects last up to 24 hours.

Methadone has similar risk as OPIATES for DEPENDENCE and ADDICTION. In the United States methadone is a schedule 2 DRUG doctors prescribe primarily to treat HEROIN addiction. It works by blocking opiate receptors in the brain, which prevents other opiates such as heroin from doing so. Though methadone is itself addictive, withdrawal symptoms are less severe than withdrawal from heroin. As a drug of abuse methadone has effects similar to those of heroin. Doctors also occasionally prescribe methadone as an analgesic, often to treat CHRONIC PAIN.

See also ANALGESIC MEDICATIONS; DETOXIFICATION; ILLICIT DRUG USE; SCHEDULED DRUGS; SUBSTANCE ABUSE TREATMENT; WITHDRAWAL SYNDROME.

methamphetamine A very potent DRUG that is a CENTRAL NERVOUS SYSTEM stimulant. Though one formulation of methamphetamine is available for therapeutic use to treat a certain type of NARCOLEPSY, in the United States methamphetamine is primarily illicit and classified as a schedule 2 drug; its possession and therapeutic uses are extremely limited. Highly addictive, methamphetamine produces euphoria and a sense of invincibility. The drug stays active in the body for an extended time, making repeated use dangerously toxic; fatal OVERDOSE is a significant risk.

Though relatively simple from a chemistry perspective, which gives rise to proliferate clandestine "meth labs," the manufacture of methamphetamine is also quite toxic. Meth labs require only rudimentary equipment and supplies. However, the methamphetamine production process is so harmful that it renders uninhabitable or unusable any structures (including homes, apartments, and motels) used for meth labs.

Chronic, long-term methamphetamine abuse causes serious and permanent damage to many body systems. Classic indications of such abuse include rotted and missing TEETH, emaciated appearance, open sores on the face, and patchy HAIR loss. Continuous picking at the SKIN reflects damage to BRAIN neurons; PARANOIA and SCHIZO-PHRENIA are common with chronic methampheta-mine abuse. DETOXIFICATION and maintaining SOBRIETY are difficult.

HEALTH RISKS OF METHAMPHETAMINE ABUSE

Short Term

altered reactions and reaction time	disordered thinking
	DYSPHORIA as effect wears off
excitability and hyperactivity	rapid mood swings
unpredictable and violent behavior	

Long Term

ADDICTION	HALLUCINATION
MALNUTRITION	PSYCHOSIS
rotted TEETH	SCHIZOPHRENIA
sores on the face and body	unhealthy weight loss

See also HALLUCINOGENS; ILLICIT DRUG USE; SCHED-ULED DRUGS; STIMULANTS; SUBSTANCE ABUSE TREATMENT; WITHDRAWAL SYNDROME.

methylenedioxymethamphetamine   (MDMA)

An illicit DRUG that acts on the CENTRAL NERVOUS SYSTEM to produce hallucinogenic and stimulant effects. A designer drug, MDMA is best known by its slang name ecstasy. MDMA is chemically simi-lar to amphetamine, a stimulant, and mescaline, a hallucinogen. The drug's risks for DEPENDENCE and ADDICTION are very high. In the United States MDMA is a schedule 1 drug with no therapeutic uses.

The desired effects of MDMA are euphoria, increased energy, heightened sensory perceptions, and intensified sexual interest and experiences. The undesired side effects of MDMA may have long-lasting or permanent consequences, includ-ing ARRHYTHMIA, organ damage or failure, and damage to BRAIN neurons. Cravings for MDMA can continue long after stopping the drug. As well, because MDMA is an illicit drug it is often con-taminated with other drugs, commonly amphet-amine compounds, though underground chemists use a variety of substances as fillers. These sub-stances may interact with each other or have toxic consequences of their own.

HEALTH RISKS OF MDMA (ECSTASY) ABUSE

Short Term

disturbed thought processes	erratic body temperature
HYPERTENSION	hyperthermia
increased or irregular HEART RATE (ARRHYTHMIA)	memory impairment

Long Term

ADDICTION	BRAIN damage
cognitive dysfunction	organ damage

See also AMPHETAMINES; CLUB DRUGS; COGNITIVE FUNCTION AND DYSFUNCTION; HALLUCINOGENS; MEMORY AND MEMORY IMPAIRMENT; NEURON; SCHEDULED DRUGS; STIMULANTS; SUBSTANCE ABUSE PREVENTION; SUBSTANCE ABUSE TREATMENT.

N

naltrexone A medication to treat opiate ADDICTION. Naltrexone binds with opiate receptors in the BRAIN, preventing opiate drugs from binding. This action can block further effect of OPIATES already in the body or prevent the effect of opiates taken after naltrexone is in the body. Naltrexone is a treatment for addiction to opiates including prescription NARCOTICS and illicit drugs such as HEROIN. Naltrexone also helps reduce ALCOHOL cravings in some people who are recovering from ALCOHOLISM. Naltrexone is most effective in people who have strong desire to remain abstinent from DRUG or alcohol use and when starting DETOXIFICATION as part of a comprehensive SUBSTANCE ABUSE TREATMENT program.

See also ILLICIT DRUG USE; LEVO-ALPHA ACETYL-METHADOL (LAAM); METHADONE; PRESCRIPTION DRUG ABUSE; WITHDRAWAL SYNDROME.

narcotics Drugs that produce insensitivity to physical sensation, often altering perception and the level of CONSCIOUSNESS. Many narcotics subject to abuse are legitimate drugs that have therapeutic uses such as to relieve PAIN, stop COUGH, and treat DIARRHEA. Anesthesiologists use some narcotics to initiate or provide ANESTHESIA. Some narcotics are illicit, produced in clandestine labs by people who have rudimentary knowledge of chemistry. All narcotics have high risk for DEPENDENCE and ADDICTION. Accordingly narcotics are SCHEDULED DRUGS in the United States and many other countries, restricting their legal use and possession.

Narcotics act on neuroreceptors in the CENTRAL NERVOUS SYSTEM (BRAIN and SPINAL CORD) called opiate receptors, which researchers discovered in 1973. These specialized proteins regulate the brain's perceptions about and responses to pain signals as well as certain aspects of mood and consciousness. Opiate receptor binding also influences the rate of BREATHING (respiratory rate). The gastrointestinal tract contains some opiate receptors, which is why certain types of narcotics are useful for treating diarrhea and others cause CONSTIPATION as an undesired SIDE EFFECT.

There are two general classifications of narcotics: OPIATES, which come from natural sources, and synthetics, which are produced from chemicals in laboratories. Opiates derive from opium, the sap from the *Papaver somniferum* poppy plant. Synthetic narcotics, sometimes called opioids because they act in an opiate-like manner in the body, are chemical formulas designed in the laboratory to bind with specific types of opiate receptors for a lower risk of dependence and addiction. Opiate receptors rapidly become tolerant to the actions of narcotics, resulting in higher doses being necessary to achieve the same effect.

Narcotics come in forms for all ROUTES OF ADMINISTRATION: oral (liquids, tablets, capsules), rectal (suppositories), sublingual (under the tongue), intravenous injection (with a needle into a VEIN), intramuscular injection (with a needle into a MUSCLE), subcutaneous (with a needle under the SKIN), transdermal (patches, for absorption through the skin), and mucosal (sprays or lozenges, for absorption through the mucous membranes of the MOUTH or NOSE). Some narcotics do not absorb well through the gastrointestinal tract and are available only for injection, whereas for other narcotics injection offers the most rapid effect. The most commonly used methods for abuse are oral and injectable. As well, in circumstances of narcotic abuse a person may add a powdered narcotic to a cigarette and smoke it, which allows absorption through the LUNGS.

The short-term health risks of narcotic use include

- drowsiness
- reduced alertness or consciousness
- NAUSEA, VOMITING, and constipation

Health risks that may occur with long-term use of narcotics include

- TOLERANCE, dependence, and addiction
- INFECTION through shared needles among those who inject the drugs
- depressed respiration and RESPIRATORY FAILURE leading to death as the boundary between effective and toxic dosages grows increasingly narrow

Narcotic antagonists are drugs that have greater affinity for opiate receptors than do narcotics; they are able to "bump" opioids from the receptors. These drugs are often effective for treating narcotic OVERDOSE and addiction. DETOXIFICATION from narcotic addiction often entails numerous withdrawal symptoms that are more severe the longer a person has taken or abused the drugs.

COMMON NARCOTICS

Opiates (Narcotics of Natural Origin)

codeine	HEROIN
hydrocodone	hydromorphone
morphine	oxycodone
paregoric (opium)	thebaine

Synthetics (Opioids)

BUPRENORPHINE	butorphanol
dextropropoxyphene	fentanyl
meperidine	METHADONE
pentazocine	

See also ANALGESIC MEDICATIONS; ILLICIT DRUG USE; NARROW THERAPEUTIC INDEX (NTI); PRESCRIPTION DRUG ABUSE; SUBSTANCE ABUSE PREVENTION; SUBSTANCE ABUSE TREATMENT; WITHDRAWAL SYNDROME.

needle exchange programs See INJECTING DRUGS, RISKS OF.

nicotine The primary psychoactive DRUG in tobacco and SMOKING CESSATION products. Nicotine has stimulant as well as vasoconstrictive effects and is highly addictive. Many health experts consider nicotine at least as addictive as COCAINE and HEROIN. Most tobacco users, particularly smokers, attempt to quit numerous times before they achieve long-term success. Nicotine crosses the BLOOD–BRAIN BARRIER within seconds of tobacco use, where it affects the presence and activity of several BRAIN neurotransmitters, notably DOPAMINE and acetylcholine. These actions set in motion a cascade of events throughout the body that affect multiple functions, ranging from mood to cardiovascular activity.

Common sources of nicotine include

- cigarettes
- cigars
- NICOTINE REPLACEMENT products
- smokeless (chewing) tobacco
- snuff

HEALTH RISKS OF NICOTINE ABUSE

Short Term

activation of STRESS RESPONSE HORMONAL CASCADE
elevated BLOOD PRESSURE
increased HEART RATE
vasoconstriction

Long Term

ADDICTION
ARTERIOSCLEROSIS
chronic HYPERTENSION
health complications associated with tobacco use
inability to focus without nicotine in the BLOOD circulation

As a stimulant nicotine can heighten a person's mental focus and cognitive capability. However, tolerance develops rapidly such that with continued use (nicotine ADDICTION) this effect diminishes. Nicotine, through its effect on acetylcholine in the brain, activates the STRESS RESPONSE HORMONAL CASCADE, increasing the flow of EPINEPHRINE and NOR-

EPINEPHRINE in the body. This causes immediate changes in the walls of the arteries, causing them to stiffen and narrow. With long-term use of nicotine-containing substances these changes become permanent and alter cardiovascular function, contributing to serious HEART conditions such as HYPERTENSION (high BLOOD PRESSURE) and HEART FAILURE. The cardiovascular changes also affect the body's tiniest arteries, which can result in restricted circulation in the fingers and toes (RAYNAUD'S SYN-DROME) and of the blood flow to the PENIS, resulting in ERECTILE DYSFUNCTION. The only therapeutic use for nicotine is in nicotine replacement products to treat nicotine addiction (SMOKING CESSATION).

See also ANTISMOKING EFFORTS; CANCER RISK FACTORS; CARCINOGEN; ENVIRONMENTAL CIGARETTE SMOKE; NEUROTRANSMITTER; SMOKING AND CANCER; SMOKING AND CARDIOVASCULAR DISEASE (CVD); SMOKING AND HEALTH; WITHDRAWAL SYNDROME.

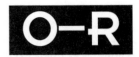

opiates Drugs derived from opium, the dried sap of the *Papaver somniferum* poppy plant. *P. somniferum* is the only one of about 120 species in the *Papaver* family of poppy plants that produces opium; other species are common ornamental flowering annuals or perennials. In the United States opiates are SCHEDULED DRUGS, restricting legal use and possession to physician prescription. HEROIN, which derives from morphine, is a schedule 1 drug, a classification that prohibits possession and use. Opiates have moderate to high risk for TOLERANCE, DEPENDENCE, and ADDICTION.

Most opiates are NARCOTICS used for analgesia (PAIN relief) or ANESTHESIA (loss of sensation). Opium is the main ingredient in the medication paregoric, sometimes used to treat DIARRHEA. Because opiates suppress the COUGH REFLEX, prescription antitussive medications often contain them (notably codeine and hydrocodone). The most effective opiate for significant pain relief, such as pain after surgery or terminal pain, is morphine, which became available in sustained-release tablets in the 1990s. The most commonly used opiates are hydrocodone and codeine, which appear in numerous products to relieve moderate pain and also for cough relief.

COMMON OPIATES

alfentanil	butorphanol
codeine	dextropropoxyphene
fentanyl	HEROIN
hydrocodone	hydromorphone
meperidine	METHADONE
morphine	oxycodone
pentazocine	sufentanil

See also ANALGESIC MEDICATIONS; DEXTROMETHORPHAN; ILLICIT DRUG USE; INJECTING DRUGS, RISKS OF; LEVO-ALPHA ACETYLMETHADOL (LAAM); NALTREXONE; PRESCRIPTION DRUG ABUSE; SUBSTANCE ABUSE PREVENTION; SUBSTANCE ABUSE TREATMENT; WITHDRAWAL SYNDROME.

organic solvents Petroleum distillates found in gasoline and some paints, paint thinners, aerosols, household cleaners, and glues. When inhaled in small quantities organic solvents produce a sense of INTOXICATION and mild HALLUCINATION. Inhaling the vapors into the LUNGS allows rapid absorption into the BLOOD circulation. However, the margin between intoxication and neurologic toxicity is very narrow and inhaled solvents can cause rapid death. The highest rate of organic solvent abuse is among children between 9 and 13 years of age.

Short-term health risks of inhaling organic solvents include

- slurred speech and uncoordinated movement
- HEADACHE
- NAUSEA and VOMITING
- panic attacks
- erratic mood and behavior
- DEPRESSION
- ASPIRATION of the substance into the lungs
- asphyxiation (suffocation) resulting in death

Long-term abuse of inhalants has significant health risks including

- RENAL FAILURE
- LIVER damage
- cognitive dysfunction
- memory impairment
- HEART FAILURE

Because numerous products contain organic solvents, preventing inhalant abuse is challenging. The very fact that these products are ordinary and common perpetuates the mistaken belief that inhaling them is harmless. Many parents are unaware of the practice of sniffing or huffing such products. Substance abuse experts urge parents to read product labels to identify those products that contain organic solvents to minimize the amount of such products in the home. Indications a child may be abusing substances containing organic solvents include

- RASH around the NOSE and MOUTH
- wheezing and coughing (new and unrelated to upper respiratory INFECTION)
- red, teary eyes
- unpredictable and erratic behavior

COMMONLY ABUSED ORGANIC SOLVENTS

acetone	benzene
methanol	methyl butyl ketone
methyl ethyl ketone	methylene chloride
toluene	trichloroethane
trichloroethylene	

See also ALKYL NITRITES; ILLICIT DRUG USE; PANIC DISORDER.

performance-enhancing substances Drugs, hormones, herbs, and nutritional supplements an individual takes to improve athletic capability or that results in an unfair competitive advantage. Performance-enhancing substances present health risks because they alter the body's functions or structure.

Athletic organizations in the United States and internationally prohibit the use of performance-enhancing substances at all levels of participation and competition, though the kinds of substances banned varies with the sport and level of competition. However, use and abuse of performance-enhancing substances remains a particular concern among younger athletes who compete at levels where testing for banned substances is infrequent or does not occur. PEER PRESSURE and perceptions that such substances are necessary to excel (win) may also be factors.

CAFFEINE is perhaps the most commonly used performance-enhancing substance. Coffee, tea, and cola drinks contain caffeine as do many energy drinks, gels, and food bars. Energy products also commonly contain GINSENG and other herbs that act as STIMULANTS. Some contain ma huang, a Chinese herb whose active ingredient is ephedra, a stimulant that is no longer legal in the United States. Other commonly available products used for their stimulant actions to enhance performance are decongestants such as pseudoephedrine. Illicit performance-enhancing substances include ANABOLIC STEROIDS AND STEROID PRECURSORS, ERYTHROPOIETIN (EPO), human growth hormone (hGH), and prescription stimulants.

See also BLOOD DOPING; DESIGNER DRUGS; HORMONE; MUSCLE.

phencyclidine (PCP) A veterinary anesthetic that causes varied and unpredictable effects when used as a substance of abuse. A single use may result in long-term psychiatric disorders such as PARANOIA, PSYCHOSIS, mood disorders, and SCHIZOPHRENIA. Though the risks for DEPENDENCE and ADDICTION are high with chronic use, the unpredictability and unpleasantness of PCP's effects tend to limit its use. PCP is a schedule 2 drug in the United States. However, no manufacturers currently produce it so it is nearly always an illicit drug. The most common method of use is to sprinkle the powder on a cigarette or onto marijuana and smoke it.

HEALTH RISKS OF PHENCYCLIDINE ABUSE

Short Term

amnesia	dissociation
extreme anxiety	HALLUCINATION
involuntary MUSCLE activity	loss of physical coordination
slurred speech	violent behavior

Long Term

GENERALIZED ANXIETY DISORDER (GAD)	mood disorders
	movement disorders
PARANOIA	PSYCHOSIS
SCHIZOPHRENIA	

See also ILLICIT DRUG USE; HALLUCINOGENS; KETAMINE; STIMULANTS; SUBSTANCE ABUSE PREVENTION; SUBSTANCE ABUSE TREATMENT.

prescription drug abuse The misuse of drugs prescribed for therapeutic purposes. Most prescription DRUG abuse begins unintentionally and may become intentional as psychologic DEPENDENCE or ADDICTION develops. The most commonly abused prescription drugs are NARCOTICS, BENZODIAZEPINES, and STIMULANTS. In the context of abuse, possession and use of the drugs may be illicit when the

means of obtaining the drugs is illicit, such as through altered or forged prescriptions, or obtaining drugs through unlicensed sources.

See also ANALGESIC MEDICATIONS; ILLICIT DRUG USE; OPIATES; SCHEDULED DRUG; SUBSTANCE ABUSE PREVENTION; SUBSTANCE ABUSE TREATMENT.

Rohypnol   See FLUNITRAZEPAM.

S

sobriety The state of abstinence from ALCOHOL and drugs. Sobriety is a marker of success in SUBSTANCE ABUSE TREATMENT. Individuals who are in recovery keep track of the length of time they remain sober. When treatment and sobriety are ordered through the courts, such as in connection with the breaking of laws in regard to use or possession of alcohol or drugs, it may be necessary for the person to prove sobriety through BLOOD and URINE tests that check for the presence of prohibited substances. Sobriety begins when the body is clear of alcohol or drugs, which may take days to weeks, depending on the substance, and continues for as long as it remains so.

See also DETOXIFICATION; ILLICIT DRUG USE; INTOXICATION; PRESCRIPTION DRUG ABUSE.

stimulants Drugs that stimulate the CENTRAL NERVOUS SYSTEM, producing heightened awareness and alertness. Stimulants have therapeutic uses as treatments for ATTENTION DEFICIT HYPERACTIVITY DISORDER (ADHD), NARCOLEPSY, sinus congestion, and weight loss. All central NERVOUS SYSTEM stimulants belong to the same general DRUG classification, sympathomimetic amines, and elicit the same kinds of responses though at varying levels. Stimulants have moderate to high risk for DEPENDENCE and ADDICTION.

Over-the-Counter Stimulants

Numerous stimulants are commonly available without a doctor's prescription, such as

- CAFFEINE, found in coffee, tea, cola, and energy drinks, gels, and food bars as well as in OVER-THE-COUNTER (OTC) DRUGS for weight loss, alertness, and PAIN relief

- NICOTINE, the primary active ingredient of tobacco

- pseudoephedrine and phenylephrine, decongestants found in OTC cold remedy and allergy relief products

- GINSENG, guarana, and kola nut, which are common ingredients in energy products

Though OTC and herbal products containing stimulants are readily available, they are not inherently safe. Herbal products, which are not subject to regulation as drugs in the United States, often contain numerous and sometimes poorly identified ingredients that may interact with each other or are of inconsistent potency and purity. Ephedrine and phenylpropanolamine are formerly common decongestants that are now banned in the United States, though herbal products manufactured in other countries sometimes contain them. Ma huang, a common Chinese herb, is a natural source of ephedra, an ephedrine alkaloid. Many states also limit the sale of pseudoephedrine, once the most commonly used decongestant, because of its use in illicitly manufacturing METHAMPHETAMINE, to which it has key chemical similarities.

Prescription and Illicit Stimulants

Federal law in the United States regulates most stimulant drugs as SCHEDULED DRUGS; possession and use require a physician's prescription. Prescription stimulants most commonly abused include AMPHETAMINES, dextroamphetamine, and methylphenidate. Illicit stimulants most commonly abused are COCAINE and METHAMPHETAMINE. These drugs all have high risk for psychologic dependence and addiction as well as for withdrawal symptoms when stopping them. A unique risk of cocaine use is that of SUDDEN CARDIAC DEATH due to the drug's unpredictable effects on the HEART and cardiovascular system.

COMMON STIMULANTS

AMPHETAMINES	benzphetamine
CAFFEINE	COCAINE
dextroamphetamine	diethylpropion
ephedra	ephedrine
mazindol	METHAMPHETAMINE
methcathinone	methylphenidate
modafinil	NICOTINE
phendimetrazine	phentermine
phenylephrine	pseudoephedrine

See also ILLICIT DRUG USE; PRESCRIPTION DRUG ABUSE; SUBSTANCE ABUSE PREVENTION; SUBSTANCE ABUSE TREATMENT.

substance abuse treatment   A method for helping people stop abusing drugs (including ALCOHOL), overcome ADDICTION, and maintain SOBRIETY. The acute stage of substance abuse treatment is DETOXIFICATION, which is most often a health circumstance that requires medical care until the person's body is completely free from the drug (typically 72 hours to 10 days). This stage of treatment is often inpatient though may be outpatient.

The follow-up treatment may last weeks to months, depending on the nature of the addiction and the person's individual situation. This stage may have require inpatient treatment with follow-up outpatient care or may be entirely outpatient. There are numerous methods for substance abuse treatment. The two main structured approaches are the 12-step programs and BEHAVIOR MODIFICATION THERAPY.

12-Step Programs
The original 12-step program, started in the 1930s, is Alcoholics Anonymous, which today has more than two million members worldwide. As well there are numerous similar programs for other addictions. The basic premise of the 12-step program is that addiction is an incurable disease from which a person is in ongoing recovery no matter how long he or she has maintained sobriety.

A fundamental tenet of the 12-step approach is anonymity for members within a structure of regular meetings that provide consistent peer support. There are no requirements for membership in 12-step groups other than agreement to follow the 12 steps; and there are no fees, charges, or dues. Each group determines the ways in which its members support the group's functions and expenses. There are also 12-step support programs, such as Al-Anon, for the family members and friends of people who have addictions.

Behavior Modification Therapy
Behavior modification therapy is formally structured care through a licensed psychologist or substance abuse professional and takes the approach that a person can change the ways he or she thinks and acts in regard to alcohol and drugs of abuse. Methods may include incentives, setting and then working to meet goals, behavior substitution skills, PSYCHOTHERAPY to help the person understand his or her reasons for abusing drugs or alcohol, education about drugs and addiction, and techniques for coping with situations that present high risk for relapse. Behavior modification therapy builds on the premises that the individual is responsible for his or her behavior, behaviors are learned, and learning new behaviors is always possible.

Related Health Care and Lifestyle Issues
Many people recovering from addiction have other health conditions that need appropriate medical attention, from NUTRITIONAL DEFICIENCY to damage resulting from abused drugs or alcohol. Recovery from substance abuse must also include treatment for such health conditions. Some conditions, such as HEPATITIS or other bloodborne infections, may require medications or extended treatment. Other conditions, such as LIVER disease or CARDIOVASCULAR DISEASE (CVD), may need ongoing medical care.

Nutritional eating is particularly important because nutritional deficiencies are common. Many people need vitamin and mineral supplements. Eating foods that are enjoyable provide a source of pleasure. Regular physical exercise is also important to maintain overall health as well as help stabilize mood, reduce cravings for drugs or alcohol, and provide a sense of purpose and routine.

Long-Term Outlook

Though many people successfully maintain sobriety and a drug-free lifestyle, relapse into addiction is not uncommon. Maintaining sobriety is an ongoing effort that requires continuous attention that many people find more challenging than they can manage. The more skills a person acquires for finding alternatives to drugs and alcohol—jobs, education, community involvement, sports and athletics, and other activities that provide a productive, fulfilling experience of everyday life—the more likely he or she will also create long-term success with treatment.

Support from family members and friends is also essential. Many people who relapse do so because they do not separate from the circumstances and relationships that supported their addictions. Underlying or co-existing psychiatric disorders or psychologic conditions often contribute to relapse. When considering and evaluating potential substance abuse treatment programs, it is important to ask what about the program's rate of success and how the program measures it.

See also ALCOHOLISM; EXERCISE AND HEALTH; ILLICIT DRUG USE; NUTRITION AND HEALTH; PRESCRIPTION DRUG ABUSE; SUBSTANCE ABUSE PREVENTION; SUPPORT GROUPS.

tobacco A plant cultivated as a crop in the southern United States and regions around the world with similar climate. In the United States federal and state laws regulate the sale and possession of tobacco products, with most states restricting sales to people age 18 or older (age 19 in a few states). Further restrictions on smoking affect the use of tobacco throughout the United States.

Though tobacco releases hundreds of chemicals when it burns, its primary psychoactive ingredient is NICOTINE, a powerful stimulant and vasoconstrictor (narrows and stiffens the BLOOD vessels). Nicotine enters the blood circulation within seconds of the first inhalation of cigarette smoke and remains active in the body for up to two hours after the person finishes smoking the cigarette. Its primary route is via absorption in the LUNGS, though the mucous membranes of the MOUTH (oral mucosa) and NOSE also absorb nicotine from the smoke. Mucosal absorption is the primary route for nicotine and tobacco's other chemicals to enter the blood circulation with cigar smoking and forms of tobacco other than cigarettes, such as chewing tobacco and snuff.

No form of tobacco or tobacco product is safe to use. Any use of tobacco, smoked or oral, can cause numerous health conditions. Smoking tobacco further exposes others to health risks.

Nicotine is one of the most addictive substances known. It rapidly crosses the BLOOD–BRAIN BARRIER to act directly on neurotransmitters and neuroreceptors in the BRAIN, affecting primarily DOPAMINE and acetylcholine. Dopamine has numerous functions related to mood, emotion, and sensations of pleasure; researchers believe dopamine plays a key role in addiction not only to nicotine but to most psychoactive drugs. Acetylcholine affects the release of other neurotransmitters in the brain and hormones in the body, notably EPINEPHRINE and NOREPINEPHRINE. These chemicals stimulate brain activity as well as increase BLOOD PRESSURE and HEART RATE. Though cigarette smoking provides the most rapid release of nicotine with tobacco use, oral forms of tobacco (chewing tobacco and snuff) deliver significantly higher concentrations of nicotine into the blood circulation and thus have high risk for addiction though many people perceive them to have fewer health risks.

Dozens of the chemicals in tobacco are carcinogenic (cause cancer). Many are most potent when burning, such as smoking a cigarette or cigar, releases them. Tobacco use, primarily cigarette smoking, is the leading cause of CARDIOVASCULAR DISEASE (CVD), LUNG CANCER, laryngeal cancer, and CHRONIC OBSTRUCTIVE PULMONARY DISEASE (COPD). Chewing tobacco and snuff cause nearly all oral cancers (cancers of the mouth); cigar smoking also causes oral cancers. Smoked forms of tobacco also expose other people to carcinogenic chemicals.

See also ANTISMOKING EFFORTS; CANCER RISK FACTORS; CARCINOGEN; ENVIRONMENTAL CIGARETTE SMOKE; SMOKING AND CANCER; SMOKING AND CARDIOVASCULAR DISEASE (CVD); SMOKING AND HEALTH; SMOKING CESSATION; WITHDRAWAL SYNDROME.

tolerance The need for increasing amounts of a DRUG to reach the same level of effectiveness. Tolerance is an expected physiologic effect with many drugs; for some, the therapeutic benefits rely on it. Tolerance accounts for the ability of long-time users to take doses of drugs that might otherwise be harmful.

In the context of substance abuse, tolerance is a factor in the development of DEPENDENCE, in which body biochemistry changes in response to the drug's presence so that the body depends on the drug for a particular way of functioning, and in ADDICTION, in which the drive to use the drug (irrespective of dependence) is all-consuming so that most efforts in daily life focus on obtaining and using the drug. Dependence and addiction may have physiologic or psychologic components, or both; tolerance is physiologic and may occur without dependence or addiction.

Tolerance develops at an unpredictable rate with psychoactive drugs (drugs that affect the mind, mood, and emotions) and NARCOTICS. It may be necessary to wean from, or gradually taper the DOSAGE of, these drugs so a person may stop taking them without adverse effects.

See also DETOXIFICATION; ILLICIT DRUG USE; PRESCRIPTION DRUG ABUSE; SUBSTANCE ABUSE TREATMENT; WITHDRAWAL SYNDROME.

withdrawal syndrome The physical and psychologic symptoms that may occur with DETOXIFICATION from substance abuse, DEPENDENCE, or ADDICTION. The symptoms of withdrawal vary, depending on the substances of dependence and addiction. Because substance abuse often involves multiple drugs, there is wide variation in the specific symptoms individuals experience during detoxification. Among the more common symptoms are

- NAUSEA and VOMITING
- shivering or trembling ("the shakes")
- abdominal cramping or PAIN
- intense cravings for the drugs of abuse
- HALLUCINATION

ALCOHOL withdrawal, especially from long-term alcohol abuse, may result in DELIRIUM TREMENS, a severe and potentially fatal complex of symptoms that requires medical treatment and monitoring until the body completely detoxifies from alcohol. Withdrawal from BARBITURATES also requires close medical supervision and usually medications to relieve withdrawal symptoms; suddenly stopping barbiturates can result in lethal complications, resulting from NEUROTRANSMITTER imbalances in the BRAIN. Withdrawal from STIMULANTS typically causes profusely runny NOSE because stimulants have a decongestant action through constricting the BLOOD vessels in the nose. Withdrawal from OPIATES results in sometimes severe coughing because opiates suppress the COUGH REFLEX; removing this suppression causes rebound coughing until opiate receptors re-acclimate.

Doctors typically use medications such as BENZODIAZEPINES to ease withdrawal symptoms until detoxification is complete. Subsequent treatment to maintain SOBRIETY may include medications such as disulfiram and NALTREXONE for alcohol addiction and METHADONE, NALTREXONE, or LEVO-ALPHA ACETYLMETHADOL (LAAM) for narcotic addiction. Many people trying to stop smoking benefit from NICOTINE REPLACEMENT products to wean from NICOTINE addiction. When PRESCRIPTION DRUG ABUSE of NARCOTICS for CHRONIC PAIN relief results in dependence or addiction, subsequent treatment incorporates alternative methods of pain relief. Though withdrawal symptoms end when the substances of abuse are no longer present in the body, continued treatment for addiction remains key for preventing relapse.

See also ALCOHOLISM; ILLICIT DRUG USE; SMOKING CESSATION; SUBSTANCE ABUSE PREVENTION; SUBSTANCE ABUSE TREATMENT.

EMERGENCY AND FIRST AID

This section, "Emergency and First Aid," provides brief and basic instructional information for common health emergencies, directed at the average person who has minimal medical knowledge or training. The structure and presentation of the content in this section differs from other sections of *The Facts On File Encyclopedia of Health and Medicine* in having such an instructional focus. Other sections contain content that gives detailed information about the health conditions.

This content does not substitute for appropriate and timely medical attention from trained medical personnel. Nearly always, the most appropriate first step in an emergency is to call 911 to summon medical assistance.

Three basic rules govern emergency and first aid response for the average person in nearly every type of situation.

Rule One: First Summon Emergency Personnel

In the United States, cellular telephones and the 911 network have revolutionized emergency response. The first action for the first person on the scene of a medical emergency should be to call 911 to summon emergency medical personnel. If the responder does not have a cell phone odds are high that the person in need of assistance does; cell phones have become ubiquitous in American society. Except for the most remote areas, the 911 network coordinates response to all emergencies.

When calling 911 to report an emergency and request aid, certain basic information helps get the right assistance to the right location in the shortest amount of time.

- Where is the site or scene? If a home, provide the address. If a business, provide the name and address. When at a home or business, calling 911 from a land line (regular telephone) displays location information for 911 dispatchers. When at the scene of a traffic accident, try to note key location markers such as street names and intersections, highway numbers, exit ramp numbers, or milepost markers.

- What happened and is it still happening? Though most emergency dispatch includes law enforcement, fire, and medical personnel, knowing what has happened helps the 911 dispatcher send an appropriate balance and number of personnel. A motor vehicle accident, a fire, and a shooting situation require different blends of emphasis, personnel, and equipment.

- How many people are involved and what kinds of injuries or medical crises do they appear to have? Just the basics—bleeding, BURNS, HEART ATTACK, not BREATHING, not conscious—help the 911 dispatcher determine an appropriate level of medical response (evacuation helicopter or ambulance, for example).

Rule Two: Self-Protection

The natural tendency is to rush to provide assistance. But however strong the urge to leap into the situation, the first responder must not become another victim. Self-protection has two components: situational safety and personal safety.

Before moving to provide aid to the person in need, the responder must determine whether the situation continues to hold risk. If this is a fire, is it still burning? If a motor vehicle accident, is there traffic, are there downed power poles or trees, or are any of the involved vehicles unstable or at risk for fire? If an apparent heart attack, are there any indications of ELECTROCUTION such as power tools, electrical appliances, or downed power lines? Is there any evidence of toxic chemicals?

Next, the responder must protect his or her personal safety. This includes acting within the boundaries of personal expertise as well as safeguarding oneself from exposure to bloodborne pathogens. For example, a person who does not have training in water rescue should not enter the water to save someone who is drowning; being a strong swimmer is often not enough. Rushing into a burning building or automobile is heroic and may save a life otherwise lost; however, the risk is far greater that such action will result instead in losing another life. The success of such rescues often requires expertise, experience, and specialized equipment.

Exposure to pathogens through contact with body fluids is an unfortunately common means of contracting serious infections such as HEPATITIS, HIV/AIDS, and TUBERCULOSIS. Two essential items of personal protection that ideally all adults should have easily accessible are latex or latex-type gloves and CARDIOPULMONARY RESUSCITATION (CPR) shields. These items are widely available in disposable, key-chain-size packets. Medical response professionals encourage everyone to carry these two personal protection items in their vehicles, first aid kits, backpacks, purses, briefcases, or whatever they often have with them.

Rule Three: Do No Further Harm

Because emergency medical personnel can reach the scene of a medical emergency within minutes in most locations, often the most appropriate actions for the first responder to take are only those necessary to safeguard the person's life. Often the full extent of a person's injuries is not apparent.

For example, it is often better to leave a person injured in an auto accident in the vehicle until emergency personnel arrive, unless removing the person is essential to save his or her life. The tremendous forces of impact in MOTOR VEHICLE ACCIDENTS may cause head and SPINAL CORD trauma such that improperly moving the person could result in permanent PARALYSIS. As well, the pressure of being wedged in the vehicle may be containing an injury in ways that are temporarily beneficial, such as bracing a FRACTURE or slowing bleeding. Even an apparently obvious circumstance, such as near-drowning or heart attack, may have hidden injuries. More appropriate actions on the part of the first responder might be to turn off the vehicle's ignition and kick dirt or gravel over any gasoline or oil that has leaked from the vehicle, for example, or to cover the person with blankets or coats to keep him or her warm and dry.

Learn More

All teens and adults should receive emergency first aid and CPR training. Many high schools include these classes as part of the health curriculum. Many employers also provide such classes, often with content specific to health hazards encountered on-the-job. Public agencies in such as fire departments, police departments, public safety departments, health departments, community centers, and hospitals in most communities offer such classes for nominal or no cost.

Basic first aid and CPR are easy to learn; the investment of a few hours' time for classes may save countless lives. As well, many employers and public safety agencies conduct first responder training, typically a 40- to 60-hour curriculum that teaches advanced medical assistance and emergency response techniques. Companies and communities may then call on certified first responders in emergency situations.

First Response

The responses and actions of the first person who arrives on the scene of an emergency, commonly called the first responder, are crucial. This person must rapidly assess the nature of the situation, the safety of the site, and the possible injuries and treatment needs for those involved in the emergency. In many situations the most appropriate first response is to call 911 to summon medical assistance and provide comfort for those who are injured. In other circumstances the first responder may need to stop bleeding, perform CARDIOPULMONARY RESUSCITATION (CPR), or stabilize a possible FRACTURE.

The essential and most crucial first action for the first person to arrive on the scene of an emergency is to safeguard his or her own safety and protection. This means conducting a rapid but thorough SITE AND SITUATION ASSESSMENT to determine:

- What happened?
- Does the cause of the situation still exist as a risk for further harm?
- How many people appear to be involved?
- What is the nature of injuries or medical need?

The next action for the first responder is to summon aid. Though it is a natural tendency to rush to the aid of the person who needs care, the few seconds it will take to call 911 are more likely to save lives by getting trained and equipped rescue personnel to the scene. This is especially critical when the emergency is a HEART ATTACK; people who receive advanced cardiac care in a hospital within one hour of the heart attack's onset have a significantly higher chance of survival. As well, taking a few moments to survey the scene and the situation helps the responder focus and become calm.

The situation and circumstances determine the first responder's subsequent actions, which may include administering first aid, removing the person from danger, directing traffic or the activities of others who arrive to help, or simply comforting the person until medical and rescue personnel arrive. Because responding aid personnel may have questions about what happened or the circumstances under which the first responder happened upon the scene, the first responder should check with them before leaving the site.

body substance isolation Procedures for safely handling and disposing of body fluids and tissues such as BLOOD, SPUTUM, URINE, and feces. Body fluids can transmit bacterial and viral infections to others. Cuts and scrapes on the responder's body can allow pathogens to enter, risking INFECTION. Other possible points of entry are the responder's eyes, NOSE, and MOUTH.

Everyone who provides assistance to those who are injured or ill should wear latex or latex-type gloves and use barrier protection when performing resuscitation BREATHING to protect against direct contact with body fluids. Commercial first aid kits such as many people carry in their cars typically contain gloves. When gloves or resuscitation shields are not available, the responder must carefully consider his or her personal risk for infection before proceeding with any contact. The natural tendency when first arriving on the scene of an emergency to arrive at the scene of an emergency is to perform the necessary first aid procedures without consideration for personal risk. Materials such as clothing, towels, and other substances provide some protection from direct contact when the situation is life threatening. When emergency aid personnel are on the way a minimal response may be both adequate and most appropriate.

Should direct contact with body fluids occur, the responder should wash the area of contact thoroughly (rinse extensively with water if the eyes or mouth) and promptly seek a doctor's advice and appropriate prophylaxis (preventive measures). Prophylaxis is available to reduce the risk for contracting infections such as HEPATITIS and TUBERCULOSIS. However, there are currently no methods to prevent infection with HIV (human immunodeficiency virus), the virus that causes AIDS (acquired immunodeficiency syndrome).

See also ACCIDENTAL INJURIES; BLEEDING CONTROL; CARDIOPULMONARY RESUSCITATION (CPR); HIV/AIDS; MULTIPLE TRAUMA; PATHOGEN; RESPONDER SAFETY AND PERSONAL PROTECTION; SITE AND SITUATION ASSESSMENT; SYMPTOM ASSESSMENT AND CARE TRIAGE.

confidentiality   The requirement to maintain the personal privacy of individuals who require emergency assistance or first aid. Though laws regarding confidentiality apply to people employed in fields such as health care, law enforcement, and firefighting, any person who responds to provide assistance should similarly respect the privacy of those involved in the situation. Such respect includes not discussing details of the situation with anyone, including media or press, other than those involved in the subsequent care of the person. A good rule of thumb is for the responder to consider whether he or she would want the information divulged were the responder the one who received assistance. As well, it is possible for there to be legal repercussions should information made public turn out to be erroneous.

See also GOOD SAMARITAN LAWS.

Good Samaritan laws   Legal protections in the United States that states enact to shelter people who provide emergency assistance and first aid from legal liability for outcomes that may result from their actions. Such laws primarily affect individuals (other than those who work in public safety or health care jobs) who stop to help at MOTOR VEHICLE ACCIDENTS, when a person suffers a HEART ATTACK, or in other crisis situations. The premise is that the person providing aid is doing

so with good intent and due prudence. These laws do not prevent legal action, however.

See also CONFIDENTIALITY; FIRST RESPONSE; SITE AND SITUATION ASSESSMENT; SYMPTOM ASSESSMENT AND CARE TRIAGE.

responder safety and personal protection   Items and methods responders should use when providing emergency assistance and first aid. The personal safety and protection of responders is essential. At a minimum, personal protection items should include

- latex gloves (or medical-grade, latex-free gloves for people who have latex allergies)
- a resuscitation shield or mask when performing RESCUE BREATHING or CARDIOPULMONARY RESUSCITATION (CPR)

Most commercial first aid kits now contain these items. If the responder does not have them, the person in need of medical attention might have them in a home or auto first aid kit. When these items are not available and the situation is a dire one in which the person is likely to die without immediate aid that risks exposure to body fluids, the responder can reduce such exposure by using clothing to establish a barrier.

The other fundamental dimension of responder safety and personal protection is quick but thorough SITE AND SITUATION ASSESSMENT to determine what, if any, risks exist that pose hazards for the responder. Key among these risks are the possibilities of

- fire, explosion, or ELECTROCUTION
- drowning, when the person needing assistance is in or near the water
- direct harm, when the situation is one of VIOLENCE such as a shooting
- hazardous conditions such as traffic or unstable terrain
- toxic chemical exposure

When these risks are present or uncertain, they put the responder at great peril.

See also ACCIDENTAL INJURIES; HEPATITIS PREVENTION; HIV/AIDS; INFECTION; PATHOGEN; SYMPTOM ASSESSMENT AND CARE TRIAGE; TUBERCULOSIS PREVENTION.

site and situation assessment The first action a responder should take when arriving at a situation that requires emergency assistance or first aid. The assessment must be brief but thorough enough to determine potential hazards for the responder as well as the condition of the person who needs assistance. Site and situation assessment should consider, at minimum

Nature of the emergency

- How many people are involved?
- Is anyone bleeding?
- Is anyone not BREATHING?
- Is the cause of the emergency still an active hazard?
- Are those who need aid safe from further harm?

Risk of fire

- Are flames visible?
- Is there a smell of smoke?
- Is there a smell of gasoline, diesel, oil, or natural gas?
- Are the engines of any vehicles still running after involvement in a collision or accident?
- Are there downed power lines?

Risk of ELECTROCUTION

- Are or were there power tools in use?
- Are there downed trees, power poles, or power lines?

Risk of drowning

- Is the person in water?
- Does the responder have training in water rescues?

Multiple hazards are often present, such as traffic attempting to pass through the scene of a motor vehicle accident or water on the surface when power lines are down. Less obvious hazards may include dogs in the home or at the scene of a motor vehicle accident whose behaviors to protect their owners threaten responders, power tools that have caused injury and remain plugged in, or gasoline leaking from a vehicle involved in an accident. Often the most appropriate response for the person first on the site is to summon emergency personnel and follow their instructions after they arrive for providing further assistance.

See also ACCIDENTAL INJURIES; MOTOR VEHICLE ACCIDENTS; RESPONDER SAFETY AND PERSONAL PROTECTION; SYMPTOM ASSESSMENT AND CARE TRIAGE.

symptom assessment and care triage A methodic approach to quickly determining the nature and severity of injuries so as to provide appropriate FIRST RESPONSE. A responder's ability to provide symptom assessment depends on the responder's level of knowledge and training.

Medical emergency personnel use various systems to triage patients—that is, determine the severity of injuries, type of care the injuries need, and likelihood for survival within the context of the medical resources immediately available. Emergency personnel will conduct such an assessment when they arrive at the site. In the meantime, the person who is first on the scene of a medical emergency that involves more than one person, or one person with multiple injuries, needs to determine how to provide the most appropriate attention to those who need care until medical emergency personnel arrive.

The most important and fundamental assessment is whether the person's life is in imminent danger. These four basic steps help make a rapid determination; the findings direct the responder's subsequent actions. Because time is crucial when the injuries or circumstances (such as HEART ATTACK) are life threatening, the basic assessment should take no more than 30 seconds.

1. **Is the person conscious?** If so ask, "Where do you hurt?" CONSCIOUSNESS, especially right after an injury or medical crisis such as heart attack, is not of itself an indication of whether the situation is life threatening.

2. **Is the person BREATHING?** Look for bluish gray discoloration of the lips, fingers, and SKIN overall. Watch to see if the person's chest rises and falls. Feel for air coming out of the NOSE or MOUTH.

3. **Is the person's HEART beating?** Feel for a PULSE in the side of the neck, two finger-widths below the notch toward the back of the lower jaw. Listen, with the EAR against the chest, for a heart beat.

4. **Is the person bleeding severely?** External bleeding is generally obvious; look at the person's front and back. Indications of internal bleeding include unusual or rapid swelling.

It is essential to assess all four life-threatening factors as well as the context of the situation before initiating emergency care because the findings determine the most appropriate response. Multiple life-threatening injuries present a complicated situation, especially when there is only one responder and he or she may have to make rapid decisions about what to do. It may be necessary to stop severe bleeding before proceeding to CARDIOPULMONARY RESUSCITATION (CPR), for example. The first action of the responder—call 911 to summon emergency aid—is often the most crucial.

See also BLEEDING CONTROL; RESPONDER SAFETY AND PERSONAL PROTECTION; SITE AND SITUATION ASSESSMENT.

Burns, Bleeding, Breaks

The most common types of injuries that require emergency medical assistance are BURNS, LACERATIONS (cuts) that result in external bleeding, BLUNT TRAUMA that results in internal bleeding, and fractures (broken bones). Many such injuries are mild to moderate in severity; mild burns and lacerations often require only self-care. Fractures and moderate injuries may need medical attention to assess their severity, especially burns and lacerations that may extend deep into the tissues.

Burns and bleeding have the highest risk for being life threatening. Traumatic injury to the chest can result in the loss of 25 percent of the body's BLOOD supply within minutes. A second- or third-degree burn that covers 36 percent of the body's surface results in extensive fluid and heat loss. Both circumstances cause rapid SHOCK. Though fractures are not as likely to be life threatening, an open FRACTURE exposes body tissues to high risk for INFECTION. As well, the BONE ends may sever blood vessels, resulting in hemorrhage.

These types of injuries present the highest risk of bloodborne infection, such as HEPATITIS and HIV/AIDS, for first responders. Latex or latex-type gloves are essential; the responder should be wearing them before touching the injured person. There is also the risk for injury to the responder, such as in a fire or explosion or when injuries result from VIOLENCE.

abrasions Scrape wounds that remove the outer layers of SKIN to expose the dermis and sometimes the subcutaneous layer beneath. Abrasions are common sports- and activity-related injuries resulting from falling or sliding on hard surfaces such as sidewalks, pavement, artificial turf, and hard-packed dirt.

Abrasions often look raw and may bleed; they usually hurt because they expose nerves and BLOOD vessels. Small abrasions are more nuisance than health problem. Large, deep abrasions may leave scars after they heal though most abrasions do not damage the dermis, the innermost layer of skin. Most abrasions require only minor first aid and heal uneventfully within two weeks.

These are the recommended steps for treating abrasions:

- Gently but thoroughly flush all dirt and debris from the abrasion with normal saline or a wound cleansing solution. Do not use soap and water or hydrogen peroxide; these formerly popular approaches delay scab formation and HEALING.

- Apply a topical antibiotic ointment and cover the abrasion completely with a bandage.

- Change the bandage daily or when it gets wet, applying fresh antibiotic ointment with each bandage change.

- Keep antibiotic ointment and a bandage on the abrasion until it heals, typically 7 to 10 days.

A health-care provider should assess and débride (clear away debris and damaged tissue) large abrasions to minimize the risk of scarring and INFECTION.

See also ANTIBIOTIC MEDICATIONS; LACERATIONS; SCAR.

avulsion An injury of force that tears away a body structure such as a TOOTH, segment of finger or toe, piece of tissue, or fragment of BONE. A major avulsion may involve a limb. Avulsion may be, though is not always, a type of TRAUMATIC AMPUTATION. Surgeons can replant some avulsed structures, such as teeth and bone fragments. The force that creates the separation often causes significant and irreparable damage to the tissues, however.

Site and situation assessment The responder should identify what caused the avulsion and if necessary neutralize its ability to do further damage. This includes turning off the power to any machinery or equipment that caused an avulsion injury.

Responder personal protection measures Latex gloves, which the responder should put on before approaching the injured person, are essential for personal protection from bloodborne pathogens as nearly always there is moderate to heavy bleeding with avulsions.

First response actions Substantial bleeding is likely at the site of the avulsion. The first person to respond should take every practical effort to stop the bleeding. When possible, salvage the avulsed body part and protect it by wrapping it in sterile gauze moistened with sterile water or saline, if possible, and placing it in a plastic bag or container. Put the container in a portable cooler with ice around it and transport it to the hospital with the wounded person. Time is of the essence, however; the longer the avulsed part remains separated from the body the less likely the surgeon will be able to successfully replant it.

Follow-through An avulsion injury requires a physician's prompt evaluation and treatment, usually surgery either to replant the body part or surgically débride and repair the avulsion site.

See also BLEEDING CONTROL; BLOOD; PATHOGEN.

bleeding control The measures necessary to stop bleeding. Bleeding occurs when an injury damages the walls of the BLOOD vessels, allowing blood to escape.

Though profusely flowing blood may rapidly become life threatening, the amount of blood present or obvious is not always a good indication of the injury's severity. ABRASIONS (scrapes) and minor LACERATIONS (cuts) may appear to bleed extensively when they damage large numbers of the tiny blood vessels in the dermis (middle layer of the SKIN) and the subcutaneous layer, as these tissues contain a rich supply of blood. Wounds to the face and head tend to bleed especially profusely though often are not serious or life threatening. Injuries to the inside of the MOUTH not only bleed extensively but the blood also mixes with SALIVA, appearing as though there were even more blood. A nosebleed (EPIS-TAXIS) may also appear to produce a large amount of bleeding. However, the amount of blood lost with these types of injuries is usually minor.

BLOOD that spurts or surges from the wound comes from an ARTERY or major VEIN. Immediately apply pressure firmly enough to compress the blood vessel and maintain the pressure until emergency medical personnel take over.

Injuries that damage major veins or arteries can result in rapid loss of blood with risk for SHOCK and possible death. Bleeding in such circumstances is heavy and may spurt, gush, or surge from the injury. Life-threatening bleeding from the injury may also occur internally or as the result of BLUNT TRAUMA. Indications of INTERNAL BLEEDING include rapid swelling in the area of the bleeding and signs of shock in the injured person.

Site and situation assessment Situations of criminal VIOLENCE are often not safe for the first person who arrives to do any more than summon emergency aid. When injuries are due to animal bites, the responder must determine that the animal is no longer present or a threat. MOTOR VEHICLE ACCIDENTS may result in multiple injuries to the same person or to multiple people. Rapid SYMPTOM ASSESSMENT AND CARE TRIAGE is essential to determine whether any injuries appear life threatening.

Responder personal protection measures Latex gloves, which the responder should put on before approaching the injured person, are essential for personal protection from bloodborne pathogens as well as to prevent BACTERIA on the responder's hands from causing INFECTION in the wound.

First response actions Bleeding frightens most people, those who are injured and those who are providing FIRST RESPONSE alike, especially when there appears to be a lot of blood. It is important for the responder to act calmly and comfortingly as well as quickly.

Use these measures to stop bleeding from an external injury such as an abrasion or laceration:

- Put on latex or latex-type gloves.
- Cover the injury with gauze bandages, a washcloth or towel, or even a wadded piece of clothing and apply firm, steady pressure.

- If the injury bleeds through the covering material, add more but do not remove the original covering.
- Maintain pressure until emergency medical personnel arrive.

Use these measures to stop a nosebleed:

- Put on latex or latex-type gloves.
- Have the person sit upright, holding the head tipped slightly toward the chest.
- Firmly squeeze both nostrils with the thumb and forefinger.
- Hold pressure in this way for at least 10 minutes.
- If bleeding starts again after releasing the pressure, repeat the procedure.

Follow-through A health-care provider should evaluate most bleeding injuries to cleanse them and determine whether sutures (stitches) or other treatments are necessary. Nosebleeds require medical attention when they persist or frequently recur.

See also GASTROINTESTINAL BLEEDING; IMPALEMENT; PUNCTURE WOUND; SYMPTOM ASSESSMENT AND CARE TRIAGE.

burns Injuries resulting from exposure to fire, intense heat, extremely hot water, electricity (including lightning), radiation (including ultraviolet radiation from sunlight or tanning systems), or caustic chemicals. The severity of a burn depends on the depth of penetration into the tissues (first degree, second degree, and third degree) and the amount of surface area the burn covers (percentage). SHOCK is a significant risk with any burn.

Medical personnel often use a method called the "rule of nines" to assess the body surface area a burn covers. This method assigns a percentage of 9 or 18 percent to regions of the body. For example, each arm is 9 percent, as is the head; the legs, back, and chest are each 18 percent. The surface area a burn covers may have more significant health consequences than the burn's depth. A first-degree (superficial) burn that covers an extensive area is often more serious than a third-degree burn that covers a very small area.

Heat and explosion burns on the upper body, face, and head may indicate the person also has burns to the MOUTH, NOSE, or upper airway (INHALATION BURNS). Such burns are potentially life threatening because swelling may close the airway, blocking the flow of oxygen to the LUNGS and compromising the ability to breathe.

Site and situation assessment Risk for injury to the first person to respond is very high when the source of the burn remains. In situations of active fire, risk for explosion, lightning, downed power lines, or chemical or radioactive contamination, the only response that may be safe for the responder is to provide as detailed information as possible when summoning emergency aid to help dispatchers send the appropriate equipment and trained personnel.

Responder personal protection measures Latex gloves, which the responder should put on before

BURN SEVERITY		
Burn Classification	**Extent of Burn**	**Symptoms**
first degree or superficial thickness	burn penetrates only into the epidermis (outer layer of SKIN)	redness, PAIN, slight swelling
second degree or partial thickness	burn penetrates into the dermis (middle layer of skin)	blisters, pain, moderate swelling
third degree or full thickness	burn penetrates into the subcutaneous layer (innermost layer of skin) and possibly into underlying tissues	open wound or charring, may be no pain

approaching a person who has burns, are essential for personal protection from bloodborne pathogens as well as to prevent BACTERIA on the responder's hands from causing INFECTION in the burn wounds.

First response actions If the person's clothing is on fire, get the person on the ground and smother the flames by rolling or covering with a blanket, rug, jacket, or other object that can block the flow of air. Burns require specialized care from medical personnel trained in burn care. The most appropriate actions for an untrained responder first on the scene are to keep the person warm and comfort the person until medical personnel arrive. Most important:

- Do *not* put anything on the burns.
- Do *not* pull clothing or debris from the burns.
- Do *not* pop BLISTERS or pull the SKIN off blisters that spontaneously rupture.

Cool water, such as from a water faucet, is appropriate first aid to soothe small, minor burns. Promptly cooling a small first- or second-degree burn relieves PAIN and reduces swelling. However, the burn may still require medical attention.

Follow-through A health-care provider should evaluate and treat most second- and third-degree burns as well as first-degree burns that cover 36 percent or more of the body. Infection is a significant risk with second- and third-degree burns; any indications (FEVER, increased pain or swelling) require prompt medical assessment.

See also SITE AND SITUATION ASSESSMENT; SUNBURN; SYMPTOM ASSESSMENT AND CARE TRIAGE.

closed fracture A broken BONE that does not protrude through the surface of the SKIN. A closed FRACTURE most commonly results from a blow that delivers intense energy to small or limited area, causing the bone beneath to break. The bone ends may remain relatively aligned or may cause significant soft tissue damage even though the ends do not penetrate through the skin. Although the ends of the bones with a closed fracture do not break the skin, they may still do considerable damage to tissues and structures around the area of the break. Fractures require prompt evaluation and treatment from a health-care provider.

Do *not* move a person who may have a FRACTURE of the back or neck. Brace the person with rolled towels and blankets or other objects and keep him or her still until emergency medical personnel arrive.

The most appropriate action for the responder is to immobilize the limb, as well as the joints above and below the point of the fracture when possible, and obtain immediate medical attention. Splints are effective for fractures of the fingers, arms, and legs. Commercial first aid kits may include soft or inflatable splints. As well, the responder can use many common objects to fashion an improvised splint: towels, pillows, cardboard, and folded newspapers or magazines. A sling to support the arm on the side of the injury helps immobilize a fractured clavicle (collarbone) or shoulder blade (scapula). Scarves, belts, towels, and even a long-sleeve jacket or shirt with the sleeve pinned to the upper part of the garment are among the items the responder can use to make a sling.

See also ACCIDENTAL INJURIES; ATHLETIC INJURIES; OPEN FRACTURE; SYMPTOM ASSESSMENT AND CARE TRIAGE

dislocations Injury to the ligaments at a JOINT that allows the ends of the bones to separate. Often the responder cannot determine whether an injury is a dislocation or a CLOSED FRACTURE; FIRST RESPONSE treats them the same.

Do *not* attempt to "pop" a dislocated JOINT back into place.

The primary first response action is to immobilize the joint using a splint, or, in the case of a dislocated shoulder, a sling. A health-care provider should evaluate a dislocation to determine if there is a FRACTURE (which requires an X-RAY) and whether surgery is necessary to repair the ligaments.

See also ACCIDENTAL INJURIES; ATHLETIC INJURIES; BONE; LIGAMENT; SPRAINS AND STRAINS; SURGERY BENEFIT AND RISK ASSESSMENT.

impalement A wound in which an object penetrates a part of the body and remains embedded there. Impalement injuries may occur when a person falls into a stationary object such as a fence rail or tree branch. Nail guns are responsible for numerous impalement injuries. Such injuries may penetrate a hand or foot in such a way as to nail it to a surface. Because nail guns expel nails under tremendous force, a nail may penetrate the skull or sternum to cause potentially life threatening injury. Impalement injuries may also occur when falling on an object such as a pencil.

Do *not* attempt to remove an impaled object from any part of the body. Immobilize the part as quickly as possible and summon emergency medical personnel.

Site and situation assessment Generally there are no risks to others at the site of an impalement injury. An exception might be in the circumstance of a nail gun, in which the responder must determine the nail gun is inactive.

Responder personal protection measures Latex gloves, which the responder should put on before approaching the injured person, are essential for personal protection from bloodborne pathogens as there is often bleeding from an impalement injury.

First response actions It is crucial to avoid moving a person who is impaled on an immobile object and to provide as much information as possible about the object to the 911 dispatcher. The responder should stabilize the person to support the body or impaled body part and attempt to comfort and calm the person until emergency personnel arrive.

Follow-through Impalement injuries require a physician's assessment and medical treatment.

See also INFECTION; PUNCTURE WOUND; SITE AND SITUATION ASSESSMENT; SYMPTOM ASSESSMENT AND CARE TRIAGE; TRAUMA TO THE EYE.

inhalation burns Thermal or chemical BURNS of the upper airway (TRACHEA) that result from BREATHING extreme heat (as in a fire) or toxic fumes. There may also be burns to the lips, tongue, and inside of the MOUTH and NOSE. Inhalation burns may cause rapid swelling of the airway, blocking the flow of air and presenting a life threatening situation. As emergency intubation or

tracheotomy (invasive methods to bypass the upper airway to get air to the LUNGS) may be the only measures to save the person's life, the need for care from appropriate medical personnel is urgent.

Site and situation assessment The risk for injury to rescuers and others is high if there is still a burning or smoldering fire or a chemical exposure remains uncontained. A situation that requires personal protective equipment is one the first person to arrive should not enter.

Responder personal protection measures The responder should use a resuscitation shield if CARDIOPULMONARY RESUSCITATION (CPR) or RESCUE BREATHING is necessary.

First response actions Most inhalation burns are critical injuries that require advanced life support care well beyond the scope of untrained medical response. The most effective action on the part of the first person at the site is to rapidly summon emergency personnel.

Follow-through Inhalation burns require urgent medical treatment from physicians and other personnel trained and experienced in treating such injuries. Emergency transportation to a hospital or trauma center is often crucial.

See also ACUTE RESPIRATORY DISTRESS SYNDROME (ARDS); INHALED TOXINS; SHOCK.

lacerations Cuts or tears of the skin and tissues. Lacerations may be fairly superficial or extend deep into the body. The risk for damage to nerves and BLOOD vessels is high. A large or deep laceration may bleed profusely, requiring immediate BLEEDING CONTROL efforts. A responder providing first aid for a laceration should put on latex or latex-type gloves approaching the injured person, are essential for personal protection from bloodborne pathogens as well as to prevent BACTERIA from the responder's hands from causing INFECTION in the wound.

To treat a mild laceration (less than ½ inch in length):

- Apply a bandage or gauze pad and hold it in place to stop any bleeding.
- When the bleeding stops, remove the bandage and apply an antibiotic ointment and a clean bandage.

- Change the bandage daily or when it gets wet, applying free antibiotic ointment with each bandage change.

- Continue to treat the laceration until its edges completely heal together (typically 7 to 10 days).

A laceration that is jagged or longer than ½ inch, or whose edges do not stay together, requires medical treatment. These are the recommended steps for the first responder to take to help protect the wound until the person can receive such treatment:

- Stop the bleeding; apply a bandage or other covering and hold it firmly enough to exert pressure.

- When the bleeding stops place gauze or tape to hold the bandage in place. Do *not* remove the bandage. If bleeding persists, add more bandage.

- Immobilize the area of the laceration to minimize and further damage.

Minor lacerations often heal well with self-treatment. When the edges of a laceration will not stay together on their own, the wound needs sutures (stitches). A jagged or deep laceration may require debridement, a procedure in which a doctor or physician's assistant numbs the area with a local anesthetic and trims away all loose tissue and cleans out any debris that contaminates the wound. The provider may suture the wound if it is clean enough or allow it to heal on its own, a process called granulation in which new tissue grows from the inside to the outside of the wound.

See also ABRASIONS; ANTIBIOTIC MEDICATIONS; AVULSION; SCAR.

open fracture A FRACTURE in which the broken BONE protrudes through the surface of the SKIN, creating an open wound that may bleed profusely. There is high risk for the bone ends to significantly damage nerves, BLOOD vessels, and other tissues in the area around the fracture.

Site and situation assessment Open fractures result from significant trauma as may occur in MOTOR VEHICLE ACCIDENTS, industrial accidents in which a heavy object falls on the person, falls, or collisions (such as when bicycling, skiing, or skateboarding). A person who has an open fracture may have multiple injuries or there may be multiple people involved in the accident who have various injuries. Possible site hazards that present risk of injury for responders, particularly the responder first to arrive, include downed power lines, unstable terrain or structures, and traffic.

Responder personal protection measures Latex gloves, which the responder should put on before approaching the injured person, are essential for personal protection from bloodborne pathogens as nearly always there is moderate to heavy bleeding from open fractures.

First response actions Necessary actions from the first responder may include BLEEDING CONTROL, fracture stabilization, and comforting the injured person. Open fractures are serious injuries and moving the person is likely to require technical expertise as well as multiple rescuers. Often the most important role for the first responder is to keep the injured person calm, warm, and dry until rescue and emergency medical personnel arrive.

Follow-through Open fractures require urgent medical treatment and surgery to clean the injury and repair the fracture and damage to the surrounding tissues.

See also BODY SUBSTANCE ISOLATION; LACERATION; SHOCK; SYMPTOM ASSESSMENT AND CARE TRIAGE.

puncture wound An injury in which an object penetrates through the SKIN and into the underlying structures, sometimes deeply, with the wound closing with the object's withdrawal. There may be little or no external bleeding with a puncture wound. However, the risk for INFECTION is extremely high. First aid measures include rinsing debris and BLOOD from the wound and applying a bandage to protect it from exposure to further pathogens. A health-care provider should evaluate the wound promptly as it might be necessary to incise it (cut it open under sterile conditions) to clean it and irrigate it with antibiotic solution. The health-care provider is also likely to prescribe ANTIBIOTIC MEDICATIONS to treat bacterial INFECTION. The injured person should receive a tetanus toxoid booster if the last one was more than 10 years ago.

See also BODY SUBSTANCE ISOLATION; GUNSHOT WOUNDS; IMPALEMENT; NECROTIZING FASCIITIS; PATHOGEN; SITE AND SITUATION ASSESSMENT; SYMPTOM ASSESSMENT AND CARE TRIAGE; TRAUMA TO THE EYE.

shock Life-threatening cardiovascular collapse. Shock occurs when BLOOD PRESSURE drops below the level necessary to pump BLOOD to the tissues (peripheral perfusion), depriving them of oxygen (HYPOXIA). The symptoms of shock may include

- clammy or bluish SKIN (CYANOSIS)
- confusion, anxiety, or disorientation
- diminished or loss of CONSCIOUSNESS
- rapid BREATHING (TACHYPNEA) and HEART RATE (tachycardia)
- difficulty BREATHING (DYSPNEA)

Urgent medical treatment is essential. While waiting for emergency medical personnel to arrive, the responder first on the scene should perform whatever emergency aid measures are appropriate for the person's circumstances. It is also important to keep the person warm and calm and to have the injured person lie as horizontally as is possible with the feet and legs elevated about 12 inches to help blood flow back to the HEART.

CIRCUMSTANCES THAT CAN RESULT IN SHOCK	
ANAPHYLAXIS	BURNS
ELECTROCUTION	GUNSHOT WOUNDS
HEART ATTACK	HEAT STROKE
hemorrhage	MULTIPLE TRAUMA
OPEN FRACTURE	poisoning
severe DEHYDRATION	SPINAL CORD INJURY
TRAUMATIC AMPUTATION	TRAUMATIC BRAIN INJURY (TBI)

See also CARDIOPULMONARY RESUSCITATION (CPR); MULTIPLE TRAUMA; RESCUE BREATHING; SITE AND SITUATION ASSESSMENT; SYMPTOM ASSESSMENT AND CARE TRIAGE.

soft tissue injuries Injuries to muscles, tendons, and ligaments that occur as a result of sudden excessive tension, causing the tissue to tear or stretch. Soft tissue injuries are common and may occur during everyday activities as well as during athletic activities. Soft tissue injuries tend to hurt and swell fairly immediately. Ice to the injured area is the most effective FIRST RESPONSE to reduce both PAIN and swelling. Immobilization, such as with elastic bandage wraps, splints, or slings, helps prevent further damage.

In general, a soft tissue injury requires evaluation and treatment from a doctor or other health-care provider when:

- the person cannot bear weight on a lower extremity or use an upper extremity
- swelling significantly distorts the appearance of the injured part
- over-the-counter (OTC) ANALGESIC MEDICATIONS such as acetaminophen or NONSTEROIDAL ANTI-INFLAMMATORY DRUGS (NSAIDS) fail to relieve pain

Though most soft tissue injuries are minor and heal with self-care measures in two to six weeks, severe injuries may require surgical repair, especially tears.

COMMON SOFT TISSUE INJURIES	
ACHILLES TENDON INJURY	ANKLE INJURIES
groin pull	KNEE INJURIES
MUSCLE tears and pulls	SPRAINS AND STRAINS

See also ATHLETIC INJURIES; CLOSED FRACTURE; DISLOCATIONS; FRACTURE; HERNIA; INFLAMMATION; OPEN FRACTURE; SPRAINS AND STRAINS; SYMPTOM ASSESSMENT AND CARE TRIAGE.

Drowning

More than 4,000 Americans die from drowning each year. About 15,000 are revived and survive. The most common causes of drowning are swimming, boating, and scuba diving accidents. Though a person may struggle in the water for an extended time, the threshold for remaining submerged is only about three minutes, after which the BRAIN can no longer function and the person loses CONSCIOUSNESS.

When the head goes under the water a sequence of physiologic changes are activated, sometimes called the diving REFLEX, that alter the body's cardiovascular system to reserve BLOOD and the oxygen it carries to maintain the body's vital functions. The HEART RATE slows, BLOOD PRESSURE decreases, peripheral blood vessels constrict, blood supply to vital organs increases, and body temperature drops. These changes rapidly slow METABOLISM (the rate at which the body uses energy), significantly cutting the body's need for oxygen, which is one of the two fuel sources for cells (the other being GLUCOSE) throughout the body and the only fuel source for brain cells. When water enters the airway, the larynx severely spasms, closing off the TRACHEA. This laryngeal SPASM reflex is so intense that most people who die of drowning die from asphyxiation (lack of oxygen). In only about 10 percent of drownings does water enter the LUNGS.

The urge to save someone who is drowning is so strong that many would-be rescuers rush to jump into the water. However, water rescues are difficult. A person who is still struggling will often fight with the rescuer as a survival reaction, even to the extent of pushing the rescuer under the water. All too often the outcome is two drownings rather than a rescue. An unconscious drowning victim is easier to pull from the water, though nonetheless there is great risk for the rescuer who does not know water rescue techniques. Being a strong swimmer is not enough. Public pools, water parks, and swimming beaches typically have lifeguards and rescue equipment. Poles, rescue flotation rings, and other devices can allow a first responder to begin helping a drowning victim while waiting for trained rescue personnel to reach the scene.

cold water drowning Drowning that occurs when the water temperature is below 50°F. Survival is somewhat higher with cold water drowning because the cold temperature of the water seems to further depress METABOLISM, dramatically lowering the body's oxygen needs. Though in general a person who has been submerged in cold water for longer than 10 minutes has a poor chance for revival, some people have survived being under frigid water for 40 minutes. Rescue experts recommend initiating resuscitation efforts for all cold water drownings.

Site and situation assessment Important aspects of the situation include the type of water (pool, lake, river), how long the person has been under water, and whether other injuries are possible. SPINAL CORD INJURY or head injury is likely when diving into the water, for example.

Responder personal protection measures Essential responder personal protection items include latex or latex-style gloves and a resuscitation shield.

First response actions When the person is still in the water and is conscious, the responder should use items such as ropes, poles, and flotation devices to attempt to help the person rather than jumping into the water, unless the responder has training in water rescues. RESCUE BREATHING or CARDIOPUL-

MONARY RESUSCITATION (CPR) may be necessary when the person is brought to shore or the pool's edge.

Follow-through Emergency medical personnel typically transport cold water drowning victims to a hospital emergency department or trauma center even when resuscitative efforts appear unsuccessful because there is the possibility for revival when body temperature returns to normal. A doctor should thoroughly assess a person who survives, as secondary complications may occur.

See also RESPONDER SAFETY AND PERSONAL PROTECTION; SITE AND SITUATION ASSESSMENT; SYMPTOM ASSESSMENT AND CARE TRIAGE; WARM WATER DROWNING.

rescue breathing A method to revive a person who has stopped BREATHING (RESPIRATORY FAILURE) but who still has a HEART beat (PULSE). Rescue breathing may be necessary in drowning, poisoning, ELECTROCUTION, and other circumstances in which the respiratory failure occurs suddenly and the first response is rapid. The BRAIN begins to experience irreversible damage after about 6 minutes of oxygen deprivation, so urgent response is essential.

Site and situation assessment Risks for the first responder may include the continued presence of the cause of the person's respiratory failure, such as live electricity.

Responder personal protection measures Essential responder personal protection items include latex or latex-style gloves and a resuscitation shield.

First response actions Position the person to lie flat on his or her back and tilt the head back. Sometimes this action is sufficient to clear the airway and the person begins to breathe. Check for a PULSE (press two fingers against the side of the neck just beneath the notch at the back of the lower jaw) and watch and feel for signs of air movement. **When there is also no heart beat, CARDIOPULMONARY RESUSCITATION (CPR) is necessary.** CPR adds chest compressions to pump the heart to push BLOOD through the body. If there is a pulse but no evidence of air movement, begin rescue breathing:

1. Quickly look (and feel, if wearing latex gloves) inside the person's MOUTH for any objects that could block air from entering the airway (such as dentures, food, vomitus, or blood).

2. Place a resuscitation shield over the person's mouth, pinch the nostrils closed, and breathe with normal intensity into the shield (or the person's mouth) until the chest rises.

3. Give one breath about every five seconds. Pull away from the shield to allow air to leave the LUNGS.

4. Continue rescue breathing until the person resumes breathing independently or emergency medical personnel arrive and take over.

Follow-through A person who stops breathing requires urgent evaluation and treatment from a physician at a hospital emergency department or trauma center.

See also ANAPHYLAXIS; COLD WATER DROWNING; POISON PREVENTION; RESPONDER SAFETY AND PERSONAL PROTECTION; SITE AND SITUATION ASSESSMENT; SYMPTOM ASSESSMENT AND CARE TRIAGE; WARM WATER DROWNING.

warm water drowning Drowning that occurs when the water temperature is higher than 60°F. Most warm water drownings take place in swimming pools and shallow lakes. The risk for death is very high when the person has been underwater longer than three minutes, thus rapid response is essential. However, there is great risk for the responder in an attempted rescue when the responder does not have training in water rescues.

Site and situation assessment Important aspects of the situation include the type of water (pool, lake, river), how long the person has been under water, and whether injuries in addition to drowning are possible. SPINAL CORD INJURY or head injury is likely when diving into the water, for example.

Responder personal protection measures Essential responder personal protection items include latex or latex-style gloves and a resuscitation shield.

First response actions When the person is still in the water and is conscious, the responder should use items such as ropes, poles, and flotation devices to attempt to help the person rather than jumping into the water, unless the responder has training in water rescues. RESCUE BREATHING or CARDIOPULMONARY RESUSCITATION (CPR) may be necessary when the person is brought to shore or the pool's edge.

Follow-through Emergency medical personnel may decide whether to continue resuscitative efforts after they arrive and evaluate the situation.

A physician should thoroughly assess a person who revives, as secondary complications may occur.

See also CARDIAC ARREST; COLD WATER DROWNING; RESPONDER SAFETY AND PERSONAL PROTECTION; SITE AND SITUATION ASSESSMENT; SYMPTOM ASSESSMENT AND CARE TRIAGE.

Cardiac Arrest

Cardiac arrest—any circumstance in which the HEART stops beating—is immediately life-threatening. The BRAIN can survive only four to six minutes without oxygen, after which brain cells begin to die. Their loss is permanent. After 10 minutes without oxygen brain death occurs. The American Heart Association (AHA) identifies four actions, called the cardiac chain of survival, as crucial:

1. Call 911 to summon emergency medical aid.
2. Start CARDIOPULMONARY RESUSCITATION (CPR) to restore circulation.
3. Defibrillate (shock) the heart to restore functional electrical activity.
4. Get the person to a hospital for advanced cardiac life support care.

The first person to come upon a person who is in cardiac arrest sets this chain in motion and may perform the first two or three actions, depending on whether there is an AUTOMATED EXTERNAL DEFIBRILLATOR (AED) at the scene. The speed with which the first responder acts establishes the likelihood of survival. For optimal outcome, CPR must begin within four minutes of when the heart stops. A person who reaches step 4 within 30 minutes has the highest chance for survival.

COMMON CAUSES OF CARDIAC ARREST	
ANAPHYLAXIS	ASPHYXIATION
diabetic SHOCK	drowning
ELECTROCUTION	HEART ATTACK
hemorrhage	MULTIPLE TRAUMA
poisoning	STROKE

cardiopulmonary resuscitation (CPR) Emergency efforts to restore the function of the HEART and circulation of BLOOD through the body. CPR combines RESCUE BREATHING with cardiac compressions. The first person to respond to a situation that requires CPR must first call 911 to summon emergency medical aid. Do not stop CPR once under way, unless the person begins to COUGH or breath independently or until trained medical personnel arrive to take over.

Essential responder personal protection items include latex or latex-style gloves and a resuscitation shield. To perform CPR:

1. Listen or feel for BREATHING and check for PULSE. If absent, continue with CPR.
2. Place the person on his or her back with the head tilted back.
3. Pinch closed the nostrils and open the MOUTH. Place the resuscitation shield and breathe into the shield (or the person's mouth) until the person's chest rises.
4. Place the palm of one hand on the back of the other hand and interlace the fingers.
5. Place the hands in the center of the person's chest. (For an infant under 12 months, use the flat of the fingers on the center of the chest between the nipples.)
6. Sharply push downward to compress the chest about 2 inches. Pump the person's chest in this way at the rate of 100 compressions per minute.
7. Give 2 normal breaths every 30 compressions.

When an AUTOMATED EXTERNAL DEFIBRILLATOR (AED) is available, a second responder may add DEFIBRILLATION to the resuscitation efforts, which is the next step. The AED unit determines whether defibrillation is appropriate.

See also COLD WATER DROWNING; RESCUE BREATH-ING; RESPONDER SAFETY AND PERSONAL PROTECTION; SITE AND SITUATION ASSESSMENT; SYMPTOM ASSESSMENT AND CARE TRIAGE; WARM WATER DROWNING.

defibrillation Delivery of a controlled electrical shock, using an AUTOMATED EXTERNAL DEFIBRILLATOR (AED), to restore a functional HEART BEAT of a person who has suffered CARDIAC ARREST and whose HEART is in a state of fibrillation (rapid, disorganized, and useless contractions). Numerous public locations and businesses have AEDs.

The AED provides voice instruction for defibrillation. The AED pads, when placed on the person's chest as directed, first detect and send to the AED's computer the heart's electrical signals. If the rhythm is one that could respond to defibrillation, the AED prepares to deliver a preset electrical shock. If the heart is not beating or has a rhythm for which defibrillation is inappropriate the AED advises the responder what to do, which may be to perform CARDIOPULMONARY RESUSCITATION (CPR).

As with any life-threatening situation, the responder should first call 911 to summon emergency medical personnel.

See also HEART ATTACK; RESPONDER SAFETY AND PERSONAL PROTECTION; SITE AND SITUATION ASSESSMENT; SUDDEN CARDIAC DEATH; SYMPTOM ASSESSMENT AND CARE TRIAGE.

electrocution Injury resulting from electrical shock. Typically a person who experienced electrocution is not BREATHING and may not have a HEART beat, which is a life-threatening circumstance. The person is also likely to have electrical BURNS.

Do *not* approach a person who has suffered electrocution until certain the source of electricity is no longer active. Do *not* try to move a person who remains in contact with a high-voltage power line.

Site and situation assessment The scene of an electrocution is extremely hazardous. The first person to respond must determine whether the source of electricity remains "live." Indications of this include downed power lines and plugged in power tools or appliances. Water, including wet surfaces, increases the risk to the responder as water conducts electricity. There may also be risk for explosion or fire.

Responder personal protection measures Latex gloves, which the responder should put on before approaching the injured person, are essential for personal protection from bloodborne pathogens. A resuscitation shield is necessary for personal protection when performing RESCUE BREATHING or full CARDIOPULMONARY RESUSCITATION (CPR).

First response actions When certain there is no live electricity at the scene, determine whether the person is breathing and has a heart beat. When necessary, begin rescue breathing or CPR. When these measures are not necessary, provide basic FIRST RESPONSE for burns and any other apparent injuries.

Follow-through The person requires urgent transportation to a trauma center or hospital emergency department. Burns are usually more severe than they appear and other injuries are likely.

See also PATHOGEN; RESPONDER SAFETY AND PERSONAL PROTECTION; SHOCK.

Heimlich maneuver A method to dislodge a foreign object from the upper airway that blocks the flow of air. The most common substances that become stuck and block BREATHING are incompletely chewed foods, especially meats, and small foods such as grapes, nuts, and hard candies. Young children may choke on nearly any food as well as small toys and other objects they pick up and put in their mouths.

To perform the Heimlich maneuver:

1. Confirm that the person is choking by asking him or her to speak. If the person cannot speak, the airway is blocked.

2. Stand behind the person, with the person standing.

3. Reach around the person and place one hand formed into a fist just above the person's belly button, thumb-side of the fist toward the person's body.

4. Grab the fist with the other hand and give a sharp pull inward and upward.

5. For an infant or small child, hold the infant in a sitting position. Use two or three fingers placed just above the belly button and jab sharply.

6. Repeat until the force of air pressure in the airway expels the object.

Rapid response is essential. Most people are fine once the object dislodges and they can breathe again. An object that does not come out with the Heimlich maneuver, or a person who loses CONSCIOUSNESS, requires further emergency care from trained medical personnel.

See also CARDIOPULMONARY RESUSCITATION (CPR); COUGH; RESCUE BREATHING; SWALLOWING DISORDERS.

Heat and Cold Injuries

Heat and cold injuries most often occur in response to environmental exposure to extremes in temperature. Environmental temperatures that are above or below the body's normal temperature require the body to implement actions to compensate. When the external temperature is higher than body temperature, these actions include peripheral vasodilation (BLOOD vessels in the extremities relax to increase the flow of blood), which moves greater quantities of blood closer to the body's surface where the temperature is somewhat cooler, and sweating, which cools the SKIN through evaporation.

When the external temperature is lower than body temperature, the body's compensatory mechanisms include peripheral vasoconstriction (blood vessels in the extremities narrow to decrease the flow of blood), which pulls more blood within the body core where temperature is somewhat warmer, and shivering, which increases energy output that in turn raises body temperature. When either set of mechanisms fails to achieve an acceptable body temperature, body chemistry and METABOLISM begin to change, altering vital body activities such as neurologic (BRAIN), cardiovascular (HEART rhythm and BLOOD PRESSURE), and renal (kidney) functions.

A person's body size and composition and activity level also influence the rate at which the body retains or loses heat. A person who has fairly high body fat loses body heat more slowly; he or she may have better tolerance for exposure to cold and less tolerance for exposure to heat. For a person who has low body fat, the reverse is the case: He or she often has better tolerance for exposure to heat and less for exposure to cold.

Moisture further influences the extent to which such exposure is tolerable or becomes a health concern. In cold water or when wearing wet clothing a person loses body heat at a rate up to 20 times that which occurs in cold air. Wind also influences the effects of cold; a calculation called the wind-chill factor represents the effect.

Moisture similarly affects the consequences of heat. High humidity in combination with high temperature intensifies the risk for heat injury; a calculation called the heat index represents the effect. HEAT EXHAUSTION and HEAT STROKE, the two types of heat-related injuries, most often occur in people who are engaged in intense physical activity in circumstances of combined high temperature and high humidity. DEHYDRATION can occur rapidly with heat injuries, further complicating health concerns.

Untreated, progressive heat or cold injury has high risk for permanent tissue and organ damage or death.

dehydration Insufficient water intake or excessive water loss resulting in electrolyte imbalance within the body. Though there are numerous possible causes for dehydration, the most common first aid scenario for dehydration occurs with athletic activities, sporting events, intense physical labor (especially in hot conditions), and extremely hot weather.

Early symptoms of dehydration include thirst, light-headedness, and dry SKIN. Drinking cool water, to 6 ounces every 15 minutes, is often adequate treatment for mild dehydration. Symptoms of moderate dehydration may include mild MUSCLE cramps, mental confusion, and disorientation. Though drinking water may improve moderate dehydration as a first aid response, intravenous fluids are often necessary to restore electrolyte balance. Severe dehydration may result in loss of CONSCIOUSNESS, rapid or irregular HEART RATE (tachycardia or ARRHYTHMIA), rapid BREATHING, severe muscle cramps, and SHOCK. Severe dehydration requires urgent treatment from a hospital emergency department or trauma center.

COMMON CAUSES OF DEHYDRATION

acute GASTROENTERITIS	DIABETES
excessive diuretic use	excessive laxative use
heavy sweating	inadequate drinking
persistent DIARRHEA	persistent VOMITING
strenuous exercise	sustained FEVER

See also HEAT EXHAUSTION; HEAT STROKE.

heat exhaustion Overheating of the body in conditions of extreme heat or heavy physical activity. Symptoms of heat exhaustion come on suddenly and may include blanched SKIN, heavy sweating, NAUSEA, and lightheadedness. Get the person into a cool environment, such as a shaded area or an air-conditioned location, as quickly as possible. Loosen clothing, offer cool water or cool sports drinks (nothing iced), and spray or moisten the skin with cool water. When these measures are effective, the person improves dramatically and does not need further medical care.

Though heat exhaustion is mild and nearly always improves with appropriate interventions such as these, untreated heat exhaustion may progress to HEAT STROKE, a potentially life-threatening disturbance of body temperature. Call 911 to summon emergency medical aid if the person's temperature is higher than 102°F or the person has seizures.

See also DEHYDRATION; FEVER; SPORTS DRINKS AND FOODS.

heat stroke A life-threatening emergency in which the body is unable to lower body temperature. Heat stroke most commonly develops when there is a combination of intense physical activity and high environmental temperature. Though most people who develop heat stroke first experience HEAT EXHAUSTION, symptoms of heat stroke may appear suddenly. Such symptoms include

- hot, flushed SKIN
- absence of sweating
- HEADACHE

- rapid HEART RATE (tachycardia)
- HALLUCINATION
- disorientation, agitation, or loss of CONSCIOUSNESS
- seizures

Body temperature is usually above 102°F. Urgent treatment is necessary to avert permanent BRAIN and other neurologic damage. Call 911 to summon emergency medical aid, then get the person into an air-conditioned location, if possible, and remove outer layers of clothing. Spray a mist of water or apply cool, wet washcloths to the skin. If possible, place ice packs or extremely cold objects under the armpits and at the groin; at these locations large volumes of BLOOD circulate near the skin's surface. Position the person lying on his or her back with feet and legs elevated about 12 inches (SHOCK position). Emergency medical personnel may have cooling blankets and will begin intravenous fluids, then transport the person to a hospital or trauma center for further care.

See also DEHYDRATION; FEVER.

hypothermia The sustained loss of body heat resulting in low body temperature. Hypothermia occurs with extended exposure to cold external temperatures. Cool, wet conditions may also result in hypothermia. The key symptom of mild hypothermia, in which body temperature is no lower than 95°F, is intense shivering. Attempt to warm the person getting him or her into a warm location, removing wet clothing and wrapping in warm blankets, and offering warm fluids to drink.

When body temperature drops below 95°F in moderate hypothermia, the body loses the ability to shiver and the rate of heat loss increases. HEART RATE slows, BLOOD PRESSURE drops, and METABOLISM slows. The person is often confused or agitated, may paradoxically feel warm, and feels increasingly sleepy. Emergency response includes warming efforts as well as calling 911 to summon emergency aid personnel. Moderate hypothermia often requires further medical care to stabilize body temperature.

The lower body temperature drops, the less likely recovery becomes. Body temperature below 90°F, severe hypothermia, is very precarious.

Organ systems, especially the cardiovascular and neurologic, become exceedingly fragile. The risk for life-threatening ARRHYTHMIA (irregular heart beat) and especially VENTRICULAR FIBRILLATION is already high because of the body's altered metabolic and biochemical state; jostling the person during movement can rapidly destabilize the HEART and cardiovascular function. Severe hypothermia significantly slows neurologic function, causing UNCONSCIOUSNESS. The pupils are often fixed (non-responsive to light). CARDIOPULMONARY RESUSCITATION (CPR) is necessary if the person is not BREATHING and has no PULSE. As with COLD WATER DROWNING, aggressive resuscitation efforts may revive someone who has had very low body temperature for an extended time.

See also FROSTBITE; HEAT EXHAUSTION; HEAT STROKE; RAYNAUD'S SYNDROME; SITE AND SITUATION ASSESSMENT.

Major Trauma

Major trauma is a circumstance of a single catastrophic injury, such as GUNSHOT WOUNDS or BURNS, or multiple injuries that affect multiple body systems in such a fashion that without urgent medical intervention death is likely. Major trauma most often results from events such as MOTOR VEHICLE ACCIDENTS, fires, serious falls, occupational accidents, and other situations in which the body encounters multiple hazards. Situations of major trauma are often more than an individual first responder can adequately assess. The top priority of FIRST RESPONSE is to get emergency personnel and equipment to the scene and prevent further injuries to the person or to others who are involved in the situation or arrive at the scene.

blunt trauma Injury that results from a strong blow or force. The injury may not be initially obvious because there may be no outward signs such as LACERATIONS or bruises. However, blunt trauma may cause internal bleeding or rupture of upper abdominal organs such as the SPLEEN or PANCREAS. Blunt trauma to the head may cause TRAUMATIC BRAIN INJURY (TBI).

Site and situation assessment MOTOR VEHICLE ACCIDENTS, industrial accidents, and collisions with stationary objects (such as a skier running into a tree) are among the situations that may result in multiple trauma.

Responder personal protection measures Latex gloves, which the responder should put on before approaching the injured person, are essential for personal protection from the possibility of acquiring INFECTION through contact with body fluids.

First response actions There are few FIRST RESPONSE measures for blunt trauma beyond keeping the injured person still and calm. SHOCK may be the only indication of internal bleeding from blunt trauma, which can be serious enough to

cause rapid death. Surgery is the only means to treat internal bleeding.

Follow-through A health-care provider should evaluate blunt trauma to determine the need for further treatment.

See also CLOSED FRACTURE; SYMPTOM ASSESSMENT AND CARE TRIAGE; SITE AND SITUATION ASSESSMENT; SYMPTOM ASSESSMENT AND CARE TRIAGE.

gunshot wounds Injuries that result from bullets. Gunshot wounds are often more serious than they appear, particularly when the bullet remains lodged in the body. A bullet enters the body with high velocity and follows a trajectory of least resistance. That trajectory may carry the bullet on a direct path through soft tissue or along the path of a BONE. Gunshot wounds may be accidental or intentional, self-inflicted or inflicted by another person.

Do *not* approach a person who has a gunshot wound or the site of a shooting if there is still gunfire or the whereabouts and status of the shooter are uncertain. Use extreme caution until the situation is clear.

Site and situation assessment The most essential determination is whether gunfire presents an ongoing risk for the injured person, other people, and responders.

Responder personal protection measures Latex gloves, which the responder should put on before approaching the injured person, are essential for personal protection from bloodborne pathogens as nearly always there is moderate to heavy bleeding from gunshot injuries.

First response actions After calling 911 to summon emergency aid and then determining that the situation is safe, try to locate the entrance and exit wounds. The entrance wound is often small and is easy to overlook, especially when the exit wound is large. BLEEDING CONTROL is critical; apply direct pressure to stop or slow bleeding. Do not move the injured person unless necessary for safety, as movement may cause further damage from a lodged bullet. SHOCK is likely; help the injured person to remain calm, warm, and as comfortable as possible.

Follow-through   Gunshot wounds require urgent treatment at a hospital emergency department or trauma center.

See also MULTIPLE TRAUMA; RESPONDER SAFETY AND PERSONAL PROTECTION; SITE AND SITUATION ASSESSMENT; SYMPTOM ASSESSMENT AND CARE TRIAGE.

head and spinal cord injuries   Trauma that may cause BRAIN or neurologic damage. Common causes of head and SPINAL CORD injuries include collisions and accidents involving motor vehicles, motorcycles, bicycles, skiing, skateboarding, and diving into water. Indications of such injuries may include UNCONSCIOUSNESS, bleeding from the ears or NOSE, bruises around the eyes or behind the ears, HEADACHE, NAUSEA, and PARALYSIS.

Site and situation assessment   Determine whether the injured person is at risk for further injury, such as from traffic or drowning. MOTOR VEHICLE ACCIDENTS may involve injuries to multiple people.

Responder personal protection measures   Latex gloves, which the responder should put on before approaching the injured person, are essential for personal protection from bloodborne pathogens as often there is moderate to heavy bleeding from traumatic injuries of the head and spinal cord.

First response actions   Do *not* move a person who may have a head or SPINAL CORD INJURY. Use appropriate BLEEDING CONTROL when there are bleeding injuries. Head wounds especially can bleed profusely. To the best extent possible, brace or splint the person to immobilize the head and back. Discourage the person from attempting to move, including the arms and legs. Do *not* remove a helmet (bicycle, ski, motorcycle, football, horseback riding, or other type) unless the helmet interferes with aid attempts or the injured person's ability to breathe.

Follow-through   Head injuries require urgent medical evaluation and treatment at a hospital emergency department or trauma center.

See also ACCIDENTAL INJURIES; CONCUSSION; TRAUMATIC BRAIN INJURY (TBI); SITE AND SITUATION ASSESSMENT; SYMPTOM ASSESSMENT AND CARE TRIAGE.

motor vehicle accidents   Collisions between motor vehicles or between motor vehicles and objects. Accidental injuries are the fifth leading cause of death in the United States; motor vehicle accidents account for nearly half of those deaths. Nearly three million people receive injuries in motor vehicle accidents that require medical care. Motor vehicle accidents often result in multiple serious injuries affecting two or more people.

Site and situation assessment   The situation the first person on the scene of an accident often encounters is chaotic and panicked. The responder must remain calm and clear headed to appropriately assess the circumstances and extent of injuries. Factors to consider include

- number of vehicles and people involved
- severity of injuries
- risks such as traffic, downed power lines, dangerous terrain (woods, cliffs, water), fire, leaking gasoline

Responder personal protection measures   Latex gloves, which the responder should put on before approaching the scene, are essential for personal protection from bloodborne pathogens as nearly always there is moderate to heavy bleeding from injuries.

First response actions   The responder often must act to concurrently provide a safer site and aid to those who have injuries. Sometimes the responder must help the injured out of the vehicles. The first actions of the responder include:

- Call 911 to summon rescue personnel.
- Turn off the ignitions of any vehicles that are still running.
- Kick dirt or gravel over any spilled gasoline to reduce risk for fire or explosion.
- Check for BREATHING; perform RESCUE BREATHING or CARDIOPULMONARY RESUSCITATION (CPR) when necessary.

- Stop bleeding.
- Speak calmingly and comfortingly to those involved in the accident.

Unless there is risk for fire or further injury, or it is necessary to remove the person from the vehicle to provide lifesaving first aid, it is usually best to wait for emergency personnel to safely evacuate or extricate people from their vehicles. Even injuries that appear mild may involve more serious damage that incorrectly moving the person could exacerbate.

Follow-through People who have moderate to severe injuries need further medical assessment and care. Medical aid personnel typically perform minimal treatment at the accident scene to stabilize the injured person's condition, with the goal of transporting the person to a hospital or trauma center within one hour of the accident. People who have mild injuries may desire to follow-up with their regular health-care providers.

See also BLEEDING CONTROL; BODY SUBSTANCE ISOLATION; CLOSED FRACTURE; MULTIPLE TRAUMA; OPEN FRACTURE; RESPONDER SAFETY AND PERSONAL PROTECTION; SITE AND SITUATION ASSESSMENT; SYMPTOM ASSESSMENT AND CARE TRIAGE.

multiple trauma Numerous significant injuries such as may occur in MOTOR VEHICLE ACCIDENTS, shooting incidents, falls from high places, and fires. Multiple trauma is often life threatening and beyond the ability of the first responder to take much action beyond comforting the injured person until emergency medical personnel arrive.

Site and situation assessment Multiple trauma situations require rapid assessment of the nature and extent of the injuries, especially when numerous people are injured. The first person to respond to the scene of multiple trauma should also determine what risks are present that threaten responders and emergency personnel, such as unstable terrain, traffic, and crime scenes. Other important details include the number of people involved and the nature and seriousness of injuries.

Responder personal protection measures Latex gloves, which the responder should put on before approaching the scene or the injured person, are essential for personal protection from bloodborne pathogens as nearly always there is heavy bleeding with multiple trauma.

First response actions Multiple trauma is a difficult circumstance for an individual first responder to handle. After calling 911 to summon emergency personnel, priorities include checking the injured person's BREATHING and HEART beat, looking for bleeding, and providing basic first aid for SHOCK. CARDIOPULMONARY RESUSCITATION (CPR) and BLEEDING CONTROL may be necessary.

Follow-through A person who has multiple trauma is often gravely wounded and requires urgent medical care at a hospital emergency department or trauma center.

See also ACCIDENTAL INJURIES; BLEEDING CONTROL; BODY SUBSTANCE ISOLATION; BLUNT TRAUMA; GUNSHOT WOUNDS; RESPONDER SAFETY AND PERSONAL PROTECTION; SITE AND SITUATION ASSESSMENT; SYMPTOM ASSESSMENT AND CARE TRIAGE.

trauma to the eye Penetrating or blunt force injuries to the EYE or the structures around the eye, flash BURNS, and chemical burns. Such injuries can cause partial or complete loss of vision as well as loss of the eye itself. Do only what is necessary to minimize movement and prevent further injury.

Do *not* remove an object that penetrates into the EYE, the eyelid, or the tissues around the eye.

For FIRST RESPONSE for eye trauma, cover the injured eye with a small paper cup or similar item to prevent contact with the eye or any object that might be penetrating the eye. Cover the uninjured eye with a bandage or cloth; covering both eyes prevents movement that could further damage the injured eye. Talk reassuringly and steadily to the person; being unable to see is disorienting and often frightening. Conversation helps the injured person maintain contact with his or her surroundings and know what is going on.

An ophthalmologist (physician who specializes in care of the eyes) should evaluate most eye injuries, even those that appear minor. Bacterial INFECTION in ABRASIONS and small LACERATIONS on the surface of the eye can threaten vision. Significant injuries to the eye require urgent ophthalmologic care.

See also ACCIDENTAL INJURIES; BLACK EYE; CONJUNCTIVITIS; ENUCLEATION; IMPALEMENT; SYMPTOM ASSESSMENT AND CARE TRIAGE; VISION IMPAIRMENT.

traumatic amputation The accidental or unintended severance of a body part. Fingers are the body parts most often lost to traumatic AMPUTATION. When the amputation is clean, such as may occur with a sharp object, surgeons may be able to reattach the amputated part. Avulsions (tearing of the structures) are often jagged and do considerable damage to the tissues, and the amputated part may not be intact enough to recover. Traumatic amputations typically bleed heavily and cause extreme PAIN. SHOCK is a significant risk.

Site and situation assessment It is important to salvage the amputated part and take it to the hospital with the injured person. A person who remains entangled in machinery remains at high risk for further injury unless properly extricated by emergency personnel trained in such situations. Power tools and appliances that remain plugged in create a hazard for further injury to the person or injury to the responder as well as the risk for ELECTROCUTION. The injured person may

have MULTIPLE TRAUMA, depending on the cause of the traumatic amputation.

Responder personal protection measures Latex or latex-type gloves, which the responder should put on before approaching the injured person, are essential for personal protection from bloodborne pathogens as nearly always traumatic amputation results in heavy bleeding.

First response actions A major traumatic amputation is a difficult circumstance for an individual responder to handle. Call 911 to summon emergency medical aid, then attempt to control the bleeding. As with other bleeding injuries, direct pressure to the injury is the most effective method. Continue adding bandages, cloths, or other materials to establish bulk with the pressure. BLOOD loss may rapidly be substantial Try to keep the person warm and calm.

Follow-through Traumatic amputation typically requires emergency surgery to stop the bleeding, repair tissue damage, and reattach the amputated part when possible.

See also ACCIDENTAL INJURIES; AVULSION; BLEEDING CONTROL; BODY SUBSTANCE ISOLATION; MOTOR VEHICLE ACCIDENTS; RESPONDER SAFETY AND PERSONAL PROTECTION; SITE AND SITUATION ASSESSMENT; SYMPTOM ASSESSMENT AND CARE TRIAGE.

Poisoning

Many substances are toxic when used inappropriately or through accidental exposure. Personal protection and safety are crucial for the first responder, who must first determine that there is no risk for becoming another victim of the same exposure. This is especially of concern with poisonous BITES AND STINGS, CONTACT TOXINS, and INHALED TOXINS. Though the FIRST RESPONSE should always be to call 911 to summon emergency medical aid, contact with a poison control telephone hotline can provide specific advice for the first responder until emergency medical personnel arrive. In the United States, there is a nationwide toll-free telephone hotline available 24 hours a day, 7 days a week.

**US national poison control hotline:
1-800-222-1222
Available 24 hours a day, 7 days a week, from anywhere in the United States. The number is toll-free.**

---

bites and stings Poisoning or HYPERSENSITIVITY RESPONSE (allergic reaction) to insect and reptile venoms. Though numerous insects sting and spiders and snakes bite, most are not poisonous (harmful beyond local discomfort at the site of the sting or bite). Rapid FIRST RESPONSE efforts can often reduce the severity of the resulting injury from poisonous stings and bites.

Remove rings, watches, and other jewelry in the area of a bite or sting to prevent further injury if swelling occurs. Significant swelling is especially common with poisonous snake bites.

Hymenoptera stings The most common stings come from wasps, hornets, yellow jackets, honey bees, and fire ants, collectively known as the Hymenoptera order. For the two million Americans who are allergic to the venom of these insects, the sting is far more significant than irritation or discomfort. Severe hypersensitivity response can cause swelling of the THROAT that blocks the airway; anaphylactic SHOCK is a life-threatening circumstance.

First response for Hymenoptera stings:

1. Gently scrape the stinger out of the wound with the edge of an object such as a credit card. Do *not* grasp the stinger with tweezers or fingernails as this squeezes the venom sack and forces more venom into the wound.

2. Apply ice until the area is numb.

3. Make a paste of baking soda and water and liberally spread it over the area of the sting. (Alternately, apply a small amount of hydrocortisone cream or diphenhydramine cream.)

4. Seek further evaluation and treatment from a health-care provider when PAIN persists or worsens, or when the person stung has a hypersensitivity response (allergic reaction).

Poisonous spider bites and scorpion stings There are only two types of poisonous spiders in North America, the widows (of which the black widow is the most notorious species) and the brown recluse. There is one species of poisonous scorpion, *Centruroides sculpturatus,* found in the southwestern United States (particularly Arizona) and northern Mexico. The venom of a widow spider is a neurotoxin that produces pain and swelling at the site of the bite and systemic effects that may include generalized discomfort or pain, MUSCLE CRAMP, and muscle SPASM. It may also elevate BLOOD PRESSURE (HYPERTENSION). Many people do not notice the bite of the brown recluse spider for up to a week, when the toxin begins to cause tissue necrosis (death) at the site of the bite. The sting of the *C. sculpturatus* scorpion is also a neurotoxin; pain is immediate and later systemic response is common. Though unpleasant, these bites and stings are seldom fatal.

First response for poisonous scorpion stings and spider bites:

1. Apply ice to the bite.
2. Minimize movement of the bitten area; splint if possible.
3. Seek immediate medical care at a hospital emergency department. ANTIVENIN is available for widow spider and *C. sculpturatus* scorpion bites.

Poisonous snake bites There are four types of poisonous snakes in North America (see table), the bites of which are all capable of causing death. Antivenin is available for each type. Bites from poisonous snakes require urgent medical treatment at a hospital emergency department.

First response for snake bite:

1. Loosely splint or otherwise immobilize the area of the bite, and keep it lower than the HEART.
2. Keep the bitten person calm and still.
3. If it will be longer than 30 minutes before the bitten person can get to a hospital, wrap a bandage (or improvise with a scarf or other item of clothing) firmly but not tightly three to four inches above the bite, between the bite and the heart. The tightness of the wrap should be such that the responder's finger can fit under it. After placing such a bandage, do *not* remove it for any reason. Doing so will release a surge of venom into the person's BLOOD circulation.

Stings from stingrays, jellyfish, and sea urchins Numerous species common in the oceans in the coastal United States can deliver a significant sting. Stingrays and sea urchins sting with spines coated in venom. The spines may break off under the SKIN, continuing to release venom. They also present very high risk for bacterial INFECTION. Heat inactivates the venom and vinegar dissolves the spines. First response for stingray and sea urchin stings:

1. Soak the area of the sting in water as hot as the person stung can tolerate for at least 30 minutes.
2. After the hot water soak, place gauze pads soaked in vinegar over the sting area.
3. Repeat these measures until symptoms improve or the stung person reaches a hospital for further treatment.

Jellyfish and related creatures such as sea anemones and Portuguese man-o-war have clusters of long tentacles covered with stinging cells. First response for these stings:

1. Flush the area of the sting with seawater.
2. Place gauze pads soaked in vinegar over the sting area for at least 30 minutes.
3. Use gloved hands or tweezers to remove tentacles.
4. Repeat steps 2 and 3 until all tentacles are gone and pain subsides.
5. Seek treatment at a hospital emergency department.

See also ALLERGY; POISON PREVENTION.

contact toxins Substances, such as chemicals, that cause symptoms upon coming in contact with the SKIN. Many contact toxins cause mild symptoms such as contact DERMATITIS; some can cause chemical BURNS that require urgent or prompt medical care, depending on their severity. Rapid FIRST RESPONSE minimizes the severity of injury and prevents further absorption of the toxin through the skin and into the BLOOD circulation, if the toxin is one that absorbs in such of a way.

Site and situation assessment Determine the severity of symptoms and the toxin. When a chemical, take the container (with due caution to avoid contact with the ingredients) or label.

Responder personal protection measures Latex or latex-style gloves are essential to prevent responder contact with the toxin.

First response actions Call 911 to summon emergency medical personnel when situation appears significant or call the poison control hotline (in the United States: 1-800-222-1222) for guidance. Further first response actions:

POISONOUS SNAKES IN THE UNITED STATES

Type of Snake	Geographic Range	Characteristics of Bite
copperhead	much of United States from Texas to Rhode Island and the southern coast to the Ohio River valley	PAIN, swelling, and discoloration at the site of the bite that expand progressively systemic effects can cause significant illness bites of some species more toxic with risk of death treatment may require ANTIVENIN
coral snake	2 species in the US southeast, 1 species in the US southwest	venom is a powerful neurotoxin rapid systemic symptoms that may include NAUSEA, sleepiness, excessive drooling, difficulty BREATHING, and sometimes PARALYSIS high risk for death without prompt treatment antivenin need is urgent
cottonmouth, also called water moccasin	southern United States from eastern Texas to the northeast Maryland shore and inland to southern Missouri and western Tennessee	pain, swelling, and discoloration at the site of the bite that expand progressively systemic effects can cause significant illness bites of some species more toxic with risk of death treatment may require antivenin
rattlesnake	20 species diversely throughout United States and Mexico	pain, swelling, and discoloration at the site of the bite that expand progressively systemic effects can cause significant illness bites of some species more toxic with risk of death treatment may require antivenin

1. Remove any clothing contaminated by the toxin.
2. If the toxin is a dry powder, use gauze or a piece of fabric or a small brush to brush the powder off the skin.
3. After the powder is completely gone and for all other contact toxins, flush the area of contact (including the eyes if the toxin is in the eyes) with large amounts of water for at least 20 minutes. Hold or position the injured area such that the runoff water does not spread the toxin to other body parts or to the responder.

Follow-through Most poisonings resulting from contact poisons require further medical care to provide relief from symptoms such as itching, swelling, or PAIN. Chemical burns that form blisters (second-degree BURNS) or cover 10 percent or more of body surface require evaluation and treatment at a hospital emergency department or urgent care facility.

COMMON CONTACT TOXINS

ammonia	bleach
drain cleaners	gardening and yard products
household cleaning products	industrial solvents
lye	pesticides
poison ivy, oak, and sumac	stinging nettles

See also ACCIDENTAL INJURIES; POISON PREVENTION; RESPONDER SAFETY AND PERSONAL PROTECTION; SITE AND SITUATION ASSESSMENT; SYMPTOM ASSESSMENT AND CARE TRIAGE; WORK AND OCCUPATIONAL SAFETY.

ingested toxins Substances, that when swallowed, can cause systemic poisoning. Ingestion may be intentional or accidental. Accidental ingestion of medications is the most common form of poisoning in children. Children may also eat or drink other substances not intended for consumption such as cleaning products, nail polish remover, and plants. Injury may range from gastrointestinal upset to life-threatening cardiovascular, kidney, LIVER, or neurologic damage. Appropriate FIRST RESPONSE is often crucial.

Site and situation assessment Determine, to the best extent possible, what and how much of it the person has swallowed, as well as when. Take the container or label when it is present.

Responder personal protection measures Latex or latex-style gloves are essential to prevent responder contact with the toxin as well as body fluids from the injured person. A resuscitation shield is necessary for RESCUE BREATHING or CARDIOPULMONARY RESUSCITATION (CPR).

First response actions Call 911 to summon emergency medical personnel when the situation appears significant or call the poison control hotline (in the United States: 1-800-222-1222) for guidance. Further first response actions:

1. If the person is conscious, give small, frequent drinks of water.

2. Do *not* give anything else and do *not* induce vomiting unless emergency medical or poison control personnel so instruct.

3. If the person is unconscious, position the person to lie on a side with the head somewhat down in case of VOMITING. If vomiting occurs, clear vomitus from the MOUTH to maintain an open airway.

4. If the person is not BREATHING, begin rescue breathing.

5. If the person is not breathing and does not have a PULSE, begin CPR.

Follow-through People who have ingested toxic substances or overdoses of medications require urgent treatment at a hospital emergency department or trauma center.

See also BODY SUBSTANCE ISOLATION; OVERDOSE; POISON PREVENTION; RESPONDER SAFETY AND PERSONAL PROTECTION; SITE AND SITUATION ASSESSMENT; SUICIDE IDEATION AND SUICIDE; SYMPTOM ASSESSMENT AND CARE TRIAGE.

inhaled toxins Substances that, when breathed, can injure the airways and LUNGS as well as cause systemic poisoning. Inhaled toxins require urgent medical care.

Site and situation assessment Attempt to determine the toxin and whether it remains present in the environment. There may be multiple

COMMON INHALED TOXINS		
Toxin	**Common Sources**	**Characteristics**
carbon monoxide	poorly ventilated furnaces or stoves automobiles or gas power tools running in enclosed area such as garages	odorless symptoms include intense sleepiness progressing to loss of consciousness, bright redness to face
propane gas; natural gas	heating and cooking appliances	sulfuric odor ("rotten egg" smell) added to help detect leaks symptoms include disorientation and confusion progressing to loss of consciousness
ammonia gas	fertilizer products for commercial agricultural use industrial exposures	strong, pungent odor small exposure is highly toxic symptoms include severe respiratory irritation, intense coughing, and chemical BURNS to the nasal passages and airways
chlorine gas	pool cleaning products industrial exposures	strong, bleachlike odor symptoms include intense irritation to eyes, nose, and respiratory tract

people injured with environmental toxins such as chemical leaks.

Do *not* approach or enter an area where the possibility of environmental presence of the toxin exists.

Responder personal protection measures Latex or latex-style gloves are essential to prevent responder contact with the toxin as well as body fluids from the injured person. A resuscitation shield or mask is necessary for RESCUE BREATHING or CARDIOPULMONARY RESUSCITATION (CPR).

First response actions Call 911 to summon emergency medical personnel or call the poison control hotline (in the United States: 1-800-222-1222) for guidance. Many situations of inhaled toxins require self-contained BREATHING apparatus, protective clothing, and specialized training to safely rescue injured people. In such situations the first responder can only summon help. Do *not* perform rescue breathing or CPR without a resuscitation shield or mask, as doing so exposes the responder to the toxin.

Follow-through People exposed to inhaled toxins require urgent medical evaluation and treatment at a hospital emergency department or trauma center.

See also INHALATION BURNS; ORGANIC SOLVENTS; RESPONDER SAFETY AND PERSONAL PROTECTION; SITE AND SITUATION ASSESSMENT; SYMPTOM ASSESSMENT AND CARE TRIAGE.

injected toxins Poisons that enter a person's body through injection with a needle subcutaneously (beneath the SKIN), intramuscularly (into a MUSCLE), or intravenously (into a VEIN). Most circumstances of injected toxins are inadvertent DRUG OVERDOSE resulting from ILLICIT DRUG USE. Illicit drugs may also contain poisons used as fillers or to dilute the drug.

Site and situation assessment Attempt to determine the drug or substance injected. Collect any vials, syringes, and other apparatus that may help identify the substance (handle these items only if wearing latex or latex-style gloves).

Responder personal protection measures Latex or latex-style gloves are essential to prevent responder contact with the toxin as well as body fluids from the injured person. A resuscitation shield or mask is necessary for RESCUE BREATHING or CARDIOPULMONARY RESUSCITATION (CPR). The risk for exposure to HEPATITIS, HIV/AIDS, and TUBERCULOSIS is very high when illicit drug abuse is the cause of the injected toxin poisoning.

First response actions Call 911 to summon emergency medical personnel and call the poison control hotline (in the United States: 1-800-222-1222) for guidance. Further first response actions:

1. If the person is conscious, try to keep him or her awake and moving.

2. If the person is unconscious, position the person to lie on a side with the head somewhat down in case of VOMITING. If vomiting occurs, clear vomitus from the MOUTH to maintain an open airway.

3. If the person is not BREATHING, begin rescue breathing using a resuscitation shield or mask.

4. If the person is not breathing and does not have a PULSE, begin CPR using a resuscitation shield or mask.

Follow-through Overdose or poisoning due to injected toxins requires urgent medical assessment and treatment at a hospital emergency department.

See also INJECTING DRUGS, RISKS OF; POISON PREVENTION; RESPONDER SAFETY AND PERSONAL PROTECTION; SITE AND SITUATION ASSESSMENT; SYMPTOM ASSESSMENT AND CARE TRIAGE.

Radiation and Biochemical Injuries

Acts of terrorism using radiation, biologic pathogens, and chemical toxins became a heightened worldwide concern in the latter decades of the 20th century. Such acts have the potential to affect large numbers of people. Because the toxicity of these methods is very high, even FIRST RESPONSE requires a sophisticated public health approach. Injuries resulting from radiation, biologic, or chemical exposure may also occur through industrial accidents. RESPONDER SAFETY AND PERSONAL PROTECTION are crucial.

Radiation injuries Radiation injuries occur when there is exposure to radiation that exceeds the recommended safe limits. The exposure may be chronic (small exposure over time) or acute (sudden, massive exposure). Exposure to massive radiation doses results in acute radiation syndrome, which is often fatal. Radioactive substances that pose the greatest risk for radiation injuries include radionuclides, diethylenetriaminepentaacetate (DTPA), Neupogen, potassium iodide, and Prussian blue.

Biologic injuries Biologic injuries that occur when there is exposure to pathogens (BACTERIA and viruses) for which immunity is low are often serious or life-threatening illnesses. Among the pathogens of concern for intentional harm through biologic injury are those that cause ANTHRAX, BOTULISM, plague, and SMALLPOX.

Chemical injuries Chemical injuries that occur through intentional exposure to highly toxic chemicals, typically through inhalation or contact, often cause serious or fatal neurologic and pulmonary injury. Among the chemicals of concern are ammonia, arsenic, benzine, chlorine, cyanide, mercury, mustard gas, nitrogen mustard, osmium tetroxide, phosphine, ricin, sarin, tabun, thallium, and VX.

See also BODY SUBSTANCE ISOLATION; CHEMOTHERAPY; CONTACT TOXINS; ENVIRONMENTAL HAZARD EXPOSURE; HEAVY-METAL POISONING; INFECTION; INHALED TOXINS; PATHOGEN; POISON PREVENTION; RADIATION THERAPY; SITE AND SITUATION ASSESSMENT; SYMPTOM ASSESSMENT AND CARE TRIAGE.

APPENDIXES

APPENDIX I
VITAL SIGNS

Vital signs are the observable, objective measures of a person's basic health status. The four standard vital signs are PULSE (HEART RATE), BLOOD PRESSURE, RESPIRATION RATE (BREATHING rate), and body temperature. Within a range of normal measurements, these signs vary among individuals and according to age, gender, aerobic condition, and level of physical activity. Health conditions further affect vital signs. A person may have vital signs that are outside the parameters of "normal" in a general context though are consistent for him or her.

VITAL SIGNS				
	Heart Rate (Pulse)	**Blood Pressure**	**Breathing Rate**	**Body Temperature**
adult	60 to 89 beats per minute at rest	systolic < 120 millimeters of mercury (mm Hg) diastolic < 80 mm Hg	12 to 18 breaths per minute	97.8° to 99.1°F
child, 1 to 8 years	80 to 100 beats per minute at rest	systolic <110 mm Hg	15 to 30 breaths per minute	97.8° to 99.1°F
infant, 1 to 12 months	100 to 120 beats per minute at rest	systolic 70 to 100 mm Hg	25 to 50 breaths per minute	97.8° to 99.1°F
infant, birth to 30 days	120 to 160 beats per minute at rest	systolic > 60 mm Hg	40 to 60 breaths per minute	97.8° to 99.1°F

APPENDIX II
ADVANCE DIRECTIVES

Advance directives are instructions a person prepares that state his or her desires and preferences for end-of-life care. Typically advance directives consist of two legal documents

- a living will, which specifies the person's intentions in regard to medical treatment and resuscitative efforts
- a durable power of attorney for health care, also called durable medical power of attorney, which authorizes another individual (called a health-care agent or proxy) to make medical decisions on behalf of a person in the circumstance of a medical crisis when the person is unable to make such decisions

Advance directives are valid in all states in the United States, though each state has unique laws, regulations, and procedures for implementing advance directives. Documents should be updated, renewed, and resigned every few years to ensure currency. Information for obtaining and completing advance directive forms for each state is available through

**National Hospice and Palliative
Care Organization (NHPCO)**
1700 Diagonal Road, Suite 625
Alexandria, VA 22314
703-837-1500
www.nhpco.org

APPENDIX III
GLOSSARY OF MEDICAL TERMS

afferent Moving inward or toward the body's center.

anastomosis A natural or surgically created connection between two structures.

arterial blood gases Measurement of the levels of oxygen (partial pressure of oxygen, Po_2) and carbon dioxide (partial pressure of carbon dioxide, Pco_2) in a sample of blood drawn from an artery. Tests may also measure the level of carbon monoxide and the blood's acidity (pH).

benign Harmless.

biopsy Removal of a tissue or fluid sample from the body to conduct pathologic examination for diagnostic purposes.

cabbage Pronunciation of the acronym "CABG," which stands for coronary artery bypass graft.

carcinogenic Capable of causing cancer.

complete blood count (CBC) Measure of the numbers and types (differentiation) of blood cells present in a sample drawn from a vein.

computed tomography (CT) scan A diagnostic imaging procedure that uses a computer to generate three-dimensional images from multiple, segmental X-rays. A CT scan may include ingestion or injection of a contrast medium to increase the density of structures, making them more visible via X-ray.

cyst An enclosed, saclike structure that may contain liquid or solid material.

dark adaptation test A test that assesses the ability to see in a dimly lighted environment.

deformity An abnormality of structure. Deformities, also called defects, may be congenital (present at birth) or acquired (result from injury or disease).

diagnosis The identification of a health condition, disorder, or disease.

diagnostic imaging Procedures that allow visualization of internal organs, structures, or processes to diagnose health conditions or monitor the progress of treatment. Common diagnostic imaging procedures include X-ray, ultrasound, computed tomography (CT) scan, and magnetic resonance imaging (MRI).

disease A health condition for which there are signs (objective and observable evidence) though the person may experience no symptoms (subjective perceptions).

donor A person who gives a structure or substance (blood, tissue, organ) to another person, the recipient.

dorsal The back, or spinal, surface.

efferent Moving outward or away from the body's center.

electrocautery The use of electrical current to generate heat capable of fusing bleeding blood vessels or eliminating tissue.

electromyography (EMG) A diagnostic procedure that uses electrodes attached to tiny needles inserted into selected muscles or placed on the surface of the skin, to measure the electrical activity in muscles to assess their function.

electronystagmography A diagnostic procedure that measures the electrical activity of the muscles that move the eyes.

fatigue Extended, persistent loss of physical, mental, and emotional energies and abilities.

fissure A natural division or channel in an organ or an abnormal split in a tissue.

fistula An abnormal opening between two structures.

fluoroscopy An imaging procedure that uses a steady stream of X-rays viewed on a monitor (television screen) to provide real-time, moving images during diagnostic or therapeutic procedures such as cardiac catheterization.

fundus The base or body of a hollow organ.

graft Tissue, including whole organs, that a surgeon places within a person's body to treat a disease, defect, or deformity.

hematocrit A blood test to determine the percentage of red blood cells (erythrocytes) in a blood sample drawn from a vein.

hemorrhage Rapid and significant loss of blood.

home health care Medical providers such as nurses and physical therapists who provide treatment and care at the person's home.

hospice Care and support for a person who is terminally ill. Hospice providers may care for the person at home or in a hospice center.

humor Fluid within the body (from Latin, meaning "wet").

illness The perception of being unwell; the experience of symptoms.

in situ In the natural position or surroundings (in the body as opposed to in a test tube, for example).

in utero Contained within the uterus during pregnancy.

inferior Below or beneath.

integumentary A covering or cloak; refers to the skin.

ischemia Deprived of oxygen, usually as a consequence of restricted blood flow.

lap choly Medical shorthand for "laparoscopic cholecystectomy" (surgical removal of the gallbladder).

latent Delayed.

lateral Side.

lavage To rinse, wash, or flush with fluid.

lesion An abnormal growth of cells that are similar to, though altered from, the tissue from which they arise. Some injuries are also called lesions.

lifestyle Habits and practices in which a person chooses to engage that influence health and disease.

lobe A distinctive, defined section of an organ or gland.

localized Confined to a distinct area.

magnetic resonance imaging (MRI) A diagnostic imaging procedure that uses very powerful magnets to provide images of internal structures and organs. The MRI machine first emits a pulse of radiofrequency energy that causes the hydrogen atoms in the body to align in a uniform pattern. When the hydrogen atoms return to their normal alignment they send out electromagnetic signals that the MRI machine's magnets detect. A computer translates the signals into visual images.

malignant Capable of causing harm.

medically necessary A product, device, substance, or treatment that a person needs to recover from, accommodate to, or prevent injury or disease.

membrane A thin layer of tissue that covers or lines a structure or organ.

mucus A somewhat thick (viscous) fluid that glands or membranes produce.

occlusion Blockage.

organ A distinctive structure of tissues that performs a complex function within the body.

positron emission tomography (PET) scan A diagnostic imaging procedure that uses radionuclides, also called radioisotopes, to "see" cellular metabolism. The radionuclides (radioactive particles that rapidly disintegrate) enter cells attached to glucose molecules, which the cells use for energy. The rate at which the cells use the glucose, measured by tracking the rate of radionuclide disintegration, indicates whether the cells' function is normal; abnormal function may indicate disease such as cancer.

post After (in the context of time, as in postoperative).

primary Occurring without underlying cause.

prognosis The anticipated course of a health condition, disorder, or disease.

prone The position of lying with the chest and belly on the surface, with arms at the sides and legs outstretched.

recipient A person who receives a structure or substance (blood, tissue, organ) from another person, the donor.

resection The surgical removal of part of an organ or structure.

risk factor A circumstance that contributes to the likelihood for developing a disease.

Schirmer's test A procedure to assess the amount of tears the tear glands produce. The test involves placing tiny pieces of special paper at the edges of the eyelids, with the eyes closed, for five minutes and then measuring the amount of fluid the paper absorbs.

scope of practice The legal, professional, and conventional responsibilities and duties of a health-care provider.

secondary Occurring as a consequence of another health condition, injury, disorder, disease, or treatment.

sensory perception Information the brain receives through the five senses: vision, hearing, smell, taste, and touch.

sign An objective observation of a body function or dysfunction.

single photon emission computed tomography (SPECT) scan A diagnostic imaging procedure that uses radionuclides to generate three-dimensional images of internal organs, structures, and functions. A special camera detects the presence of the radionuclides (rapidly disintegrating radioactive particles) in cells and tissues. Normal cells and tissues take up the radionuclides at known rates; unusual cell activity results in variations from these rates that may indicate health conditions such as infection or cancer.

speculum An instrument to hold apart the walls of an opening or hollow organ within the body to allow its examination.

spirometry A measure of the amount of air a person is capable of breathing in and breathing out, performed to assess basic pulmonary (lung) function.

standard of care The customary practices in diagnosis, treatment, and follow-up care as determined by professional health organizations.

superior Above.

supine The position of lying on the back with arms at the sides and legs outstretched.

suture A thread or wire used to hold closed the edges of a wound. Also called a stitch.

symptom A subjective perception of a body function or dysfunction.

syndrome A collection of symptoms, signs, and diagnostic findings that occurs in a particular pattern.

system Organs and structures of the body that work together to perform related, coordinated functions and activities.

teratogenic Capable of causing birth defects in a developing fetus.

tissue An organized group of cells that work collectively to perform a specific function.

transposition Body structures that are present but switched or exchanged in location or position; also called transposed.

tumor An abnormal growth of cells that are unique from the tissue from which they arise; also called a neoplasm.

ultrasound A diagnostic imaging procedure that uses focused sound waves to generate images of internal organs, structures, or functions. The sound waves reflect, or echo, from objects they encounter. A computer translates the echoes into electrical signals, which are displayed on a monitor screen as visual images.

vag hyst Medical short hand for "vaginal hysterectomy" (surgical removal of the uterus).

ventral The front, or belly, surface.

watchful waiting A planned treatment approach of observation and regular physician visits to monitor the status of a health condition.

APPENDIX IV
ABBREVIATIONS AND SYMBOLS

AA	Alcoholics Anonymous
ac	before eating (*ante cibum;* Latin)
ACTH	adrenocorticotropic hormone
ADH	antidiuretic hormone
ADHD	attention-deficit hyperactivity disorder
AED	automated external defibrillator
AFP	alpha-fetoprotein
AHA	alphahydroxy acid; American Heart Association
AIDS	acquired immunodeficiency syndrome
ALS	amyotrophic lateral sclerosis
AMC	arthrogryposis multiplex congenita
ANCA	antineutrophil cytoplasmic antibody
APLS	antiphospholipid syndrome
ARDS	adult respiratory distress syndrome
ARMD	age-related macular degeneration
ART	assisted reproductive technology
ASA	aspirin (acetylsalicylic acid)
ATC	certified athletic trainer
AuD	doctor of audiology
AV	atrioventricular
AVM	arteriovenous malformation
BALT	bronchus-associated lymphoid tissue
BCP	birth control pill
BID/bid	twice a day (*bis in die;* Latin)
BiPAP	bilevel positive airway pressure
BM	bowel movement
BMI	body mass index
BP	blood pressure
BPH	benign prostatic hyperplasia; benign prostatic hypertrophy
BPPV	benign paroxysmal positional vertigo
BSE	breast self-examination
BUN	blood urea nitrogen
$\bar{c}$	with (*cum;* Latin)
Ca	cancer
CABG	coronary artery bypass graft

CAD	coronary artery disease
CBC	complete blood count
cc	cubic centimeter
CDA	certified dental assistant
CDC	US Centers for Disease Control and Prevention
CEA	carcinoembryonic antigen
CICU	cardiac intensive care unit
CIN	cervical intraepithelial neoplasia
CIS	carcinoma in situ (cancer in the cell)
CJD	Creutzfeldt-Jakob disease
CLS/MT	clinical laboratory scientist/medical technologist
CMA	certified medical assistant
CMV	cytomegalovirus
CNM	certified nurse midwife
CNS	central nervous system
COPD	chronic obstructive pulmonary disease
CP	cerebral palsy
CPAP	continuous positive airway pressure
CPhT	certified pharmacy technician
CPR	cardiopulmonary resuscitation
CRC	certified rehabilitation counselor
CRH	corticotropin-releasing hormone
CRNA	certified registered nurse anesthetist
CRNP	certified registered nurse practitioner
CRT	certified respiratory therapist
CSA	certified surgical assistant
CSF	cerebrospinal fluid; colony-stimulating factor
CST	certified surgical technologist
CST/CFA	certified surgical technologist/certified first assistant
CT	computed tomography
CTCL	cutaneous T-cell lymphoma
CTRS	certified therapeutic recreational specialist
CVD	cardiovascular disease

CVID	common variable immunodeficiency		GH	growth hormone
CVS	chorionic villi sampling		GHB	gamma hydroxybutyrate
D&C	dilation and curettage (also dilatation and curettage)		GHRH	growth hormone–releasing hormone
			GIFT	gamete intrafallopian transfer
DASH	dietary approaches to stop hypertension		GnRH	gonadotropin-releasing hormone
			GPI	gastric inhibitive polypeptide
DC	doctor of chiropractic		HAART	highly active antiretroviral therapy
DDS	doctor of dental surgery		Hg	mercury
DEA	US Drug Enforcement Agency		HGE	human granulocytic ehrlichiosis
DES	diethylstilbestrol		HHV	human herpesvirus
DHEA	dehydroepiandrosterone		HIV	human immunodeficiency virus
DIC	disseminated intravascular coagulation		HLA	human leukocyte antigen
			HME	human monocytic ehrlichiosis
dL (dl)	deciliter		HNPCC	hereditary nonpolyposis colorectal cancer
DLE	discoid lupus erythematosus			
DMARD	disease-modifying antirheumatic drug		HPV	human papillomavirus
DMD	doctor of dental medicine		HRT	hormone replacement therapy
DNA	deoxyribonucleic acid		IABP	intra-aortic balloon pump
DO	doctor of osteopathy		IBD	inflammatory bowel disease
DRE	digital rectal examination		IBS	irritable bowel syndrome
DrPH	doctor of public health		ICD	implantable cardioverter defibrillator
DTH	delayed-type hypersensitivity		ICSI	intracytoplasmic sperm injection
DUB	dysfunctional uterine bleeding		IgA	immunoglobulin A
DVT	deep vein thrombosis		IgD	immunoglobulin D
EBCT	electron beam computed tomography		IgE	immunoglobulin E
ECC	emergency cardiovascular care		IgG	immunoglobulin G
ECG	electrocardiogram		IgM	immunoglobulin M
ECT	electroconvulsive therapy		IM	intramuscular
EECP	enhanced external counterpulsation		IND	investigational new drug
EEG	electroencephalogram		ITP	immune thrombocytopenic purpura
EENT	eyes, ears, nose, throat		IUI	intrauterine artificial insemination
EKG	electrocardiogram		IV	intravenous
EMG	electromyogram		IVF	in vitro fertilization
EMT	emergency medical technician		IVP	intravenous pyelogram
EPO	erythropoietin		L (l)	liter
EPS	electrophysiology study		LAAM	levo-alpha acetylmethadol
ERCP	endoscopic retrograde cholangiopancreatography		LAc	licensed acupuncturist
			LAVH	laparoscopically assisted vaginal hysterectomy
ESRD	end-stage renal disease			
ESRF	end-stage renal failure		LH	luteinizing hormone
ESWL	extracorporeal shock wave lithotripsy		LP	lumbar puncture
FAP	familial adenomatous polyposis		LPN	licensed practical nurse
FDA	US Food and Drug Administration		LPT	licensed physical therapist
FOBT	fecal occult blood test		LQTS	long QT syndrome
FSH	follicle-stimulating hormone		LSD	lysergic acid diethylamide
GABA	gamma-aminobutyric acid		LSW	licensed social worker
GAD	generalized anxiety disorder		LVEF	left ventricular ejection fraction
GALT	gut-associated lymphoid tissue		LVN	licensed vocational nurse
GERD	gastroesophageal reflux disorder		m	meter

MAb (Mab)	monoclonal antibody
MAF	macrophage-activating factor
MALT	mucosa-associated lymphoid tissue
MD	doctor of medicine
MDMA	methylenedioxymethamphetamine
MEN	multiple endocrine neoplasia
MET	metabolic equivalent
MHC	major histocompatibility complex
MI	myocardial infarction
mL (ml)	milliliter
mm	millimeter
mm Hg	millimeters of mercury
MMR	measles/mumps/rubella (vaccine)
MRA	magnetic resonance angiography
MRI	magnetic resonance imaging
MS	multiple sclerosis
mtDNA	mitochondrial deoxyribonucleic acid
mtRNA	mitochondrial ribonucleic acid
NCCAM	National Center for Complementary and Alternative Medicine
ND	doctor of naturopathy
NDV	Newcastle disease virus
NIH	US National Institutes of Health
NK	natural killer
NPO	nothing by mouth (*non per os;* Latin)
NSAID	nonsteroidal anti-inflammatory drug
NTI	narrow therapeutic index
OC	oral contraceptives
OCD	obsessive–compulsive disorder
OCT	optical coherence tomography
OD	doctor of optometry
OMT	osteopathic manipulative treatment
OR	operating room
OTC	over the counter
OTR	registered occupational therapist
PA-C	certified physician assistant
PAT	paroxysmal atrial tachycardia
Pb	lead
pc	after eating (*post cibum;* Latin)
PCA	patient-controlled analgesia
PCID	partial combined immunodeficiency
PCOS	polycystic ovary syndrome
PCP	phencyclidine
PCTA	percutaneous transluminal coronary angioplasty
PDD	pervasive developmental disorder
PE	pulmonary embolism
PERP	positive end-respiratory pressure
PET	positron emission tomography
PharmD	doctor of pharmacy
PID	pelvic inflammatory disease
PKU	phenylketonuria
PMS	premenstrual syndrome
PNS	peripheral nervous system
PO	by mouth (*per os;* Latin)
POF	premature ovarian failure
PPI	proton pump inhibitor
PRN	as is needed (*pro re nata;* Latin)
PSA	prostate-specific antigen
PT-PTT	prothrombin time and partial thromboplastin time
PTA	physical therapy assistant
PTK	phototherapeutic keratectomy
PTSD	post-traumatic stress disorder
PUVA	psoralen and ultraviolet A
PVC	premature ventricular contraction
PVD	peripheral vascular disease
QD	once a day (*quaque die;* Latin)
QID	four times a day (*quartar in die;* Latin)
QN	once a night (*quaque noc;* Latin)
QOD	every other day (*quaque altera die;* Latin)
RA	rheumatoid arthritis
RBC	red blood count
RD	registered dietitian
RDH	registered dental hygienist
Rh	Rhesus (factor blood type)
RICE	rest, ice, compression, elevation
RN	registered nurse
RNA	ribonucleic acid
RPh	registered pharmacist
RRA	registered radiology assistant
RT	radiology technologist
$\bar{s}$	without (*sans;* Latin)
SA	sinoatrial; surface area; surgeon's assistant
SAD	seasonal affective disorder
SALT	skin-associated lymphoid tissue
SAMe	S-adenosylmethionine
SARS	severe acute respiratory syndrome
SC	subcutaneous
SCI	spinal cord injury
SCID	severe combined immunodeficiency
SIDS	sudden infant death syndrome
sig	as instructed (*signa;* Latin)
SLE	systemic lupus erythematosus
SNP	single nucleotide polymorphism
SOB	shortness of breath

SPECT	single photon emission computed tomography	TPMT	thiopurine methyltransferase
SPF	sun protection factor	TRH	thyrotropin-releasing hormone
SQ	subcutaneous	TSE	testicular self-examination
SSRI	selective serotonin reuptake inhibitor	TSH	thyroid-stimulating hormone
STAT	immediately (*statim;* Latin)	TTP	thrombotic thrombocytopenic purpura
STD	sexually transmitted disease	UA	urinalysis
T_3	triiodothyronine	URI	upper respiratory infection
T_4	thyroxine	URR	urea reduction ratio
TBI	traumatic brain injury	USP	United States Pharmacopeia
TCA	trichloroacetic acid	UTI	urinary tract infection
TCM	traditional Chinese medicine	UVA	ultraviolet A
TENS	transcutaneous electrical nerve stimulation	UVB	ultraviolet B
		VAD	ventricular assist device
TGF	transforming growth factor	VALT	vascular-associated lymphoid tissue
TIA	transient ischemic attack	VBAC	vaginal birth after cesarean
TID/tid	three times a day (*ter in die;* Latin)	vCJD	variant Creutzfeldt-Jakob disease
TMLR	transmyocardial laser revascularization	VIP	vasoactive intestinal peptide
		WBC	white blood count
TNF	tumor necrosis factor	ZIFT	zygote intrafallopian transfer

APPENDIX V
MEDICAL SPECIALTIES AND ALLIED HEALTH FIELDS

MEDICAL PRACTITIONERS AND SPECIALTIES

Practitioner	Specialty	Practitioner	Specialty
anesthesiologist	anesthesiology; anesthesia during surgery, pain management	neonatologist	neonatology; newborns
		nephrologist	nephrology; kidney conditions
bariatrician	bariatrics; obesity	neurologist	neurology; nervous system
cardiologist	cardiology; heart and blood vessels	obstetrician	obstetrics; pregnancy and childbirth
chiropractor	chiropractic; spine and back	oncologist	oncology; cancer
dermatologist	dermatology; integumentary system (skin, hair, nails)	ophthalmologist	ophthalmology; eyes
		optometrist	optometry; vision correction
endocrinologist	endocrinology; endocrine glands	orthopedist	orthopedics; musculoskeletal system
epidemiologist	epidemiology; trends in health and disease	otolaryngologist	otolaryngology; ear, nose and throat
		pathologist	pathology; tissue examination
family practitioner	family practice; medical and surgical care, children and adults	pediatrician	pediatrics; children (birth through adolescence)
gastroenterologist	gastroenterology; gastrointestinal system	physiatrist	physiatry; physical and rehabilitative medicine
geneticist	genetics; inherited and metabolic diseases	podiatrist	podiatry; feet
		psychiatrist	psychiatry; mental disorders
geriatrician	geriatrics; elderly	psychologist	mental health counseling
gynecologist	gynecology; women's reproductive system	pulmonologist	pulmonology; lungs
		radiologist	radiology; diagnostic and therapeutic radiologic and nuclear medicine procedures
hematologist	hematology; blood and circulation		
hospitalist	care for hospitalized patients		
immunologist	immunology; immune system conditions and allergies	rheumatologist	rheumatology; rheumatic diseases
		surgeon	surgery; surgical operations
internist	internal medicine; adult health care (except surgery)	urologist	urology; urologic system, male reproductive system

APPENDIX VI
RESOURCES

The resources cited in this section offer up-to-date treatment and research information. Most have access through written communication, telephone, and Web sites. As Internet access becomes more available, many organizations find the World Wide Web to be the most efficient means for providing current and varied information. Consequently, some organizations are shifting their point of contact entirely to their Web sites. Though the contact information for these resources is current at the time of *The Facts On File Encyclopedia of Health and Medicine's* publication, it is subject to change. For additional resource material, please see the section "Bibliography and Further Reading."

GENERAL

Administration for Children and Families (ACF)
US Department of Health and Human Services (HHS)
370 L'Enfant Promenade SW
Washington, DC 20447
www.acf.hhs.gov

Administration on Aging (AoA)
US Department of Health and Human Services (HHS)
Washington, DC 20201
202-619-0724
www.aoa.gov

Agency for Healthcare Research and Quality (AHRQ)
US Department of Health and Human Services (HHS)
Office of Communications and Knowledge Transfer
540 Gaither Road, Suite 2000
Rockville, MD 20850
www.ahcpr.gov

American Academy of Family Physicians (AAFP)
PO Box 11210
Shawnee Mission, KS 66207-1210
913-906-6000 / 800-274-2237
www.aafp.org

American Academy of Pediatrics (AAP)
141 Northwest Point Boulevard
Elk Grove Village, IL 60007-1098
847-434-4000
www.aap.org

American Board of Medical Specialties (ABMS)
1007 Church Street, Suite 404
Evanston, IL 60201-5913
847-491-9091
www.abms.org

American Medical Association
515 North State Street
Chicago, IL 60610
800-621-8335
www.ama-assn.org

Centers for Medicare & Medicaid Services (CMS)
US Department of Health and Human Services (HHS)
7500 Security Boulevard
Baltimore, MD 21244
800-MEDICARE (800-633-4227)
TTY: 877-486-2048
www.cms.hhs.gov

ClinicalTrials.gov
US National Institutes of Health (NIH)
www.clinicaltrials.gov

Health Resources and Services Administration (HRSA)
US Department of Health and Human Services (HHS)
Parklawn Building
5600 Fishers Lane
Rockville, MD 20857
www.hrsa.gov

Indian Health Service (IHS)
US Department of Health and Human Services
The Reyes Building
801 Thompson Avenue, Suite 400
Rockville, MD 20852
www.ihs.gov

National Center for Health Statistics (NCHS)
US Centers for Disease Control and Prevention (CDC)
3311 Toledo Road
Hyattsville, MD 20882
301-458-4000 / 866-441-NCHS (866-441-6247)
www.cdc.gov/nchs/

National Center on Minority Health and Health Disparities (NCMHD)
US National Institutes of Health (NIH)
6707 Democracy Boulevard, Suite 800, MSC 5465
Bethesda, MD 20892-5465
301-402-1366
TTY: 301-451-9532
www.ncmhd.nih.gov

National Institute on Aging (NIA)
US National Institutes of Health (NIH)
Building 31, Room 5C27
31 Center Drive, MSC 2292
Bethesda, MD 20892
301-496-1752
TTY: 800-222-4225
www.nia.nih.gov

National Library of Medicine (NLM)
US National Institutes of Health (NIH)
8600 Rockville Pike
Bethesda, MD 20894
301-594-5983 / 888-346-3656
www.nlm.nih.gov

National Organization for Rare Disorders (NORD)
55 Kenosia Avenue, PO Box 1968
Danbury, CT 06813-1968
203-744-0100
TDD: 203-797-9590
www.rarediseases.org

Office of the Surgeon General
US Department of Health and Human Services (HHS)
5600 Fishers Lane, Room 18066
Rockville, MD 20857
301-443-4000
www.surgeongeneral.gov

Office on Women's Health
US Department of Health and Human Services (HHS)
200 Independence Avenue SW, Room 712E
Washington, DC 20201
202-690-7650
www.womenshealth.gov

US Department of Health and Human Services
200 Independence Avenue SW
Washington, DC 20201
202-619-0257 / 877-696-6775
www.hhs.gov

US Food and Drug Administration (FDA)
5600 Fishers Lane
Rockville, MD 20857-0001
888-INFO-FDA (888-463-6332)
www.fda.gov

US National Institute of Environmental Health Sciences (NIEHS)
PO Box 12233
Research Triangle Park, NC 27709
919-541-3345
www.niehs.nih.gov

US National Institutes of Health (NIH)
9000 Rockville Pike
Bethesda, MD 20892
301-496-4000
TTY: 301-402-9612
www.nih.gov

US Social Security Administration (SSA)
Office of Public Inquiries
Windsor Park Building
6401 Security Boulevard
Baltimore, MD 21235
800-772-1213
www.ssa.gov

VOLUME 1

The Ear, Nose, Mouth, and Throat

Alexander Graham Bell Association for the Deaf and Hard of Hearing (AG Bell)
3417 Volta Place NW
Washington, DC 20007-2778
202-337-5220 / 866-337-5220
TTY: 202-337-5221
www.agbell.org

American Society for Deaf Children (ASDC)
PO Box 3355
Gettysburg, PA 17325
717-334-7922 / 800-942-ASDC (800-942-2732)
www.deafchildren.org

American Speech-Language-Hearing Association (ASHA)
10801 Rockville Pike
Rockville, MD 20852
301-897-5700 / 800-638-8255
TTY: 301-897-0157
www.asha.org

National Association of the Deaf (NAD)
814 Thayer Avenue, Suite 250
Silver Spring, MD 20910-4500
301-587-1788
TTY: 301-587-1789
www.nad.org

National Institute on Deafness and Other Communication Disorders (NIDCD)
US National Institutes of Health (NIH)
31 Center Drive, MSC 2320
Bethesda, MD 20892-2320
800-241-1044
TTY: 800-241-1055
www.nidcd.nih.gov

The Eyes

American Academy of Ophthalmology
PO Box 7424
San Francisco, CA 94120
415-561-8500
www.aao.org

American Optometric Association
243 North Lindbergh Boulevard
St. Louis, MO 63141
314-991-4100
www.aoanet.org

American Society of Ophthalmic Plastic and Reconstructive Surgery
1133 West Morse Boulevard, #201
Winter Park, FL 32789
407-647-8839
www.asoprs.org

Lighthouse International
111 East 59th Street
New York, NY 10022-1202
800-829-0500
www.lighthouse.org

National Eye Institute (NEI)
US Institutes of Health (NIH)
2020 Vision Place
Bethesda, MD 20892-3655
301-496-5248
www.nei.nih.gov

Prevent Blindness America
500 East Remington Road
Schaumburg, IL 60173
847-843-2020 / 800-331-2020
www.preventblindness.org

The Integumentary System

American Society for Dermatologic Surgery
5550 Meadowbrook Drive, Suite 120
Rolling Meadows, IL 60008
847-956-0900
asds-net.org

International Pemphigus Foundation
The Atrium Plaza, Suite 210
828 San Pablo Avenue
Albany, CA 94706
510-527-4970
www.pemphigus.org

**National Organization for Albinism and
    Hypopigmentation (NOAH)**
PO Box 959
East Hampstead, NH 03826-0959
603-887-2310 / 800-473-2310
www.albinism.org

National Pediculosis Association, Inc.
50 Kearney Road
Needham, MA 02494
781-449-NITS (781-449-6487)
www.headlice.org

National Psoriasis Foundation
6600 Southwest 92nd Avenue, Suite 300
Portland, OR 97223-7195
503-244-7404 / 800-723-9166
www.psoriasis.org

The Nervous System

**Alzheimer's Disease Education & Referral
    Center (ADEAR)**
PO Box 8250
Silver Spring, MD 20907-8250
800-438-4380
www.alzheimers.org

American Academy of Neurology
1080 Montreal Avenue
St. Paul, MN 55116
651-695-2717 / 800-879-1960

American Parkinson Disease Association
135 Parkinson Avenue
Staten Island, NY 10305
718-981-8001 / 800-223-2732
www.apdaparkinson.org

Huntington's Disease Society of America
505 Eighth Avenue, Suite 902
New York, NY 10018
212-242-1968 / 800-345-HDSA (800-345-4372)
www.hdsa.org

International Dyslexia Association
8600 LaSalle Road
Chester Building, Suite 382
Baltimore, MD 21286-2044
410-296-0232 / 800-ABCD123 (800-222-3123)
www.interdys.org

Learning Disabilities Association of America
4156 Library Road, Suite 1
Pittsburgh, PA 15234-1349
412-341-1515
www.ldaamerica.org

**Michael J. Fox Foundation for Parkinson's
    Research**
Grand Central Station
PO Box 4777
New York, NY 10163
800-708-7644
www.michaeljfox.org

**Multiple Sclerosis Association of America
    (MSAA)**
706 Haddonfield Road
Cherry Hill, NJ 08002
856-488-4500
www.msaa.com

National Center for Learning Disabilities
381 Park Avenue South, Suite 1401
New York, NY 10016
212-545-7510 / 888-575-7373
www.ld.org

**National Institute of Neurological Disorders
    and Stroke (NINDS)**
US Institutes of Health (NIH)
PO Box 5801
Bethesda, MD 20824
301-496-5751 / 800-352-9425
TTY: 301-468-5981
www.ninds.nih.gov

National Multiple Sclerosis Society
733 Third Avenue
New York, NY 10017
800-FIGHT-MS (800-344-4867)
www.nationalmssociety.org

National Parkinson Foundation
1501 Northwest 9th Avenue/Bob Hope Road
Miami, FL 33136-1494
00-327-4545
www.parkinson.org

Parkinson's Disease Foundation
1359 Broadway, Suite 1509
New York, NY 10018
212-923-4700 / 800-457-6676
www.pdf.org

United Cerebral Palsy
1660 L Street NW, Suite 700
Washington, DC 20036
202-776-0406 / 800-872-5827
TTY: 202-973-7197
www.ucp.org

The Musculoskeletal System

American Association of Orthopaedic Surgeons (AAOS)
6300 North River Road
Rosemont, IL 60018-4262
847-823-7186 / 800-346-AAOS (800-346-2267)
www.aaos.org

Arthritis Foundation
1330 West Peachtree Street, Suite 100
Atlanta, GA 30309
404-872-7100
800-568-4045
www.arthritis.org

Muscular Dystrophy Association (MDA)
3300 East Sunrise Drive
Tucson, AZ 85718
800-FIGHT-MD (800-344-4863)
www.mdausa.org

National Institute of Arthritis and Musculoskeletal and Skin Diseases (NIAMS) Information Clearinghouse
US National Institutes of Health (NIH)
1 AMS Circle
Bethesda, MD 20892-3675
301-495-4484 / 877-226-4267

TTY: 301-565-2966
www.niams.nih.gov

National Institute of Dental and Craniofacial Research (NIDCR)
US National Institutes of Health (NIH)
45 Center Drive, Room 4AS19, MSC 6400
Bethesda, MD 20892-6400
301-496-4261
www.nidcr.nih.gov

National Osteoporosis Foundation
1232 Twenty-second Street NW
Washington, DC 20037-1292
202-223-2226
www.nof.org

Pain and Pain Management

American Chronic Pain Association (ACPA)
PO Box 850
Rocklin, CA 95677-0850
916-632-0922 / 800-533-3231
www.theacpa.org

American Council for Headache Education
19 Mantua Road
Mt. Royal, NJ   08061
856-423-0258 / 800-255-ACHE (800-255-2243)
www.achenet.org

American Pain Foundation
201 North Charles Street
Suite 710
Baltimore, MD 21201
888-615-PAIN (888-615-7246)
www.painfoundation.org

National Chronic Pain Outreach Association (NCPOA)
PO Box 274
Millboro, VA 24460
540-862-9437
www.chronicpain.org

National Foundation for the Treatment of Pain
PO Box 70045
Houston, TX 77270
713-862-9332
www.paincare.org

National Headache Foundation
820 North Orleans, Suite 217
Chicago, IL 60610-3132
773-388-6399 / 888-NHF-5552 (888-643-5552)
www.headaches.org

VOLUME 2

The Cardiovascular System

American College of Cardiology
Heart House
9111 Old Georgetown Road
Bethesda, MD 20814-1699
301-897-5400 / 800-253-4636, ext. 694
www.acc.org

American Heart Association
7272 Greenville Center
Dallas, TX 75231
800-AHA-USA1 (800-242-8721)
www.americanheart.org

American Stroke Association
7272 Greenville Avenue
Dallas, TX 75231
888-4STROKE (888-478-7653)
www.strokeassociation.org

The Mended Hearts, Inc.
7272 Greenville Avenue
Dallas TX 75321
214-706-1442 / 888-HEART99 (888-432-7899)
www.mendedhearts.org

The Blood and Lymph

American Association of Blood Banks (AABB)
8101 Glenbrook Road
Bethesda, MD 20814-2749
301-907-6977
www.aabb.org

National Heart, Lung, and Blood Institute (NHLBI) Health Information Center
National Institutes of Health
PO Box 30105
Bethesda, MD 20824-0105
301-592-8573
www.nhlbi.nih.gov

The Pulmonary System

American Lung Association/American Thoracic Society
1740 Broadway
New York, NY 10019-4374
800-LUNG-USA
www.lungusa.org

The Immune System and Allergies

Allergy and Asthma Network/Mothers of Asthmatics, Inc.
3554 Chain Bridge Road, Suite 2000
Fairfax, VA 22030
800-878-4403
www.podi.com/health/aanma

American Academy of Allergy, Asthma and Immunology
611 East Wells Street
Milwaukee, WI 53202
800-822-ASMA
www.aaaai.org

American College of Allergy, Asthma and Immunology
85 West Algonquin Road, Suite 550
Arlington Heights, IL 60005
800-842-7777
www.allergy.mcg.edu

American College of Rheumatology
1800 Century Place, Suite 250
Atlanta, GA 30345
404-633-3777
www.rheumatology.org

Asthma and Allergy Foundation of America
1125 Fifteenth Street NW, Suite 502
Washington, DC 20036
202-466-7643 / 800-7ASTHMA
www.aafa.org

Food Allergy and Anaphylaxis Network
10400 Eaton Place, Suite 107
Fairfax, VA 22030
800-929-4040
www.foodallergy.org

JAMA Asthma Information Center
American Medical Association
515 North State Street
Chicago, IL 60610
www.ama-assn.org/asthma

Lupus Foundation of America, Inc.
2000 L Street NW, Suite 710
Washington, DC 20036
202-349-1155 / 800-558-0121
www.lupus.org

Parents of Asthmatic/Allergic Children
1412 Marathon Drive
Ft. Collins, CO 80524
303-842-7395

Scleroderma Foundation
12 Kent Way, Suite 101
Byfield, MA 01922
800-722-4673
www.scleroderma.org

Sjögren's Syndrome Foundation
366 North Broadway
Jericho, NY 11753
516-933-6365 / 800-475-6473
www.sjogrens.org

Infectious Diseases

National Institute of Allergy and Infectious Diseases (NIAID)
US National Institutes of Health
Bethesda, MD 20892
www.niaid.nih.gov

Cancer

American Cancer Society (ACS)
1599 Clifton Road NE
Atlanta, GA 30329
800-ACS.2345 (800-227-2345)
www.cancer.org

National Cancer Institute (NCI)
US National Institutes of Health (NIH)
NCI Public Inquiries Office
6116 Executive Boulevard, Room 3036A
Bethesda, MD 20892-8322

800-4-CANCER (800-422-6237)
www.cancer.gov

National Comprehensive Cancer Network (NCCN)
500 Old York Road, Suite 250
Jenkintown, PA 19046
215-690-0300 / 888-909-NCCN (888-909-6226)
www.nccn.org

VOLUME 3

The Gastrointestinal System

American College of Gastroenterology (ACG)
PO Box 342260
Bethesda, MD 20827-2260
301-263-9000
www.acg.gi.org

American Gastroenterological Association (AGA)
4930 Del Ray Avenue
Bethesda, MD 20814
301-654-2055
www.gastro.org

National Institute of Diabetes and Digestive and Kidney Diseases (NIDDK)
US National Institutes of Health (NIH)
Office of Communications and Public Liaison
Building 31, Room 9A04
31 Center Drive, MSC 2560
Bethesda, MD 20892-2560
www.niddk.nih.gov

The Endocrine System

American Diabetes Association
National Call Center
1701 North Beauregard Street
Alexandria, VA 22311
800-DIABETES (800-342-2383)
www.diabetes.org

American Thyroid Association
6066 Leesburg Pike, Suite 500
Falls Church, VA 22041
703-998-8890 / 800-THYROID (800-849-7643)
www.thyroid.org

National Diabetes Education Program
One Diabetes Way
Bethesda, MD 20814-9692
301-496-3583
www.ndep.nih.gov

The Urinary System

National Kidney Foundation
30 East 33rd Street
New York NY 10016
800-622-9010
www.kidney.org

The Reproductive System

Alan Guttmacher Institute (AGI)
120 Wall Street, 21st Floor
New York, NY 10005
212-248-1111
800-355-0244
www.agi-usa.org

American College of Obstetricians and Gynecologists (ACOG)
409 Twelfth Street SW, PO Box 96920
Washington, DC 20090-6920
www.acog.org

Kinsey Institute for Research in Sex, Gender, and Reproduction
Morrison 313, Indiana University
Bloomington, IN 47405
812-855-7686
www.kinseyinstitute.org

La Leche League International
1400 North Meacham Road
Schaumburg, IL
847-519-7730
www.lalecheleague.org

March of Dimes
1275 Mamaroneck Avenue
White Plains, NY 10605
www.marchofdimes.com

National Institute of Child Health and Human Development (NICHD)
US National Institutes of Health (NIH)
PO Box 3006

Rockville, MD 20847
800-370-2843
TTY: 888-320-6942
www.nichd.nih.gov

National Women's Health Information Center
US Department of Health and Human Services (HHS)
Office on Women's Health
800-994-9662
TTD: 888-220-5446
www.4women.gov

North American Menopause Society
5900 Landerbrook Drive, Suite 195
Mayfield Heights, OH 44124
440-442-7550
www.menopause.org

Planned Parenthood Federation of America
434 West 33rd Street
New York, NY 10001
212-541-7800
www.plannedparenthood.org

Psychiatric Disorders and Psychologic Conditions

American Academy of Child and Adolescent Psychiatry (AACAP)
3615 Wisconsin Avenue NW
Washington, DC 20016-3007
202-966-7300
www.aacap.org

American Psychiatric Association (APA)
1000 Wilson Boulevard, Suite 1825
Arlington, VA 22209
703-907-7300
www.healthyminds.org

Depression and Bipolar Support Alliance (DBSA)
730 North Franklin Street, Suite 501
Chicago, IL 60610-7224
800-826-3632
www.dbsalliance.org

National Alliance for the Mentally Ill (NAMI)
Colonial Place Three
2107 Wilson Boulevard, Suite 300
Arlington, VA 22201-3042

800-950-NAMI (6264)
www.nami.org

National Institute of Mental Health (NIMH)
US National Institutes of Health (NIH)
Public Information and Communications
6001 Executive Boulevard, Room 8184, MSC 9663
Bethesda, MD 20892-9663
301-443-4513 / 866-615-6464
TTY: 301-443-8431 / 866-415-8051
www.nimh.nih.gov

National Mental Health Association (NMHA)
2001 North Beauregard Street, 12th Floor
Alexandria, VA 22311
800-969-NMHA (6642)
www.nmha.org

VOLUME 4

Preventive Medicine

Agency for Toxic Substances and Disease Registry (ATSDR)
Division of Toxicology
US Centers for Disease Control and Prevention (CDC)
1600 Clifton Road NE, Mailstop F-32
Atlanta, GA 30333
888-42-ATSDR (888-422-8737)
www.atsdr.cdc.gov

Healthy People 2010
www.healthypeople.gov

National Center for Injury Prevention and Control
US Centers for Disease Control and Prevention (CDC)
4770 Buford Highway NE, Mailstop K65
Atlanta, GA 30341-3724
770-488-1506
www.cdc.gov/ncipc

National Institute for Occupational Safety and Health (NIOSH)
US Centers for Disease Control and Prevention (CDC)
4676 Columbia Parkway
Mail Stop C-18

Cincinnati, OH 45226
800-356-4674
www.cdc.gov/niosh

National Safety Council
1121 Spring Lake Drive
Itasca, IL 60143-3201
630-285-1121
www.nsc.org

Occupational Safety & Health Administration (OSHA)
US Department of Labor
200 Constitution Avenue
Washington DC 20210
202-693-1999 / 800-321-OSHA (6742)
www.osha.gov

US Centers for Disease Control and Prevention (CDC)
1600 Clifton Road
Atlanta, GA 30333
404-639-3534 / 800-311-3435
www.cdc.gov

US Environmental Protection Agency (EPA)
Ariel Rios Building
1200 Pennsylvania Avenue NW
Washington, DC 20460
202-272-0167
www.epa.gov

Alternative and Complementary Approaches

American Association of Naturopathic Physicians (AANP)
3201 New Mexico Avenue NW #350
Washington, DC 20016
202-895-1392 / 866-538-2267
www.naturopathic.org

National Center for Complementary and Alternative Medicine (NCCAM)
NCCAM Clearinghouse
PO Box 7923
Gaithersburg, MD 20898
888-644-6226
TTY: 866-464-3615
www.nccam.nih.gov

Genetics and Molecular Medicine

National Human Genome Research Institute (NHGRI)
US National Institutes of Health (NIH)
Building 31, Room 4B09
31 Center Drive, MSC 2152
9000 Rockville Pike
Bethesda, MD 20892-2152
301-402-0911
www.genome.gov

National Institute of General Medical Sciences (NIGMS)
US National Institutes of Health (NIH)
45 Center Drive, MSC 6200
Bethesda, MD 20892-6200
301-496-7301
www.nigms.nih.gov

United Mitochondrial Disease Foundation
8085 Saltsburg Road, Suite 201
Pittsburgh, PA 15239
412-793-8077
www.umdf.org

Drugs

National Council on Patient Information and Education (NCPIE)
4915 Saint Elmo Avenue, Suite 505
Bethesda, MD 20814-6082
301-656-8565
www.talkaboutrx.org

Nutrition and Diet

American Dietetic Association
216 West Jackson Boulevard
Chicago, IL 60606-6995
800-877-1600
www.eatright.org

US Department of Agriculture (USDA)
1400 Independence Avenue SW
Washington DC 20250
www.usda.gov

Fitness: Exercise and Health

American College of Sports Medicine (ACSM)
401 West Michigan Street
Indianapolis, IN 46202-3233
317-637-9200
www.acsm.org

President's Council on Physical Fitness and Sports
US Department of Health and Human Services (HHS)
Department W
200 Independence Avenue SW, Room 738-H
Washington, DC 20201-0004
202-690-9000
www.fitness.gov

Human Relations

APA Lesbian, Gay, and Bisexual Concerns Program
American Psychiatric Association
750 First Street NE
Washington, DC 20002
202-336-6050
www.apa.org/pi/lgbc/

National Gay and Lesbian Task Force
2320 Seventeenth Street
Washington, DC 20009
202-332-6483
www.thetaskforce.org

Parents, Families and Friends of Lesbians and Gays (PFLAG)
1726 M Street NW, Suite 400
Washington, DC 20036
202-467-8180
www.pflag.org

Sexuality Information and Education Council of the United States (SIECUS)
130 West 42nd Street, Suite 350
New York, NY 10036
212-819-9770
www.siecus.org

Surgery

American Academy of Cosmetic Surgery
737 North Michigan Avenue, Suite 2100
Chicago, IL 60611-5405
312-981-6760
www.cosmeticsurgery.org

American Academy of Facial Plastic and Reconstructive Surgery (AAFPRS)
310 South Henry Street
Alexandria, VA 22314
703-299-9291 / 800-332-FACE (800-332-3223)
www.aafprs.org

Lifestyle Variables: Smoking and Obesity

American Obesity Association
1250 Twenty-fourth Street NW, Suite 300
Washington, DC 20037
202-776-7711
www.obesity.org

SmokeFree.gov
A Web-based partnership of the American Cancer Society (ACS), CDC Office on Smoking and Health, and the National Cancer Institute (NCI).
800-QUITNOW (800-784-8669)
TTY: 800-332-8615
www.smokefree.gov

Tobacco Control Research Branch
NCI Division of Cancer Control and Population
Sciences National Cancer Institute
US National Institutes of Health (NIH)
6130 Executive Boulevard, Room 6134
Executive Plaza North
Rockville, MD 20852
301-594-6776
www.tobaccocontrol.cancer.gov

Tobacco Information and Prevention Source (TIPS)
Office on Smoking and Health (OSH)
National Center for Chronic Disease Prevention and
  Health Promotion
US Centers for Disease Control and Prevention (CDC)
www.cdc.gov/tobacco/index.htm

Substance Abuse

National Council on Alcoholism and Drug Dependence, Inc.
22 Cortlandt Street, Suite 801
New York, NY 10007-3128
212-269-7797
www.ncadd.org

National Institute on Alcohol Abuse and Alcoholism (NIAAA)
US National Institutes of Health (NIH)
5635 Fishers Lane, MSC 9304
Bethesda, MD 20892-9304
www.niaaa.nih.gov

National Institute on Drug Abuse (NIDA)
US National Institutes of Health (NIH)
6001 Executive Boulevard, Room 5213
Bethesda, MD 20892-9561
301-443-1124
www.nida.nih.gov

Substance Abuse and Mental Health Services Administration
US Department of Health and Human Services (HHS)
1 Choke Cherry Road
Room 8-1036
Rockville, MD 20857
crisis hotline: 800-273-8255
TTY crisis hotline: 800-799-4889
www.samhsa.gov

Emergency and First Aid

American Red Cross
2025 East Street NW
Washington, DC 20006
202-303-4498
www.redcross.org

APPENDIX VII
BIOGRAPHIES OF NOTABLE PERSONALITIES

Auenbrugger, [Josef] Leopold (1722–1809) Austrian physician, also known as Leopold von Auenbrugg, who developed chest percussion as a diagnostic method. Auenbrugger recognized that fluid accumulations in the tissues changed the densities of the structures and consequently their tonal qualities. The method became a mainstay of diagnosis for cardiomyopathy (enlargement of the heart characteristic of heart failure) and lung conditions such as pulmonary edema, pneumonia, and tuberculosis.

Avicenna (980–1037) Persian physician and philosopher, also known as Ibn Sina, who earned recognition and fame before he turned 20 for his gifts as a healer. Among Avicenna's numerous writings was *The Canon of Medicine (Canticum de medicina)*, 14 volumes that covered health, disease, treatment, and prevention. *The Canon of Medicine* was a primary medical text throughout Europe from the 11th to the 17th century.

Axelrod, Julius (1912–2004) American research scientist who discovered the reuptake process of the brain neurotransmitters epinephrine and norepinephrine, work for which he received a share of the Nobel Prize for Physiology or Medicine in 1970. Axelrod also conducted key research of the pineal gland, contributing to understanding of the hormone melatonin, and of analgesic medications (pain relievers), contributing to the discovery of acetaminophen.

Banting, Frederick (1891–1941) Canadian physician and researcher who, with medical student Charles Best and physician John Macleod, discovered insulin and its connection to diabetes. Banting and Macleod shared the Nobel Prize in Physiology or Medicine in 1923 for this discovery.

Barnard, Christiaan (1922–2001) South African surgeon who performed the first human heart transplant operation in 1967. Barnard transplanted the heart of a young woman who received fatal injuries in an auto accident, Denise Darvall, into the chest of Louis Washkansky, a 55-year-old dentist in the end stages of heart failure. Washkansky lived only 18 days with his new heart before dying of pneumonia; however, by the 1990s heart transplantation became the standard of care for end-stage heart failure. During his career Barnard pioneered numerous surgical techniques and devices for heart surgery.

Beaumont, William (1785–1853) US Army surgeon who studied the workings of the stomach through a healed gunshot wound that left an opening into the stomach of his patient Alexis St. Martin. Beaumont used the opening to observe the processes of the stomach's stages of digestion. Beaumont collected samples of "gastric juices" and analyzed them, discovering the chemical composition of stomach acid to be primarily hydrochloric acid. Beaumont detailed his experiments and findings in his book *Experiments and Observations on the Gastric Juice and the Physiology of Digestion* published in 1833.

Bernard, Claude (1813–1878) French physiologist who studied and documented numerous dimensions of human physiology, key among them the functions of the pancreas in digestion and the discovery of vasomotor nerves (nerves that cause blood vessels to dilate or constrict). Bernard's most significant postulation was that the interior environment of the human body remained stable relative to the external environment. This postulation became the foundation for the contemporary concept of homeostasis.

Best, Charles (1899–1978) Canadian medical student whose work with physician Frederick Banting resulted in the discovery of insulin.

Though Best did not receive a share of the Nobel Prize in Physiology or Medicine in 1923 awarded to Banting and another collaborator, John Macleod, Banting protested and shared his portion of the award money with Best. Best pursued a career in medical research that resulted in numerous other honors including induction into the Canadian Medical Hall of Fame.

Blackwell, Elizabeth (1821–1910)   First woman to earn a medical degree from an American medical school. Blackwell was born in England and came with her family to the United States in 1832. She graduated with a doctor of medicine degree from Geneva Medical College in New York in 1849. Though she wanted to become a surgeon, an infection that cost her the vision in one eye forced her to change direction to specialize in obstetrics and gynecology. Blackwell founded the New York Infirmary for Women and Children in 1857 and 10 years later opened an affiliated medical school for women. During her career Blackwell wrote several influential medical texts about women's health and diseases.

Blalock, Alfred (1899–1964)   American heart surgeon who pioneered numerous techniques, devices, and instruments to repair congenital heart defects. Blalock's interest in the heart came about as a result of his research to investigate and find treatments for cardiovascular shock. Blalock and his assistant, Vivien Thomas, subsequently turned their interest and methods to create surgical repairs for otherwise fatal "blue baby" heart defects, notably tetralogy of Fallot. Blalock performed the first successful such operation in 1944 on a patient of pediatrician Helen Taussig. Blalock's collaborations with other researchers resulted in operations for coarctation of the aorta and transposition of the great arteries, two other severe congenital heart defects.

Broca, Pierre Paul (1824–1880)   French surgical pathologist and medical researcher best known for his study of brain anatomy and physiology. Broca identified the region of the brain's frontal lobe that controls speech, now known as Broca's area. Broca also studied correlations between brain structure and intelligence, developing numerous methods for measuring the convolutions and size of human and other primate brains, and was a prolific writer.

Chain, Ernst (1906–1979)   German-born biochemist who shared the Nobel Prize in Physiology or Medicine in 1945 with Alexander Fleming and Howard Florey. The award honored the work of the three in the discovery and uses of penicillin. Chain developed methods to analyze natural antibacterial substances and discovered the process by which penicillin killed bacteria.

Charcot, Jean Martin (1825–1893)   French physician who identified multiple sclerosis.

Cooley, Denton (b. 1920)   American cardiovascular surgeon renowned for his skill and innovation in operations on the heart. As an intern Cooley assisted pediatric heart surgeon Alfred Blalock in the first operation to correct a congenital heart malformation ("blue baby" syndrome). Cooley spent much of his surgical career perfecting techniques that would extend the ability to surgically repair such defects. He was one of the first American cardiovascular surgeons to perform a human heart transplantation (in 1968) and to implant an artificial heart as a bridge to transplantation (in 1969). Cooley also pioneered and perfected coronary artery bypass graft (CABG).

Crick, Francis (1916–2004)   British scientist who co-discovered, with American zoologist James Watson, the structure of DNA in 1953. Crick and Watson, along with biophysicist Maurice Wilkins, received the Nobel Prize in Physiology or Medicine in 1962 for the discovery. Crick devoted the remainder of his research career to studies of protein synthesis and genetic code.

de Graaf, Regnier (1641–1673)   Dutch anatomist who published the first detailed studies of the male and female reproductive systems. The egg-bearing follicles on the ovaries, which de Graaf identified and described, are called Graafian follicles.

de Luzzi, Mondinus (1275–1326)   Italian anatomist whose book *Anathomia*, published in 1316, was the first detailed textbook of anatomy of what medical historians consider modern Western medicine. Though heavily framed within the teachings of Galen, *Anathomia* presented de Luzzi's observations from the numerous autopsies he performed as a professor at Bologna.

DeVries, William (b. 1943)   American heart surgeon best known for implanting the first artificial heart into retired dentist Barney Clark in

1982, an experimental procedure that unfolded in full public scrutiny via television. People around the world were simultaneously captivated and repulsed during the four months Clark survived with the device in his chest attached by six feet of tubing to an external and noisy pump the size of a washing machine. DeVries worked closely with Robert Jarvik, the pump's designer, and physician-inventor Willem Kolff, on the mechanical heart's design. After Clark, DeVries implanted mechanical hearts into four other people. DeVries retired from cardiovascular surgery in 1999.

Ehrlich, Paul (1854–1915) German bacteriologist and physician whose extensive research on immunity resulted in developing salvarsan, the first successful treatment for syphilis, and earned him the Nobel Prize for Physiology or Medicine in 1908. Ehrlich's studies of cell structure and function later became the foundation of chemotherapy as a treatment for cancer.

Einthoven, Willem (1860–1927) Dutch physician and scientist whose penultimate achievement was the development of the electrocardiogram (ECG) in 1903. The importance of this device for measuring and visually representing the electrical activity of the heart became apparent over the next two decades. Einthoven received the Nobel Prize in Physiology or Medicine in 1924 to honor the discovery.

Elion, Gertrude (1918–1999) American chemist who developed the first chemotherapy agents successful in treating childhood leukemia, an achievement for which she received the Nobel Prize in Physiology or Medicine in 1988 (shared with her collaborator, chemist George H. Hitchings, and chemist James W. Black who won for his work to develop beta blockers and histamine H_2 blockers). Elion developed other drugs that, although ineffective as treatments for leukemia, became therapies for immunosuppression (azathioprine) and gout (allopurinol).

Fleming, Alexander (1881–1955) Scottish bacteriologist credited with the discovery of penicillin and its actions to kill pathogenic microbes. Fleming shared, with Ernest Chain and Howard Florey, the Nobel Prize in Physiology or Medicine in 1945 for his work with penicillin. Fleming devoted his career to the study of antisepsis and wrote prodigiously of his work.

Florey, Howard Walter (1898–1968) Australian research pathologist whose work to investigate the actions of penicillin earned him a share of the Nobel Prize in Physiology or Medicine in 1945, with Alexander Fleming and Ernest Chain. Florey worked to produce large quantities of penicillin for use as an antibiotic at the end of World War II. He co-authored numerous books during his career.

Freud, Sigmund (1856–1939) Austrian psychiatrist who developed the method of psychoanalysis. As a physician Freud specialized in emotional disorders, such as neurosis, and became intrigued with the nature of the unconscious mind. He studied dreams, forgetfulness, and inadvertent comments ("Freudian slips")—all of which he perceived as insights into the workings of the mind. Freud also correlated much of the mind's functions with sexuality. Freud wrote extensively of his findings and theories, some of which remain controversial and highly debated even today. However, Freud remains the founder of psychiatry, and his work continues to provide insights for medical researchers interested in understanding the link between body and mind.

Galen, Claudius (129–199) A physician and philosopher, also called Galen of Pergamum, whose observations and study of the human body framed the practice of medicine until the Middle Ages. Galen drew much of his information from dissections of animals such as pigs and apes, however, which resulted in some fundamental errors in understanding of human anatomy and physiology. Galen also embraced the premise of the four humors (blood, phlegm, yellow bile, and black bile), in which illness and disease resulted from imbalances among these vital substances.

Gibbon, John H. Jr. (1904–1973) American physician and thoracic surgeon who developed the cardiopulmonary bypass machine, the first successful use of which took place in 1953. Gibbon continued to perfect the design and methods for using cardiopulmonary bypass, making possible the many advances in surgical operations on the heart that occurred through the latter half of the 20th century.

Gray, Henry (1825–1861) English physician, anatomist, and physiologist best known for his landmark work *Gray's Anatomy.* This extraordinary detailed description of the human body's structure and function was first published in 1864 and remains the standard text today for medical students and other students of the medical arts. Gray taught at St. George's Hospital Medical School in London and originally produced his anatomy book to serve as a textbook for his students.

Hales, Stephen (1677–1761) English physiologist who developed a method for measuring arterial blood pressure. Hales's method required inserting a glass tube into an artery and measuring the level to which blood rose within it. Though this method was not practical from a clinical perspective, doctors soon realized the value of blood pressure as a diagnostic marker and researchers developed less intrusive methods for its measurement. Hales also conducted the first measure of a heart's capacity by filling the chambers of a freshly slaughtered sheep's heart with molten wax.

Hall, Marshall (1790–1857) English physician who discovered capillaries and their role in blood circulation. Hall also developed the first method of resuscitation for drowning victims.

Harvey, William (1578–1657) English physician who determined the flow of blood through the body's circulation to be a closed system, with the heart and lungs at its core. Harvey broke with the Galenic understanding that defined medical knowledge at the time, testing his theories extensively before releasing them in the 1628 manuscript that profoundly changed understanding of the human body: *Exercitatio Anatomica de Motu Cordis et Sanguinis in Animalibus (An Anatomical Exercise on the Motion of the Heart and Blood in Animals)*.

Havers, Clopton (1650–1701) English physician and physiologist who was the first to document detailed microscopic descriptions of the tubular structure of compact bone, now known as the Haversian system.

Hippocrates (460–400 B.C.E.) Greek physician widely credited with establishing the tenets of modern medicine. A keen observer, Hippocrates developed numerous diagnostic and therapeutic methods and the philosophy that the physician "first and foremost, do no further harm" when treating patients. Hippocrates advanced the premise of treating the body as a whole rather than isolating and treating its symptoms.

Ibn Al-Nafis (1213–1288) Islamic physician who discovered the circulation of the blood, though his writings did not emerge into the mainstream of Western medicine for several centuries because there was little contact between East and West during his lifetime.

Ingrassias, Giovanni (1510–1580) Italian physician and anatomist who identified the smallest bone in the body, the inner ear's stapes, and a pair of small bones at the back of the eye socket that bear his name, the processes of Ingrassias.

Jarvik, Robert (b. 1946) American physician and researcher who developed a series of mechanical hearts in the 1970s and 1980s. In the first operation of its kind cardiac surgeon William DeVries implanted a Jarvik-7 mechanical heart (which Jarvik developed in collaboration with heart surgeon Willem Kolff) into retired dentist Barney Clark in 1982. Though heart surgeons eventually implanted Jarvik-7 mechanical hearts into about six dozen people, complications were extensive and quality of life was poor. In 1990 the US Food and Drug Administration (FDA) withdrew approval for human use of the mechanical heart.

Jenner, Edward (1749–1823) British physician who developed the smallpox vaccine and the process of vaccination in 1796. A country doctor in rural England, Jenner observed that dairymaids who recovered from cowpox infection did not again get the disease and furthermore did not get smallpox, a deadly or disfiguring infection that researchers later identified as being caused by a related virus. At the time the process for inducing immunity to smallpox, called variolation, was nearly as hazardous as the disease itself. Jenner instead variolated people with cowpox, a milder disease. This form of vaccination rapidly replaced variolation and became mandatory in England, significantly reducing smallpox infection and leading to improved vaccination methods that would eventually eradicate smallpox worldwide.

Jerne, Niels (1911–1994) Danish immunologist who proposed the theories that led to the development of methods to produce monoclonal antibodies (MAbs), specifically targeted immune substances now used as treatment for certain cancers and other diseases. Jerne received a share of the Nobel Prize in Physiology or Medicine in 1984 for his work.

Julian, Percy (1899–1975) African American research chemist who developed a method to synthesize (create in the laboratory) cortisone, a natural hormone of the adrenal glands. Julian's methods also made possible the synthesis of other hormones for therapeutic applications, such as oral contraceptives (birth control pills) and immunosuppressive drugs.

Jung, Carl (1875–1961) Swiss psychiatrist, once a protégé of Austrian psychiatrist Sigmund Freud, who developed a theory of personality based on the premise of a collective unconscious, a pool of inborn recognitions and experiences. The collective unconscious, in Jung's view, explained commonalities across human populations in dreams, mythology, and religion. Jung identified these commonalities as archetypes, which he defined as unlearned experiences.

Koch, [Heinrich Herman] Robert (1843–1910) German bacteriologist who discovered the pathogenic nature of bacteria and the bacterium responsible for causing tuberculosis. Koch received the Nobel Prize in Physiology or Medicine in 1905 for his work in understanding the infectious mechanisms of tuberculosis. Koch made further numerous contributions to the discovery of the role of pathogenic microbes and disease.

Kolff, Willem J. (b. 1911) Physician and medical inventor who founded the first European blood bank during World War II and developed the first artificial kidney a few years later. A pioneer in devices for the heart, Kolff devised an implantable mechanical heart in 1955 and an intra-aortic balloon pump in 1957. In the 1970s and 1980s Kolff collaborated with Robert Jarvik to develop a series of mechanical hearts. Heart surgeon William DeVries implanted one model, the Jarvik-7, into the chest of retired dentist Barney Clark in 1982. Clark lived for four months on the artificial heart. Kolff also developed a portable kidney dialysis unit.

Laënnec, René (1781–1826) French physician who invented the stethoscope to listen to the heart and lungs. Laënnec's early stethoscopes were straight tubes carved of wood. Later models incorporated brass fittings to better hear certain ranges of sounds.

Landsteiner, Karl (1868–1943) Austrian scientist who discovered the antigens on the surfaces of blood cells that led to the identification of blood types. The discovery earned Landsteiner the 1930 Nobel Prize for Physiology or Medicine.

Lister, Joseph (1827–1912) British surgeon responsible for implementing methods of antisepsis to prevent infection during and after surgical operations. Lister built on the foundations that Louis Pasteur's work established, implementing a routine of cleaning surgical and traumatic wounds with carbolic acid to kill any bacteria present. He also applied antiseptic methods to cleaning surgical instruments and maintaining a clean operating field, turning surgery from an approach of last resort to a successful therapeutic method.

Macleod, John James Richard (1876–1935) Co-discoverer, with Frederick Banting and Charles Best, of insulin. Macleod and Banting won the Nobel Prize in Physiology or Medicine in 1923 for their research. While Banting shared his Nobel Prize money with Charles Best, whom he felt was slighted in being not similarly honored, Macleod shared his with the young chemist James Bertram (J.B.) Collip, who had acquired a steady supply of insulin for the team's research.

Maimonides, Moses (1135–1204) Jewish physician and rabbi, also known as Moshe ben Maimon, who was the first of four generations of his family to serve as court physician for the sultans of Egypt. Maimonides established a practice of medicine that integrated body, mind, and spirit, blending the most advanced scientific knowledge of his time with meditation and prayer.

Paré, Ambroise (1510–1590) French battlefield surgeon considered the father of trauma surgery. Paré developed numerous techniques for rapid and humane treatment with an orientation toward eventual recovery and return to productivity through the use of prosthetic limbs and other devices. Paré served as court surgeon to four French kings.

Pasteur, Louis (1822–1895) French biochemist who recognized that pathogenic microbes, notably bacteria, caused infection. Pasteur developed what became known as the germ theory of disease, establishing an understanding of the causes of infection fundamental to developing methods for treating and preventing infection. Pasteur's work became the foundation for antisepsis, vaccination, and pasteurization, all methods for preventing infection. Pasteur further discovered the bacterial cause of rabies and developed the first vaccine to prevent the fatal infection in dogs, the primary source of rabies in his time, as well as in people bitten by rabid dogs.

Pavlov, Ivan (1849–1936) Russian scientist best known for his research on conditioned reflexes, in which he trained dogs to expect food when he rang a bell. Pavlov observed that after a time the dogs began to salivate when they heard the bell ring, altering the body's normal physiologic response to salivate at the sight and smell of food. Pavlov also used surgical gastric fistulas in dogs (operations to create openings into the stomach) to study the physiology of digestion, research for which he won the 1904 Nobel Prize in Physiology or Medicine.

Piaget, Jean (1896–1980) Swiss psychologist who developed numerous theories about human intelligence, the foundation of which centered around his belief of intelligence as a process of adaptation within genetically defined frameworks. Piaget defined this process through four stages beginning at birth and culminating in adolescence, with completion of one stage crucial to entering the next.

Prusiner, Stanley (b. 1942) American neurologist and biochemist who discovered prions, infectious protein fragments that cause progressive, degenerative brain diseases such as kuru disease, Creutzfeldt-Jakob disease (CJD), and variant CJD (vCJD) arising from infection with bovine spongiform encephalopathy (BSE; commonly called mad cow disease). Prusiner received the Nobel Prize in Physiology or Medicine in 1997 for his discovery and work in understanding the infectious mechanisms of prions.

Roëntgen, Wilhelm (1845–1923) German physicist who discovered X-rays and the process for using them to create images, called roentgenograms, which revealed internal structures of density such as the bones. Roëntgen received the Nobel Prize in Physiology or Medicine in 1901 for his discoveries.

Sabin, Florence (1871–1953) American physician who was the first woman to become a full professor at Johns Hopkins Medical School. Sabin conducted research that resulted in significant findings about the structure of the brain, fetal development of the lymphatic system, and tuber-

culosis infection. In the latter years of her medical career Sabin turned her efforts to public health in her home state of Colorado.

Salk, Jonas (1914–1995) American physician who developed the first polio vaccine, released in 1955 after eight years of research. Polio vaccination has eradicated poliomyelitis, once one of the most debilitating and often fatal infections, from much of the world.

Semmelweis, Ignaz Philipp (1818–1861) Hungarian physician who recognized the connection between puerperal fever (childbirth fever) and the then-common practice physicians followed of moving between autopsies on women who died and women who had just given birth. Semmelweis implemented stringent antisepsis procedures at the hospital where he worked, requiring physicians to wash their hands with chlorinated lime before examining patients. As a result the death rate dropped to nearly zero. Though the established medical community was slow to embrace this revolutionary change, antiseptic hand washing eventually became standard practice.

Soper, Fred (1893–1977) American epidemiologist who organized vector-eradication programs worldwide to eliminate diseases such as malaria, yellow fever, and hookworm infestation.

Taussig, Helen (1898–1986) American pediatrician and cardiologist who worked with heart surgeon Alfred Blalock and surgical researcher Vivien Thomas to develop an operation to correct severe congenital defects of the heart. The first such operation, the Blalock-Taussig procedure, was a shunt that restored the flow of blood through the lungs in defects such as tetralogy of Fallot. Taussig overcame a severe hearing loss suffered in childhood as well as bias that prevented women from obtaining medical degrees at most medical schools in the United States.

Thomas, Vivien (1910–1985) African American researcher who collaborated with heart surgeon Alfred Blalock and pediatrician Helen Taussig to develop the operative procedures and instruments to correct congenital heart defects. Intending himself to become a physician, Thomas lost his savings in the stock market crash of 1929 that ushered in the American Great Depression. By the time he recovered financially, changing educational standards and racial discrimination in combination proved too formidable for Thomas to follow his dream. Blalock nonetheless insisted that Thomas assist him in the operating room, and often Thomas guided Blalock through difficult aspects of the operations Thomas devised.

van Leeuwenhoek, Antonie (1632–1723) Dutch amateur scientist who built his own microscopes. His studies were among the earliest to detail the structures and functions of blood cells, bacteria, and sperm. The work of van Leeuwenhoek also established the role of bacteria in causing illness, providing the foundation for the research more than a century later of Robert Koch and Joseph Lister.

Vesalius, Andreas (1514–1564) Flemish anatomist whose book *De Humanis Corporis Fabrica (On the Workings of the Human Body)* was the foundation of human anatomy for centuries. Through a friendship with a judge, Vesalius gained access to the bodies of executed criminals for dissection. Many of Vesalius's discoveries contradicted the teachings of Galen, still popular at the time. Key among them were that the heart had four chambers, not two as Galen asserted, and that the major blood vessels arose from the heart, not the liver. Vesalius also provided correct and detailed drawings of the gastrointestinal structures.

von Behring, Emil Adolf (1854–1917) Prussian physician whose research on toxins and antitoxins led to the development of tetanus and diphtheria vaccines, established the foundation for serum therapy, and earned the first Nobel Prize for Physiology or Medicine awarded in 1901.

Waksman, Selman (1888–1973) Biochemist who discovered the antibiotic medications streptomycin, the first antibiotic effective for treating tuberculosis, and neomycin. Waksman received the 1952 Nobel Prize in Physiology or Medicine in recognition of his work.

Watson, James (b. 1928) American scientist who co-discovered, in collaboration with British researcher Francis Crick, the double helix structure of DNA in 1953. Watson and Crick shared the 1962 Nobel Prize in Physiology or Medicine for their work. Watson conducted much research on the role of RNA in viruses and served as director of the Human Genome Project from 1989 to 1992. He wrote several books, among them the 1968 best-seller *Double Helix,* which chronicled the discovery of DNA.

Yalow, Rosalyn (b. 1921) American physicist who developed techniques to use radioisotopes to measure the amount of peptide hormones such as insulin in the blood, which are present in very small quantities. These techniques became known as radioimmunoassays (RIAs) and are today the basis for such measurements. Yalow received a share of the Nobel Prize in Physiology or Medicine in 1977 for her work.

APPENDIX VIII
DIAGNOSTIC IMAGING PROCEDURES

Diagnostic imaging procedures offer noninvasive approaches for visualizing the structure and function of internal organs. Though each procedure has specific applications and diagnostic value, doctors often use procedures in combination with one another to give detailed information to help diagnose health conditions as well as monitor the effectiveness of treatment. Some procedures involve the injection or consumption of radio-opaque contrast media (special dyes) or radioisotopes to create dimensional images.

The entries in this appendix discuss procedures that have broad application across body systems and health conditions. Entries for diagnostic imaging procedures specific to a particular body system are in the section of *The Facts On File Encyclopedia of Health and Medicine* that covers that body system. For example, MAMMOGRAM—X-RAY of the breast—appears in the section "The Reproductive System" and INTRAVENOUS PYELOGRAM (IVP)—imaging of the KIDNEYS—appears in the section "The Urinary System."

computed tomography (CT) scan A radiologic procedure that uses multiple X-RAY images to create multi-dimensional pictures of the structure of internal organs. The CT scanner takes numerous X-ray "slices" that a computer then assembles into an image of the organ or structure. The X-ray tube rotates within the scanner, moving around area of the body being scanned. A CT scan may be done with or without contrast media, depending on the reason for the procedure. CT scan of the abdomen may require a bowel prep (laxative or enema). Most other CT scans do not require any advance preparation.

The scan itself is painless, though some people may feel claustrophobic when inside the scanner. Some CT scanners are open, which reduces the sense of being closed in. Most often it is necessary to change out of regular clothing into a hospital gown for the scan, to prevent interference from objects such as zippers and buttons. A CT scan generally takes between 15 minutes and an hour, depending on the type of images the doctor desires. No recovery is necessary; when the radiologist is satisfied with the quality of images, the person may get dressed and leave.

There is a slight risk of an adverse or allergic reaction to contrast dye, which is iodine-based. CT scan does expose a person to ionizing radiation, though for most procedures the level of exposure is within the established safety boundaries. Frequent CT scans or complex CT scans, such as cardiac multislice CT (CMCT), result in significantly higher exposure, however. It is important to discuss the potential risks of such exposure before undergoing the procedure.

Doctors may order CT scans to evaluate STROKE and TRAUMATIC BRAIN INJURY (TBI), complex or questionable BONE fractures, internal masses that could be tumors, and damage to the HEART after HEART ATTACK. Certain surgeries that require extraordinary precision, such as operations on the BRAIN (for example, THALAMOTOMY and PALLIDOTOMY), may use CT scan to guide the placement of surgical instruments.

magnetic resonance imaging (MRI) An imaging procedure that uses powerful magnetic energy to visualize internal organs and structures. MRI does not involve exposure to radiation. The nuclei of hydrogen atoms (a component molecule of water) align themselves in a known pattern within the body's natural magnetic field. The MRI machine emits a strong pulse of electromagnetic energy, also called radiofrequency (RF) energy, causing the hydrogen nuclei to temporarily realign themselves. The MRI machine then detects the rate at which the nuclei return to their natural alignment. A computer constructs multidimensional images based on this data.

MRI is particularly effective for detecting abnormal tissue within the body, such as tumors, tears to muscles, and neurologic injury or deterioration. Because of the electromagnetic disruption the MRI machine temporarily causes, people who have implanted pacemakers and other devices, metal hardware (such as to repair fractures), permanent prostheses (such as an artificial eye or COCHLEAR IMPLANT), and certain other circumstances cannot undergo MRI. It is essential to remove all clothing and items that may contain metal; the person wears a hospital gown during the procedure.

MRI is painless and takes 15 minutes to an hour depending on the area of the body being scanned. Sometimes the doctor may choose to administer an intravenous injection of a contrast medium to enhance the images the MRI produces. The MRI machine is very loud and surrounds the person during the procedure. Some people find the experience of the procedure disconcerting because of these factors. The technologist performing the MRI can provide methods to minimize this. MRI does not have any adverse side effects.

radionuclide scan A nuclear medicine procedure that measures the rate of deterioration of low-level radioactive isotopes to present images of the cellular function of organs such as the BRAIN, BONE, LIVER, THYROID GLAND, and GALLBLADDER. Radionuclide scans involve exposure to radiation. Before the scan, the person receives an intravenous injection of a small amount of fluid, typically a glucose (sugar) solution, "tagged" with the appropriate radioisotope (the radionuclide). Cells throughout the body uptake, or take in, the tagged glucose molecules. The attached radioisotope molecules deteriorate as the body uses the glucose.

Cells in various organs and structures use glucose at known rates; measuring the rate helps doctors to determine whether there is abnormal function such as tumors or healing (increased glucose use). Slowed uptake may indicate degenerative disorders or problems with healing.

During the scan the person lies on a procedure table and the gamma camera or other device passes over the area of the body being evaluated. The procedure may take 15 to 90 minutes. There is usually no need to change out of regular clothes. The risks of radionuclide scans are minimal. The radioisotopes dissipate rapidly, so the radiation does not remain in the body very long. Specialized types of radionuclide scans include positron emission tomography (PET) scan and single photon emission computed tomography (SPECT).

ultrasound Also called ultrasonography, a diagnostic procedure that uses high-frequency sound waves (beyond the frequency human hearing can detect) to create images of internal organs and structures. Ultrasound does not involve exposure to radiation. Ultrasound is painless and is especially effective for evaluating hollow structures within the body such as the GALLBLADDER, urinary BLADDER, and arteries and veins. Doppler ultrasound is a technique that presents moving images, such as the flow of BLOOD or the movement of a FETUS within a pregnant woman's uterus. Ultrasound is also useful for detecting cysts and tumors in structures such as the OVARIES, TESTICLES, BREASTS, and PROSTATE GLAND. Doctors sometimes use ultrasound to guide the placement of biopsy instruments.

Ultrasound typically requires no advance preparation, though pelvic ultrasound may require a full urinary bladder. The procedure is painless. During the procedure, the sonographer applies a warm gel to the surface of the skin over the area being scanned. The gel improves the conductivity of sound signals. The sonographer gently presses a transducer against the skin and moves it in a particular pattern. The transducer emits ultrasound waves, which "echo" from the structures within the body. The transducer then picks up the echoes and transmits them back to the ultrasound machine, which creates representational images from them.

Some ultrasound procedures involve placing the transducer within a natural body opening such as the VAGINA, RECTUM, or ESOPHAGUS to provide focused examination of key structures that are deeper within the body. Transesophageal ultrasound, for example, can provide close examination of the heart. ECHOCARDIOGRAM is another type of ultrasound that specifically examines the HEART.

X-ray A radiologic procedure to evaluate the structure of dense organs within the body such as bone. X-ray involves exposure to ionizing radiation. An X-ray machine emits a beam of ionizing radiation that tissues within the body absorb. The more dense the tissue, the more radiation it absorbs. Solid structures such as bone absorb high amounts of radiation; thus X-ray is particularly effective for detecting injuries and other abnormalities of the bones. X-ray can also detect the presence of many types of tumors because their tissues have different density than normal structures, as well as the presence of abnormal air or fluid (such as in the lungs or abdomen).

Most X-ray procedures require removing clothing that could interfere with the X-ray image, such as items that have buttons and zippers. Some X-ray procedures, such as BARIUM ENEMA, require advance preparation and the use of contrast media. Some X-ray procedures require awkward positions or holding the breath, which may be temporarily uncomfortable. Most X-ray procedures are painless, though people may feel pain from the injuries being evaluated during the procedure. Infrequent X-rays pose very little risk to health. People who need frequent X-rays should discuss the risk of radiation exposure with their doctors.

APPENDIX IX
FAMILY MEDICAL TREE

A family medical tree can help your doctor determine inherited and genetic health risks. Optimally a family medical tree includes information about the causes of death and significant medical conditions for as many family generations as possible. The most significant health information is that for first-degree relatives (siblings, parents, and children) and second-degree relatives (nephews, nieces, cousins, aunts, uncles, and grandparents). Some health information may be vague or use antiquated terminology (for example, consumption to identify tuberculosis or dropsy to identify congestive heart failure).

It is especially important to know the cause of death whenever possible, as this provides clues to underlying health conditions. For deaths occurring within the past few decades, this information appears on the death certificate. Other useful information includes any history of

- HEART disease, such as STROKE, HEART ATTACK (MYOCARDIAL INFARCTION), sudden (or unexplained) cardiac death, ATHEROSCLEROSIS, ARTERIOSCLEROSIS, CARDIOMYOPATHY (enlarged heart), congestive HEART FAILURE, PERIPHERAL VASCULAR DISEASE (PVD), DEEP VEIN THROMBOSIS (DVT), INTERMITTENT CLAUDICATION, LONG QT SYNDROME (LQTS), and ARRHYTHMIA

- congenital heart defects or disorders, including treatments (such as surgery) to repair or treat them

- CANCER, especially BREAST CANCER, COLORECTAL CANCER, OVARIAN CANCER, PROSTATE CANCER, and childhood cancers such as LEUKEMIA or WILMS'S TUMOR

- neurologic disorders such as ALZHEIMER'S DISEASE, HUNTINGTON'S DISEASE, and PARKINSON'S DISEASE

- known GENETIC DISORDERS or CHROMOSOMAL DISORDERS such as HEMOPHILIA, DOWN SYNDROME, TURNER'S SYNDROME, KLINEFELTER'S SYNDROME, or generalized BIRTH DEFECTS

- SEASONAL ALLERGIES, allergies to medications or foods, ASTHMA, or MIGRAINE HEADACHE

- INFLAMMATORY BOWEL DISEASE (IBD), SYTEMIC LUPUS ERYTHEMATOSUS (SLE), HYPOTHYROIDISM, type 1 DIABETES, RHEUMATOID ARTHRITIS, or other AUTOIMMUNE DISORDERS

- INFERTILITY, PREMATURE OVARIAN FAILURE (POF), MISCARRIAGE (spontaneous ABORTION), STILLBIRTH, breech presentation, or other difficulties with PREGNANCY and CHILDBIRTH

- type 2 DIABETES, OBESITY, or INSULIN RESISTANCE

- DEPRESSION, GENERALIZED ANXIETY DISORDER (GAD), BIPOLAR DISORDER, SCHIZOPHRENIA, SEASONAL AFFECTIVE DISORDER (SAD), LEARNING DISORDERS, or intellectual deficiency (mental retardation)

- ALCOHOLISM, SUBSTANCE ABUSE, or CIGARETTE SMOKING

- HEMOCHROMATOSIS, WILSON'S DISEASE, PHENYLKETONURIA (PKU), and other disorders of METABOLISM

- MUSCULAR DYSTROPHY or CYSTIC FIBROSIS

A family history of health conditions does not necessarily point to a personal history with the same conditions. However, it provides important clues about a person's possible predilection for such conditions. The most accurate method to compile a family medical tree is to ask key family members, such as parents and grandparents, about health conditions. However, some people are reluctant to discuss health problems. Sometimes it is helpful to mention to the doctor that a particular health condition affects more than one first degree relative or multiple second degree relatives.

Record family health information, and give a copy of the document to the family or regular physician as well as other family members.

APPENDIX X
IMMUNIZATION AND
ROUTINE EXAMINATION SCHEDULES

Preventive health examinations and immunizations are crucial for optimal health and disease resistance across the spectrum of life. Recommended schedules, examination procedures, and immunizations change as knowledge grows and new developments become available. The information in this appendix represents a composite of common recommendations current at the time of publication. Recommendations may differ according to age and between men and women.

Preventive Health Care for Infants and Children
Most health experts recommend well child examinations for basic preventive health care on a schedule frequent enough for early detection of physical or mental developmental delays and concerns. Well child exams should include age-appropriate general health measures such as

- length/height

- weight

- head circumference (infants)

- reflexes

- vital signs (heart rate, breathing rate, blood pressure, body temperature)

- basic vision and hearing screening

- scoliosis detection

- coordination, balance, and gait

- nutritional status

- appropriate immunizations

WELL CHILD EXAMINATION SCHEDULE RECOMMENDATIONS BY AGE

Infancy

2 to 4 days after birth	10 days after birth

Early Childhood

2 months	4 months
6 months	9 months
12 months	15 months
18 months	24 months

Middle Childhood

3 years	4 years
5 years	6 years
8 years	10 years

Adolescence

12 years	14 years
16 years	18 years

Immunizations and immunization schedules change as new vaccines become available. The American Academy of Pediatrics (AAP) establishes and updates recommendations. The most current immunizations and their schedules are available on the AAP's Web site (www.aap.org) as well as through public health departments and public and private health organizations.

Immunization schedules for children vary according to the age at which the child receives the first dose of a multidose vaccination series. For some immunizations there is a window of opportune timing. The pediatrician adjusts each child's schedule for appropriate timing of doses, including "catch-up" scheduling for children who begin immunizations later than recommended. Timing and doses for each vaccine are crucial for the body's process of developing immunity. Nearly all children should receive all recommended immunizations; public schools throughout the United States require certain immunizations for school registration unless there are extenuating circumstances. Such factors vary among states.

Preventive Health Care for Adults

Preventive health-care examinations for adults vary according to gender and age. Adults also require certain immunizations. Most adults should receive a tetanus-diphtheria booster every 10 years, hepatitis B vaccine if not immunized in childhood, and influenza vaccination (flu shot) and every year.

PREVENTIVE HEALTH EXAMINATION RECOMMENDATIONS: ADULTS

Age	Well Exam Frequency	Exam Includes
19 to 39	men: every 5 years women: every 3 years	health risk screening: cholesterol, blood pressure, diabetes, sexually transmitted diseases (STDs) height/weight vital signs men: testicular exam women: breast exam, pelvic exam, Pap test
40 to 49	men: every 5 years women: every 3 years	health risk screening: cholesterol, blood pressure, diabetes, STDs, heart disease, cancer height/weight vital signs fecal occult blood test (FOBT) men: testicular exam, baseline prostate exam women: breast exam, pelvic exam, Pap test, baseline mammogram
50 to 64	men: every 3 to 5 years women: every 2 to 3 years	health risk screening: cholesterol, blood pressure, diabetes, STDs, heart disease, cancer, thyroid height/weight vital signs FOBT baseline colonoscopy, repeat every 10 years men: testicular exam, prostate exam women: breast exam, pelvic exam, Pap test annual mammogram
65 and older	men and women: every year	health risk screening: cholesterol, blood pressure, diabetes, STDs, heart disease, cancer, thyroid height/weight vital signs FOBT colonoscopy every 10 years men: prostate exam women: breast exam, pelvic exam, mammogram

APPENDIX XI
MODERN MEDICINE TIMELINE

TIMELINE OF MODERN MEDICINE

Date	Discovery	Date	Discovery
1950	penicillin, the first broad-spectrum antibiotic, became available	1976	single photon emission computed tomography (SPECT) scan; coronary artery bypass graft (CABG)
1952	polio vaccine; isoniazid developed to treat tuberculosis; first published link between cigarette smoking and lung cancer	1978	first in vitro fertilization infant born; radionuclides for diagnostic imaging
1953	first open heart surgery using a heart–lung bypass machine; DNA decoded; medical ultrasound	1980	magnetic resonance imaging (MRI); smallpox declared eradicated worldwide; first laparoscopic appendectomy
1954	first living donor kidney transplantation	1981	first heart–lung combined transplantation; hepatitis B vaccine
1959	first drug to treat leukemia	1982	acquired immunodeficiency syndrome (AIDS) identified; first permanent artificial heart implanted; first use of monoclonal antibodies (MAbs) to treat cancer
1960	first oral contraceptive (birth control pill) becomes available in the United States		
1962	oral polio vaccine	1983	human immunodeficiency virus (HIV) identified as cause of AIDS
1963	first cadaveric donor kidney transplantation		
1964	measles vaccine; first US Surgeon General's report on smoking and health	1984	first cochlear implant
1965	US Congress passes laws to establish Medicare and Medicaid programs, require warning labels on cigarette packages	1985	positron emission tomography (PET) scan
		1986	first double-lung transplantation
		1987	first small bowel transplantation
1966	first pancreas–kidney combined transplantation; first mammography machine	1988	first split-liver transplantation
1967	first human heart transplantation; first liver transplantation; mumps vaccine; kidney dialysis machine	1989	first living donor liver transplantation
		1990	first living donor lung transplantation
1970	rubella vaccine	1994	robotic laparoscopy
1973	DNA cloning	1995	blood substitute
1974	first disposable syringe	1999	first human chromosome sequenced
1975	chorionic villi sampling (CVS)	2003	human genome mapping completed

APPENDIX XII
NOBEL LAUREATES IN PHYSIOLOGY OR MEDICINE

Alfred Nobel (1833–1896), a successful Swedish businessman who invented dynamite, established the Nobel Prize in his will. Nobel intended for the prize to honor "those who, during the preceding year, shall have conferred the greatest benefit on mankind." Nobel stipulated five areas of award: physics, chemistry, physiology or medicine, literature, and peace.

The Nobel Assembly at Karolinska Institutet in Stockholm, Sweden accepts nominations—up to several hundred each year—and selects the laureates. Up to three people, working independently or in collaboration, may share the Nobel Prize in Physiology or Medicine each year. No Nobel Prize in Physiology or Medicine was awarded in 1915, 1916, 1917, 1918, 1921, 1925, 1940, 1941, and 1942.

Complete information about Nobel laureates in all categories appears on the Nobel Prize Web site (nobelprize.org).

LAUREATES, NOBEL PRIZE IN PHYSIOLOGY OR MEDICINE

Year	Laureate(s)	Discovery
2005	Barry J. Marshall (b. 1951; Australia) J. Robin Warren (b. 1937; Australia)	*Helicobacter pylori* as the cause of peptic ulcer disease
2004	Richard Axel (b. 1946; USA) Linda B. Buck (b. 1947; USA)	mechanisms through which the sense of smell (olfactory system) recognizes and organizes odors
2003	Paul C. Lauterbur (b. 1929; USA) Sir Peter Mansfield (b. 1933; UK)	magnetic resonance imaging (MRI)
2002	Sydney Brenner (b. 1927; UK) H. Robert Horvitz (b. 1947; USA) John E. Sulston (b. 1942; UK)	how genes regulate organ development and cell apoptosis (natural cell death)
2001	Leland H. Hartwell (b. 1939; USA) Tim Hunt (b. 1943; UK) Sir Paul Nurse (b. 1949; UK)	mechanisms that control the life cycle of cells and cell division
2000	Arvid Carlsson (b. 1923; Sweden) Paul Greengard (b. 1925; USA) Eric R. Kandel (b. 1929; USA)	mechanisms by which neurotransmitters carry nerve impulses among brain neurons
1999	Günter Blobel (b. 1999; Germany)	intrinsic signals that direct proteins to their target locations within cells

Year	Laureate(s)	Discovery
1998	Robert F. Furchgott (b. 1916; USA) Louis J. Ignarro (b. 1941; USA) Ferid Murad (b. 1936; USA)	role of nitric oxide in the functions of the heart and blood vessels
1997	Stanley B. Prusiner (b. 1942; USA)	infectious prions
1996	Peter C. Doherty (b. 1940; Australia) Rolf M. Zinkernagel (b. 1944; Switzerland)	mechanisms through which the immune system recognizes and attempts to contain cells infected with viruses
1995	Edward B. Lewis (1918–2004; USA) Christiane Nüsslein-Volhard (b. 1942; Germany) Eric F. Wieschaus (b. 1947; USA)	mechanisms through which genes control the development of cells and tissues into specialized structures and organs in the embryo
1994	Alfred G. Gilman (b. 1941; USA) Martin Rodbell (1925–1998; USA)	G-proteins, which regulate how cells receive and use other protein signals
1993	Richard J. Roberts (b. 1943; UK) Phillip A. Sharp (b. 1944; USA)	split, or segmented, genes
1992	Edmond H. Fischer (b. 1920; USA) Edwin G. Krebs (b. 1918; USA)	roles of the enzymes kinase and phosphatase to attach and remove molecules for energy (glucose) release and storage
1991	Erwin Neher (b. 1944; Germany) Bert Sakmann (b. 1942; Germany)	single ion channels and their functions in cell electrical activity
1990	Joseph E. Murray (b. 1919; USA) E. Donnall Thomas (b. 1920; USA)	organ transplantation to treat diseases such as kidney failure and heart failure, including management of the immune response to prevent organ rejection and host vs. graft disease
1989	J. Michael Bishop (b. 1936; USA) Harold E. Varmus (b. 1939; USA)	origin of oncogenes is within cells that become cancerous
1988	Sir James W. Black (b. 1924; UK) Gertrude B. Elion (1918–1999; USA) George H. Hitchings (1905–1998; USA)	Black: mechanisms by which drugs are effective in treating diseases such as heart disease and cancer Elion and Hitchings: mechanisms of RNA function resulting in new drugs to treat various diseases such as leukemia, malaria, and organ rejection after transplantation
1987	Susumu Tonegawa (b. 1939; Japan)	role of genes in the production and function of antibodies
1986	Stanley Cohen (b. 1922; USA) Rita Levi-Montalcini (b. 1909; Italy)	nerve growth factor (NGF) and epidermal growth factor (EGF), substances that regulate cell growth and differentiation
1985	Michael S. Brown (b. 1941; USA) Joseph L. Goldstein (b. 1940; USA)	mechanisms that regulate cholesterol metabolism

Year	Laureate(s)	Discovery
1984	Niels K. Jerne (1911–1994; Denmark) Georges J. F. Köhler (1946–1995; Germany) César Milstein (1927–2002; Argentina)	Jerne: regulatory mechanisms of antibody production and function Köhler and Milstein: monoclonal antibodies (MAbs)
1983	Barbara McClintock (1902–1992; USA)	mobile genetic elements and genetic instability
1982	Sune K. Bergström (1916–2004; Sweden) Bengt I. Samuelsson (b. 1934; Sweden) John R. Vane (1927–2004; UK)	prostaglandins
1981	Roger W. Sperry (1913–1994; USA) David H. Hubel (b. 1926; USA) Torsten N. Wiesel (b. 1924; Sweden)	Sperry: specialized differences in the functions of the brain's hemispheres Hubel and Weisel: mechanisms through which the brain's visual cortex receives and interprets visual signals
1980	Baruj Benacerraf (b. 1920; USA) Jean Dausset (b. 1916; France) George D. Snell (1903–1996; USA)	genetic regulation of major histocompatibility complex (MHC) antigens
1979	Allan M. Cormack (1924–1998; USA) Godfrey N. Hounsfield (1919–2004; UK)	computed tomography (CT) scanning
1978	Werner Arber (b. 1929; Switzerland) Daniel Nathans (1928–1999; USA) Hamilton O. Smith (b. 1931; USA)	restrictive enzymes and their roles in genetic functions
1977	Roger Guillemin (b. 1924; USA) Andrew V. Schally (b. 1926; USA) Rosalyn Yalow (b. 1921; USA)	Guillemin and Schally: hypothalamus production of "releasing hormones" that direct the functions of other endocrine glands Yalow: radioimmunoassays to detect levels of peptide hormones in the blood circulation
1976	Baruch S. Blumberg (b. 1925; USA) D. Carleton Gajdusek (b. 1923; USA)	mechanisms through which infectious diseases originate and perpetuate
1975	David Baltimore (b. 1938; USA) Renato Dulbecco (b. 1914; USA) Howard M. Temin (1934–1994; USA)	mechanisms by which viruses interact with cell DNA and RNA to cause transformations that result in tumor development and growth
1974	Albert Claude (1899–1983; Belgium) Christian de Duve (b. 1917; Belgium) George E. Palade (b. 1912; USA)	cell components and composition and their effects on cell structure and function
1973	Karl von Frisch (1886–1982; Germany) Konrad Lorenz (1903–1989; Austria) Nikolaas Tinbergen (1907–1988; UK)	patterns of personal behaviors and social interactions as they relate to healthy and unhealthy psychosocial states
1972	Gerald M. Edelman (b. 1929; USA) Rodney R. Porter (1917–1985; UK)	chemical structures of antibody molecules

Year	Laureate(s)	Discovery
1971	Earl W. Sutherland Jr. (1915–1974; USA)	mechanisms through which hormones function in the body
1970	Sir Bernard Katz (1911–2003; UK) Ulf von Euler (1905–1983; Sweden) Julius Axelrod (1912–2004; USA)	neurotransmitters and their roles in the mechanisms through which nerve cells communicate with other cells in the body
1969	Max Delbrück (1906–1981; USA) Alfred D. Hershey (1908–1997; USA) Salvador E. Luria (1912–1991; USA)	genetic structure and replication mechanisms of viruses
1968	Robert W. Holley (1922–1993; USA) H. Gobind Khorana (b. 1922; USA) Marshall W. Nirenberg (b. 1927; USA)	role of genes in protein synthesis
1967	Ragnar Granit (1900–1991; Sweden) Haldan K. Hartline (1903–1983; USA) George Wald (1906–1997; USA)	biochemical and physiologic mechanisms involved in the eye's processing of visual input and information
1966	Peyton Rous (1897–1970; USA) Charles B. Huggins (1901–1997; USA)	Rous: viruses that cause tumors to develop Huggins: effect of therapeutic hormones on prostate cancer
1965	François Jacob (b. 1920; France) André Lwoff (1902–1994; France) Jacques Monod (1910–1976; France)	role of genes in regulating enzyme synthesis and virus replication
1964	Konrad Bloch (1912–2000; USA) Feodor Lynen (1911–1979; Germany)	relationship between metabolism of fatty acids and formation of cholesterol in the body
1963	Sir John Eccles (1903–1997; Australia) Alan L. Hodgkin (1914–1998; UK) Andrew F. Huxley (b. 1917; UK)	role of ions and ion channels in the conduction of electrical impulses through nerve cells
1962	Francis Crick (1916–2004; UK) James Watson (b. 1928; USA) Maurice Wilkins (1916–2004; UK)	double helix structure of DNA and its role in transmitting genetic and molecular information
1961	Georg von Békésy (1899–1972; USA)	mechanisms of function of the cochlea
1960	Sir Frank Macfarlane Burnet (1899–1985; Australia) Peter Medawar (1915–1987; UK)	characteristics and development of acquired immunity
1959	Severo Ochoa (1905–1993; USA) Arthur Kornberg (b. 1918; USA)	synthesis of RNA and DNA
1958	George Beadle (1903–1989; USA) Edward Tatum (1909–1975; USA) Joshua Lederberg (b. 1925; USA)	Beadle and Tatum: biochemical mechanisms of gene activity Lederberg: genetic recombination

Year	Laureate(s)	Discovery
1957	Daniel Bovet (1907–1992; Italy)	mechanisms through which certain drugs can block the actions and effects of endogenous substances
1956	André F. Cournand (1895–1988; USA) Werner Forssmann (1904–1979; Germany) Dickinson W. Richards (1895–1973; USA)	use of cardiac catheterization to diagnosis diseases of the heart and blood vessels
1955	(Axel) Hugo (Theodor) Theorell (1903–1982; Sweden)	mechanisms through which enzymes that cause oxidation function
1954	John F. Enders (1897–1985; USA) Thomas H. Weller (b. 1915; USA) Frederick C. Robbins (1916–2003; USA)	laboratory culture of the poliomyelitis virus in different kinds of tissues
1953	Hans Krebs (1900–1981; UK) Fritz Lipmann (1899–1986; USA)	Krebs: metabolic process within the cell that converts nutrients to energy (now called the Krebs cycle) Lipmann: coenzyme A and its role in cellular metabolism
1952	Selman A. Waksman (1888–1973; USA)	streptomycin, first antibiotic to treat tuberculosis
1951	Max Theiler (1899–1972; South Africa)	mechanisms of and treatment for yellow fever
1950	Edward C. Kendall (1886–1972; USA) Tadeus Reichstein (1897–1996; Switzerland) Philip S. Hench (1896–1965; USA)	isolation and functions within the body of cortisone and other hormones of the adrenal cortex
1949	Walter Hess (1881–1973; Switzerland) Egas Moniz (1874–1955; Portugal)	Hess: activities of the midbrain as they regulate the body's autonomic vital functions Moniz: prefrontal leucotomy (surgery to sever connections between regions of the brain responsible for intense emotional responses, notably anger) to treat schizophrenia
1948	Paul Müller (1899–1965; Switzerland)	use of the organic pesticide DDT to eradicate insects responsible for transmitting disease
1947	Carl Cori (1897–1984; USA) Gerty Cori (1897–1957; USA) Bernardo Houssay (1887–1971; Argentina)	Cori and Cori: conversion of glycogen to glucose Houssay: role of the hypophysis in carbohydrate metabolism and diabetes
1946	Hermann J. Muller (1890–1967; USA)	capability of X-rays to cause gene mutations
1945	Sir Alexander Fleming (1881–1955; UK) Ernst B. Chain (1906–1979; UK) Sir Howard Florey (1898–1968; Australia)	penicillin and its ability to cure infectious diseases
1944	Joseph Erlanger (1874–1965; USA) Herbert S. Gasser (1888–1963; USA)	varying conductivity and function of single fibers within nerves

Year	Laureate(s)	Discovery
1943	Henrik Dam (1895–1976; Denmark) Edward A. Doisy (1893–1986; USA)	isolation and biochemical actions of vitamin K
1939	Gerhard Domagk (1895–1964; Germany)	antibacterial actions of prontosil, particularly against streptococcal bacteria
1938	Corneille Heymans (1892–1968; Belgium)	functions of the cardio-aortic and carotid sinus areas in regulating the rate of respiration (breathing)
1937	Albert von Szent-Györgyi Nagyrapolt (1893–1986; Hungary)	metabolic functions of vitamin C
1936	Sir Henry Dale (1875–1968; UK) Otto Loewi (1873–1961; Austria)	role of neurotransmitters and other biochemicals in conducting nerve impulses
1935	Hans Spemann (1869–1941; Germany)	embryonic organizer areas that regulate how cells form tissues, organs, and structures within the developing embryo
1934	George H. Whipple (1878–1976; USA) George R. Minot (1885–1950; USA) William P. Murphy (1892–1987; USA)	consumption of animal liver as treatment for anemia
1933	Thomas H. Morgan 1866–1945; USA)	chromosomes as primary units of heredity
1932	Sir Charles Sherrington (1857–1952; UK) Edgar Adrian (1889–1977; UK)	structures and functions of neurons and nerves (afferent and efferent conductivity)
1931	Otto Warburg (1883–1970; Germany)	identification and function of hydrogen-transferring enzymes in respiration
1930	Karl Landsteiner (1868–1943; Austria)	human blood groups
1929	Christiaan Eijkman (1858–1930; Netherlands) Sir Frederick Hopkins (1861–1947; UK)	Eijkman: role of vitamins in diseases such as beriberi Hopkins: role of vitamins in growth
1928	Charles Nicolle (1866–1936; France)	transmission of typhus by the body louse
1927	Julius Wagner-Jauregg (1857–1940; Austria)	inoculation with malaria as a treatment, by inducing fever high enough to alter brain function, for psychoses
1926	Johannes Fibiger (1867–1828; Denmark)	*Spiroptera carcinoma*, a burrowing worm capable of causing cancerous tumors
1924	Willem Einthoven (1860–1927; Netherlands)	electrocardiogram (ECG)
1923	Frederick G. Banting (1891–1941; Canada) John Macleod (1876–1935; Canada)	insulin

Year	Laureate(s)	Discovery
1922	Archibald V. Hill (1886–1977; UK) Otto Meyerhof (1884–1951; Germany)	muscle metabolism and the ability of muscle activity to generate heat
1920	August Krogh (1874–1949; Denmark)	neuromuscular mechanisms that regulate capillary constriction and dilation
1919	Jules Bordet (1870–1961; Belgium)	immunity and infectious diseases
1914	Robert Bárány (1876–1936; Austria)	vestibular apparatus (receptors located within the inner ear that detect the body's position relative to the external environment)
1913	Charles Richet (1850–1935; France)	mechanisms of anaphylaxis (severe hypersensitivity reaction)
1912	Alexis Carrel (1873–1944; France)	transplantation of blood vessels and organs
1911	Allvar Gullstrand (1862–1930; Sweden)	refractive functions and errors of the eye (physiologic dioptrics)
1910	Albrecht Kossel (1853–1927; Germany)	role of proteins and nucleic acids in cellular function
1909	Theodor Kocher (1841–1917; Switzerland)	function and dysfunction of the thyroid gland
1908	Ilya Mechnikov (1845–1916; Russia) Paul Ehrlich (1854–1915; Germany)	Mechnikov: function of phagocytosis in the immune response Ehrlich: salvarsan as the first effective treatment for syphilis
1907	Alphonse Laveran (1845–1922; France)	role of protozoa in causing diseases such as malaria
1906	Camillo Golgi (1843–1926; Italy) Santiago Ramón y Cajal (1852–1934; Spain)	structure of the nervous system, notably the spinal cord and spinal nerves
1905	Robert Koch (1843–1910; Germany)	isolation and cultivation of the tubercle bacillus responsible for causing tuberculosis and the mechanisms of tuberculosis infection
1904	Ivan Pavlov (1849–1936; Russia)	physiology of digestion
1903	Niels Ryberg Finsen (1860–1904; Denmark)	therapeutic use of sunlight to treat conditions of the skin such as lupus vulgaris
1902	Ronald Ross (1857–1932; UK)	transmission of malaria by mosquito bites
1901	Emil von Behring (1854–1917; Germany)	serum antitoxin to treat diphtheria

SELECTED BIBLIOGRAPHY AND FURTHER READING

The books listed in this section can provide comprehensive information about health and medical subjects. Many are reference books that publishers periodically update and may be available in newer editions than those listed here. "Appendix VI: Resources" contains Web sites and other sources that provide the most current information about health topics, including research.

Aging and Health

Fries, James. *Living Well: Taking Care of Yourself in the Middle and Later Years*. 4th ed. Cambridge, MA: Da Capo Press, 2004.

Kandel, Joseph, and Christine Adamec. *Senior Health and Well-Being*. New York: Facts On File, 2003.

Kausler, Donald H., and Barry C. Kausler. *The Graying of America: An Encyclopedia of Aging, Health, Mind, and Behavior Second Edition*. Champaign: University of Illinois Press, 2001.

Morley, John E., and Lucretia van den Berg, eds. *Endocrinology of Aging*. Totowa, NJ: Humana Press, 2000.

Peterson, Elisabeth. *Voices of Alzheimer's: Courage, Humor, Hope, and Love in the Face of Dementia*. Cambridge, MA: Da Capo Press, 2004.

Weil, Andrew T. *Healthy Aging: A Lifelong Guide to Your Physical and Spiritual Well-Being*. New York: Knopf, 2005.

Cardiovascular and Pulmonary Health and Conditions

Crapo, James D., Jeffrey L. Glassroth, Joel B. Karlinsky, and Talmadge E. King, eds. *Baum's Textbook of Pulmonary Diseases*. 7th ed. New York: Lippincott Williams & Wilkins, 2003.

Frownfelter, Donna, and Elizabeth Dean. *Cardiovascular and Pulmonary Physical Therapy: Evidence and Practice*. 4th ed. New York: Mosby Elsevier, 2006.

Klabunde, Richard E. *Cardiovascular Physiology Concepts*. New York: Lippincott Williams & Wilkins, 2004.

Levitzky, Michael G. *Pulmonary Physiology*. 6th ed. New York: McGraw-Hill, 2002.

Mohrman, David E., and Lois Jane Heller. *Cardiovascular Physiology*. 5th ed. New York: McGraw-Hill, 2002.

West, John B. *Respiratory Physiology: The Essentials*. 7th ed. New York: Lippincott Williams & Wilkins, 2004.

Children's Health

Brazelton, T. Berry. *Touchpoints, The Essential Reference: Your Child's Emotional and Behavioral Development*. Cambridge, MA: Da Capo Press, 1992.

Hays, William W. Jr., Myron J. Levin, Judith R. Sondheimer, and Robin R. Deterding, eds. *Current Pediatric Diagnosis and Treatment*. 17th ed. New York: McGraw-Hill, 2004.

Pantell, Robert H., James F. Fries, and Donald M. Vickery. *Taking Care of Your Child: A Parent's Illustrated Guide to Complete Medical Care*. 7th ed. Cambridge, MA: Da Capo Press, 2005.

Shelov, Steven P. *Caring for Your Baby and Young Child: Birth to Age 5*. 5th ed. New York: Bantam Books, 1998.

Drugs and Medicines

Deglin, Judith Hopfer, and April Hazard Vallarand. *Davis's Drug Guide for Nurses*. 9th ed. Philadelphia: F. A. Davis, 2004.

Griffin, H. Winter. *Complete Guide to Prescription and Nonprescription Drugs. Edition 2005*. Rev. and updated by Stephen Moore. New York: Berkeley Publishing Group, 2004.

Katzung, Bertram G. *Basic and Clinical Pharmacology*. 9th ed. New York: McGraw-Hill, 2003.

Olson, James. *Clinical Pharmacology Made Ridiculously Simple*. 2nd ed. Miami: Medmaster, 2003.

Silverman, Harold M. *The Pill Book: The Illustrated Guide to the Most Prescribed Drugs in the United States*. 11th ed. New York: Bantam, 2004.

Skidmore-Roth, Linda. *2006 Mosby's Nursing Drug Reference*. New York: Mosby Elsevier, 2005.

Emergency and First Aid

Field, John, Mary Fran Hazinski, and David Gilmore, eds. *Handbook of Emergency Cardiovascular Care for Healthcare Providers*. Dallas: American Heart Association, 2006.

Forgey, William W. *Wilderness Medicine: Beyond First Aid*. 5th ed. Guilford, CT: Globe Pequot Press, 2000.

Krohmer, Jon R. *American College of Emergency Physicians First Aid Manual*. 2nd ed. New York: DK Publishing, 2004.

Stone, C. Keith, and Roger L. Humphries. *Current Emergency Diagnosis and Treatment*. 5th ed. New York: McGraw-Hill, 2003.

Endocrine and Hormonal Health and Conditions

Bode, Bruce, ed. *Medical Management of Type 1 Diabetes*. 4th ed. Alexandria, VA: American Diabetes Association, 2003.

Burant, Charles F., ed. *Medical Management of Type 2 Diabetes*. 5th ed. Alexandria, VA: American Diabetes Association, 2004.

Margioris, Andrew N., and George P Chrousos, eds. *Contemporary Endocrinology: Adrenal Disorders*. Totowa, NJ: Humana Press, 2001.

Melmed, Shlomo, ed. *The Pituitary*. 2nd ed. Malden, MA: Blackwell Science, 2002.

Nieschlag, Eberhard, and Hermann M. Behre, eds. *Testosterone: Action, Deficiency, Substitution*. 3rd ed. New York: Cambridge University Press, 2004.

Porterfield, Susan P. *Endocrine Physiology*. 2nd ed. St. Louis, MO: C. V. Mosby, 2000.

Rothfeld, Glenn S., and Deborah S. Romaine. *Thyroid Balance: Traditional and Alternative Methods for Treating Thyroid Disorders*. Avon, MA: Adams Media, 2001.

Ruderman, Neil, John T. Devlin, Stephen H. Schneider, and Andrea M. Kriska, eds. *American Diabetes Association Handbook of Exercise in Diabetes*. Alexandria, VA: American Diabetes Association, 2001.

Wales, Jerry K. H. *Clinician's Guide to Growth Disorders*. New York: Oxford University Press, 2001.

Gastroenterologic, Renal, and Urologic Health and Conditions

Eaton, Douglas C., and John P. Pooler, eds. *Vander's Renal Physiology*. 6th ed. New York: McGraw-Hill, 2004.

Danovitch, Gabriel M., ed. *Handbook of Kidney Transplantation*. 3rd ed. New York: Lippincott Williams & Wilkins, 2001.

Daugirdas, John T., Peter Gerard Blake, and Todd S. Ing, eds. *Handbook of Dialysis*. 3rd ed. New York: Lippincott Williams & Wilkins, 2000.

Friedman, Scott L., Kenneth R. McQuaid, and James H. Gendell. *Current Diagnosis and Treatment in Gastroenterology*. 2nd ed. New York: McGraw-Hill, 2002.

Greenberg, Arthur, ed. *Primer on Kidney Diseases*. 4th ed. Philadelphia: W. B. Saunders, 2005.

Hanno, Philip M., Alan J. Wein, and S. Bruce Malkowicz. *Clinical Manual of Urology*. 3rd ed. New York: McGraw-Hill, 2001.

Johnson, Leonard R., and Thomas A. Gerwin, eds. *Gastrointestinal Physiology*. 6th ed. St. Louis: C. V. Mosby, 2001.

Koeppen, Bruce M., and Bruce A. Stanton, eds. *Renal Physiology*. 3rd ed. St. Louis: C. V. Mosby, 2001.

Tanagho, Emil A., and Jack W. McAninch, eds. *Smith's General Urology*. 16th ed. New York: McGraw-Hill, 2004.

Yamada, Tadataka, William L. Hasler, John M. Inadomi, Michelle A. Anderson, and Robert S. Brown, eds. *Handbook of Gastroenterology*. 2nd ed. New York: Lippincott Williams & Wilkins, 2005.

General Health and Medicine

Anderson, Douglas M., ed. *Mosby's Medical Dictionary*. 7th ed. New York: Mosby Elsevier, 2005.

Beers, Mark H., and Robert Berkow, eds. *The Merck Manual of Diagnosis and Therapy*. 17th ed. White House Station, NJ: Merck Research Laboratories, 1999.

Beers, Mark H., and Thomas V. Jones, eds. *The Merck Manual of Health and Aging*. White House Station, NJ: Merck Research Laboratories, 2004.

Blau, Sheldon, and Dodi Shultz. *Living with Lupus: The Complete Guide*. 2nd ed. Cambridge, MA: Da Capo Press, 2004.

Dorland's Illustrated Medical Dictionary. 30th ed. Philadelphia: W. B. Saunders, 2003.

Gray, Henry. *Gray's Anatomy: The Classic Collector's Edition*. New York: Gramercy Books, 1988.

Griffith, H. Winter. *Complete Guide to Symptoms, Illness, and Surgery*. 4th ed. Rev. and updated by Stephen Moore and Kenneth Yoder. New York: Berkeley Publishing Group, 2000.

Guyton, Arthur C., and John E. Hall, eds. *Textbook of Medical Physiology*. 11th ed. Philadelphia: Elsevier Saunders, 2005.

Kasper, Dennis L., Eugene Braunwald, Anthony Fauci, Stephen Hauser, Dan Longo, and J. Larry Jameson, eds. *Harrison's Principles of Internal Medicine*. 16th ed. McGraw-Hill, 2004.

Komaroff, Anthony L., ed.-in-chief. *Harvard Medical School Family Health Guide*. New York: Simon & Schuster, 1999.

Leikin, Jerrold B., and Martin S. Lipsky, medical eds. *American Medical Association Complete Medical Encyclopedia.* New York: Random House, 2003.

Margolis, Simeon, medical editor. *The Johns Hopkins Consumer Guide to Medical Tests: What You Can Expect, How You Should Prepare, What Your Results Mean.* New York: Rebus, 2001.

Moore, Keith L, and Arthur F. Dalley. *Clinically Oriented Anatomy.* 5th ed. Baltimore: Lippincott Williams & Wilkins, 2005.

Parker, Steven. *Human Body* (Eyewitness Science Series). New York: Dorling Kindersley, Inc., 1993.

Schlossberg, Leon, and George D. Zuidema, *The Johns Hopkins Atlas of Human Functional Anatomy.* 4th ed. Baltimore: The Johns Hopkins University Press, 1997.

Stedman's Medical Dictionary. 28th ed. New York: Lippincott Williams & Wilkins, 2005.

Tierney, Lawrence M., Stephen J. McPhee, and Maxine Papadakis, eds. *2006 Current Medical Diagnosis and Treatment.* 45th ed. New York: McGraw-Hill, 2006.

Venes, Donald, *Taber's Cyclopedic Medical Dictionary.* 20th ed. Philadelphia: F. A. Davis, 2005.

Vickery, Donald, and James Fries. *Take Care of Yourself: The Complete Illustrated Guide to Medical Self-Care.* 8th ed. Cambridge, MA: Da Capo Press, 2003.

Genetics and Molecular Medicine

Gelehrter, Thomas D., Francis S. Collins, and David Ginsburg. *Principles of Medical Genetics.* 2nd ed. New York: Lippincott Williams & Wilkins, 1998.

Nussbaum, Robert L., Roderick R. McInnes, and Huntington F. Willard, eds. *Thompson and Thompson Genetics in Medicine.* 6th rev. ed. Philadelphia: W. B. Saunders, 2004.

Pierce, Benjamin. *Genetics: A Conceptual Approach.* 2nd ed. New York: W. H. Freeman, 2004.

Ross, Dennis W. *Introduction to Molecular Medicine.* 3rd ed. New York: Springer, 2002.

Shawker, Thomas H. *Unlocking Your Genetic History: A Step-by-Step Guide to Discovering Your Family's Medical and Genetic Heritage.* Nashville, TN: Rutledge Hill Press, 2004.

Trent, R. J. *Molecular Medicine.* 3rd ed. Burlington, MA: Elsevier Academic Press, 2005.

History of Medicine

Fenster, Julie M. *Mavericks, Miracles, and Medicine: The Pioneers Who Risked Their Lives to Bring Medicine into the Modern Age.* New York: Barnes & Noble Books, 2005.

Friedman, Meyer, and Gerald W. Friedland. *Medicine's 10 Greatest Discoveries.* New Haven, CT: Yale University Press, 1998.

Lyons, Albert S., and R. Joseph Petrucelli II. *Medicine: An Illustrated History.* New York: Abradale Press/Harry N. Abrams, 1987.

Magner, Lois. *A History of Medicine.* New York : Marcel Dekker, 1992.

Immune Health and Disorders, Allergies, and Infectious Diseases

Adkinson, N. Franklin, John W. Yunginger, William W. Busse, Bruce S. Bochner, Stephen T. Holgate, and Estelle R. Simons, eds. *Middleton's Allergy: Principles and Practice.* 6th ed. 2 vols. St. Louis: C. V. Mosby, 2003.

Cassell, Dana K., and Noel R. Rose. *The Encyclopedia of Autoimmune Diseases.* New York: Facts on File, 2003.

Ewald, Paul W. *Evolution of Infectious Disease.* New York: Oxford University Press, 1996.

Fanta, Christopher H., Lynda M. Cristiano, and Kenan Haver, with Nancy Waring. *The Harvard Medical School Guide to Taking Control of Asthma: A Comprehensive Prevention and Treatment Plan for You and Your Family.* New York: Simon & Schuster, 2003.

Fireman, Philip, M.D., ed. *Atlas of Allergies and Clinical Immunology.* 3rd ed. St. Louis MO: C.V. Mosby, 2005.

Fisher, Margaret C., ed.-in-chief. *Immunizations and Infectious Diseases: An Informed Parent's Guide.* Washington DC: American Academy of Pediatrics, 2005.

Gladwin, Mark, and Bill Trattler. *Clinical Microbiology Made Ridiculously Simple.* 3rd ed. Miami, FL: Medmaster, 2004.

Gorbach, Sherwood L., John G. Bartlett, and Neil R. Blacklow, eds. *Infectious Diseases.* 3rd ed. New York: Lippincott Williams & Wilkins, 2003.

Hill, Stuart, and Michael A. Palladino, eds. *Emerging Infectious Diseases.* San Francisco: Benjamin Cummings, 2005.

Karlen, Arno. *Man and Microbes: Disease and Plagues in History and Modern Times.* New York: Simon & Shuster, 1996.

Lahita, Robert G., ed. *Systemic Lupus Erythematosus.* 4th ed. Burlington, MA: Elsevier Academic Press, 2004.

Leung, Donald Y. M., Hugh A. Sampson, Raif S. Geha, and Stanley J. Szefler. *Pediatric Allergy: Principles and Practice.* St. Louis: C. V. Mosby, 2003.

Mandell, Gerald L., John E. Bennett, and Raphael Dolin, eds. *Principles and Practice of Infectious Diseases.* 6th ed. 2 vols. New York: Churchill Livingstone, 2004.

Nelson, Kenrad E., Carolyn Masters Williams, and Neil M.H. Graham, eds. *Infectious Disease Epidemiology: Theory and Practice.* Sudbury, MA: Jones and Bartlett, 2003.

Wessner, David, and Michael A. Palladino, eds. *HIV and AIDS.* San Francisco: Benjamin Cummings, 2005.

Integrative, Complementary, and Alternative Health

Cowan, Eliot. *Plant Spirit Medicine.* Columbus, NC: Swan Raven, 1995.

Rothfeld, Glenn S., and Suzanne Levert. *The Acupuncture Response: Balance Energy and Restore Health—A Western Doctor Tells You How.* New York: Contemporary Books, 2002.

Wansink, Brian. *Marketing Nutrition: Soy, Functional Foods, Biotechnology, and Obesity.* Champaign: University of Illinois Press, 2005.

Weil, Andrew, *Health and Healing: The Philosophy of Integrative Medicine and Optimum Health.* Rev. ed. New York: Houghton Mifflin, 2004.

Weil, Andrew, *Natural Health, Natural Medicine: The Complete Guide to Wellness and Self-Care for Optimum Health.* Rev. ed. New York: Houghton Mifflin, 2004.

Mental Health, Alcoholism, and Substance Abuse

Fehr, Scott Simon. *Introduction to Group Therapy: A Practical Guide.* 2nd ed. Binghamton, NY: Haworth Press, 2003.

Johnson, Bankole A., Pedro Ruiz, and Marc Galanter, eds. *Handbook of Clinical Alcoholism Treatment.* New York: Lippincott Williams & Wilkins, 2003.

Sadock, Benjamin J., and Virginia A. Sadock. *Kaplan and Sadock's Synopsis of Psychiatry: Behavioral Sciences/Clinical Psychiatry.* 9th ed. New York: Lippincott Williams & Wilkins, 2002.

Substance Abuse and Mental Health Services Administration (SAMHSA). *Overview of Findings from the 2004 National Survey on Drug Use and Health* [NSDUH Series H-27, DHHS Publication No. SMA 05-4061]. Rockville, MD: Office of Applied Studies, 2005.

Neurologic and Neuromuscular Health and Conditions

Aminoff, Michael J., Robert R. Simon, and David Greenburg, eds. *Clinical Neurology.* 6th ed. New York: McGraw-Hill, 2005.

Compston, Alastair, Ian R. McDonald, John Noseworthy, Hans Lassmann, David H. Miller, Kenneth J. Smith, Hartmut Wekerle, and Christian Confavreux. *McAlpine's Multiple Sclerosis.* 4th ed. New York: Churchill Livingstone, 2005.

Donaghy, Michael, ed. *Brain's Diseases of the Nervous System.* 11th ed. New York: Oxford University Press, 2001.

Fox, Michael J. *Lucky Man: A Memoir.* New York: Hyperion, 2002.

Jankovic, Joseph, and Eduardo Tolosa, eds. *Parkinson's Disease and Movement Disorders.* New York: Lippincott Williams & Wilkins, 2004.

Latchaw, Richard, John Kucharczyk, and Michael Moseley, eds. *Imaging of the Nervous System: Diagnostic and Therapeutic Applications.* New York: Mosby Elsevier, 2004.

Mosley, Anthony D., and Deborah S. Romaine. *The Encyclopedia of Parkinson's Disease.* New York: Facts On File, 2004.

Noback, Charles R., Norman L. Strominger, Robert J. Demarest, and David A. Ruggiero. *The Human Nervous System: Structure and Function.* 6th ed. Totowa, NJ: Humana Press, 2005.

Sanes, Dan H., Thomas A. Reh, and William A. Harris. *Development of the Nervous System.* 2nd ed. Burlington, MA: Elsevier Academic, 2005.

Scheld, Michael W., Richard J. Whitley, and Christina M. Marra, eds. *Infections of the Central Nervous System.* 3rd ed. New York: Lippincott Williams & Wilkins, 2004.

Watts, Ray L., and William C. Koller. *Movement Disorders: Neurologic Principles and Practice.* 2nd ed. New York: McGraw-Hill, 2004.

Nutrition and Diet

Duyff, Roberta Larson. *American Dietetic Association Complete Food and Nutrition Guide.* 2nd ed. Hoboken, NJ: John Wiley & Sons, 2002.

Mahan, L. Kathleen, and Sylvia Escott-Stump. *Krause's Food, Nutrition, and Diet Therapy.* Philadelphia: W. B. Saunders, 2003.

McArdle, William D., Frank I. Katch, and Victor L. Katch. *Sports and Exercise Nutrition.* New York: Lippincott Williams & Wilkins, 1999.

Whitney, Eleanor Noss, and Sharon Rady Rolfes. *Understanding Nutrition.* 10th ed. Belmont, CA: Wadsworth/Thomson Learning, 2004.

Williams, Melvin H. *Nutrition for Health, Fitness, and Sport.* 7th ed. New York: McGraw-Hill, 2004.

Orthopedics, Sports Medicine, and Exercise

Anderson, Marcia K. *Fundamentals of Sports Injury Management.* 2nd ed. New York: Lippincott Williams & Wilkins, 2002.

Baechle, Thomas R., and Roger W. Earle, eds. *Essentials of Strength Training and Conditioning.* 2nd ed. Champaign, IL: Human Kinetics, 2000.

Bahr, Roald, and Sverre Maehlum, eds. *Clinical Guide to Sports Injuries: An Illustrated Guide to the Management of Injuries in Physical Activity.* Champaign: Human Kinetics, 2003.

Dutton, Mark. *Orthopaedic Examination, Evaluation, and Intervention.* New York: McGraw-Hill, 2002.

Emery, Alan E. H., ed. *The Muscular Dystrophies*. New York: Oxford University Press, 2002.

Griffin, Letha Yurko, ed. *Essentials of Musculoskeletal Care*. Rosemont, IL: American Academy of Orthopaedic Surgeons, 2005.

Hislop, Helen J., and Jacqueline Montgomery. *Daniels and Worthington's Muscle Testing: Techniques of Manual Examination*. 7th ed. Philadelphia: W. B. Saunders, 2002.

Kisner, Carolyn, and Lynn Allen Colby. *Therapeutic Exercise: Foundations and Techniques*. 4th ed. Philadelphia: F. A. Davis, 2002.

Levangie, Pamela K., and Cynthia C. Norkin. *Joint Structure and Function: A Comprehensive Analysis*. 4th ed. Philadelphia: F. A. Davis, 2005.

Robergs, Robert A., and Steven J. Keteyian. *Fundamentals of Exercise Physiology: For Fitness, Performance, and Health*. New York: McGraw-Hill, 2005.

Sahrmann, Shirley A. *Diagnosis and Treatment of Movement Impairment Syndromes*. St. Louis: C. V. Mosby, 2001.

Reproductive and Sexual Health

Anderson, Barbara A. *Reproductive Health: Women and Men's Shared Responsibility*. Sudbury, MA: Jones and Bartlett, 2005.

Armstrong, Lance, and Sally Jenkins. *It's Not about the Bike: My Journey Back to Life*. New York: Penguin Putnam, 2000.

Aronson, Diane and the staff of RESOLVE. *Resolving Infertility*. New York: HarperCollins, 2001.

Blute, Michael, ed. *Mayo Clinic on Prostate Health*. New York: Kensington Publishing, 2003.

Bostwick, David G., *American Cancer Society's Complete Guide to Prostate Cancer*. Atlanta, GA: American Cancer Society, 2004.

DeCherney, Alan H., and Lauren Nathan. *Current Obstetric and Gynecologic Diagnosis & Treatment*. 9th ed. New York: McGraw-Hill, 2002.

Ganschow, Pamela S., Frances E. Norlock, Elizabeth A. Jacobs, and Elizabeth A. Marcus, eds. *Breast Health and Common Breast Problems: A Practical Approach*. Philadelphia: American College of Physicians, 2004.

Grimm, Peter D., John C. Blasko, and John E. Sylvester, eds. *The Prostate Cancer Treatment Book*. New York: Contemporary Books, 2003.

Holmes, King K., ed. *Sexually Transmitted Diseases*. 4th ed. New York: McGraw-Hill, 2006.

Love, Susan, *Dr. Susan Love's Breast Book*. 4th ed. Cambridge, MA: Da Capo Press, 2005.

Moore, Keith L., and T. V. N. Persaud, eds. *The Developing Human: Clinically Oriented Embryology*. 7th ed. Philadelphia: W. B. Saunders, 2003.

Murkoff, Heidi, Arlene Eisenburg, and Sandee Hathaway. *What to Expect When You're Expecting*. 3rd ed. New York: Workman Publishing, 2002.

Northrup, Christiane, M.D. *The Wisdom of Menopause: Creating Physical and Emotional Health and Healing during the Change*. Rprnt. New York: Bantam Books, 2001.

Northrup, Christiane. *Women's Bodies, Women's Wisdom: Creating Physical and Emotional Health and Healing*. Rprnt. New York: Bantam Books, 2002.

Rothfeld, Glenn S., and Deborah S. Romaine. *The Encyclopedia of Men's Health*. New York : Facts On File, 2005.

Stanley, Deborah A., ed. *Sexual Information for Teens: Health Tips about Sexual Development, Human Reproduction, and Sexually Transmitted Diseases*. Detroit, MI: Omnigraphics, 2003.

Stoppard, Miriam. *Woman's Body: A Manual for Life*. New York: Dorling Kindersley, 1994.

Skin Health and Conditions

Habif, Thomas P., James L. Campbell, Jr., M. Shane Chapman, James G. H. Dinulos, and Kathryn A. Zug, eds. *Skin Disease: Diagnosis and Treatment*. 2nd ed. New York: Mosby-Year Book, 2005.

McNally, Robert Aquinas. *Skin Health Information for Teens: Health Tips about Dermatological Concerns and Skin Cancer Risks*. Detroit, MI: Omnigraphics, 2003.

Rigel, Darrell, Robert Friedman, Leonard M. Dzubow, Douglas Reintgen, Jean-Claude Bystryn, and Robin Marks. *Cancer of the Skin*. Philadelphia: W. B. Saunders, 2004.

Sheen, Barbara. *Acne*. San Diego, CA: Lucent Books, 2004.

Turkington, Carol, and Jeffrey S. Dover. *Skin Deep: An A–Z of Skin Disorders, Treatments, and Health*. New York: Facts On File, 1996.

Hywel C. Williams, ed. *Atopic Dermatitis: The Epidemiology, Causes and Prevention of Atopic Eczema*. New York: Cambridge University Press, 2000.

Wolff, Klaus, Richard A. Johnson, and Dick Suurmond, eds. *Fitzpatrick's Color Atlas and Synopsis of Clinical Dermatology*. 5th ed. New York: McGraw-Hill, 2005.

MEDICAL ADVISORY REVIEW PANEL

Kyra J. Becker, M.D., is codirector of the University of Washington Stroke Center in Seattle, Washington. She is also an associate professor of neurology and neurological surgery at the University of Washington School of Medicine. Dr. Becker provides patient care through her practice at Harborview Medical Center and is a primary investigator on several stroke-related research studies.

Dr. Becker received her bachelor of science (B.S.) degree in biology *summa cum laude* from Virginia Tech in Blacksburg, Virginia, and her doctor of medicine (M.D.) degree from Duke University School of Medicine in Durham, North Carolina. She completed her internship in internal medicine, residency in neurology, and clinical fellowship in critical care neurology all at Johns Hopkins Hospital in Baltimore, Maryland. Dr. Becker is board-certified in neurology and psychiatry with a special certification in vascular neurology.

James C. Blair, III, PA-C, is director of Madrona Hill Urgent Care Center in Port Townsend, Washington. Mr. Blair is a physician assistant certified with special recognition in primary care and surgery. He is an advanced cardiac life support (ACLS) instructor and has worked much of his career to provide emergency services in small hospitals and clinical care settings in rural communities.

Mr. Blair received his associate of science degree in nursing from Wenatchee Valley College in Wenatchee, Washington, and completed the MEDEX Northwest Physician Assistant Program at the University of Washington School of Medicine in Seattle, Washington.

Alexa Fleckenstein, M.D., writes books and conducts lectures and workshops about natural health topics. Educated in Germany and the United States, she has extensive experience in natural therapies and integrative medicine. Dr. Fleckenstein is board-certified in internal medicine.

Dr. Fleckenstein received her medical degree from Universität Hamburg, Germany. She completed her internship and residency in primary care medicine at Carney Hospital in Boston, Massachusetts, and a fellowship in ambulatory medicine at VA Brockton, Massachusetts. Her subspecialty certification in natural medicine is from Ärztekammer Hamburg (German Board).

Nancy A. Lewis, Pharm.D., is a clinical pharmacist and medical science liaison for MGI Pharma, Inc., a biopharmaceutical company specializing in oncology and acute care products. Dr. Lewis frequently conducts workshops and focused training presentations. She is an active member of the Washington-Alaska Cancer Pain Initiative.

Dr. Lewis received her bachelor of science (B.S.) in pharmacy and her doctor of pharmacy (Pharm.D.) degrees from the University of Washington in Seattle, Washington. She serves on the clinical faculty at the University of Washington in Seattle, Washington and on the adjunct faculty at Washington State University in Pullman, Washington.

Gary R. McClain, Ph.D., is a psychologist, counselor, and consultant in New York City. Dr. McClain has more than 25 years of experience as a mental health professional and in the business world. The focus of his practice is healthcare and wellness.

Dr. McClain's graduate studies were in clinical psychology and education, with a focus on adult personality development and learning. He received his doctor of philosophy (Ph.D.) from the

University of Michigan. Dr. McClain has coauthored or edited 14 books and frequently conducts workshops.

Maureen Ann Mooney, M.D., is a clinical, surgical, and cosmetic dermatologist in private practice in Puyallup, Washington, where she specializes in treating skin cancer. Dr. Mooney is trained to perform Mohs' Micrographic Surgery. Dr. Mooney is board-certified in dermatology and dermatopathology.

Dr. Mooney received her bachelor of science (B.S.) degree in biology *summa cum laude* from the University of Minnesota College of Biological Sciences in St. Paul, Minnesota, and her doctor of medicine (M.D.) degree from the University of Minnesota School of Medicine in Minneapolis, Minnesota. She completed her internship at Hennepin County Medical Center in Minneapolis, Minnesota, and her residency in dermatology at New Jersey Medical School in Newark, New Jersey. Dr. Mooney also completed fellowships in Dermatopathology at New Jersey Medical School and Mohs' Micrographic Surgery at Louisiana State University Healthcare network in New Orleans, Louisiana.

Margaret J. Neff, M.D., M.Sc., is attending physician, pulmonary and critical care medicine, at Harborview Medical Center in Seattle, Washington. Dr. Neff is a medical monitor for the Cystic Fibrosis Therapeutic Diagnostics Network, co-chair of one of the biomedical committees of the University of Washington Institutional Review Board, and a clinical investigator on several research studies. She is board-certified in internal medicine, pulmonary disease, and critical care medicine.

Dr. Neff earned her bachelor's degree in biological sciences (B.S.) and medical degree (M.D.) from Stanford University in Stanford, California, and her master of science (M.S.) degree in epidemiology from the University of Washington in Seattle, Washington. She completed her internship and residency in internal medicine and a fellowship in intensive care at Stanford University and a fellowship in pulmonary/critical care at the University of Washington. Dr. Neff is an assistant professor of medicine in the division of pulmonary and critical

care medicine at the University of Washington School of Medicine, Seattle, Washington.

Maureen Pelletier, M.D., C.C.N., F.A.C.O.G., is board-certified in obstetrics and gynecology as well as in clinical nutrition. A former aviation medical examiner, Dr. Pelletier is also licensed as a medical acupuncturist and is a DAN! (Defeat Autism Now!) physician. She is in private practice in Cincinnati, Ohio, with an emphasis on integrative medicine.

Dr. Pelletier received her medical degree (M.D.) from Tufts University School of Medicine in Boston, Massachusetts, and completed her residency in obstetrics and gynecology at the University of Cincinnati. She received clinical training in mind-body medicine at the Mind-Body Institute at Harvard University and completed the integrative medicine program at the University of Arizona School of Medicine. Dr. Pelletier is a national and international lecturer.

Otelio S. Randall, M.D., F.A.C.C., is director of the preventive cardiology program, hypertension and clinical trials, and the Cardiovascular Disease Prevention and Rehabilitation Center at Howard University Hospital in Washington, D.C. Dr. Randall is widely published in peer-reviewed journals and has authored two books. He has received numerous awards during his career, including the 2004 Outstanding Faculty Research Award from Howard University School of Medicine.

Dr. Randall received his bachelor's degree (B.S.) in chemistry from Howard University and his medical degree (M.D.) from the University of Michigan Medical School in Ann Arbor, Michigan. He completed his internship at the State University of New York at Brooklyn, residencies in internal medicine at Baylor College of Medicine in Houston, Texas, and University of Michigan Hospital, and a fellowship in cardiology at the University of Michigan Hospital. Dr. Randall is designated a specialist in hypertension by the ASH specialists program in affiliation with the American Society of Hypertension (ASH).

Susan D. Reed, M.D., M.P.H., is program director for the Women's Reproductive Health Research Program at the University of Washington in Seattle, Washington. She is a clinician at Harborview

Medical Center and University of Washington Medical Center. Dr. Reed is also an affiliate investigator at the Center for Health Studies and Fred Hutchinson Cancer Research Center, and an associate professor of obstetrics and gynecology, and an adjunct professor in epidemiology at the University of Washington School of Medicine. Dr. Reed's areas of clinical and research interest are gynecologic issues for women with genetic diseases, cross-cultural medicine, and management of menopause.

Dr. Reed received her master's degree (M.S.) in human genetics from Sarah Lawrence College in Bronxville, New York, her medical degree (M.D.) from Stanford University Medical Center in Stanford, California, and her Master of Public Health (M.P.H.) degree from the University of Washington School of Public Health. Dr. Reed is a licensed genetic counselor and board-certified in obstetrics and gynecology.

Jerry Richard Shields, M.D., is an ophthalmologist in private practice in Tacoma, Washington. He sees general ophthalmology patients and performs laser correction and cataract surgery. Dr. Shields is board-certified in ophthalmology and VISIX-certified.

Dr. Shields received his bachelor of science (B.S.) degree in biology *cum laude* from Wake Forest University in Winston-Salem, North Carolina, and his medical degree (M.D.) from the Medical College of Georgia in Augusta, Georgia. He completed his internship in internal medicine and his residency in ophthalmology at the University of Washington in Seattle, Washington.

Christina M. Surawicz, M.D., is gastroenterology section chief of at Harborview Medical Center in Seattle, Washington. She is also professor of medicine and assistant dean for faculty development at the University of Washington School of Medicine in Seattle. Dr. Surawicz is widely published in peer-reviewed journals and has authored, edited, and contributed to dozens of books.

Dr. Surawicz received her undergraduate degree, a bachelor of arts (B.A.) in biology, from Barnard College in New York City and her medical degrees (M.D.), awarded with honors, from the University of Kentucky College of Medicine in Lexington, Kentucky. She completed her medical internship, medical residency, and gastroenterology fellowship at the University of Washington in Seattle. Dr. Surawicz is board-certified in internal medicine and gastroenterology.

Denise L. Wych, R.N. C.M., is a cardiac nurse case manager at Palmetto Health-Richland Heart Hospital in Columbia, South Carolina, where she integrates clinical and medical appropriateness criteria in discharge planning and resource utilization within the framework of an interdisciplinary health-care team. She has worked in medical-surgical, intensive care unit, newborn, school nursing, and home health.

Ms. Wych received her diploma in nursing from Providence School of Nursing in Sandusky, Ohio. She served 10 years as an officer in the US Navy Nurse Corps, during which she was twice awarded the Navy Achievement Medal.

CUMULATIVE INDEX
TO VOLUMES 1–4

Volume numbers appear in **bold** followed by a colon and the relevant volume page reference. Pages in **bold** indicate major treatment of a topic. Pages with a *t* indicate tables.